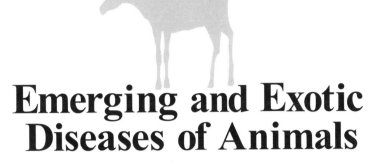

Emerging and Exotic Diseases of Animals

Edited by:
Anna Rovid Spickler, DVM, PhD
James A. Roth, DVM, PhD, DACVM

Project Management:
Jane Galyon, MS
Gayle B. Brown, DVM, PhD
Glenda Dvorak, DVM, MS, MPH
Travis Engelhaupt, BS

Disease Images:
Steven D. Sorden, DVM, PhD, DACVP
Claire B. Andreasen, DVM, PhD, DACVP

Graphic Design:
Clint May, BFA
Travis Engelhaupt, BS
Sara Hall, BS

Institute for International Cooperation in Animal Biologics
An OIE Collaborating Center for the Diagnosis of Animal Diseases and
Vaccine Evaluation in the Americas

Iowa State University College of Veterinary Medicine
Ames, Iowa

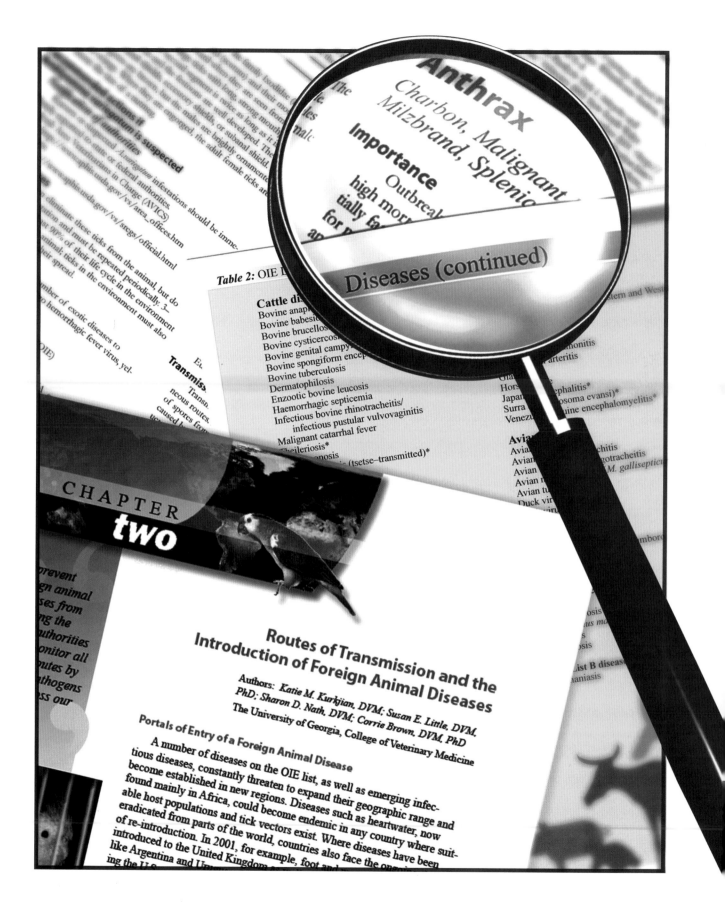

Preface

This is the third edition of Emerging and Exotic Diseases of Animals, published by Iowa State University, Institute for International Cooperation in Animal Biologics (IICAB). In addition to updated overview chapters, a new chapter on the role of response teams in animal health emergencies, and updated fact sheets for 81 diseases, we are pleased to add 261 annotated images for 36 important animal diseases.

A majority of the materials for this book are derived from an Internet-based course entitled Emerging and Exotic Diseases of Animals (EEDA) which was originally developed with funding from the USDA Cooperative State Research, Education, and Extension Service (CSREES) Higher Education Challenge Grants program (grant number 00384119278). Faculty from three colleges of veterinary medicine with past leadership in EEDA and international animal health issues worked to design the Internet-based course (Iowa State University—James Roth and Eldon Uhlenhopp; the University of California, Davis—David Hird and Janine Kasper; and the University of Georgia – Corrie Brown and Susan Little). The three universities provided matching funds for the project. USDA APHIS personnel (Aida Boghossian and Paula Cowen) collaborated on the project.

Image acquisition was funded by a USDA CSREES Higher Education Challenge Grant "A Digital Image Database to Enhance Foreign Animal Disease Education" (grant number 2005-38411-15859) to Claire Andreasen, Steven Sorden and James Roth at Iowa State University in 2005.

In 2002, the Center for Disease Control and Prevention provided a three year grant (E11/CCE721850) to establish the Center for Food Security and Public Health (CFSPH) at Iowa State University. The fact sheets were updated and maintained by individuals supported through the CFSPH.

In 2005, under the leadership of Dr. Aida Boghossian, the USDA APHIS Emergency Management group provided funds to update overview sections of this textbook and the EEDA course and to distribute a copy of this textbook to senior veterinary students at all the U.S. colleges of veterinary medicine. In addition, the USDA APHIS has provided a grants program to encourage veterinary colleges to use the EEDA Internet course. The Internet course also includes interactive scenarios of EEDA outbreaks. These scenarios do not lend themselves to inclusion in a book. In 2006, 22 of the 28 U.S. colleges of veterinary medicine will offer this course. The course is offered to veterinary students and practicing veterinarians through the Veterinary Information Network (http://www.vin.com)

As new disease outbreaks occur, new fact sheets will be added and current fact sheets updated. These will be available at www.cfsph.iastate.edu/DiseaseInfo. Additional annotated images will also be available on the same website.

For more information, contact James A. Roth, DVM, PhD, Executive Director, Institute for International Cooperation in Animal Biologics, Iowa State University, College of Veterinary Medicine, Ames Iowa 50011; Phone: 515 294 7189; Fax: 515 294 8259; Email: iicab@iastate.edu

Introduction

James A. Roth, DVM, PhD, DACVM

The purpose of this book is to provide veterinarians and veterinary students with an overview of exotic (foreign) and emerging animal diseases, their methods of introduction and spread, and the role of local, state, federal and international agencies in control of these diseases (Section 1). It is also meant to serve as a ready resource for information. Because these diseases either do not exist in North America, or are rare, veterinarians have had little exposure to them and may not be familiar with their important characteristics. The disease fact sheets (Section 2) have a standard outline so that critical information related to the diseases can be found quickly. For the third edition of this book, we have added images for a number of important diseases (Section 3).

The need for continuing education for veterinarians in exotic diseases of animals is widely recognized. U.S. agriculture is highly vulnerable to the introduction of exotic animal diseases. The risk for accidental introduction of these diseases grows as international travel and trade increases. There is also increasing concern regarding the threat of intentional introduction of exotic agents. Seventy-five percent of the Centers for Disease Control and Prevention designated bioterrorism agents affect domestic animals as well as man. Veterinarians will need to take an active role in any response to bioterrorism. There is also concern about the intentional introduction of disease agents targeted at livestock or poultry (agroterrorism). The accidental or intentional introduction of exotic diseases into the North American livestock or companion animal population could have devastating effects on public and animal health, agriculture, and the economy.

The last 25 years has seen the emergence of new diseases affecting man and animals, including AIDS, *E. coli* O157:H7, bovine spongiform encephalopathy and new variant Cruetzfeld-Jacob disease, hantavirus, Nipah virus, West Nile virus, SARS, monkeypox, and zoonotic H5N1 avian influenza. The factors leading to the emergence of new diseases are still present and in many cases are accelerating. We should expect the emergence of additional diseases with similar impact in the next 25 years.

The Iowa State University (ISU) College of Veterinary Medicine has been working to meet educational needs in emerging and exotic diseases for many years. The Institute for International Cooperation in Animal Biologics (IICAB) was established in 1995 by ISU and the USDA Animal and Plant Health Inspection Service (APHIS). The IICAB is a World Organization for Animal Health (OIE)–Collaborating Center for Diagnosis of Animal Disease and Vaccine Evaluation in the Americas with the USDA APHIS National Veterinary Services Laboratories and Center for Veterinary Biologics in Ames, Iowa. The IICAB activities center around veterinary biologics training, immunology and vaccinology. The Center for Food Security and Public Health (CFSPH) was established in 2002 by the Centers for Disease Control and Prevention (CDC). The CFSPH is a CDC Center for Public Health Preparedness in Veterinary Medicine and Zoonotic Diseases and is the only such Center to address veterinary medicine. The CFSPH activities focus on awareness education, biological risk management, and giving veterinarians the tools and knowledge they need to recognize and appropriately respond to unusual animal diseases. The IICAB and CFSPH are administered together.

Together, these two organizations have developed a library of resources on exotic and emerging animal diseases. These resources are available at no cost on the CFSPH website: www.cfsph.iastate.edu All of the fact sheets and images in this book are available on the website. More than 35 additional fact sheets on important zoonotic diseases (many with images) are also on the website. A "mobile" version of the CFSPH website has been created, so that individuals using a Blackberry, Palm, or Pocket PC can easily access the fact sheets and images.

The CFSPH has also developed more than 50 PowerPoint presentations for the diseases with bioterrorism or agroterrorism potential. These presentations are available on the same website as the fact sheets and images. All PowerPoint presentations have speaker notes for each slide and can be downloaded and individualized. The CFSPH developed these presentations for use by veterinarians as part of a train the trainer program. Over 330 veterinarians were trained to use these materials to educate their colleagues and the general public. Overview PowerPoint presentations addressing agroterrorism and bioterrorism are available at: http://www.cfsph.iastate.edu/TrainTheTrainer/resources.htm

The CFSPH website also contains the following web-based continuing education courses for veterinarians:
- Foreign Animal Disease Awareness (developed for USDA APHIS employees)
- Program Diseases (developed for USDA APHIS employees)
- Incident Command System 100 & 200 (developed and distributed by USDA)
- National Incident Management System (developed and distributed by USDA)

Veterinarians have been trained to recognize exotic and emerging diseases, to appropriately respond if they suspect an exotic disease, and to protect the public, their staff, clients, family, and themselves from those diseases that are zoonotic. We hope that the information in this book and on the CFSPH website will assist them in carrying out these important responsibilities.

Emerging & Exotic Diseases of Animals

•Table of Contents•

Section 2-Fact Sheets for Emerging and Exotic Diseases of Animals
Section 3-Images of Emerging and Exotic Diseases of Animals

CHAPTER one

Foreign Animal Diseases and the Consequences of their Introduction

Authors: *Sharon D. Nath, DVM; Corrie Brown, DVM, PhD; Katie M. Kurkjian, DVM; Susan E. Little, DVM, PhD*

The University of Georgia, College of Veterinary Medicine

A foreign animal disease could devastate naïve livestock or poultry populations through high morbidity or mortality.

The United States produces approximately $250 billion in agricultural products annually. Through exportation to other nations, the market for U.S. agricultural sales is greatly expanded; thus a major mission of the United States Department of Agriculture (USDA) is to protect existing export markets and investigate future expansion into new markets. If a foreign animal disease enters the U.S., there may be extensive market losses and even more costly export barriers, causing severe economic impacts.

The risks of introduction today are greater than ever because of expanding international trade and travel. The amount of agricultural imports has doubled in the 1990's and, in the climate of free trade, will certainly continue to grow. A highly transmissible foreign animal disease can spread ferociously if undetected or not reported. Animal production today is very intensified and specialized, with fewer farms raising more animals. Also, animals today are transported extensively throughout the nation. For instance, it is common for a steer to cross several state lines between birth and slaughter—born in one state, weaned in a second, fattened in a third, and slaughtered in a fourth. At each of these waystations there is possibility of contact with numerous other animals, with tremendous potential for disease spread and dissemination.

The Consequences of
Introducing a Foreign Animal Disease

What are foreign animal diseases and why the potential for such devastation? A **foreign animal disease (FAD)** is an important transmissible livestock or poultry disease believed to be absent from the United States and its territories. Many diseases which are considered foreign were present in the U.S. at one time, but have been eradicated. Foreign animal diseases are sometimes called **exotic animal diseases. Transboundary disease** is a new term used in many international documents to describe a FAD. A foreign animal disease introduced into the United States could have far-reaching impacts on the health of livestock, pets and poultry, as well as on the economy.

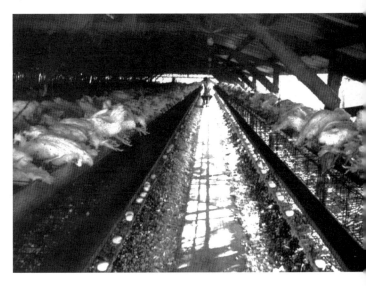

A foreign animal disease could devastate naïve livestock or poultry populations through high morbidity or mortality. In 1997, an outbreak of classical swine fever, a highly contagious and often fatal systemic disease of pigs, occurred in the Netherlands. To eradicate this exotic disease from their swine population, the Dutch were forced to slaughter approximately eight million pigs.

The presence of a foreign animal disease in the U.S. is likely to result in export bans on animals and related animal products because other countries want to protect their agricultural industry. In 1998, exotic Newcastle disease, a foreign animal disease that causes diarrhea and death in poultry, was found in game chickens in downtown Fresno, California. Rapid recognition and response limited the spread of the disease, and commercial poultry operations remained free of the disease; however, even this limited presence caused poultry exports to be seriously curtailed, costing a minimum of $400 million (USD) in lost revenue because of embargoes levied by countries concerned about importing the disease in meat products. During another Newcastle disease outbreak in 2002-2003, the virus was discovered in backyard game fowl near Los Angeles, California but spread to Nevada and Arizona before it was contained. As of September 19, 2003, the direct trade losses in this outbreak were estimated to be $121 million.

Millions or possibly billions of dollars could be spent to control or eradicate the disease, even if it is localized to a small region. Estimates of the cost of a foreign animal disease outbreak are staggering. In 1983-84, an epizootic of highly pathogenic avian influenza occurred in Pennsylvania and neighboring states. The highly pathogenic strains of the avian influenza virus, which cause a severe and often fatal illness in poultry, are exotic to the U.S. and can devastate commercial poultry

In 1983-84, an outbreak of highly pathogenic avian influenza in Pennsylvania, New Jersey and Virginia took the lives of 17 million birds and cost taxpayers $63 million in control measures.
Source: USDA

Foreign Animal Disease (FAD)—an important transmissable livestock or poultry disease believed to be absent from the United States and its territories

Exotic Animal Disease (EAD)—animal diseases which are unusual, including foreign animal diseases

Transboundary Diseases—a new term used in many international documents to describe FADs

Emerging Infectious Diseases—diseases that have the potential for significant health impacts in animals or humans, and whose incidence has recently increased or is likely to increase

operations. Over six months, all infected chickens were depopulated and the premises decntaminated, with a price tag of $63 million paid by the federal government. Other foreign animal diseases could be even more costly. It is estimated that if foot and mouth disease entered the U.S. and spread for any length of time, it would cost at least $2 billion to depopulate and disinfect. Lost trade costs during the detection and clean-up process have been estimated at $27 billion.

A foreign animal disease could spread into a susceptible wildlife population, which would complicate, or worse, prohibit eradication of the disease. The West Nile virus, which was discovered in the eastern United States in 1999, is an example of a foreign animal disease that has now become established in wildlife populations. Humans, horses, many species of birds, and other wild animals are hosts for the virus, which can cause severe encephalitis and even death in susceptible species. The virus is particularly devastating to our corvid bird populations, especially crows. To date, millions of dollars have been spent to investigate the disease and its geographic sprawl. A special West Nile virus surveillance program operates through partnerships with the Centers for Disease Control and Prevention, U.S. Department of Agriculture, U.S. Geological Survey, Department of Defense, Environmental Protection Agency, state and local health departments, state veterinarians and wildlife biologists. Data are continually collected to determine the prevalence and transmission of the virus in human, animal, wild bird, and mosquito populations. Over the last few years, this surveillance has seen the West Nile virus spread into all of the 48 contiguous U.S. states.

Other diseases could also become established in the U.S. s a vector-borne disease of particular concern. This foreign animal disease, caused by *Cowdria ruminantium,* is an important tick-transmitted disease of livestock in Africa. Heartwater can affect all ruminants, causing fever, respiratory distress, and neurologic signs. There are serious concerns that *C. ruminantium* could be introduced into the U.S. at any moment, carried on a tick-infested wild bird. If it is not detected at the earliest possible incursion, heartwater is likely to become established in the wild deer population, in which case it will be impossible to eradicate.

The World Organization for Animal Health and Its Role in Preventing the Spread of Disease

World Organiation for Animal Health, or Office International des Epizooties (OIE)—an international animal health organization that informs goverment veterinary services of disease outbreaks that could endanger animal or human health.

All foreign animal diseases are not of equal concern to the United States. Currently, the U.S. has the diagnostic capability for approximately 50 different FADs; the most important of these are on a list maintained by an international animal health organization, the **World Organization for Animal Health (OIE)**. This group was formed early in the 20th century, after an outbreak of rinderpest. Rinderpest is a severe, often fatal, viral disease of cattle and other cloven-hooved animals. In 1920, rinderpest was introduced into Belgium when zebus, originating in India and destined for Brazil, passed through the port of Antwerp. The outbreak soon spread to other countries in Europe. The desire to prevent future outbreaks of this and other diseases led 24 countries to form the Office International des Epizooties in 1924. Although the English name of this organization was changed in 2002 to the World Organization for Animal Health, its acronym remained as OIE. Over the last 20 years, the OIE has expanded and is indeed a global organization; as of May 2004, it contained 167 member nations, each with equal representation.

The purpose of the OIE is to help countries coordinate animal disease information and decrease the potential for epizootics. Its most important function is to inform governmental veterinary services of the occurrence and course of epizootics that could endanger animal or human health. The OIE maintains a list of infectious diseases of particular concern in international trade. These animal diseases were formerly divided into two lists based on their relative socio-economic and public health significance. The fifteen List A diseases had the highest priority for exclusion. They were defined as "transmissible diseases [with] the potential for very serious and rapid spread, irrespective of national borders,…of serious socio-economic or public health consequence and…of major importance in the international trade of animals and animal products." List A diseases included African horse sickness, African swine fever, bluetongue, classical swine fever, contagious bovine pleuropneumonia, foot and mouth disease, highly pathogenic avian influenza, lumpy skin disease, Newcastle disease, peste des petits ruminants, Rift Valley fever, rinderpest, sheep and goat pox, swine vesicular disease, and vesicular stomatitis. List B diseases were defined by the OIE as "transmissible diseases ... of socio-economic and/or public health importance within countries and... significant in the international trade of animals and animal products." In 2004, List B contained approximately 90 diseases. In May 2004, OIE member countries approved the merging of List A and List B into a single list of diseases reportable to the OIE. As of November 2005, this list (Table 1) contained approximately 130 diseases of cattle, sheep, goats, horses, swine, birds, lagomorphs, fish, crustaceans, molluscs, and bees. It also includes leishmaniasis, a disease that most often affects humans and canids.

The OIE's warning system, which allows member countries to take rapid action when outbreaks occur, is based on the list of reportable diseases. Within 24 hours of the first confirmed case of a listed disease, the affected country must report the incident to the OIE Central Bureau. When the disease appears to be eradicated, this is also reported to the OIE. If any new cases occur afterward, the OIE is again informed. Member nations must also immediately report emerging diseases that are either zoonotic or have significant morbidity or mortality rates in animals. In addition, they must inform the OIE of any changes in endemic diseases on the list. These changes might include a new strain of the pathogen, a sudden and unexpected increase in morbidity or mortality rates, or changes in epidemiology such as an expansion of the agent's host range or an increase in its pathogenicity. The OIE disseminates the reported information to its member countries via alerts published on its Web site and an electronic distribution list sent to member nations, OIE Reference Laboratories and Collaborating Centers, international and regional organizations, and others. Information on past outbreaks is also available on the OIE Web site. In addition, the OIE promotes and coordinates research into the surveillance and control of animal diseases throughout the world.

Another important function of the OIE is to set the standards for diagnostic methods and vaccine methodologies in international trade. In the world economy, the unimpeded flow of international trade in animals and animal products requires veterinary regulations designed to prevent the spread of transmissible diseases to animals and to human beings. To avoid unjustified trade barriers, these requirements must be harmonized between countries. The advent of the World Trade Organization (WTO) in 1995 has expanded the influence and importance of the OIE. The WTO was established as the implementing body for the Sanitary and Phytosanitary Measures Agreement (SPS Agreement) of the General Agreement on Tariffs and Trade (GATT). Member nations of the WTO must respect the SPS Agreement, which defines the requirements for food safety and animal and plant health as they relate to international trade. Any country that feels that its products are being unreasonably blocked by another country may appeal to the WTO. To decide the merits of a case, the WTO relies on the standards set by the OIE. Consequently, policies and decisions by the OIE can have reverberating consequences for international trade. Barriers to trade must now be scientifically justified and must not arbitrarily or unjustifiably discriminate among nations.

Table 1: Diseases Reportable to OIE as of January 23, 2006 *(formerly Lists A and B)*

Multiple species diseases

Anthrax
Aujeszky's disease
Bluetongue
Brucellosis (*Brucella abortus*)
Brucellosis (*Brucella melitensis*)
Brucellosis (*Brucella suis*)
Crimean Congo haemorrhagic fever
Echinococcosis/hydatidosis
Foot and mouth disease
Heartwater
Japanese encephalitis
Leptospirosis
New world screwworm
   (*Cochliomyia hominivorax*)

Old world screwworm (*Chrysomya bezziana*)
Paratuberculosis
Q fever
Rabies
Rift Valley fever
Rinderpest
Trichinellosis
Tularemia
Vesicular stomatitis
West Nile fever

Cattle diseases

Bovine anaplasmosis
Bovine babesiosis
Bovine genital campylobacteriosis

Bovine spongiform encephalopathy
Bovine tuberculosis
Bovine viral diarrhoea
Contagious bovine
    pleuropneumonia
Enzootic bovine leukosis
Haemorrhagic septicaemia
Infectious bovine rhinotracheitis/
    infectious pustular vulvovaginitis
Lumpky skin disease
Malignant catarrhal fever
Theileriosis
Trichomonosis
Trypanosomosis (tsetse-transmitted)

Sheep and goat diseases

Caprine arthritis/encephalitis
Contagious agalactia
Contagious caprine
    pleuropneumonia
Enzootic abortion of ewes
    (ovine chlamydiosis)
Maedi-visna
Nairobi sheep disease
Ovine epididymitis (*Brucella ovis*)
Peste des petits ruminants
Salmonellosis (*S. abortusovis*)
Scrapie
Sheep pox and goat pox

Equine diseases

African horse sickness
Contagious equine metritis
Dourine
Equine encephalomyelitis (Eastern)
Equine encephalomyelitis (Western)
Equine infectious anaemia
Equine influenza
Equine piroplasmosis
Equine rhinopneumonitis
Equine viral arteritis
Glanders
Surra (*Trypanosoma evansi*)
Venezuelan equine
    encephalomyelitis

Swine diseases

African swine fever
Classical swine fever

Nipah virus encephalitis
Porcine cysticercosis
Porcine reproductive and
    respiratory syndrome
Swine vesicular disease
Transmissible gastroenteritis

Avian diseases

Avian chlamydiosis
Avian infectious bronchitis
Avian infectious laryngotracheitis
Avian mycoplasmosis
    (*M. gallisepticum*)
Avian mycoplasmosis (*M. synoviae*)
Duck virus hepatitis
Fowl cholera
Fowl typhoid
Highly pathogenic avian influenza
Infectious bursal disease
    (Gumboro disease)
Marek's disease
Newcastle disease
Pullorum disease
Turkey rhinotracheitis

Lagomorph diseases

Myxomatosis
Rabbit haemorrhagic disease

Bee diseases

Acarapisosis of honey bees
American foulbrood of honey bees
European foulbrood of honey bees
Small hive beetle infestation
    (*Aethina tumida*)
Tropilaelaps infestation of honey bees
Varroosis of honey bees

Fish diseases

Epizootic haematopoietic necrosis
Infectious haematopoietic necrosis
Spring viraemia of carp
Viral haemorrhagic septicaemia
Infectious pancreatic necrosis
Infectious salmon anaemia
Epizootic ulcerative syndrome
Bacterial kidney disease
    (*Renibacterium salmoninarum*)
Gyrodactylosis (*Gyrodactylus salaris*)

Red sea bream iridoviral disease
Koi herpesvirus disease

Mollusc diseases

Infection with *Bonamia ostreae*
Infection with *Bonamia exitiosa*
Infection with *Marteilia refringens*
Infection with *Mikrocytos mackini*
Infection with *Perkinsus marinus*
Infection with *Perkinsus olseni*
Infection with
    Xenohaliotis californiensis

Crustacean diseases

Taura syndrome
White spot disease
Yellowhead disease
Tetrahedral baculovirosis
    (*Baculovirus penaei*)
Spherical baculovirosis (*Penaeus
    monodon-type baculovirus*)
Infectious hypodermal and
    haematopoietic necrosis
Necrotising hepatopancreatitis
Infectious myonecrosis

Other diseases

Camelpox
Leishmaniosis

Emerging Infectious Diseases

In addition to the foreign animal diseases on the OIE list, the U.S. is concerned about a number of **emerging infectious diseases**. Emerging infectious diseases are diseases that may have significant health impacts in animals or humans, and whose incidence has recently increased or is likely to increase. These emerging diseases are, in general, not yet found on the official OIE list. Examples of emerging diseases include postweaning multisystemic wasting syndrome (PMWS) in pigs and avian vacuolar myelinopathy in wild waterfowl and bald eagles. Some emerging diseases such as Hendra, Nipah, and bovine spongiform encephalopathy cause disease in both animals and humans while others —for example, hantaviruses, Ebola, Marburg, and *E. coli* O157:H7—seem to mainly threaten humans and related primates.

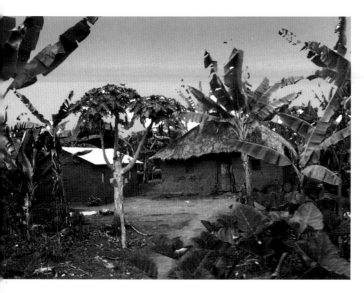

Emerging diseases are often seen where human settlements or agriculture expand into previously undeveloped areas. Here, humans and their domestic animals come into increasing contact with wildlife and their pathogens.
Source: Phil Hart
www.philhart.com

A variety of factors, often in combination, can result in an emerging disease. Sometimes new diseases are recognized when a pathogen enters a new host or becomes more virulent as the result of a mutation. New hosts are often infected as a result of increased contact with insect vectors, animal reservoirs, or environmental reservoirs for the pathogen. For this reason, emerging diseases are sometimes seen when human settlements or agriculture expand into previously undeveloped areas. The emerging disease may appear as sporadic cases, in limited outbreaks, or as a massive epidemic. In 1994, 1995, and 1999, Australia experienced small outbreaks of a new respiratory disease in horses; in all, 23 horses became ill and 16 of these animals died. Three humans in contact with the sick horses also became infected and two died as the result of their illness. The pathogen, called the Hendra virus, seems to have spread to the horses from flying foxes (a type of fruit bat). The Nipah virus in Malaysia also appears to have entered pigs from fruit bats; however, this virus was recognized when it caused an epizootic of respiratory and neurologic disease in pigs and an epidemic of fatal encephalitis in humans. To control the outbreak, more than a million pigs were culled and pig farming was banned in some parts of the country. Other emerging diseases that seem to result from contact with a pathogen's natural host include hantaviruses, which are contracted from various rodent hosts, and Ebola and Marburg, which spread to humans and other primates from unknown natural hosts.

In some cases, emerging diseases may be diseases that were simply not recognized before. It is quite possible that cases of Hendra, Nipah, or even Ebola occurred before the syndrome was described and the pathogen isolated. Bovine spongiform encephalopathy was recognized only in the mid-1980s but appears to have existed in cows since the 1970s. Emerging diseases also include infections that have expanded their geographic range and appeared in a new region; the West Nile virus, which entered the U.S. in 1999, can be considered an emerging pathogen.

Bioterrorism

Exotic diseases are usually introduced accidentally into a country or emerge as the result of natural factors. However, pathogens could also be introduced deliberately. **Bioterrorism**, or biological warfare, is defined as the intentional use of microorganisms or biological toxins in an effort to cause death or disease in humans, other animals, or plants in civilian settings. Chemical weapons, in contrast, are human-made poisonous substances that kill or incapacitate. In veterinary medicine, we are also concerned about **agroterrorism**, a specific form of bioterrorism in which the biological weapons target animal or crop agriculture to cause economic damage and instability. Some but not all of the agents that could be used in agroterrorism are foreign animal diseases.

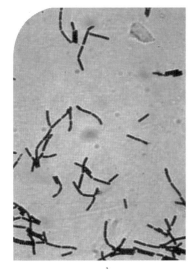

Anthrax bacteria can be used by bioterrorists to cause disease in humans or in animals.
Source: Texas Department of Health

The consequences of bioterrorist attacks directed at humans differ considerably from consequences of agroterrorist attacks. The effects of an attack directed against public health would be measured in human morbidity and mortality as well as the costs associated with decontamination, surveillance, control, and eradication if possible. The effects of an attack directed at the health of livestock or poultry would be measured in animal morbidity and mortality and associated clean up costs as for human diseases. In addition, astronomical costs associated with disruption of animal and animal product exports would likely accrue. If the biological agent used were a zoonotic agent, both sets of costs could be incurred, and the situation could be far worse. *Bacillus anthracis* is an example of a zoonotic agent. This spore-forming bacterium causes anthrax, a potentially fatal disease that can affect most mammals, including humans. The spores of *B. anthracis* can be used by bioterrorists to cause illness in humans or animals, spread fear, and disrupt the economy. During World War II, the German military allegedly used anthrax to contaminate horses and mules in Mesopotamia and France. In a more recent situation, anthrax spores sent through the U.S. mail caused fatal inhalation anthrax in several people and spread panic throughout the country.

One alarming aspect of bioterrorism is the relative ease of availability of pathogens and biological toxins and the lack of complicated equipment and technology required to use them. Bioterrorists could introduce the pathogen itself, infected animals or animal products, or insect vectors. How likely a pathogen is to be used as a bioterrorism agent is dictated by how easily it can be acquired as well as by its innate infectiousness, contagiousness, virulence, and pathogenicity. However, the magnitude of

Bioterrorism or biological warfare—the intentional use of microorganisms or toxins derived from living organisms or viruses to cause death or disease in humans, other animals, or plants in civilian settings

Agroterrorism—a specific form of bioterrorism in which the biological weapons target animal or crop agriculture to cause economic damage and instability

a bioterrorist attack is most heavily influenced by how quickly the agent is recognized, a response mobilized, and the agent contained, as well as by the availability of control and treatment options. Below are two lists of biological agents and diseases that are thought to pose the greatest threat to animal and public health. Although some agents are common to both lists, most of them are not. It is important to remember that the agents useful to the agroterrorist are primarily those that detrimentally impact agricultural trade, whereas the agents used in bioterrorist attacks against humans are chosen to elicit human mortality and cause fear.

Table 2: USDA and HHS Select Agent and Toxins (7 CFR Part 331, 9 CFR Part 121, and 42 CRF Part 73)

USDA

African horse sickness virus
African swine fever virus
Akabane virus
Avian influenza virus (highly pathogenic)
Bluetongue virus (exotic)
Bovine spongiform encephalopathy agent
Camel pox virus
Classical swine fever virus
Cowdria ruminantium (Heartwater)
Foot and mouth disease virus
Goat pox virus
Japanese encephalitis virus
Lumpy skin disease virus
Malignant catarrhal fever virus (exotic)
Menangle virus
Mycoplasma capricolum /*M.F38/M. mycoides capri*
    (contagious caprine pleuropneumonia)
Mycoplasma mycoides mycoides
    (contagious bovine pleuropneumonia)
Newcastle disease virus (VVND)
Peste des petits ruminants virus
Rinderpest virus
Sheep pox virus
Swine vesicular disease virus
Vesicular stomatitis virus (exotic)

USDA/HHS OVERLAP

Bacillus anthracis
Botulinum neurotoxins
Botulinum neurotoxin producing
    species of *Clostridium*
Brucella abortus
Brucella melitensis
Brucella suis
Burkholderia mallei
Burkholderia pseudomallei

Clostridium perfringens epsilon toxin
Coccidioides immitis
Coxiella burnetii
Eastern equine encephalitis virus
Francisella tularensis
Hendra virus
Nipah virus
Rift Valley fever virus
Shigatoxin
Staphylococcal enterotoxins
T-2 toxin
Venezuelan equine encephalitis virus

HHS

Abrin
Cercopithecine herpesvirus 1 (Herpes B virus)
Coccidioides posadasii
Conotoxins
Crimean-Congo haemorrhagic fever virus
Diacetoxyscirpenol
Ebola virus
Lassa fever virus
Marburg virus
Monkeypox virus
Reconstructed 1918 influenza virus
Ricin
Rickettsia prowazekii
Rickettsia rickettsii
Saxitoxin
Shiga-like ribosome inactivating proteins
South American Haemorrhagic Fever viruses
Tetrodotoxin
Tick-borne encephalitis complex (flavi) viruses
Variola major virus (Smallpox virus)
Variola minor virus (Alastrim)
Yersinia pestis

CHAPTER

Sources of Information

The Organization for Safety and Asepsis Procedures (OPSA). Available at: http://www.osap.org/training/symp/2000/summary/bioterrorism.htm.* Accessed 2003.

The West Nile Virus Surveillance Program. Available at: http://nationalatlas.gov/virususa.html.* Accessed 2003. [Current West Nile virus surveillance is conducted by the United States Geological Survey (USGS) and is available at http://westnilemaps.usgs.gov/index.html]

U.S. Centers for Disease Control and Prevention (CDC). Available at: http://www.cdc.org. Accessed 2003.

U.S. Centers for Disease Control and Prevention (CDC). List of biological agents and diseases posing threats to the public health. Available at: http://www.bt.cdc.gov/Agent/Agentlist.asp. Accessed 2003.

United States Department of Agriculture (USDA). High consequence pathogen list. Available at: http://aphisweb.aphis.usda.gov/NCIE/pdf/agent_toxin_list.pdf.* Accessed 2003. [Information about high consequence pathogens and toxins is now available at: http://www.aphis.usda.gov/programs/ag_selectagent/index.html]

USDA Animal and Plant Health Inspection Service (APHIS). Center for Emerging Issues. Available at: http://www.aphis.usda.gov:80/vs/ceah/cei/index.htm. Accessed 2003.

USDA Animal and Plant Health Inspection Service (APHIS). Emerging disease notices. Available at: http://www.aphis.usda.gov:80/vs/ceah/cei/notices.htm.* Accessed 2003. [Emerging disease notices are now available at: http://www.aphis.usda.gov/vs/ceah/cei/EmergingDiseaseNotice_files/notices.htm]

USDA Animal and Plant Health Inspection Service (APHIS), Center for Emerging Issues (CEI), and Centers for Epidemiology and Animal Health (CEAH). Emerging disease notice update. Nipah virus, Malaysia, November 1999. Available at: http://www.aphis.usda.gov/vs/ceah/cei/EmergingDiseaseNotice_files/nipahupd.htm . Accessed 2003.The World Organization for Animal Health. Available at: http://www.oie.int/. Accessed 2003.

The World Organization for Animal Health. Diseases notifiable to the OIE. Available at: http://www.oie.int/eng/maladies/en_classification.htm. Accessed 22 Nov. 2005.

The World Organization for Animal Health. Inform on the world animal health situation in all transparency. Available at: http://www.oie.int/eng/info/en_info.htm. Accessed 22 Nov. 2005.

defunct link as of 2005

CHAPTER two

> *To prevent foreign animal diseases from entering the U.S., authorities must monitor all of the routes by which pathogens could cross our borders.*

Routes of Transmission and the Introduction of Foreign Animal Diseases

Authors: *Katie M. Kurkjian, DVM; Susan E. Little, DVM, PhD; Sharon D. Nath, DVM; Corrie Brown, DVM, PhD*
The University of Georgia, College of Veterinary Medicine

Portals of Entry of a Foreign Animal Disease

A number of diseases on the OIE list, as well as emerging infectious diseases, constantly threaten to expand their geographic range and become established in new regions. Diseases such as heartwater, now found mainly in Africa, could become endemic in any country where suitable host populations and tick vectors exist. Where diseases have been eradicated from parts of the world, countries also face the ongoing threat of re-introduction. In 2001, for example, foot and mouth disease was re-introduced to the United Kingdom as well as to other FMD-free countries like Argentina and Uruguay. To prevent foreign animal diseases from entering the U.S., authorities must monitor all of the routes by which pathogens could cross our borders. This job is made more difficult by the existence of many diverse portals of entry, including livestock and pets, wildlife, animal products, arthropod vectors, inanimate objects, and humans.

Entry in animals

Each year, the U.S. imports livestock and poultry from many countries (1.5 million cattle and 5.8 million pigs were imported in 2002). People also return to the country with pets, either following a vacation or after living abroad. These animals must be screened to ensure that diseases are not entering the U.S. as hitchhikers on a flock of sheep or the family dog. Although the system works well, occasionally a potential disease problem is missed. In one recent incident, screwworms were found in a group of horses imported from Argentina, after they had left a U.S. quarantine facility. Animals that do not pass through inspection stations, such as smuggled animals or migratory wild animals, pose an even greater risk of introducing an exotic disease. During the last 20 years, many outbreaks of Newcastle disease have been caused by psittacine birds that were illegally imported

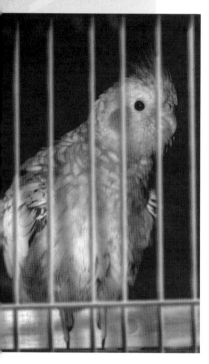

Foreign animal diseases can enter the U.S. readily in smuggled animals, which are not inspected at quarantine stations.
Source: Lisa Engelhaupt, ISU

into the U.S., bringing exotic Newcastle disease virus with them. And obviously, wild animals and birds do not stop at border inspection stations. A migratory bird carrying a bit of rabbit feces on its feet could easily stop in the U.S., depositing rabbit hemorrhagic disease in the vicinity of susceptible lagomorphs. Similarly, migrating birds with exotic poultry diseases fly freely across national borders.

Vectors and fomites

Pathogens can also enter the country on **fomites** (contaminated inanimate objects) and **vectors** (living organisms that transmit diseases from one animal to another). Vectors capable of carrying some very serious diseases of livestock have been imported on reptiles, which previously were not subject to screening by agriculture officials. *Amblyomma spp.* tick vectors of heartwater have been discovered on tortoises imported into Florida. Fomites can also carry pathogens into the country: for instance, a livestock virus could be carried across international borders on the shoe from a traveler who had walked through an infected farm.

Animal products

Each year the U.S. imports millions of tons of edible animal products. Although these shipments are screened for infectious agents, it is foolhardy to assume that the system is flawless. In addition, imported biologics such as vaccines, embryos and ova for embryo transfer, and semen for artificial insemination must be screened to ensure freedom from harmful infectious agents.

People

Humans can act as fomites or incubators to bring livestock diseases into the U.S. The foot and mouth disease virus, for example, may survive for days on clothing or shoes under cool, damp conditions. Failure to adequately disinfect outerwear contaminated by this virus could result in an epizootic within the U.S. Another human-as-fomite possibility would be carrying pork products from a country in which classical swine fever is endemic. This systemic disease of pigs, present in both the Dominican Republic and Cuba, could enter the U.S. through a discarded sausage or ham sandwich brought in by a traveler. Additionally, there are some diseases that infect both people and animals. Rift Valley fever, for instance, is a mosquito-borne viral disease that causes illness in both humans and ruminants. A human returning from a visit in an infected part of the world could be incubating Rift Valley fever on return to the U.S. and, once within our borders, develop a full-blown viremia that mosquitoes could then pick up and carry to ruminant livestock nearby.

Besides all of these unintentional means of introduction, consider the possibilities of a nefarious introduction: for instance, a bioterrorist using

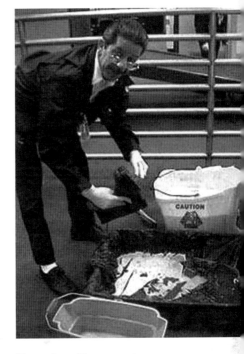

Francisco Tomas using an airport boot brush to eliminate organisms found on soiled boots.
Source: Corrie Brown

Fomites—contaminated inanimate objects

Vectors—living organisms that transmit diseases from one animal to another

a foreign animal disease agent to decimate our susceptible livestock species. Any of the routes mentioned above could be used by a bioterrorist. The economic consequences would be the same as those of an unintentional introduction and our only defense is to respond rapidly and effectively.

Definitions for Understanding the Transmission of Exotic Diseases

While many portals of entry exist for exotic diseases, each specific pathogen can use only some of these routes. To understand the characteristics of a given agent that contribute to the likelihood for introduction, we must first review some general concepts in animal disease transmission.

A **disease** is defined as any deviation from normal structure or function. Diseases may be described according to their transmission characteristics. An **infectious disease** is a disease caused by the invasion and multiplication of a living agent in or on a host. Infectious diseases can be described as viral, bacterial, mycotic, or parasitic according to the type of etiologic agent responsible. Infections may or may not result in disease. In contrast, an **infestation** is the invasion, but not multiplication, of an organism in or on a host. Because they multiply in the host, bacterial and viral diseases are considered to be infections. However, parasitic diseases can be either infestations or infections depending on the life cycle of the parasite in question. Many metazoan parasites do not multiply within the same host; the presence of these agents is most appropriately referred to as an infestation. These two terms are also commonly used to contrast the presence of organisms inside a host body (infection) with the presence of organisms on the hair, fur, feathers, or skin of the host (infestation). In Lyme disease, for example, the tick vector *Ixodes scapularis* infests a host while the bacterial pathogen *Borrelia burgdorferi* is transmitted by the tick and infects the host.

A **contagious disease** is a disease that is transmissible from one human or animal to another via direct or airborne means. Agents that cause contagious diseases can be spread from animal to animal in excretions and secretions, respiratory aerosols, scabs, and other body fluids or tissues. One example of a directly contagious disease is peste des petits ruminants, a serious viral disease of small ruminants in Africa, the Middle East, India, and the Arabian peninsula. Sheep and goats with peste des petits ruminants excrete infectious virus in their ocular, nasal, and oral secretions. Coughing and sneezing animals readily spread the virus to nearby animals in aerosols.

Infectious diseases can also be communicable without being contagious. A **communicable disease** is caused by an agent capable of transmission by direct, airborne, or indirect routes from an infected person, animal, or plant, or from a contaminated inanimate reservoir such as the soil. Indirect routes include transmission by insects or on vehicles such as food, water, clothing, and equipment. Many important communicable dis-

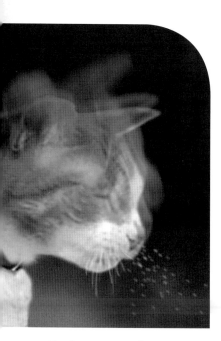

Pathogens can become aerosolized during a cough or sneeze.
Source: Clint May, ISU

Disease—any deviation from normal structure or function

Infectious disease—
a disease caused by the invasion and multiplication of a living agent in or on a host

Infestation—the invasion, but not multiplication, of an organism in or on a host

Contagious disease—
a disease that is transmissible from one human or animal to another via direct or airborne means

Communicable disease—
a disease caused by an agent capable of transmission by direct, airborne, or indirect routes from an infected person, animal, or plant, or from a contaminated inanimate reservoir

eases are not directly contagious, but are transmitted between animals by arthropod vectors. African horse sickness is one example. This disease, a severe cardiac and pulmonary disease of horses and other Equidae, is caused by an orbivirus transmitted by biting midges in the genus *Culicoides*. Infected horses can transmit the African horse sickness virus to new *Culicoides* vectors but do not spread it directly to other horses.

Understanding these terms is crucial to understanding how exotic diseases are introduced into a country. For example, if a disease is highly contagious, we know that we have to prevent close contact between possibly infected animals and those that are immunologically naïve. Such prevention may take the form of quarantining animals, possibly slaughtering infected or exposed animals, and increasing surveillance to prevent the future spread of the disease. In some cases, care must also be taken to prevent contact with inanimate objects that may harbor viable infectious organisms to prevent the spread of communicable diseases.

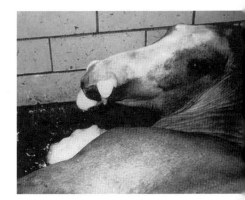

Horses with African horse sickness can develop a variety of syndromes, including pulmonary or cardiac disease. African horse sickness, which is spread by biting midges, is communicable but not contagious.
Source: Foreign Animal Diseases-The Gray Book, 1998

Routes of Transmission of Infectious Disease Agents

The most likely route of introduction of an exotic disease depends on its mode of transmission. A pathogen transmitted by mosquitoes can be spread between regions in an infected insect, while a virus that persists on fomites can enter a country on a contaminated shoe. Other, more fragile, pathogens may be able to enter new areas only in the infected host animal. A number of factors can influence the mode of introduction of a given pathogen: whether it is transmitted between unrelated animals or from parent to offspring, if an intermediate host or vector is required for transmission, how persistent the pathogen is in the environment, and whether the disease agent is immediately infectious or requires time in the environment to develop to the infectious stage. Disease agents that are more easily transmitted and spread are considered to pose a greater threat of introduction.

Vertical transmission

Vertical transmission is the transfer of a pathogen from a parent, usually the dam, to the offspring through reproduction. Infectious diseases are usually transferred from the mother to the embryo, fetus, or newborn prior to, during, or shortly after parturition. Types of vertical transmission in veterinary species include transplacental passage of pathogens to the offspring and the transmission of infectious agents through the colostrum or milk. Classical swine fever virus (CFSV) is an example of a disease agent that can

Vertical transmission—the transfer of a pathogen from a parent, usually the dam, to the offspring through reproduction.

Transmission through milk or colostrum is one form of vertical transmission.
Source: USDA

be transferred vertically. If a sow becomes infected with CSFV while she is pregnant, the virus can cross the placenta, resulting in infection of the fetus and potentially the newborn. *Toxoplasma gondii*, the causative agent of toxoplasmosis, can also be transmitted vertically through the placenta. Transplacental transmission of *T. gondii* can cause abortion in sheep and severe congenital abnormalities in humans. *Strongyloides stercoralis*, a small intestinal nematode of dogs, cats, and humans, can be transmitted via the milk from a dam to her nursing offspring.

Horizontal transmission

Horizontal transmission is the transfer of a pathogen from an infected animal to a naïve animal, independent of the parental relationship of those individuals. Horizontal transmission can occur by either direct or indirect contact. Pathogens spread by **direct contact** are transmitted directly from animal to animal; pathogens spread by **indirect contact** are transmitted through an intermediary such as a physical object or insect.

Chart 1: Horizontal Transmission

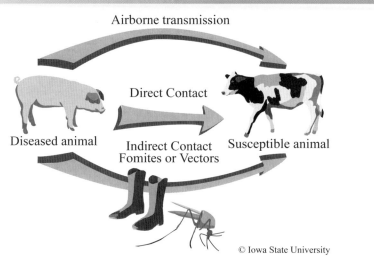

© Iowa State University

Horizontal transmission— the transfer of a pathogen from an infected animal to a naïve animal, independent of the parental relationship of those individuals

Direct contact— pathogens transmitted directly from animal to animal

Indirect contact— pathogens transmitted through an intermediary such as a physical object or insect

Airborne transmission— the transfer of a pathogen via particles in the air, usually aerosolized

Fomites— inanimate objects that can carry infectious agents from one animal to another

Disease agents transferred by direct contact may be spread by actions such as licking, rubbing, biting, and coitus. The classical swine fever virus, the causative agent of classical swine fever, is an example of an agent that can be transmitted horizontally by direct contact. This virus is spread from pig to pig primarily by oral contact with blood, tissues, secretions, and fomites. Classical swine fever is most often introduced when infected pigs are mixed with uninfected pigs; thus livestock shows and auction sales are two high-risk places for infection. **Airborne transmission** is also considered to be a form of direct horizontal transmission because pathogenic agents don't usually survive extended periods of time within aerosolized particles. Close proximity of infected and non-infected susceptible individuals is thus required for airborne transmission. Foot and mouth disease is a classic example of a disease that uses airborne transmission. The direct and indirect routes are not mutually exclusive; some agents can be spread by both routes.

Indirect contact through fomites and vectors

Pathogens transmitted by indirect contact are spread by fomites or vectors. **Fomites** are inanimate objects that can carry infectious agents from one animal to another. Examples of fomites include used needles, dirty clippers, contaminated clothing or vehicles, and contaminated food and water supplies. **Iatrogenic transmission** is a specific form of horizontal transmission by fomites in which the veterinarian or physician accidentally furthers the spread of a disease agent via routes such as contaminated instruments or vaccines. Routine procedures such as bleeding, tagging, dehorning, and vaccinating can create an opportunity for iatrogenic transmission by contaminating pieces of medical equipment, which serve as fomites for the pathogen.

The term **vector** is sometimes used in a broad sense to signify anything that allows the transport and/or transmission of a pathogen. Some sources consider fomites to be vectors. However, according to a strict, ecological definition, vector-borne transmission occurs when a living creature, because of its ecological relationship to others, acquires a pathogen from one living host and transmits it to another. Thus vector-borne transmission is a form of indirect horizontal transmission in which a biological intermediary, often an arthropod, carries a disease agent between animals. Vectors may be either biological or mechanical. A **biological vector** is a vector that supports replication of the pathogen. The disease agent and the biological vector have a long-standing ecological relationship. Biological vectors are usually persistently infected with the disease agent and may even be a required part of that organism's life cycle. A **mechanical vector**, on the other hand, is a vector that carries the pathogen but the pathogen is not altered while on the vector. Infection in mechanical vectors tends to be short-lived and a mechanical vector is considered to be little more than a flying fomite.

Bovine anaplasmosis, caused by *Anaplasma marginale,* is an example of an agent that can be transmitted by both vectors and fomites. In the western United States, *A. marginale* is transmitted by members of the hard tick genera *Dermacentor* and *Boophilus* and thus is a vector-borne disease. However, in the southeastern and midwestern U.S., mechanical transmission by biting flies and iatrogenic transmission with contaminated equipment and needles appears to be more important in maintaining this disease.

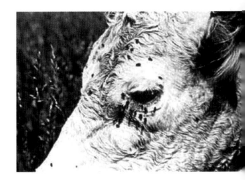

Flies feeding on a cow can transmit disease agents mechanically between animals.
Source: KY Pest News Newsletter

Iatrogenic transmission—a specific form of horizontal transmission by fomites in which the veterinarian or physician accidentally furthers the spread of a disease agent via routes such as contaminated instruments or vaccines

Vector—used in a broad sense to signify anything that allows the transport and/or transmission of a pathogen

Biological vector—a vector that supports replication of the pathogen

Mechanical vector— a vector that carries the pathogen but the pathogen is not altered while on the vector

Transstadial transmission—infection with a pathogen is maintained in the vector as it develops between life stages

Transovarial transmission—a form of vertical transmission in which the female vector passes the infectious agent through her eggs to the next generation

Transmission Dynamics within Biological Vector Populations

The two major forms of transmission within vector populations, transstadial and transovarial, can be very important in maintaining a source of infection for animals. In **transstadial transmission**, infection with a pathogen is maintained in the vector as it develops between life stages. A tick vector infected as a larva with *Borrelia burgdorferi*, the causative agent of Lyme disease, will maintain the infection when it next molts to the nymph and then the adult stage. **Transovarial transmission** is a form of vertical transmission in which the female vector passes the infectious agent through her eggs to the next generation. Eggs passed by an adult female *Boophilus* tick infected with *Babesia bigemina* will hatch infected larvae.

Transovarial transmission can be very important in maintaining a source of infection for animals. In particular, it allows pathogens to survive conditions that kill the adult vectors but allow the eggs to survive. This can be illustrated by an outbreak of vesicular stomatitis in the 1980s. Vesicular stomatitis, a livestock disease found in the Americas, causes vesicles and ulcers on the mouth and hooves of swine, cattle, and horses. The agent, the vesicular stomatitis virus, is spread by black flies and sand flies. In 1982, an outbreak of vesicular stomatitis occurred in the southwestern United States. Authorities expected this outbreak to subside upon the death of adult flies following the first winter frost. Unexpectedly, the outbreak continued throughout the winter. At the time, this continuance was attributed to the movement of infected animals and the exposure of uninfected animals to contaminated objects. However, it is now known that the vesicular stomatitis virus is transmitted transovarially in its vectors and this may have contributed to the overwintering ability of the virus.

Characteristics of Pathogens that Influence their Potential for Introduction

The innate characteristics of pathogenic organisms play a huge role in determining their modes of transmission. Understanding these characteristics is essential to preventing the introduction of a foreign animal disease and controlling or eradicating it once it has been introduced. Important characteristics that can influence the transmission of a pathogen include its persistence in the environment or in a host, the time required for it to become infective after it has been shed from a host, and other aspects of its life cycle. Some of the diseases cited below are not FADs, but serve as useful examples.

Persistence in the environment

Disease agents vary in their ability to survive outside a living host; some agents are quickly inactivated by sunlight, high temperatures, pH changes, or other environmental factors while others can withstand harsh conditions for months or even years. The **persistence** of the organism in

Persistence—the amount of time a disease agent can survive outside a living host

the environment determines how long we can expect to find the agent. Anthrax bacteria (*Bacillus anthracis*), for example, produce spores that persist in the environment for many years. Cases of anthrax can occur for decades in a contaminated pasture, in animals that have had no direct contact with an infected host. Agents that can persist in the environment for long periods of time, such as anthrax, can be particularly hard to eradicate.

Persistence in the host

Some pathogens enter the host temporarily; if they do not kill the host, they are eliminated by the immune response. Others can become permanent residents, persisting with or without symptoms for the lifetime of the animal. The maedi-visna virus, for example, usually infects a lamb or goat when it drinks contaminated milk or colostrum then becomes resident in that animal for life. Some animals infected with this virus develop dyspnea, neurologic signs, mastitis, or arthritis; however, many remain asymptomatic. These asymptomatic animals can, nevertheless, infect their offspring or other animals in close contact with them. Agents that persist in the host, such as the maedi-visna virus, can "hide" in asymptomatic hosts between clinical infections or epidemics. The asymptomatic carriers thus spread disease but are not readily detected as sources of the disease.

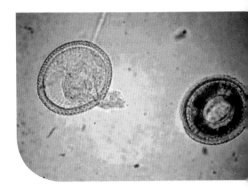

This photo shows two Toxocara canis *eggs. The one on the right contains the infectious L2 stage. The egg on the left is not embryonated, and thus is not infectious at this time.*
Source: Dr. Susan Little

Some infections are maintained in a **reservoir** population between disease outbreaks. A reservoir is an animal or group of animals that continuously contains the disease agent and can spread it to other groups. In some cases, a single animal is persistently infected throughout its lifetime. In others, the agent is maintained in a population, where it is spread from animal to animal. Reservoir hosts serve as a habitat for the pathogen to survive and may or may not become ill from the infection. Migratory waterfowl, for example, sometimes act as reservoir hosts and can spread diseases to poultry flocks when the species come into close contact.

Amount of maturation required for infectivity

Some pathogenic agents are immediately infectious to an individual and do not require time for development either within the environment or within another host or vector. The cysts of *Giardia*, a protozoan that can cause diarrhea in numerous species, are immediately infectious to animals when shed. In contrast, some organisms require time to develop into an infectious stage. *Toxocara canis*, an ascarid of wild canids and domestic dogs is a good example. The eggs of this parasite are unembryonated when shed in the feces and must develop for two to four weeks in the environment before they become infectious.

Reservoir—an animal or group of animals that continuously contains the disease agent and can spread it to other groups

The life cycle of the pathogen

Many aspects of the pathogen's life cycle, already discussed, influence how easily it can be controlled and the points at which it can be destroyed. For example, some disease agents are found only in infected animals, passing directly from animal to animal. These agents can be controlled by destroying the agent within the host or preventing it from entering new hosts. The smallpox virus, which infects only humans, was eradicated by isolating infected humans and vaccinating their contacts. This approach, however, is only successful if the pathogen does not persist for long periods in the environment or in a host that must be kept alive, and does not enter vectors. Rinderpest fits these criteria and is a candidate for worldwide eradication. The host range of the pathogen is also important. Pathogens that infect a single host species are usually easier to control than agents that infect many different host species. Infected wildlife can be particularly difficult to identify and control; once a pathogen enters native wildlife, eradication may become impossible.

Parasitic diseases present additional complications. The control of a parasitic infection is influenced by whether the parasite's life cycle is direct or indirect. Parasites with a **direct life cycle** can complete their entire developmental cycle in a single host. Parasites with an **indirect life cycle** require an intermediate host, a host in which the agent develops but does not reach sexual maturity. Most parasitic trematodes (flukes) and cestodes (tapeworms) and some nematodes have indirect lifecycles. Many species may act as intermediate hosts. For example, snails are usually the first intermediate host of trematodes. Ticks may require one, two, or three hosts to complete their life cycle. The majority of hard tick species in North America have a three-host life cycle in which the larva, nymph, and adult feed on three different hosts.

Examples of Introductions by Different Routes of Transmission

Now that you have reviewed the introductory material, we are going to investigate actual modes of introduction of exotic diseases. Exotic diseases can be introduced into a country by the movement of fomites, vectors, infected animals, animal products, or by the emergence of new diseases or new variants. The likelihood of these introduction events can be decreased through strict surveillance, precautionary practices, and improved biosecurity.

In order to enhance your understanding of the modes of introduction, we will present examples of each of these potential routes for you to review. As you work through the examples, you may wish to review the definitions and examples presented in the first half of this chapter or explore the expanded information on specific diseases provided in Section 2 of this book.

Direct life cycle—indicates a parasite that can complete their entire development within a single host

Indirect life cycle—indicates a parasite that requires an intermediary host in which to develop but does not reach sexual maturity

Fomites and the Introduction of Foot and Mouth Disease

Q: How could these filthy boots cause ulcers on the hooves of a calf?

A: By serving as a fomite that carries a pathogen from one animal to another. As you may recall, a fomite is an inanimate object on which a pathogen can be conveyed. Disease transmission occurs via shared physical contact between the object and the animal. Classic examples of fomites are contaminated footwear, veterinary equipment, needles, clothing, eating or drinking containers, cages, bedding, dander, restraint devices, and transportation vehicles. The control of fomites can be vital in preventing the spread of some diseases, such as foot and mouth disease (FMD).

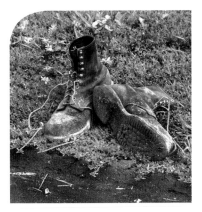

Source: Clint May, ISU

In 2001, the United Kingdom was facing a crisis of epic proportions. In February of that year, a veterinary inspector found lesions suggestive of FMD on several pigs in an abattoir. The movement of animals in the U.K. was halted and the pigs were traced back to an infected farm in Northumberland. But by this time the FMD virus had spread, resulting in an epidemic that devastated the livestock industry and economy of the U.K. Before the outbreak was finally brought under control, more than 2,000 cases of FMD had been diagnosed, more than four million animals had been slaughtered, and foci of infection had spread to France, Ireland, and the Netherlands. FMD is currently endemic in parts of Asia, Africa, the Middle East, and South America. Although the U.K. and many other countries have eradicated this disease within their borders, re-introduction of the virus can lead to massive epidemics such as the one seen in 2001. How is this disease introduced and spread to new areas?

One method of spread is by fomites. Under the right conditions, the foot and mouth disease virus can persist for days to weeks in the environment. Virus particles that contaminate footwear, clothing, transportation equipment, and other fomites can be transported long distances. Although FMD is very rarely infectious to humans, humans can carry the virus in their nasal passages for one to two days, and may transport the virus on clothing. Because of the high risk of transmission by humans and fomites, officials target people to try to prevent the introduction of the virus. Travelers who have visited FMD-positive countries and who have been on farms or contacted farm animals are required to declare this information at customs. Officials inspect their baggage and disinfect soiled footwear with bleach and detergents. Infectious virus can also be found in animal products such as meat-in-bone, milk, bones, glands, and cheese. All ruminant and swine products are confiscated and travelers are asked to wash their clothing prior to

During an epidemic, officials within FMD-positive countries may decide to vaccinate susceptible animals as an aid in controlling the outbreak. They may also work to control the outbreak by establishing free zones with border animal movement control and surveillance, slaughtering infected, recovered, and FMD-susceptible contact animals, disinfecting premises and inanimate objects that contact livestock, destroying cadavers, litter, and susceptible animal products in infected areas, and establishing strict quarantine policies.

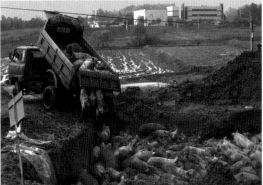

Source: Dr. John Carr, ISU

returning home to a FMD-free area. In addition, travelers are instructed to stay off all farms for at least five days after their return.

Vectors and the Introduction of West Nile Virus

Q: How could this insect cause circling, convulsions and ataxia in horses?

A: By serving as a vector for a pathogen that causes encephalitis. Vectors may be either biological vectors that are persistently infected and allow the pathogen to develop and reproduce or mechanical vectors on which the pathogen resides for a short period of time. Because they are persistently infected, biological vectors are more likely to introduce exotic disease agents to new areas than are mechanical vectors. The entry of the West Nile virus (WNV) into the United States in 1999 may have been an example of a vector-borne introduction. West Nile virus causes encephalitis in humans, horses, and some species of birds. Mosquito vectors spread this virus; in the U.S., members of both *Culex* and *Aedes* are capable of transmitting it. Until recently, West Nile encephalitis was found only in Africa, Europe, the Middle East, west and central Asia, and Oceania. In the summer and fall of 1999, West Nile virus was identified in dead birds in and around the Bronx zoo and, concurrently, in several cases of human and equine encephalitis in New York. How did West Nile virus enter the United States?

Scientists with the Centers for Disease Control and Prevention suspect that West Nile virus was present in the U.S. by at least early summer of 1999. The virus' point of origination is unclear but isolates from the U.S. most closely resemble virus strains from Israel. A possible scenario for introduction is that an infected mosquito vector from an endemic area traveled to North America on an airplane and was inadvertently released from the airplane, resulting in the introduction of the virus into native bird populations.

Various species of birds can serve as reservoirs for West Nile virus. To date, over 110 species of birds, predominately corvids (crows, ravens and their relatives), have tested positive for the virus. Birds with severe infections suffer high morbidity and mortality rates, but typically develop life-long immunity after exposure and a short viremia. Mosquitoes acquire the virus when they feed on the infected reservoir birds. Many mammals, including humans and horses, are incidental hosts that become infected when fed upon by an infected mosquito. Although mammals do not develop levels of viremia sufficient to infect mosquitoes, and thus cannot serve as reservoirs, infections in mammals may result in severe, potentially fatal meningoencephalitis. Some adult *Culex* species in the northeastern U.S. survive the winter and thus are able to overwinter the virus. Either these mosquitoes or infected birds may have been responsible for the persistence of the virus and the re-emergence of West Nile encephalitis in the sum-

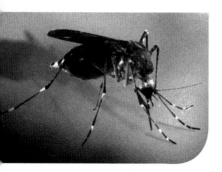

A female mosquito (Aedes trivittatus)
Source: Clint May, ISU

mers of 2000, 2001, and 2002. In spite of eradication efforts targeted at the mosquito vector, West Nile virus has become endemic in the 48 contiguous U.S. states. Additional information on the West Nile virus in the U.S. can be found in chapter 5, Descriptions of Recent Incursions of Exotic Animal Diseases.

Infected Animals and the Introduction of *Elaphostrongylus rangiferi*

Source: Phillip Greenspun

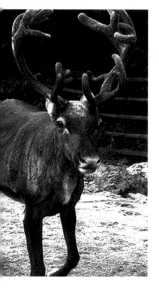

Q: How could this apparently healthy animal cause neurologic disease in caribou herds throughout Newfoundland?

A: By carrying an exotic disease agent that can become established in animal herds, the environment, or vectors native to the area. When it enters a country, a healthy-looking animal may be incubating an exotic disease or serving as an asymptomatic reservoir for a pathogen. Depending on the mode of transmission of the particular pathogen, naïve animals may then become infected by direct or indirect contact with the animal. Introduction of infected animals is thought to have been responsible for bringing cerebrospinal elaphostrongylosis to native Canadian caribou.

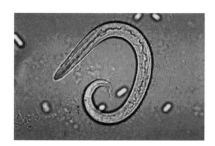

A larva of Elaphostrongylus rangiferi *found on fecal examination of an infected cervid. Larvae of* Elaphostrongylus spp. *are indistinguishable from those of the more widespread* Paralaphostrongylus spp.
Source: Susan Little

Cerebrospinal elaphostrongylosis is a severe neurological disease of cervids, sheep, and goats caused by the nematode *Elaphostrongylus rangiferi*. *E. rangiferi* has an indirect life cycle. Caribou or reindeer are the definitive hosts and shed larvae in their feces. The larvae penetrate the footpad of a snail or slug intermediate host to develop into the infective stage. Caribou or reindeer then ingest infected snails or slugs while feeding. Once in the host, the parasites migrate through the spinal cord and brain before reaching the muscles of the shoulder and hindlimbs where they mature. Eggs passed by adults are carried via the bloodstream to the lungs where they hatch into larvae, cross the alveoli, travel up the respiratory tree, are swallowed, and are then excreted in the feces.

Animals with cerebrospinal elaphostrongylosis develop a severe neurologic disease.
Source: Foreign Animal Disease-The Gray Book

Cerebral elaphostrongylosis was first recognized in Newfoundland in the 1970s. It was introduced to Newfoundland in the early 1900s when infected reindeer were imported from Norway to establish herds for food and draft animals. Once in Newfoundland, the reindeer traveled across native caribou range and some escaped, most likely commingling with caribou.

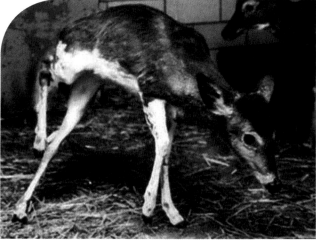

At present, most of the caribou herds in Newfoundland are infected with *E. rangiferi* although mainland herds appear to remain free of infection. To prevent introductions such as this, animals entering a country are now quarantined and tested for exotic diseases before they are allowed to mingle with native populations.

Animal Products and the
Introduction of African Swine Fever

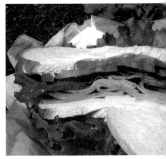

Source: Travis Engelhaupt, ISU

Q: How could this ham sandwich cause fever, anorexia, and reddened skin in pigs?

A: By carrying a pathogen that can survive for a period of time in animal products. Animal products can transmit disease agents when they are discarded near farms or are deliberately fed to susceptible animals. The practice of feeding uncooked scraps to pigs, now discouraged in many countries, is a typical route of introduction for several exotic swine diseases, including African swine fever (ASF). To prevent the introduction of African swine fever, officials tightly regulate the movement of pork products from endemic to ASF-free countries.

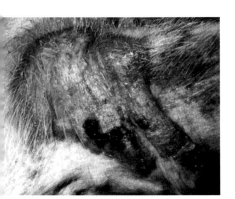

Lesions in animals with African swine fever may include reddened skin, splenomegaly, lung lobule consolidation, and skin necrosis.
Source: USDA

The African swine fever virus is a DNA virus that is newly classified in its own group, Asfarviridae but has similarities to both Iridovirus and Poxvirus. Susceptible animals include domestic and feral pigs, wart hogs, and peccaries. African swine fever is currently endemic in Sub-Saharan Africa and has been present but is now eradicated from Cuba, Haiti, and the Dominican Republic. The disease is characterized by fever, depression, occasional hemorrhagic disorders, and sometimes death. Transmission occurs via direct contact with infected animals or indirect contact via ticks, fomites, or feeding infected meat to pigs.

Preventing the introduction of African swine fever requires strict regulation of the importation of pigs and pork products. The virus is very hardy and can survive for months within pork products or in infected ticks. The virus remains infectious for 140 days in salted dried hams, for several years in frozen carcasses, and for 15 days in bone meal stored at 39°C. However, the virus can be inactivated by heating unprocessed meat to 70°C for 30 minutes. Importation of pork products from an infected herd poses the greatest risk for introduction of the disease. Official regulations control the importation of animal products from countries known to harbor OIE-regulated diseases. In addition, animal products are confiscated from travelers returning to the United States.

The Emergence of New Diseases and the Development of Bovine Spongiform Encephalopathy

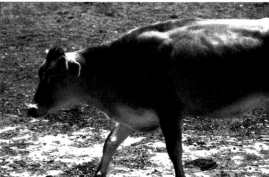

Source: Travis Engelhaupt, ISU

Q: How could this animal develop an exotic disease without exposure to any known pathogen?

A: By contracting a previously unknown animal disease. Each year new strains of pathogens are discovered, and occasionally completely novel pathogens are recognized. The transmissible spongiform encephalopathies (TSEs) are examples of a novel pathogen type that has emerged in several forms over the last few decades. Transmissible spongiform encephalopathies are fatal neurologic diseases found in a number of species including sheep, goats, cattle, elk, deer, exotic ruminants, cats, mink, and humans. Animals with TSEs develop progressive neurologic degeneration and exhibit incoordination, ataxia, nervousness or aggression, and decreased production despite continued appetite. The agents of TSEs have not been completely characterized, but the pathogen appears to be smaller than a virus. Three major theories have been put forth to describe the causative agents of TSEs: (1) the agent is a prion with an exclusively host-coded protein that is modified to a partially protease-resistant form after infection, (2) the agent is a virus with unusual characteristics, or (3) the agent is a small, noncoding regulatory nucleic acid coated with a host-derived protective protein. In most cases, TSE agents seem to be spread orally.

Some TSEs, including scrapie in sheep and chronic wasting disease in deer and elk, have been recognized for a number of years. Others appear to be new variants. Bovine spongiform encephalopathy (BSE), commonly referred to as mad cow disease, was first diagnosed in Great Britain in 1986. By the time BSE was recognized, a full-blown epidemic had begun. In spite of control measures, the number of cases escalated each year, finally peaking in 1993. Epidemiological evidence suggests that BSE developed in British cattle when they consumed feed that used contaminated meat-and-bone meal as a protein source. The relationship of BSE to other TSEs is not fully understood, but cases of new variant Creutzfeldt Jakob disease (vCJD), a human TSE, have been causally linked to exposure to BSE. In the U.K. and many other countries, the use of mammalian meat-and-bone meal in feed for all food-producing animals is now prohibited; in addition, because older animals are more likely to be infected, carcasses from animals more than 30 months of age are no longer allowed to be used as domestic animal or human food. Additional information on the BSE epidemic, including the cases recently found in the U.S., can be found in chapter 5, Descriptions of Recent Incursions of Exotic Animal Diseases.

Sources of Information

Buisch W, Hyde J, Mebus C, editors. Foreign Animal Diseases., 7th ed. Richmond, Virginia: U.S. Animal Health Association; 1998.

Personal communication, Dr. Ed Arza, Area-Veterinarian-in-Charge, APHIS-USDA, Conyers, Georgia

Personal communication, Dr. Lee Myers, State Veterinarian, Georgia. Department of Agriculture, Atlanta, Georgia

Foot and Mouth Disease:

U.S. Department of Agriculture (USDA), Animal and Plant Health Inspection Service (APHIS). Foot and mouth disease questions and answers. Available at: http://www.aphis.usda.gov/lpa/pubs/fsheet_faq_notice/faq_ahfmd.html [old URL: http://www.aphis.usda.gov/oa/pubs/qafmd301.html.*] Accessed 2003.

World Organization for Animal Health (OIE)/ Food and Agriculture Organization of the United Nations (FAO). FAO World Reference Laboratory's foot and mouth disease home page. Available at: http://www.iah.bbsrc.ac.uk/virus/Picornaviridae/Aphthovirus/fmd.htm. Accessed 2003.

World Organization for Animal Health (OIE.). Foot and mouth disease. In: Manual of diagnostic tests and vaccines for terrestrial animals. Paris: OIE; 2000.Available at: http://www.oie.int/eng/maladies/fiches/A_A010.htm. Accessed 2003.

West Nile Virus:

National Atlas of the United States, Distribution maps of West Nile virus detection in humans, mosquito, wild birds, and other animals. Available at: http://nationalatlas.gov/virususa.html.* Accessed 2003. [Current West Nile virus surveillance is conducted by the United States Geological Survey (USGS) and is available at http://westnilemaps.usgs.gov/index.html]

Sander DM. All the virology on the WWW (links to West Nile virus and other viruses). Flaviviridae – Flaviviruses. Available at: http://www.Tulane.EDU:80/~dmsander/garryfavweb12.html#Flavi. Accessed 2003.

U.S. Centers for Disease Control and Prevention. West Nile virus. Available at: http://www.cdc.gov/ncidod/dvbid/westnile/index.htm. Accessed 2003.

Cerebral Elaphostrongylosis:

Canadian Co-operative Wildlife Health Centre. Available at: http://wildlife1.usask.ca/ccwhc2003/. Accessed 2003.

The Government of Newfoundland and Labrador. Newfoundland and Labrador Agriculture Department. Available at: http://www.gov.nf.ca/agric/her&rab/BrainInfest.htm.* Accessed 2003.

African Swine Fever:

U.S. Department of Agriculture (USDA) Center for Emerging Issues. Available at: http://www.aphis.usda.gov/vs/ceah/cei/. Accessed 2003.

World Organization for Animal Health (OIE). African swine fever. In: Manual of diagnostic tests and vaccines for terrestrial animals. Paris: OIE; 2000. Available at: http://www.oie.int/eng/maladies/fiches/A_A120.HTM. Accessed 2003.

Bovine Spongiform Encephalopathy:

U.S. Department of Agriculture (USDA) Animal and Plant Health Inspection Service (APHIS). Bovine spongiform encephalopathy. Available at: http://www.aphis. usda.gov/lpa/issues/bse/bse.html. Accessed 2003.

USDA Center for Emerging Issues. Available at: http://www.aphis.usda.gov/vs/ceah/ cei/notices.htm.* Accessed 2003.

defunct link as of 2005

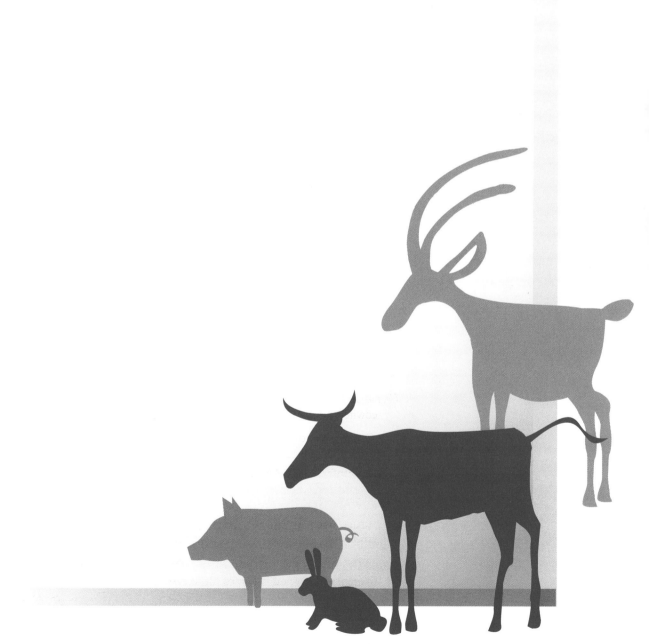

CHAPTER
three

> *Government agencies work together to prevent exotic disease agents from entering the U.S., investigate and diagnose suspicious cases, and respond to confirmed outbreaks.*

The Response to a Foreign Animal Disease Outbreak, and the Agencies Involved

Authors: *Anna Rovid Spickler, DVM, PhD*
Iowa State University

Foreign animal diseases (FADs) are a constant threat to the United States. Many diseases we consider to be exotic, such as foot-and-mouth disease, were once present in this country and could easily be re-established if surveillance, border controls, and eradication activities were relaxed. Unfortunately, FADs do occasionally enter the U.S. In 1983, an extensive epidemic of highly pathogenic avian influenza broke out in Pennsylvania and surrounding states, and lasted until 1984. Screwworms were found in a horse in Florida in 2000. Rabbit hemorrhagic disease outbreaks occurred in 2000, 2001 and 2005, and exotic Newcastle disease was found in poultry in California, Arizona, Nevada, and Texas in 2003. These outbreaks, in which the diseases were all successfully eradicated, demonstrate how vigilance and an effective response can help prevent an FAD from becoming established in a country. This chapter describes how government agencies work to prevent exotic disease agents from entering the U.S., investigate and diagnose suspicious cases, and respond to confirmed outbreaks.

The Changing Roles of Federal Agencies in Disease Eradication

At one time, responding to an FAD was mainly the responsibility of the federal government—in particular, the Animal and Plant Health Inspection Service (APHIS), an agency within the U.S. Department of Agriculture (USDA). However, the terrorist attacks of September 11, 2001 have resulted in many changes in the emergency response systems. These systems have been redesigned, and the states and industry are now expected to play bigger roles in the partnership. This approach, known as the National Response Plan (NRP), incorporates the best practices and procedures from various emergency management disciplines and integrates them into a unified structure. The NRP forms the basis of how the federal government coordinates with state, tribal, and local governments and the private sector during all incidents, including animal disease outbreaks. Under the NRP, the USDA coordinates the protection of agriculture and natural resources in all types of emergencies.

The federal government has also developed national standards to manage all types of emergencies, including animal disease outbreaks. The goal was to establish an organizational framework that would be familiar to all local, state, tribal, and federal agencies, allowing them to work together quickly and efficiently in any emergency. In March 2004, the Department of Homeland Security (DHS) issued a directive establishing a new, comprehensive national approach to incident management known as the National Incident Management System (NIMS). The three cornerstones of the NIMS are 1) a unified approach to the management of incidents of all kinds, 2) the establishment of standard command and management structures used to organize responding personnel and agencies, and 3) an emphasis on preparedness, mutual aid, and resource management.

Within APHIS, the Veterinary Services (VS) unit is primarily responsible for preventing the entry of FADs into the United States and responding to them should they occur. VS' current responsibilities include developing eradication guidelines and plans for FADs, and conducting FAD training for personnel who will be involved in disease detection or eradication. APHIS also manages import testing and quarantine, which help to ensure that live animals and animal products are not carrying diseases into the U.S.

Protecting Against the Entry of a Foreign Animal Disease— Import Requirements, Quarantine Centers and Border Patrols

The first defense against a foreign animal disease is to detect it before it ever enters the country. FADs can be transmitted in animals, including asymptomatic carriers, and animal products. APHIS has established specific importation rules, which vary by animal or product and with the diseases present in the country of origin. For example, fresh meats cannot be imported from countries that have foot and mouth disease, but meats that have been cured or heat-processed according to APHIS standards are allowed. APHIS constantly monitors OIE reports of international disease status changes, and stops imports from any countries where outbreaks have been reported. APHIS also reviews import permit applications and issues the permits.

The quarantine process is an important step in ensuring that an imported animal carrying or incubating an exotic disease will not bring it into the U.S. Any animal that can carry serious diseases or arthropod pests must be imported through a USDA Import Center. There are cur-

> *The first defense against a foreign animal disease is to detect it before it ever enters the country. FADs can be transmitted in animals, including asymptomatic carriers, and animal products.*

rently four Import Centers, located in New York, Miami, Honolulu, and Los Angeles. An APHIS port veterinarian gives the animals a preliminary examination and checks their identification, health certificates, and permits. If an animal's paperwork is in order, it is taken directly to the local quarantine facility. If any information or documentation is missing, the animal is refused entry. Animals refused entry are held at the import center until the problem is corrected or the animal is returned to its origin. At the quarantine facility, animals receive a thorough physical examination and are sprayed for external parasites. They are then taken to isolation facilities for 3, 7, 30, or 60 days, depending on the species of the animal and its country of origin. To prevent diseases from spreading within the facility, animals remain within biologically secure units with separate ventilation systems. Cattle, horses, birds, waterfowl, and zoo animals are housed separately in species-specific barns. Imported animals are also tested for any applicable diseases; these tests also vary with the animal's species and the country of origin. When all required tests are negative and the quarantine period has passed with no signs of disease, the animal is released to its owner. The receiving state is also notified that the animals are being released from quarantine.

Border patrols and inspections ensure that animals and animal products do not bypass the import and quarantine process. Until 2002, APHIS was responsible for border inspections. These employees have now been transferred to the Department of Homeland Security, Customs and Border Protection (CBP) unit. CBP Agriculture Specialists enforce the import requirements and provisions of the Bioterrorism Act. Every day, these specialists screen thousands of passengers, all types of cargo, and international mail at more than 140 ports of entry. At some ports, detector dogs search for hidden items. At others, officials use low-energy x-rays to detect the presence of organic materials such as fruit and meats.

Highly contagious, exotic diseases are held at Plum Island Laboratory.
Source: Keith Weller, USDA

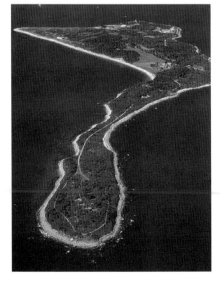

The National Veterinary Services Laboratories and the National Animal Health Laboratory Network

The primary responsibility for FAD testing belongs to the USDA APHIS National Veterinary Services Laboratories (NVSL). The NVSL consists of three laboratories in Ames, Iowa and the Foreign Animal Disease Diagnostics Laboratory (FADDL) at Plum Island, New York. Only the NVSL can confirm an outbreak of an exotic disease. Each NVSL laboratory specializes in specific diseases. The three NVSL-Ames laboratories diagnose poultry and equine diseases as well as transmissible spongiform encephalopathies (TSEs). Vesicular infections and other highly contagious exotic diseases are diagnosed at Plum Island; this laboratory, which is on an island, has particularly secure containment facilities. Research on highly contagious FADs is also conducted at Plum Island. In addition, Plum Island is where Foreign Animal Disease Diagnosticians (FADDs) are trained.

FADDs are state, USDA, or university-affiliated veterinarians who are responsible for visiting farms and other facilities where an FAD is suspected. These specialists have been trained to recognize exotic diseases, and collect samples to send to NVSL. Their roles in an outbreak are described more fully below.

The NVSL also supports export certification, as well as surveillance or eradication and control programs for domestic diseases. In addition, it certifies other laboratories to conduct diagnostic tests for regulated diseases such as equine infectious anemia, equine viral arteritis, brucellosis, and bluetongue. In the past, the NVSL conducted all FAD diagnostics and surveillance. However, exotic disease detection can be improved by increasing the number of facilities looking for FADs. The National Animal Health Laboratory Network (NAHLN) is part of a national strategy to coordinate the capabilities of federal, state, and university laboratories. By combining federal laboratory capacity with the facilities, professional expertise, and support of state and university laboratories, the NAHLN will enhance the response to animal health emergencies. During an exotic disease outbreak, these state and university laboratories assist NVSL in testing suspect herds, determining the extent of the outbreak, and conducting follow–up surveillance to determine when a state or area is disease-free. The NAHLN may also help NVSL with export certification, domestic animal disease control and eradication programs, and other services.

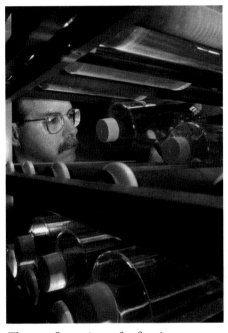

The confirmation of a foreign animal disease initiates an immediate eradication effort.
Source: USDA ARS photo

International reference laboratories can also become involved in diagnosing FADs in the U.S. This can be illustrated by the recent diagnosis of bovine spongiform encephalopathy (BSE) in a "downer" (non-ambulatory) cow born in Texas. Before the carcass of this cow was incinerated, samples were collected for routine BSE surveillance. The initial BSE screening tests were inconclusive, prompting NVSL to re-check the samples by immunohistochemistry, the usual confirmatory test. Immunohistochemistry was negative. The USDA recommended that these samples be re-tested with a second confirmatory test, immunoblotting (Western blotting). This test was positive. Faced with two contradictory tests, NVSL forwarded the inconclusive samples to Veterinary Laboratories Agency in Weybridge, England. This laboratory, a World Organization for Animal Health (OIE) Reference Laboratory with special expertise in diagnosing BSE, was able to confirm that the cow did have BSE. They also assisted NVSL with setting up new testing protocols for any inconclusive BSE tests found in the future. Similarly, international reference laboratories in the U.S. assist other countries with disease diagnosis.

Recognizing and Reporting a Possible Foreign Animal Disease

Although surveillance activities, border controls, and the import process help keep FADs out of the U.S., exotic diseases do occasionally appear in this country. If an outbreak occurs, the most important goal is to return the U.S. to a disease-free status as soon as possible. To reach this goal, the disease must be identified, an appropriate response must be implemented, and the animal industry must recover and be able to resume trade. The most critical step in this process is the rapid recognition and reporting of suspicious cases. Prompt reporting can prevent an FAD from spreading, reduce the economic costs of an outbreak, reduce the risk that the disease will become established in wildlife or arthropod reservoirs and, in some cases, prevent human disease. Conversely, delayed reporting can increase the cost and complexity of an outbreak, and increase the risk that the disease may never be eradicated. During the last few years, the number of exotic disease investigations in the United States has grown steadily, due to increasing awareness among producers and livestock owners. The number of investigations has ranged from a low of 254 in 1997 to a high of 1,013 in 2004. The peak in 2004 is related to the large number of investigations conducted in the southwestern United States in response to an outbreak of vesicular stomatitis, a livestock disease that mimics FMD.

> *Private practitioners are usually the first professionals to suspect an exotic disease; they are considered to be the first line of defense against these diseases. Practitioners who suspect an FAD should immediately contact either the State Veterinarian's office or the APHIS Area-Veterinarian-in-Charge (AVIC).*

Private practitioners are usually the first professionals to suspect an exotic disease; they are considered to be the first line of defense against these diseases. Practitioners who suspect an FAD should immediately contact either the State Veterinarian's office or the APHIS Area-Veterinarian-in-Charge (AVIC). Practitioners should never attempt to diagnose an FAD themselves; this must be left to the FADDs who will be immediately deployed by the State Veterinarian or AVIC. APHIS and the State Veterinarian's office also receive reports of possible FADs from other sources. Producers or county extension specialists may contact state and federal officials directly. Veterinary diagnostic laboratories sometimes find exotic diseases in samples submitted with the suspicion of a domestic disease. In addition, APHIS conducts routine surveillance of animals and animal products for certain FADs, such as classical swine fever, that are at a high risk of entering the U.S.

Investigating Suspicious Cases Using the Emergency Management Response System

Each state or group of states has an APHIS Area Veterinarian in Charge (AVIC), who coordinates federal animal health issues in that area. Once a suspicion of a foreign animal disease has been raised, the AVIC, State Veterinarian or designee enters the case into the computerized national Emergency Management Response System (EMRS). The purpose of this system is to track and report routine FAD and emerging disease investigations. The EMRS can also facilitate the response to outbreaks by keeping track of personnel, equipment and vehicles available to help in an emergency. The computerized case records, which are called the investigation summary, contain the herd history and any other relevant information from the referring veterinarian or owner. Each new case is given to a FADD; APHIS has FADDs within a four-hour drive of any location in the U.S. The assigned investigator contacts the affected facilities and visits the premises as soon as possible to perform a herd exam and conduct any necropsies. He or she also collects laboratory samples, ships them expeditiously to NVSL or FADDL, and informs the laboratory that they are on their way. Some high priority samples may be hand-carried. In addition, the FADD helps the producer establish biosecurity measures that will prevent the disease from spreading; in most cases, all clothing, equipment, and vehicles must be thoroughly cleaned and disinfected before leaving the premises.

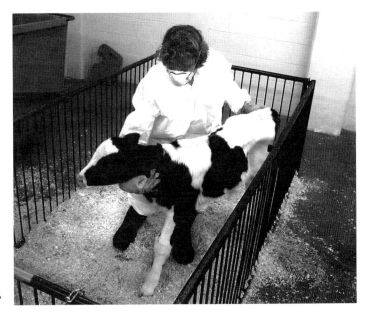

A foreign animal disease diagnostician is sent immediately to any farm where an exotic disease is suspected. The FADD collects samples from sick animals and, if necessary, establishes a quarantine of the farm.
Source: Clint May, ISU

While testing is still ongoing, APHIS VS-Emergency Management coordinates a conference call with the AVIC, FADD, State Veterinarian and other emergency personnel, to plan a response if an exotic disease is confirmed. For some FADs, final laboratory confirmation may take more than 48 hours. If the preliminary laboratory results and epidemiological evidence suggest the case is likely to be an FAD (a presumptive positive case), state or federal authorities may not wait for the final test results to begin the response and/or stop animal movements in the area. Once the confirmatory laboratory results have been received, the AVIC, FADD and State Veterinarian and VS emergency management decide whether any further examinations are needed or any other actions should be taken. A diagnosis is made in consultation with the FADD, the AVIC and any other interested parties. The owner and referring veterinarian are kept informed at all stages of this process. If the outbreak is not an exotic disease, the case is closed. The vast majority of foreign animal disease investigations do, in fact, turn out to be domestic diseases. Occasionally a case is found to be an FAD. In 2004, four of 1,013 investigations found exotic diseases; they included spring viremia of carp, white spot syndrome and Taura syndrome, all FADs of fish or crustaceans. When an FAD is diagnosed, pre-established response plans are implemented immediately.

The Response to a Confirmed Case—Informing the Participants

The responsibility for FAD prevention, preparedness, response, and recovery is shared by a variety of participants, including state and federal animal health officials, animal industry groups, and practitioners.

The states, industry groups, and other agencies have developed emergency plans for responding to an outbreak; these plans complement the federal response. These entities are notified by conference calls, electronic notification or press releases. Government participants usually include the APHIS administration, APHIS response teams for the disease, and state officials including the secretary/commissioner of agriculture, the governor, and state emergency management officials. Other federal agencies such as the Food Safety and Inspection Service (FSIS), the Office of Public Health and Science, and Centers for Disease Control and Prevention may also be involved. In addition, assistance may be requested from Department of Defense and the Federal Emergency Management Agency (FEMA) via the National Response Plan. If the outbreak involves agroterrorism, the Federal Bureau of Investigations and the Department of Homeland Security will become major participants. When a disease is zoonotic, public health officials also become involved. Industry and the universities often provide additional assistance.

Federal authorities also notify the OIE of the situation. All OIE member countries, including the U.S., are required to notify the Central Bureau within 24 hours of the confirmation of any OIE-reportable disease. OIE-reportable diseases, discussed in chapter 1, are those that could have serious repercussions on animal industries and the economy, or on public health. Outbreak reports sent to the OIE are immediately published. They are also sent directly to all member nations. In addition, U.S. officials make courtesy telephone calls to Canada, Mexico, and other major trading partners. To protect their own animal industries and human populations, other countries may then place bans on the importation of certain animals or animal products from the U.S. Similarly, the U.S. bans the importation of certain animal products from countries experiencing FAD outbreaks.

Throughout the eradication process, OIE, state, and federal officials receive continual updates on the progress of the eradication effort and the disease status of affected regions. During the outbreak, APHIS also consults with agricultural officials in other countries about the status of the outbreak, biosecurity issues, and surveillance. These updates and consultations help to ensure that U.S. trading partners will not place unnecessary restrictions on the export of disease-free animals.

The Response to an Outbreak—the Incident Command System

An exotic disease outbreak may be small or large, simple or complex, localized or widespread. Small outbreaks limited to a single farm can be controlled with a few personnel and resources. However, in a major outbreak, APHIS will need assistance from other federal, state, and local agencies, as well as industry partners. The Incident Command System (ICS) is an organizational framework used to coordinate the efforts of personnel from diverse agencies and groups. The ICS is primarily a command

and control system that establishes job responsibilities and an organizational structure, for the purpose of managing day-to-day operations in emergency incidents. One advantage to this system is that it is familiar to federal and state personnel, so that representatives from a variety of agencies find it easy to fit in. Although it was originally developed for wildfires, the ICS has been adopted by FEMA and all other emergency management organizations. It can be applied to a variety of large or small incidents, including natural disasters, and it can handle multiple, large-scale emergencies simultaneously. In 2002, APHIS VS first used an ICS system during an outbreak of low pathogenic avian influenza (LPAI) in commercial poultry in Virginia. The success of the ICS during this outbreak stimulated APHIS VS to adopt a state-based, nationally coordinated Animal Emergency Response Organization (AERO), based on ICS principles, to manage all disease outbreaks. ICS is now used by all agencies that respond to any type of disaster or outbreak.

Unlike the highly pathogenic form of avian influenza, low pathogenic avian influenza (LPAI) is not an FAD. Outbreaks of LPAI are usually managed by state agencies. However, the virus strain involved in the Virginia 2002 outbreak, H7N2, had the potential to mutate to a highly pathogenic strain and the outbreak was widespread; therefore, Virginia requested assistance from APHIS. A task force consisting mainly of VS personnel was sent to Virginia to assist the Virginia Department of Agriculture and Consumer Services. The task force included epidemiologists, veterinarians, animal health technicians, and program personnel from APHIS. They helped state personnel with disease investigations, carcass disposal, preventative measures, epidemiological investigations, and general support. A logistical support team from the Forest Service also assisted. Additional agencies that became involved included USDA's Farm Service Agency and Natural Resources Conservation Service and Virginia's Secretariat of Commerce and Trade, Secretariat of Natural Resources, and Department of Environmental Quality. All breeder birds, commercial turkeys, and broilers were tested before slaughter, and mandatory testing was required on any flocks with respiratory symptoms. Positive flocks were immediately quarantined and were destroyed, if possible, within 24 hours. The outbreak affected 197 premises and approximately 4.7 million birds were depopulated before the disease was brought under control. The task force remained in Virginia until all farms had been checked four times to ensure that the disease had been eradicated.

One of the strengths of the ICS is its adaptability. If only a local or limited response is needed, the outbreak is usually managed by regional state, federal, and industry officials, with consultation at the national level on issues such as trade and consequence management. In more extensive outbreaks, greater involvement by state and federal agencies becomes necessary and the command structure becomes more complex. The AVIC and the State Veterinarian, or his/her federal or state representative, serve as the Unified Command in the ICS. They are responsible for all outbreaks within their state. They are also responsible for establishing and training one or more Incident Management Teams for their region. These Incident Management Team(s) respond to animal health emergencies, sometimes in cooperation with other organizations. State and federal government personnel serve on Incident Management Teams. Each team contains an incident commander, incident command staff (finance, logistics, operations, and planning section chiefs), and an ICS training coordinator. The incident commander(s) are responsible for on-site coordination. An incident commander also assesses the situation and communicates the needs of the outbreak to ICS Area Command, Regional Coordination, and National Coordination personnel. In turn, they communicate with USDA and APHIS managers, so that resources can be allocated to the Incident Management Team. Off-site coordination is managed by a designated national incident coordinator and, in some cases, by personnel from other organizations. The national incident coordinator assumes overall responsibility for coordination of the outbreak, and activates multi-agency groups as needed.

In order to match the level of resources with the requirements of the emergency, the first step in the ICS is to assess a disease outbreak's complexity. Factors that are considered include the number and location of nearby livestock populations, the history of disease in the area, the current conditions, and management requirements. The complexity of an incident can be quantified using the Emergency Management and Incident Typing System. This system has five categories, with Type 5 incidents being the simplest and most easily managed, and Type 1, the most complex, resource-intensive, and long lasting. If a disease outbreak escalates, the level of complexity can be raised and additional resources can be brought in to manage it.

In a **Type 5** incident, the disease is usually contained within the premises where the first case was identified (the index premises). Typically, the outbreak can be managed with two to six people, and a complex organizational structure is not necessary.

A **Type 4** incident is usually a small outbreak or the initial response to a larger outbreak. The personnel needed for a Type 4 incident vary from one person to several, a task force, or one or more strike teams. The outbreak is usually under control within 24 hours and relatively few resources are needed. Although a more complex organization is not necessary, one or more incident commander(s) becomes responsible for managing the outbreak. Employee participation from outside the area or state is voluntary, and all regular work continues. A typical type 4 incident might be an outbreak of rabbit hemorrhagic disease.

In a **Type 3** incident, the outbreak lasts for more than a day, additional resources are needed, and additional ICS command and general staff positions may be activated. Although regular work continues and employee participation from outside the area is voluntary, a national pool of assets is made available during a type 3 incident. Type 3 incidents are organized more formally than type 4 or 5 incidents, and written action plans are used. An outbreak remains as a type 3 incident until either the outbreak is contained and controlled, or the situation is upgraded to a Type 1 or 2 incident. A screwworm outbreak would typically be one example of a Type 3 incident.

A **Type 2** incident involves a complex chain of organization under the incident commander. Up to 500 people, combined as task forces or strike teams, are usually involved. Employee participation from outside the area is mandatory and some regular work is suspended during the emergency. A national pool of assets, emergency management and veterinary reserve units are activated. Exotic Newcastle disease might typically be classified as a Type 2 incident.

A **Type 1** incident is the most complex, highly organized and intense response. More than a thousand people are usually involved, often with more than 500 people active each day. Extensive resources are needed, including a national pool of assets, and emergency management and international and/or national veterinary reserve units are activated. The command structure is highly organized, as representatives from several jurisdictions are often involved. There may be multiple Incident Command bases. Type 1 incidents represent less than 1% of all responses, but are nationally significant events. An example of a Type 1 incident would be an outbreak of foot-and-mouth disease.

The Response to an Outbreak—the Eradication Process

In an outbreak, disease eradication personnel work from a set of pre-established eradication guidelines that APHIS has developed specifically for each FAD. The response to a foreign animal disease outbreak may involve:

Quarantines and animal movement restrictions: The control of most FAD outbreaks requires movement restrictions on susceptible animals within a defined area, and quarantines on infected and exposed herds. Quarantines may be placed by the state or, once the U.S. secretary of agriculture has declared an animal health emergency, by the federal government. If the federal government does not declare an animal health emergency, it can intervene only in foreign or interstate commerce. As the disease comes under control and is eradicated from some locations, the remaining affected areas are regionalized if possible. This allows trade and transport of animals to resume in unaffected locations – an important consideration for economic reasons and sometimes for animal welfare. Animal movement restrictions and eradication activities continue inside the affected areas until the disease is gone.

Epidemiologic investigations: During a disease investigation, federal and state veterinarians trace the movements of infected animals to discover whether the disease has spread and, if so, where. The case or herd discovered first, called the index case or index herd, is used to identify other animals that may be infected. The movements of animals into and out of the affected herd are traced, and the animal's or herd's contacts with other animals are investigated. These tracebacks and trace forwards can be facilitated by a national animal identification system, which establishes a standardized animal and premises identification scheme, and records the movements of individual animals or units of animals in a central database. The goal of such a system is to be able to identify all premises that had direct contact with an FAD within two days after the disease is discovered. The U.S. has implemented a national animal identification plan for cattle, after a case of BSE was found in a cow in Washington State. Identification requirements for sheep and goats have been in place since 2001, as a part of the scrapie eradication program, and a national animal identification system for horses is under discussion.

Determining when an exotic disease has truly been eradicated is one of the most difficult aspects of control. How can we be sure the disease has not entered wildlife populations?
Source: Geoff Simpson

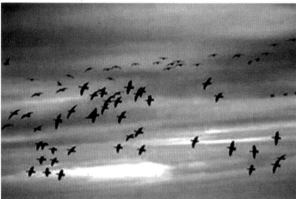

Surveillance: All potentially exposed animals must be tested for the FAD. After the initial diagnosis, these samples may be tested by NVSL, FADDL or NAHLN laboratories. Depending on the disease, susceptible animals may also be tested within a defined area; some airborne infections, for example, can be transmitted without direct contact. In any outbreak, constant reassessment is a necessity. Determining that an agent has been completely eradicated may be difficult – particularly if an agent is vector-borne, can be carried in asymptomatic animals, or can enter wildlife reservoirs. For this reason, extensive surveillance usually continues after an outbreak.

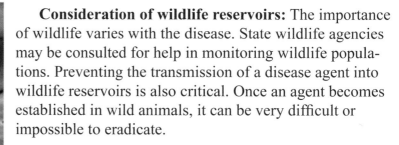

Consideration of wildlife reservoirs: The importance of wildlife varies with the disease. State wildlife agencies may be consulted for help in monitoring wildlife populations. Preventing the transmission of a disease agent into wildlife reservoirs is also critical. Once an agent becomes established in wild animals, it can be very difficult or impossible to eradicate.

Vaccination: Vaccination programs may be utilized in certain FAD outbreaks to enhance eradication activities, decrease the severity of the outbreak, or help insulate disease-free areas from affected regions. Vaccination against an FAD requires special government approval.

Humane euthanasia or treatment of affected and exposed animals: In the U.S., most FADs are eradicated by culling exposed and affected animals, a process known as humane euthanasia. The government provides affected producers with indemnity, at the fair market value, for animals that must be culled. The extent of the humane euthanasia effort depends on the disease. Most FADs are highly contagious, and entire affected and exposed herds must usually be euthanized. A few FADs are not contagious. BSE, for example, is acquired by eating contaminated feed. As BSE develops only after a very long incubation time, there is no reason to assume that other animals in the current herd are automatically infected and, typically, the rest of the herd is not culled. Similarly, horses with West Nile virus are dead end hosts and do not transmit the virus further. Treatment of FADs is rare and usually limited to exotic arthropods such as screwworms.

Carcass disposal: Either any remaining infectious agent in the carcass must be destroyed, or the carcass must be kept from coming into contact with uninfected animals while the agent is naturally deactivated. Carcasses may be disposed of by burial, incineration, rendering, composting or other means, depending on the agent and its susceptibility to destruction. Burial – which is quick and requires fewer resources than most other techniques - is often chosen for carcasses, animal products, feed, and organic wastes. However, space considerations, a high water table, or other problems may prevent burial from being practical in some cases.

Disinfection: For most FADs, the affected premises and any equipment that was exposed to the animals must be cleaned and disinfected. This prevents fomites from continuing to spread the disease agent to new animals.

Vector controls: Diseases spread by mosquitoes, ticks or other vectors require spraying programs or other vector controls, as well as surveillance of susceptible vector populations.

Public education: During an outbreak, hotlines are set up to inform the press and members of the public. Information may also be disseminated directly to specific groups such as producers or veterinarians. In addition to keeping the public informed, these information campaigns can help to raise awareness and, as a result, can identify new cases of the disease.

Funding concerns: Funding for the eradication program is initially provided by the state's agriculture department and state emergency funds. The U.S. secretary of agriculture may also declare an emergency, which allows federal funds and other federal agencies to be used.

How private practitioners can help

APHIS Veterinary Services (VS) may need temporary personnel to assist during an outbreak. APHIS maintains the National Animal Health Emergency Response Corp, a roster of private veterinarians and animal health technicians who are able to assist VS on short notice. Private practitioners may examine herds or flocks for clinical signs, vaccinate animals, do necropsies, collect laboratory samples, collect epidemiological information, and euthanize infected animals. They may also supervise the disposal of animal carcasses or inspect livestock markets and trucks. The role of private practitioners in an outbreak is addressed further in chapter 4. Interested veterinarians and animal health technicians may also call the APHIS Area Office in their state for information.

The Response to an Outbreak—Recovery

APHIS Veterinary Services works towards recovery from a disease outbreak through partnerships with local and state governments, and other organizations, including livestock industries. Recovery activities include prompt payment for euthanized livestock and destroyed materials, renegotiation of international export protocols, and federal government and industry reinforcement of consumer expectations and reassurances. The OIE's International Animal Health Code sets the standards that determine when a country will be classified as disease-free. The OIE standards, which must be satisfied before international trade resumes, serve to reassure international trading partners that trading with a country is safe.

The ultimate costs of an outbreak for a country, its producers, and affiliated industries can be high. In addition to the direct costs of eradication, there will be other losses. Trade restrictions may prevent producers from selling products from healthy animals, and the value of these products may also fall in the domestic markets. Industries such as meat packers and shipping companies as well as producers may suffer losses. In extreme cases, even industries such as tourism may be affected. Finally, every eradication effort may not be successful. The West Nile virus, which first appeared in New York City in 1999, has now become endemic throughout the 48 contiguous states. Although the U.S. made a concerted effort to eradicate this virus, it overwintered in mosquito and bird populations, reappeared in 2000 and eventually spread throughout the country. There is no way to guarantee such an event will not happen again, particularly with an arthropod-borne disease; however, the chances of another introduction can be decreased by maintaining a strong emergency management system to exclude, detect, and respond to all outbreaks.

Conclusion

An effective response to an outbreak requires prompt recognition and reporting of the initial cases, and a fast, efficient, and flexible response that can evolve with the outbreak if it grows. The current emergency management system requires cooperation between local, state, federal, and tribal agencies, as well as industry. The NIMS Incident Command System, which is being adopted by all emergency management organizations, is a framework that allows these diverse groups to work effectively together. This system provides an organizational structure for the activities important in eradication – quarantines and animal movement restrictions, epidemiologic investigations, surveillance, consideration of wildlife reservoirs, vaccination, humane euthanasia, carcass disposal, disinfection, vector controls, public education and funding considerations.

Private practitioners also have a very important role in recognizing and reporting exotic diseases. To be effective in this role, veterinarians should remember the following points*:

- Be aware of your crucial role in protecting the U.S. from a foreign animal disease. An exotic disease is easiest to control if it is diagnosed soon after it enters the country. If it looks like it might be an exotic disease, report your suspicions immediately to state or federal authorities. They have the resources to recognize and identify foreign animal diseases.

- Recognizing a foreign animal disease depends on considering it in the differential diagnosis. Become knowledgeable about the clinical signs of FADs, and remember that many FADs can resemble endemic diseases. Also be alert for subtle signs of disease: a foreign disease could make its first appearance, as, for instance, a drop in milk production or an increase in abortions. A practitioner who recognizes a drop in the normal productivity of a farm in the production records can initiate diagnostics or farm management audits. Both veterinarians and physicians are taught: "If you hear hooves, thinks horses not zebras." To prevent the spread of a foreign animal disease, keep in mind that it just might be a zebra.

- Don't unknowingly spread disease by neglecting simple biosecurity practices. Set an example for your clients, employees, and peers by taking the proper measures to safeguard your patients from transmissible diseases. Routinely clean and disinfect examination tables and equipment between patient visits and institute a policy of hand washing before handling patients. When visiting a farm or other animal facility, wear clean coveralls and boots that can be properly disinfected.

- Remember that the risk for an FAD in our nation is increasing due to rising international travel, in the U.S., intensive agricultural practices, and other factors.

*From a list originally developed by Sharon D. Nath, DVM and Corrie Brown, DVM, PhD. The University of Georgia, College of Veterinary Medicine

Baysinger AK. Private practitioners' role in outbreaks [online]. In: American Veterinary Medical Association Annual Meeting; 2000 July 22-26; Salt Lake City, UT. Available at: http://www.aphis.usda.gov/vs/ep/avma/avma-sym.html. Accessed 2 Oct 2005.

Brown C. (Department of Veterinary Pathology, University of Georgia). Threat of accidental foreign animal disease introduction [online]. In: American Veterinary Medical Association Annual Meeting; 2000 July 22-26; Salt Lake City, UT. Available at: http://www.aphis.usda.gov/vs/ep/avma/avma-sym.html. Accessed 2 Oct 2005.

Federal Emergency Management System (FEMA). National Incident Management System. NIMS and the Incident Command System. Available at: http://www.fema. gov/nims/. Accessed 27 Nov 2005.

Hamlen H. (Animal Health Branch, Animal Health and Food Safety Services, California Department of Food and Agriculture). Emergency animal disease response - The team approach [online]. In: American Veterinary Medical Association Annual Meeting; 2000 July 22-26; Salt Lake City, UT. Available at: http://www.aphis.usda.gov/vs/ep/avma/avma-sym.html. Accessed 2 Oct 2005.

Lautner EA (National Pork Producers Council). Role of industry in outbreaks [online]. In: American Veterinary Medical Association Annual Meeting; 2000 July 22-26; Salt Lake City, UT. Available at: http://www.aphis.usda.gov/vs/ep/avma/avma-sym. html. Accessed 2 Oct 2005.

U.S. Department of Agriculture, Animal and Plant Health Inspection Service [USDA APHIS]. Combining surveillance, detection and response. Available at: http://www. aphis.usda.gov/lpa/pubs/brotradc.pdf. Accessed 15 Nov 2005.

U.S. Department of Agriculture, Animal and Plant Health Inspection Service [USDA APHIS]. National Veterinary Services Laboratories. Available at: http://www.aphis. usda.gov/vs/nvsl/index.htm. Accessed 15 Nov 2005.

U.S. Department of Agriculture, Animal and Plant Health Inspection Service, Veterinary Services [USDA APHIS, VS]. APHIS-VS-emergency programs [online]. USDA APHIS, VS; 2003. Available at: http://www.aphis.usda.gov/vs/ep/. Accessed 5 Dec 2003.

U.S. Department of Agriculture, Animal and Plant Health Inspection Service, Veterinary Services [USDA APHIS, VS]. Emergency management response system [online]. USDA APHIS, VS; 2003. Available at: http://www.aphis.usda.gov/vs/ep/ emrs.html. Accessed 5 Dec 2003.

U.S. Department of Agriculture, Animal and Plant Health Inspection Service, Veterinary Services [USDA APHIS, VS]. EMRS manual for routine FAD/EDI investigations. Available at:http://www.aphis.usda.gov/vs/ep/EMRS_for_Routine_ FAD_Investigations.htm#_Toc55001051. Accessed 15 Oct 2005.

U.S. Department of Agriculture, Animal and Plant Health Inspection Service, Veterinary Services [USDA APHIS, VS]. How APHIS facilitates agricultural imports [online]. USDA APHIS, 2004 Jan. Available at: http://www.aphis.usda. gov/lpa/pubs/fsheet_faq_notice/fs_aphisimport.html (old URL: http://www.aphis. usda.gov/oa/pubs/import.html.*) Accessed 2003 & 20 Nov 2005.

U.S. Department of Agriculture, Animal and Plant Health Inspection Service [USDA APHIS].USDA announces BSE test results and new BSE confirmatory testing protocol. News Release No. 0232.05. June 24, 2005. Available at: http://www. usda.gov/wps/portal/!ut/p/_s.7_0_A/7_0_1OB/.cmd/ad/.ar/sa.retrievecontent/. c/6_2_1UH/.ce/7_2_5JM/.p/5_2_4TQ/.d/4/_th/J_2_9D/_s.7_0_A/7_0_1OB?PC_ 7_2_5JM_contentid=2005%2F06%2F0232.xml&PC_7_2_5JM_navtype=RT&PC_ 7_2_5JM_parentnav=LATEST_RELEASES&PC_7_2_5JM_navid=NEWS_ RELEASE#7_2_5JM. Accessed 14 Oct 2005.

U.S. Department of Agriculture, Animal and Plant Health Inspection Service, Veterinary Services [USDA APHIS, VS]. Identification of sheep and goats for scrapie eradication [online]. USDA APHIS, VS; 2001 Aug. Available at: http://www.ncagr. com/vet/IDSheepGoatsForScrapie.htm (old URL: http://www.aphis.usda.gov/oa/ pubs/scraera.html.*) Accessed 5 Oct 2005.

U.S. Department of Agriculture, Animal and Plant Health Inspection Service, Veterinary Services [USDA APHIS, VS]. National Animal Health Emergency Management System guidelines. Administrative procedures guidelines: Leader's guide for conducting animal emergency response using the Incident Command System. In: National Animal Health Emergency Management System. Procedural guidelines. ver 1.1. Washington, DC: U.S. Department of Agriculture; August 30, 2004. 1 CD.

U.S. Department of Agriculture, Animal and Plant Health Inspection Service, Veterinary Services [USDA APHIS, VS]. Safeguarding animal health. FY2002 annual highlights report. USDA APHIS, VS; 2002. Section 3-4, National Animal Health Reporting System provides data for confirmed diseases. Available at: http://www. aphis.usda.gov/vs/highlights/. Accessed 5 Oct 2005.

U.S. Department of Agriculture, Animal and Plant Health Inspection Service, Veterinary Services [USDA APHIS, VS]. Procedures for investigating a suspected foreign animal disease/emerging disease incident (FAD/EDI). Veterinary Services memorandum 580.4 March 30, 2004. In: National Animal Health Emergency Management System. Procedural guidelines. ver 1.1. Washington, DC: U.S. Department of Agriculture; August 30, 2004. 1 CD.

U.S. Department of Agriculture, Animal and Plant Health Inspection Service, Veterinary Services [USDA APHIS, VS]. Safeguarding animal health. FY2002 annual highlights report. USDA APHIS, VS; 2002. Section 3-10, Animal identification. Available at: http://www.aphis.usda.gov/vs/highlights/. Accessed 5 Oct 2005.

U.S. Department of Agriculture, Animal and Plant Health Inspection Service, Veterinary Services [USDA APHIS, VS]. Safeguarding animal health. FY2002 annual highlights report [monograph online]. USDA APHIS, VS; 2002. Section 3-13, Foreign animal disease investigations. Available at: http://www.aphis.usda. gov/vs/highlights/. Accessed 5 Oct 2005.

U.S. Department of Agriculture, Animal and Plant Health Inspection Service, Veterinary Services [USDA APHIS, VS]. Safeguarding animal health. FY2002 annual highlights report [monograph online]. USDA APHIS, VS; 2002. Section 4, Exclusion. Available at: http://www.aphis.usda.gov/vs/highlights/. Accessed 5 Oct 2005.

U.S. Department of Agriculture, Animal and Plant Health Inspection Service, Veterinary Services [USDA APHIS, VS]. Safeguarding animal health. FY2002 annual highlights report [monograph online]. USDA APHIS, VS; 2002. Section 5-3, NVSL: International laboratory diagnostic support. Available at: http://www.aphis. usda.gov/vs/highlights/. Accessed 5 Oct 2005.

U.S. Department of Agriculture, Animal and Plant Health Inspection Service, Veterinary Services [USDA APHIS, VS]. Safeguarding animal health. FY2002 Annual highlights report [monograph online]. USDA APHIS, VS; 2002. Section 6-6, The national animal health laboratory network. Available at: http://www. aphis.usda.gov/vs/highlights/. Accessed 5 Oct 2005.

U.S. Department of Agriculture, Animal and Plant Health Inspection Service, Veterinary Services [USDA APHIS, VS]. Safeguarding animal health. FY2002 Annual highlights report [monograph online]. USDA APHIS, VS; 2002. Section 6-7, Incident Command System: An interagency approach to emergency response. Available at: http://www.aphis.usda.gov/vs/highlights/. Accessed 5 Oct 2005.

U.S. Department of Agriculture, Animal and Plant Health Inspection Service, Veterinary Services [USDA APHIS, VS]. The significance of surveillance to safeguarding American animal health [online]. USDA APHIS, VS; 2003 July. Available at: http://www.aphis.usda.gov/lpa/pubs/fsheet_faq_notice/fs_ahsurveillance.html. Accessed 20 Sept 2005.

U.S. Department of Homeland Security. Fact sheet: National Incident Management System (NIMS). Available at: http://www.dhs.gov/dhspublic/interapp/press_release/press_release_0363.xml. Accessed 27 Nov 2005.

World Organization for Animal Health [OIE]. OIE classification of diseases [online]. OIE; 2003 Dec. Available at: http://www.oie.int/eng/maladies/en_classification.htm. Accessed 20 Nov 2003.

Low Pathogenic Avian Influenza

U.S. Department of Agriculture, Animal and Plant Health Inspection Service, Veterinary Services [USDA APHIS, VS]. Highly pathogenic avian influenza [online]. USDA APHIS, VS; 2004 March. Available at: http://www.aphis.usda.gov/lpa/pubs/fsheet_faq_notice/fs_ahavianflu.html. Accessed 15 Oct 2005.

U.S. Department of Agriculture, Animal and Plant Health Inspection Service, Veterinary Services [USDA APHIS, VS]. Managing low pathogenic avian influenza in Virginia [online]. USDA APHIS, VS; 2002 April. Available at: http://www.aphis.usda.gov/lpa/pubs/fsheet_faq_notice/fs_ahlpaiva.html. Accessed 5 Oct 2005.

U.S. Department of Agriculture, Animal and Plant Health Inspection Service, Veterinary Services [USDA APHIS, VS]. Safeguarding animal health. FY2002 annual highlights report. USDA APHIS, VS; 2002. Section 6-1, Low pathogenic avian influenza in Virginia. Available at: http://www.aphis.usda.gov/vs/highlights/. Accessed 5 Oct 2005.

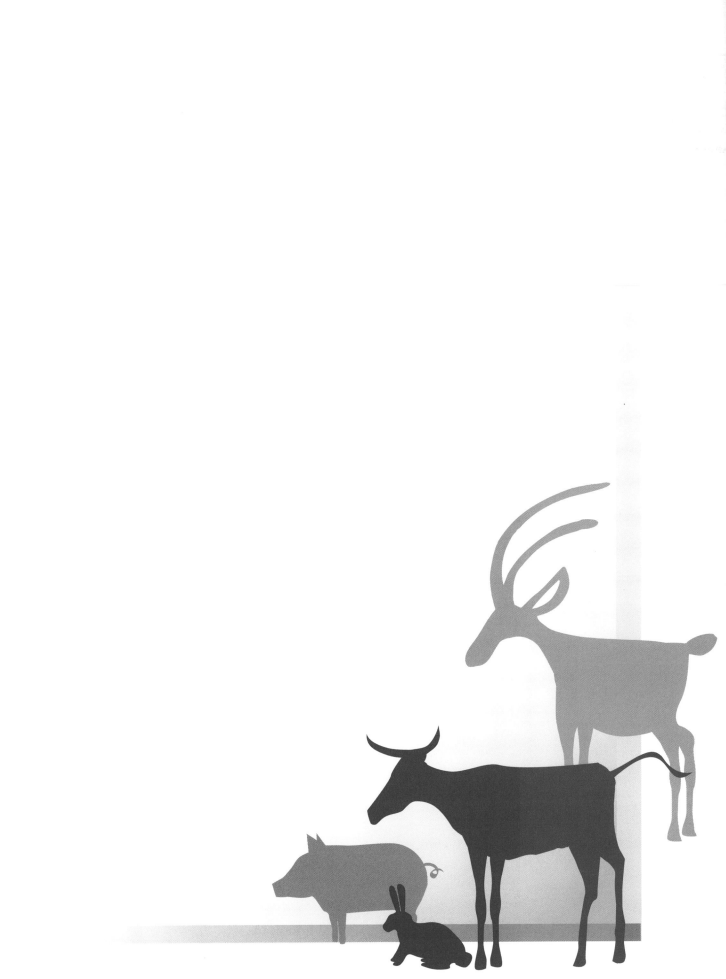

> *Veterinarians and veterinary students can use their skills to help in an animal health emergency.*

A Veterinarian's Role in an Animal Health Emergency

Author: *Jane Galyon, MS*
Iowa State University College of Veterinary Medicine

Veterinarians are important players in the response to natural disasters, manmade disasters, and animal disease outbreaks. In these emergencies, veterinarians help protect animal health, the food supply, and, in some cases, public health. This chapter describes how veterinarians and veterinary students can assist in the response effort by participating in the National Animal Health Emergency Response Corps (NAHERC), Veterinary Medical Assistance Teams (VMATs), State Animal Response Teams (SARTs), or private non-profit organizations. In addition, this chapter describes the systems used to manage emergency responses: the Incident Command System (ICS) and the National Incident Management System (NIMS).

A Foreign Animal Disease Outbreak and the
National Animal Health Emergency Response Corps

If a major outbreak of a foreign animal disease occurs in the United States, the USDA will activate its Animal Emergency Response Organization (AERO). APHIS employees will be deployed to the site of the outbreak to ensure that strategies to control and eradicate the disease are taken. A small incident may be managed easily by a few government employees. However, a large, multi-location or extended outbreak will quickly overwhelm APHIS resources and help will be needed to bring the outbreak under control. To address this need, APHIS has established a list of private and state veterinarians and veterinary technicians who can be quickly brought into federal government service and activated to the outbreak area. This group is called the National Animal Health Emergency Response Corps (NAHERC). The NAHERC was established with the assistance of the American Veterinary Medical Association and the North American Veterinary Technician Association. It is a volunteer organization. The NAHERC was first used in 2001 when volunteers were sent to the United Kingdom to help with a foot and mouth disease outbreak. It was used again in 2003 during an exotic Newcastle disease outbreak in Southern California.

Veterinarians and veterinary technicians who sign up for the NAHERC, though salaried when mobilized, are not obligated to assist in emergency situations. When an outbreak occurs and additional emergency personnel are needed, NAHERC members who are willing to participate are activated by APHIS as temporary federal personnel. Veterinarians can be asked to participate for periods of up to 30 to 60 days, or in special circumstances, up to one year. Veterinarians are considered Veterinary Medical Officers (VMOs) during the emergency and receive a salary, depending on experience, between the GS-9 and GS-11 (step 1) levels (www.opm.gov/oca/payrates/index.asp). Overtime (time and a half) is paid when employees work over 40 hours per week. All travel and per diem expenses are provided by APHIS. Activated members are covered by federal workers' compensation. They are protected under the Federal Tort Claims Act against personal liability within the scope of their temporary federal employment, and are exempt from licensure, certification, or registration requirements.

NAHERC duties for veterinarians in an outbreak may include:

- examining herds or flocks for signs of disease

- collecting specimens

- vaccinating animals

- conducting post-mortem examinations

- euthanizing animals

- supervising the disposal of animal carcasses

- collecting epidemiological information

- inspecting livestock markets, trucks and vehicles.

Veterinary students can also participate in the NAHERC. They work under the supervision of veterinarians and are classified as Animal Health Technicians or assistants. The salary for veterinary students starts at the GS-5 level and goes as high as GS-7, depending on the year in school or applicable experience, APHIS provides overtime, travel and per diem expenses, and federal workman's compensation. APHIS also gives veterinary students the same legal protections as veterinarians when they are activated.

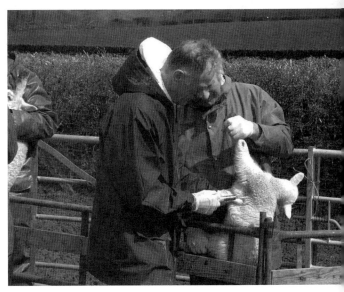

Veterinarians can have many duties in an animal health emergency.
Source: Pam Hullinger

NAHERC duties for veterinary students in an outbreak may include:

- conducting surveillance

- examining animals for signs of disease

- collecting specimens

- vaccinating animals

- conducting post-mortem examinations

- euthanizing animals

- disposing of animal carcasses

- collecting epidemiological information

- inspecting livestock markets, trucks, and vehicles

If they are activated, NAHERC members report to the incident command center and attend orientation sessions where they learn about the disease and current outbreak situation, biosecurity, personal protective equipment, and other important information specific to the outbreak. At these sessions, NAHERC members are assigned specific duties and are trained to perform these duties. During an outbreak, NAHERC members work in teams under the supervision of experienced personnel. In addition to their veterinary knowledge, volunteers in the NAHERC or other emergency response organizations are expected to have a basic understanding of how these events are managed. A poorly managed response could be devastating to our economy, the food supply, and to public health and safety. It is important that all individuals who participate in an emergency response have a basic understanding of the Incident Command System (ICS).

Biosecurity is critical in animal emergency response.
Source: Pam Hullinger

The Incident Command System

In the 1970s, a series of catastrophic wildfires in California caused 16 deaths, many injuries, and millions of dollars in property damage. Although a number of agencies responded to the wildfires, the overall response was inefficient. A government review found that the problems associated with the response were usually the result of inadequate management rather than insufficient resources or poor tactics. These problems included a lack of personnel accountability and unclear chain of command, poor communication, and failures in orderly planning. The problems could be traced to the absence of a common pre-designed management structure or method to integrate agencies from different branches of the government. In response to the review, the Forest Service, along with county and state agencies developed the ICS to ensure that future responses would be more effective.

NAHERC participants receive basic training in incident command upon arrival at the incident. However, potential NAHERC participants should consider taking web-based Incident Command level 100 and 200 courses. The USDA ICS 100 and ICS 200 level courses are available for free at www.cfsph.iastate.edu/ce. Online registration is required prior to taking the courses. All individuals who complete these courses will receive a certificate.

The Incident Command System is designed to:

- Meet the needs of incidents of any kind or size

- Be usable for routine or planned events (for example, a parade) as well as emergencies

- Allow individuals from a variety of agencies to meld rapidly into a common management structure

- Provide logistical and administrative support to operational staff

- Be cost effective by avoiding duplication of efforts

The ICS has been used for over 30 years for:

- Routine or planned events

- Fires, hazardous materials, and multiple casualty incidents

- Multi-jurisdictional and multi-agency disasters such as earthquakes, hurricanes, floods and winter storms

- Search and rescue missions

- Biological pest eradication programs

- Outbreaks and disease containment

- Acts of terrorism

The ICS is organized into five major management functions: Incident Command, Operations, Planning, Logistics, and Finance/Administration.

Chart 2: ICS Management Structure

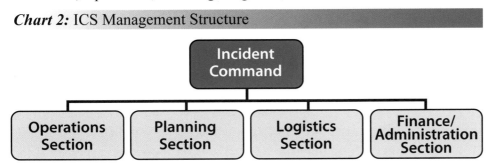

Incident Command:

The Incident Commander has the overall responsibility for managing the disease outbreak or other incident. This individual sets the incident objectives, strategies, and priorities. He or she is also responsible for ensuring the safety of the participants, providing information to internal and external stakeholders including the media, and establishing and maintaining liaisons with the other agencies involved. Small incidents may be run entirely by the Incident Commander. However, if an incident grows, the Incident Commander can assign authority to individuals based on their assigned positions. In a larger incident, for example, a Public Information Officer, Safety Officer, and Liaison Officer take over the responsibilities in each area. In addition, the Incident Commander may have one or more deputies. The Incident Commander oversees the incident at the Incident Command Post (ICP). If command is transferred during an incident, the outgoing Incident Commander provides a full briefing to the incoming Incident Commander. All personnel are notified of the change in command.

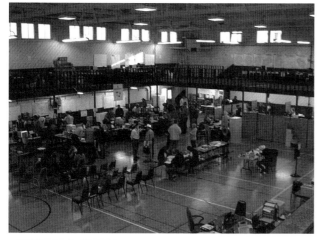

The Incident Command Headquarters during the exotic Newcastle disease outbreak in California.
Source: Don Otto, USDA

Each of the four sections under Incident Command has its own command structure. The person in charge of each section is designated as a Chief. Under the ICS structure, each person is accountable to only one designated supervisor. In addition, there is an orderly chain of command within the ICS ranks; lower levels are subordinate to and connected to higher levels. An important operating guideline, called the "span of control," specifies the number of individuals that one supervisor can effectively manage during an emergency response. One supervisor managing five individuals is the recommended ratio, but an effective span of control can vary from three to seven. Maintaining an effective span of control is especially important in incidents where safety and accountability are a top priority.

Operations Section

The Operations Section is where the tactical fieldwork is conducted. In an animal disease outbreak, for example, the Operations Section would carry out vaccination, depopulation, carcass disposal and the other activities involved in eradicating the disease. Most incident resources are assigned to this section, which is where most NAHERC participants will be working.

The Operations Section may be subdivided into groups, divisions, branches, strike teams and task forces. Groups are used to describe functional areas of operation. For example, NAHERC members assigned to help with vaccination would belong to the Vaccination Group. Each group operates under a Supervisor. In larger incidents, the Operations Section may separate an incident geographically by Divisions. Each Division responds to the incident in a specific location such as a region of the country, the floor of a building, or a specific farm. Divisions are usually identified with alphabetic characters (i.e. Division A or Division B). The person in charge of each Division is designated as a Supervisor. Divisions and Groups may both be used in an incident and are at equal levels in the Incident Command organization. Division and Group Supervisors must work together and closely coordinate their activities. Branches are used when additional organization is needed. Branches can be either geographical or functional. For example, the Vaccination Group could have a "North Branch" and a "South Branch." Branches can also be used to create supervision levels within the Operations Section. The person in charge of each Branch is called a Director.

In addition, Strike Teams or Task Forces may be established. Strike teams consist of like resources; for example, a strike team might consist of several very similar trucks, with drivers, assigned to haul carcasses. Task Forces are teams that contain mixed resources. A team that consists of an epidemiologist, a microbiologist, and a wildlife biologist with a pickup truck is considered to be a Task Force. These teams operate under the direct supervision of the Strike Team Leader or Task Force Leader, respectively.

Planning Section:

The Planning Section prepares and documents the Incident Action Plan. The Incident Action Plan gives all supervisors their instructions for each operational period (typically 12 or 24 hours). This section also collects and evaluates information and maintains documentation for incident records. In addition, the Planning Section maintains resource status by monitoring where all resources are at any given time, and keeping track of whether they are assigned, available but unassigned, or temporarily out-of-service. An example of a resource might be a person, a piece of equipment and the personnel to run it, or a team and its supervisor.

Logistics Section:

The Logistics Section provides support, resources, and all other services needed to meet the operational objectives. This unit might, for example, set up computers or provide food, lodging, and basic first aid for the ICS participants.

Financial/Administration Section:

The Finance and Administration Section monitors the costs related to the incident. This section also provides accounting and procurement services, keeps personnel/equipment time records, and conducts cost analyses.

The National Incident Management System

The Incident Command System is now a part of the National Incident Management System (NIMS). After the terrorist attacks of September 11, 2001, the federal government developed national standards to manage all types of emergencies, including animal disease outbreaks. The goal was to establish an organizational framework that would be familiar to all local, state, tribal, and federal agencies, allowing them to work together quickly and efficiently in any emergency. In March 2004, the Department of Homeland Security issued a directive establishing a new, comprehensive national approach to incident management known as the NIMS.

Other Veterinary Response Teams

Veterinarians and technicians can use their skills and knowledge in an outbreak by working with Veterinary Medical Assistance Teams (VMAT), State Animal Response Teams (SART), and non-profit groups such as the Humane Society of the United States (HSUS) and the American Society for the Prevention of Cruelty to Animals (ASPCA).

Veterinary Medical Assistance Teams

Veterinary Medical Assistance Teams (VMATs) are highly trained federal teams that provide assistance during disasters; they are part of the NRP. These mobile units can be deployed to any state or United States territory within 24-48 hours, when their assistance is requested by state officials. The teams are composed of veterinarians, veterinary technicians, epidemiologists, toxicologists, and other medical, scientific and lay support personnel who have been trained together. VMATs may treat animals affected by natural or man-made disasters or aid the USDA in the control and eradication of animal disease outbreaks. Team members carry a 3-day supply of food, water, personal living necessities, and medical supplies and equipment. Each team is capable of establishing a veterinary field hospital and can provide all veterinary services needed to support a disaster relief effort. Although the VMAT system is designed to respond to large-scale disasters, it is also flexible enough to respond to disasters of limited scope.

VMAT responsibilities during disasters include:

- Assessment of the medical needs of animals

- Treatment and stabilization of animals affected by a disaster

- Medical treatment of working dogs

- Animal decontamination

- Humane euthanasia

- Epidemiology

- Animal disease surveillance

- Biological and chemical terrorism surveillance

- Zoonotic disease surveillance and public health assessment

- Technical assistance to assure food and water quality

- Hazard mitigation

The VMAT system supplements relief efforts already underway by local veterinarians and emergency responders. Although the initial response to disasters occurs at the local level, the resources within a disaster area may be inadequate to fully cope with the effects of a major disaster, or local resources may need time to recover before assuming complete responsibility. The VMATs provide assistance during those times when the local veterinary community is overwhelmed. The ultimate goal is a cooperative animal relief effort between VMATs, state and local governments, the local veterinary community, state and local veterinary medical associations, emergency management personnel, humane groups, the American Red Cross, and search and rescue groups.

Veterinarians or veterinary technicians who are accepted in VMAT are assigned to one of the VMAT teams and are preprocessed for federal employment and issued identification cards. Students cannot serve in VMAT. VMAT members can be called to federal service for up to 14 days as "special needs" employees of the U.S. Department of Homeland Security. If activated, VMAT members are paid a salary, are covered by federal worker's compensation, and are protected under the Federal Tort Claims Act against personal liability within the scope of their temporary federal employment. They are also exempt from licensure, certification, or registration requirements. Further information about VMAT is available at www.vmat.org.

State Animal Response Teams

Veterinarians, students, and veterinary technicians can also participate in the animal emergency response teams that are being formed in many states. The State Animal Response Team (SART) concept was originally developed in North Carolina to handle natural disasters such as hurricanes. Other states including Colorado, Pennsylvania, and Florida have followed North Carolina's lead. Each state is unique in its need for these veterinary emergency response teams because of different animal populations and priorities. SART teams consist of volunteers who are willing to provide assistance if requested by local or state officials. SART teams can include veterinarians, veterinary students, veterinary technicians, animal control officers, public health officials, and Red Cross volunteers, as well as fire, sheriff, Emergency Medical Services (EMS), and other public employees.

The North Carolina SART is a public-private partnership based on the incident command system. Other states may use different terminology for their response teams and have different organization structures. Some SARTs are managed through the state veterinary medical association, and other response teams are managed through the state veterinarian's office. The following websites have information on their respective state veterinary response teams. Some state teams are currently limited to veterinarians, or veterinarians and veterinary technicians. Further information may also be available from the State Veterinarian or state veterinary medical association.

- North Carolina SART: www.ncsart.org

- Colorado SART: www.cosart.org

- Pennsylvania SART: www.pasart.org

- Nebraska Livestock Emergency Disease Response (LEDRS): www.agr.state.ne.us/division/bai/ledrs.htm

- Idaho Veterinary Emergency Response Team (IVERT): www.agri.state.id.us/Categories/Animals/emergencyMgmt/indexemergencymgmt.php

- Texas Emergency Response Team (TERT): www.tahc.state.tx.us/emergency/tert/shtml

- Minnesota Veterinary Response Corp: www.bah.state.mn.us/animals/animal_bytes/5-5-04.htm

- Iowa Veterinary Rapid Response Teams: www.agriculture.state.ia.us/IVRRT.htm

Non Profit Organizations

Private organizations such as the Humane Society of the United States (HSUS) and the American Society for the Prevention of Cruelty to Animals (ASPCA) also respond to disasters. HSUS, ASPCA and many other animal rescue groups sent personnel to respond to Hurricane Katrina in 2005. Veterinarians and veterinary students can play a role in these organizations. Further information is available from HSUS (www.hsus.org), the ASPCA (www.aspca.org), or their local or state affiliates.

Experiences in the Emergency Management Organizations

The following two stories illustrate how veterinarians and veterinary students can use their education and training to assist in animal emergencies. Pamela Kramer, a veterinary student who participated in the 2003 exotic Newcastle disease outbreak in California, and Pam Hullinger, a veterinarian who helped eradicate foot and mouth disease from the United Kingdom in 2001, share their stories in this section.

Pamela Kramer

Pamela Kramer was a first year veterinary student at Iowa State University when she learned about the opportunity to work with NAHERC on the exotic Newcastle disease (END) outbreak in southern California. The following is an account of her experience.

In January/February of 2003, I was debating what I wanted to do during the summer. I had one of two options: participate in the Merck/Merial Summer Scholars Program or join the END NAHERC. The Merck program would allow me to conduct hands-on research. The END Taskforce would teach me how to help out in disease outbreak situations. I decided to fill out the paperwork and apply for both to improve my chances of at least getting accepted into one of the programs. In March, I found out that I had been accepted into the Merck/ Merial Summer Scholars Program. I decided to accept a position in the Merck program, because I didn't really think I would be accepted by USDA-APHIS to join the END Taskforce. However, about three days after being accepted into the Merck/ Merial Summer Scholars Program, I found out that I had also been chosen to participate in the END Taskforce.

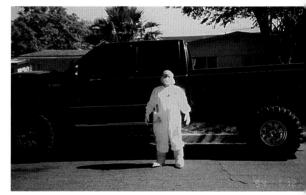

Pam Kramer at work as a NAHERC veterinary student during the exotic Newcastle disease outbreak in California.
Source: Pam Kramer

Here before me was a huge decision I had to make. Many things were going through my mind, such as…I don't know anything about birds...I have never been to California...Would I like doing research?

After speaking with some advisors, faculty and my Merck program advisor, I decided to go to California and help out with END instead. Now I am just a small town Iowa girl who didn't travel much at all, especially by myself. In spite of this, I found myself being taken to the Des Moines airport by a friend and flying to California to spend two months working with the USDA trying to eradicate END. Truthfully, I was scared but yet excited all at the same time. Scared partially because I was going somewhere that I had never been before, but for the most part I was very excited to get this once in a lifetime opportunity and get the chance to participate in a disease eradication program in California. I had the pleasure of working with veterinarians, technicians, interpreters, and clerical people in Southern California for two months -- from Memorial Day through the end of July 2003.

When I arrived in southern California, I spent the first day completing all the necessary paperwork including getting my ID card and cell phone. I had to take a defensive driving class before I could get my rental car. The USDA arranged for my hotel, and provided funds for food and related expenses.

During the first two weeks, I was assigned to the surveillance group and worked as the leader of four people. Every morning we met at Orange County headquarters at 7 a.m. to be briefed on what was going on. We were informed of new birds or premises that had tested positive or other relevant news. Following the morning briefings, each day my team received a map of a section of a community to cover. Our job was to go door to door and speak with someone at every house about pet birds and game birds. If the residents owned birds, we filled out a form indicating types and numbers of birds and whether or not they were sick. If no one was home, we left flyers about exotic Newcastle disease and a number to call if they wanted more information or if they wanted their birds tested. The USDA-APHIS would pay for all birds to be tested once. It was very interesting to go to the different neighborhoods, especially since this was my first time to California. Most of the people were very nice and didn't mind us inquiring about whether or not they had birds. However, in some areas where positive birds or flocks had been eradicated, people were hesitant to talk to us because they thought we were coming to take their birds. Surprisingly, not very many people knew much about END. The interpreters were quite helpful to have along, because in some areas, many people only spoke Spanish. We were told that if we did not feel safe in area to return to headquarters, and we would be reassigned to a different area.

For my next assignment, I worked at the Orange County APHIS headquarters for a week entering all the surveillance results in the computer database. While it may not have been the most exciting work, it gave me an understanding of what it was like to work at headquarters and the important role of the support staff in supporting an animal health emergency.

The remainder of my time with the NAHERC was spent collecting cloacal and tracheal swabs from pet birds and chickens in San Diego, Lancaster, and Santa Clarita, California. I was with a group of 15-20 people made up mainly of veterinary students, a couple interpreters and one to two veterinarians. We were trained in the field on biosecurity and collecting samples by a veterinarian. Then we were split into smaller groups consisting of two or more vet students and one to two interpreters. As with the surveillance unit, we were given maps of the area where we were to go and test birds. As a part of my daily duties, we routinely gowned up in biosecurity suits (Ty-Vex suits), boots, gloves, and masks. Each outfit was discarded into a garbage bag, sealed, and disinfected before placing it into another garbage bag after we were finished at each premise. My team started on the outside of the infection zone and worked our way in to reduce the size of the quarantine zone.

I met and worked with veterinary students from Auburn University, Colorado State, Georgia, Iowa State, Kansas State, Minnesota and Virginia/Maryland, and have maintained contact with both veterinary students and veterinarians that I worked with in California.

The most important thing I learned from this experience is how things are done in the real world. Watching the federal and volunteer teams approach each situation was really interesting. Veterinary students received a lot of respect and people listened to them. I also liked the responsibilities I was given (like being in charge of a team), not to mention free airfare, hotel accommodations, a rental car and a cell phone. We routinely worked 12-14 hour days, so overtime pay became a big benefit for all the students. But we also got some time off to interact as a group and to do a little sightseeing on holidays.

This opportunity was a once in a lifetime chance to be involved in a large scale eradication program. This was an experience that I will never forget. It was so incredible getting to know and work with other veterinary students, veterinarians, USDA-APHIS staff from all over the country. If given the opportunity to do this again, I would jump at it.

Pam Hullinger

Dr. Pam Hullinger, Veterinary Medical Officer and University Liaison with the California Department of Food and Agriculture (CDFA) worked in the United Kingdom (U.K.) assisting in the eradication of foot and mouth disease (FMD) in 2001. She initially volunteered through the CDFA and then went back to the U.K. through the NAHERC. An account of Dr. Hullinger's experience follows.

This was an experience that I will never forget. There is no substitute for firsthand experience in gaining respect for the devastation that a foreign animal disease can inflict upon on a nation. Opportunities such as this are both personally and professionally rewarding. I would encourage anyone who has even a slight interest in such work to make the time to participate.

At the time the FMD outbreak began in the U.K., I was both working for CDFA and finishing my Winter quarter in the Masters in Preventive Veterinary Medicine Program (MPVM) at UC Davis. When I found out that CDFA veterinarians might be eligible to participate in the eradication efforts I rapidly signed up. Little did I know that I would be on a plane three days later, about to begin an unforgettable adventure. It was probably the anticipation of seeing first-hand, a legendary and much feared disease, along with a sense of duty, that inspired me to act so quickly. It wasn't until I was eastbound for London that I really started to think about what I might be getting myself into and some apprehensive thoughts began to enter my mind…How would U.K. farmers react to foreign veterinarians?…How would they react when their herds or flocks had to be destroyed?…Would they let us on their farms?…Did they have guns?…Fortunately, all my apprehensions were largely unwarranted, although I did have to learn to "drive stick" with my left hand and speak (or at least understand) proper English.

My initial arrival in Carlisle (north-west England) occurred at a time when the regional Ministry of Agriculture, Fisheries and Food (now called DEFRA – Department for Environment, Food and Rural Affairs) office was expanding from a normal staff of 10-12 to well over 300 veterinarians, plus support staff. Things were very chaotic. The logistical support needed to effectively manage and support a field staff of that magnitude was mind-boggling. Acquisition of simple necessities like lodging, vehicles and cell phones was a challenge as local resources became rapidly depleted.

I had an uneasy feeling as I headed out on my first assignment, which was to inspect some potentially FMD infected cattle. While I was hoping to see "true" clinical FMD, I did not relish the thought of having to destroy the animals and/or the impact that it would undoubtedly have on the farmers. I also wondered how a "Yank" would be received by British farmers under the circumstances. I soon learned that the British farmers were an incredible group of warm, generous and gracious individuals, even in the face of personal and national tragedy. Some of these farmers and their families lost animals, herds and flocks that had been in their families for generations. Most situations were very emotional and stressful as individuals struggled with their grief and sense of hopelessness at losing their animals and their livelihoods. They say that it is not just one's experiences in life, but how they react to them, that truly defines one's character. I will forever be impressed by both the grace and the fortitude of the farmers I worked with in the United Kingdom.

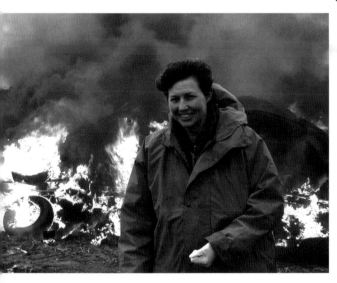

Dr. Pam Hullinger served in the NAHERC during the FMD outbreak in the U.K.
Source: Pam Hullinger

I also will never forget my initial image of Cumbria, one of the hardest hit areas of the United Kingdom. As I crested the Pennines, a central mountain/hill range (driving for the first time on the "other" side of the road) and descended toward the town of Carlisle, I entered what resembled a war zone. Smoke filled the air, burning my eyes and lungs as burning pyres of twisted cattle and sheep carcasses dotted the countryside. It was a haunting image, like nothing I could have imagined. I still can remember the smell. The challenge of disposing of up to 80,000 carcasses a day was monumental.

In the field, veterinarians were usually asked to make a decision on whether or not a flock/herd was infected based solely on clinical signs seen at the time of the initial visit (without the aid of any testing or laboratory support). The greatest challenge was in evaluating flocks of possibly infected sheep grazing coarse feed (that caused minor oral ulcerations or trauma) or flocks that may have been exposed more than three weeks prior to the initial visit (lesions would have healed on these animals). Destroying a person's livelihood, based solely on a few oral ulcers in the mouths of a few sheep without laboratory confirmation was a very uncomfortable decision. While during an outbreak one must always err on the side of caution, we now know that many uninfected animals were destroyed due to the lack of scaleable, rapid diagnostics for FMD. I hope that many have learned from that unfortunate U.K. lesson and I do believe we are now much better prepared to face the diagnostic challenges of a large scale FMD outbreak.

Most impressive was the overall magnitude and impact that FMD had on the U.K., and specifically the farming community, livestock populations and tourism industry. While the direct impact of FMD was largely regionalized within the country, the indirect effects (primarily loss of tourism) were felt throughout the U.K.. In the end, all the livestock on 9,677 farms were destroyed to control the spread of FMD. Of these, 2,030 were actually declared FMD infected premises and the remainder designated as dangerous contacts, either direct or indirect. Estimates are that from 6-10 million animals were slaughtered, approximately 10 percent of the U.K. national herd. The widespread dissemination of FMD throughout the U.K. highlighted the need for continual vigilance in both the public and private sector, and the importance of early detection of disease in minimizing the overall scale of an outbreak. Although U.K. farmers were eventually able to restock, they all suffered immeasurable personal losses that will never be quantified.

It is hard to describe the camaraderie, friendship and understanding that develops among individuals who share such an experience. There are many individuals, U.K. veterinarians, U.K. farmers and the other veterinarians (from all over the world) who I will never forget. People of great character, who unselfishly gave up personal time to help those in need. Among those who were there to first hand witness the situation and participate in the response, there is a unique bond and understanding that cannot be explained.

The time I spent working in the U.K was truly a memorable and rewarding experience. In my mind, the challenge that faces us is to take the experiences and lessons learned in the U.K. and use them to strengthen and enhance the detection, response, control and mitigation of foreign animal diseases in the U.S.

The greatest tragedy is one that nobody learns from.

CHAPTER *four*

Sources of Information

Federal Emergency Management System (FEMA). National Incident Management System. NIMS and the Incident Command System. Available at: http://www.fema.gov/nims/. Accessed 27 Nov 2005.

Federal Emergency Management System (FEMA). Basic Incident Command System for federal workers (I-100/200). Student manual. FEMA; 2005 Jan. Available at: http://training.fema.gov/EMIWeb/downloads/ICScombined/SMICS100200.doc. Accessed 7 Dec 2005.

Iowa State University, The Center for Food Security and Public Health (ISU CFSPH). USDA Incident Command 100 Training. ISU CFSPH; 2004 Aug. Available at: http://www.cfsph.iastate.edu/CE. Accessed November 2005.

Personal communication, Gordon Cleveland, DVM, APHIS Emergency Management, Riverdale, MD

Personal communication, Dr. Pam Hullinger, Veterinary Medical Officer and University Liaison with the California Department of Food and Agriculture (CDFA).[This personal account was previously published as: Hullinger P. U.S. veterinarian reflects on foot & mouth disease outbreak experience in U.K. US Animal Health Association Newsletter. Special Edition: The Nation's Plum Island Laboratories. October 2003, page 2.]

Personal communication, Pamela Kramer. Student, Iowa State University, Ames, IA.

U.S. Department of Agriculture, Animal and Plant Health Inspection Service (USDA APHIS). National Animal Health Emergency Response Corps. You can make a difference. Program Aid No. 1748. USDA APHIS; 2003 July. Available at: http://www.usda.aphis.gov/lpa/pubs/pub_ahvsreserves.html. Accessed November 2005.

U.S. Department of Agriculture, Animal and Plant Health Inspection Service, Veterinary Services (USDA APHIS, VS) Safeguarding animal health. FY2002 annual highlights report. USDA APHIS, VS; 2002. Available at: http://www.aphis.usda.gov/vs/highlights/. Accessed November 2005.

U.S. Department of Homeland Security. Emergencies and disasters, planning and prevention. National Response Plan. Available at: http://www.dhs.gov/dhspublic/interapp/editorial/editorial_0566.xml. Accessed November 2005.

U.S. Department of Homeland Security. Fact sheet: National Incident Management System (NIMS). Available at: http://www.dhs.gov/dhspublic/interapp/press_release/press_release_0363.xml. Accessed 27 Nov 2005.

U.S. Department of Homeland Security. National Incident Management System (NIMS) Online. Available at: http://www.nimsonline.com/. Accessed November 2005.

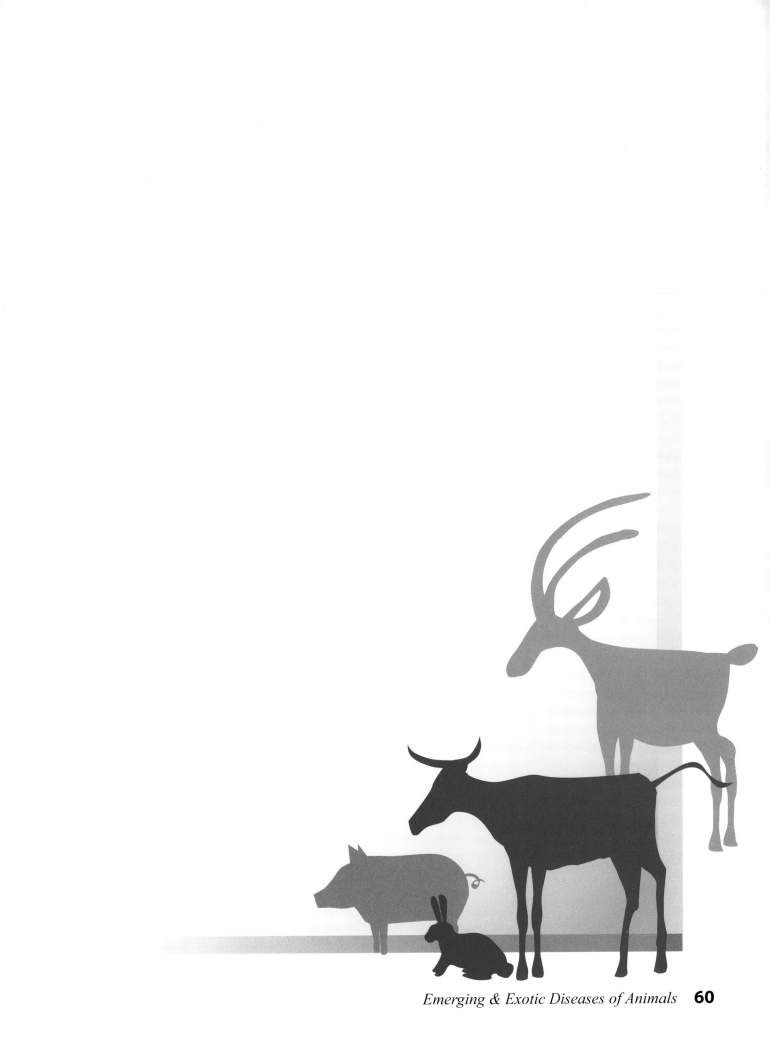

CHAPTER
five

> U.S. agriculture is very vulnerable to the introduction of a foreign animal disease. Important lessons can be learned from these examples.

Descriptions of Recent Incursions of Exotic Animal Diseases

Authors: *Jane Galyon, MS; Anna Rovid Spickler, DVM, PhD; James Roth, DVM, PhD,* Iowa State University, College of Veterinary Medicine

This overview describes recent incursions of exotic animal diseases. Important lessons can be learned from these examples. U.S. agriculture is very vulnerable to the introduction of a foreign animal disease. Outbreaks can occur when a pathogen is inadvertently introduced in contaminated material carried by an international traveler, or in imported animals or animal products. Foreign animal diseases could enter the U.S. vectored by wild animals, insects, or migratory birds or they could be intentionally introduced to cause severe economic problems or to target human health. Descriptions of recent outbreaks of foreign animal disease in various countries and the impact they had are presented here to raise understanding of the importance of these diseases and their detection, prevention, and control.

Private practitioners are the nation's first line of defense for identifying foreign animal disease outbreaks and emerging diseases. Human and animal health and the economic welfare of producers, practitioners, the feed industry, pharmaceutical and biologics industries, packers, and, ultimately, consumers depend on veterinarians.

Highly Pathogenic Avian Influenza in Hong Kong, 1997-2002, and Southeast Asia, 2003-2005

Outbreaks of highly pathogenic avian influenza occur periodically throughout the world when viruses carried in wild birds emerge into poultry. A swift response to an outbreak can eliminate the virus from poultry flocks and return trade relations to normal. Rapid eradication can also protect humans from zoonotic infections and reduce the possibility that an avian virus could become adapted to humans. Many new isolates of the influenza viruses seem to come from southern China, where farmers often mix different species of terrestrial poultry, waterfowl, and pigs – a situation that allows influenza viruses from different species to acquire gene segments from each other. Hong Kong, which maintains a comprehensive surveillance program and has a high awareness of avian influenza, is considered to be a sentinel for new viral reassortants. From 1997 to 2002, Hong Kong experienced repeated outbreaks with various H5N1 influenza viruses. These outbreaks raised the suspicion that new virulent reassortants of H5N1 were becoming established in the region. After an epidemic in 1997, during which the first serious zoonotic infections were reported, Hong Kong was diligent in maintaining surveillance for new viruses and rapidly stamping out each outbreak. The poultry population of Hong Kong was partially or completely depopulated three times in five years. In contrast, an avian influenza H5N1 virus that appeared in several Asian countries in 2003 was not immediately stamped out everywhere. As a result, this virus seems to have become endemic in Asian birds, has spread to birds in Europe, and has triggered fears of a human pandemic.

Avian influenza, a disease seen mainly in poultry, is caused by viruses in the genus influenzavirus A, family Orthomyxoviridae. The avian influenza viruses are usually spread by the fecal-oral route; they can be transmitted directly, or indirectly on fomites and mechanical vectors such as flies. They may also be transmitted in respiratory secretions when birds are in close contact. In addition, these viruses are found inside eggs; although these eggs are unlikely to hatch, they may spread the virus if they break. There are two forms of avian influenza in domestic poultry. The more common form, called low pathogenic avian influenza (LPAI), is usually a subclinical or mild infection. Typically, an infected flock has subtle signs such as decreased egg production or a somewhat increased mortality rate; serious symptoms occur only if there are concurrent diseases or stressors. In contrast, highly pathogenic avian influenza (HPAI) or 'fowl plague" is a severe disease with morbidity and mortality rates as high as 90-100%. HPAI can affect domestic poultry, game birds, and ratites; however, a HPAI virus does not necessarily affect all species equally. For instance, a virus might cause severe disease in chickens and turkeys, but minimal symptoms in ducks and quail. Typical HPAI symptoms include depression, inappetence, and respiratory signs such as coughing, nasal and ocular discharge, a swollen face, and cyanosis of the comb and wattles. The birds may also have diarrhea or neurologic signs such as paralysis. In some cases, sudden death can occur with few clinical signs. Any surviving birds are usually in poor condition.

The avian influenza viruses, which are highly variable, can be classified into subtypes based on two proteins, the hemagglutinin ('H') and neuraminidase ('N'). There are at least 16 different hemagglutinin antigens (H1 to H16) and 9 neuraminidase antigens (N1 to N9). Influenza viruses can change very quickly. Due to their poor proofreading during gene replication, they have a very high mutation rate. They also have a segmented genome, which facilitates reassortment. Reassortment can take place whenever two different influenza viruses infect the same cell;

An avian influenza H5N1 virus that appeared in several Asian countries in 2003 was not immediately stamped out everywhere. As a result, this virus seems to have become endemic in Asian birds, has spread to birds in Europe, and has triggered fears of a human pandemic.

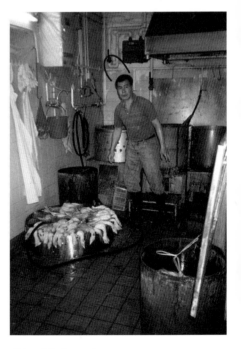

Live bird markets are popular in Hong Kong.
Source: David Swayne, USDA-ARS

when the new viruses (the 'progeny') are assembled, they may contain some genes from one parent virus and some genes from the other. Because the influenza viruses are so variable, viruses that share a subtype are not necessarily closely related and may differ greatly in their virulence, host specificity, or other factors. An avian influenza virus is classified as a LPAI or HPAI virus based on its genetic features and its virulence in poultry. HPAI viruses, which have been eradicated from poultry flocks in most developed nations, are usually H5 or H7 viruses. However, not all H5 and H7 viruses are highly virulent; many H5 and H7 LPAI viruses also exist. These LPAI viruses are also of concern, because some of them mutate and become highly pathogenic after circulating in poultry flocks for a time.

Where Do Highly Pathogenic Avian Influenza Viruses Come From?

Although avian influenza is a disease seen mainly in domestic poultry, avian influenza viruses are carried asymptomatically by a wide variety of birds. Waterfowl, which carry all of the subtypes, are considered to be the reservoir hosts. These birds shed viruses in the feces, sometimes resulting in the emergence of a virus into domestic poultry (or, rarely, mammals). Thus, outbreaks of HPAI can occur even in countries that have eradicated these viruses from their commercial poultry flocks. Many new isolates come from southern China, an area some scientists call an "epicenter" for the avian influenza viruses. Farmers there often raise different types of poultry, including domestic waterfowl, alongside each other on high-density small farms - creating a perfect breeding ground for new influenza strains. These poultry are often reared under low biosecurity conditions, and may be exposed to wild birds or water where these birds have been swimming. In addition, poultry may be raised in close contact with both pigs and people, increasing the likelihood of virus recombination and virus transmission between birds and mammals as well.

The island territory of Hong Kong, which imports large quantities of poultry from China, is considered to be a sentinel for these new viruses. China supplies over 70% of the 100,000 fresh chickens eaten in Hong Kong every day and is the territory's leading source for geese, ducks, quail, and pheasants. Unlike Mainland China, Hong Kong also has a comprehensive influenza surveillance system that allows it to quickly detect new viruses, and an established response system that allows it to respond effectively and rapidly to disease outbreaks. From 1997 to 2002, Hong Kong experienced several disquieting outbreaks with new strains of H5N1 viruses.

Avian Influenza in Hong Kong, 1997 – A Deadly Strain in Humans

The first disturbing outbreak occurred in Hong Kong poultry flocks in 1997. Before this epidemic, which began in late March, the avian influenza viruses were not thought to cause serious disease in humans. Then, in May, a H5N1 avian influenza virus was isolated from a fatal case of acute pneumonia and respiratory distress syndrome in an otherwise healthy 3-year old boy. This virus, which seemed to be transmitted by contact with sick birds, eventually killed five more Hong Kong residents and caused serious illness in 12 others. The discovery that the H5N1/97 virus was pathogenic for humans added urgency to the eradication efforts. Approximately 1.5 million chickens in live bird markets and farms were eventually slaughtered in a successful bid to stop the epidemic. Some people think this rapid response may have averted an incipient human influenza pandemic. Since 1997, sporadic human infections have been reported with other avian influenza viruses, including other isolates of H5N1 as well as H7N2, H7N3, H7N7, and H9N2 viruses. To date, human infections with the highly pathogenic viruses, particularly H5N1, seem to be more severe. Most zoonotic infections with the non-H5N1 viruses have been limited to conjunctivitis or relatively mild respiratory infections, but severe, fatal, infections have also been seen. Human cases generally seem to result from direct contact with infected poultry or fomites, although rare instances of limited person-to-person transmission have also been documented.

The H5N1/97 virus may hold clues to help researchers determine which avian influenza viruses will infect humans. When this virus was analyzed, it was found to be a reassortant that contained genes from several different species of birds. One of the 'parent' viruses was a H5N1 virus similar to one first isolated from geese in China's Guangdong province in 1996. Such viruses are known as the Goose/Guangdong/1/96 (H5N1 Gs/Gd)-like viruses. Another segment was contributed by influenza viruses found mainly in quail. The reassortment between these viruses was probably facilitated by the mixing of bird species in Hong Kong's many retail live bird markets. These markets, where poultry is bought live, and killed and plucked in front of the customer, are very popular among Hong Kong consumers. In 1997, the live bird markets contained waterfowl such as ducks and geese, and terrestrial birds such as chickens, quail, and guinea fowl. In addition to allowing new reassortant viruses to arise, these markets facilitate their spread; birds not sold at the market and returned to the farm may carry new infections with them.

To prevent the reemergence of another H5N1/97-like virus, Hong Kong established a central slaughterhouse for ducks and geese in 1998. This measure was intended to keep the influenza viruses found in these aquatic poultry separate from other parent viruses found mainly in quail. Government representatives also called for a central slaughterhouse for chickens in Hong Kong, but the industry feared that this would undermine the livelihood of its 20,000 chicken sellers. Terrestrial poultry—chickens, quail, pigeons, pheasants, and guinea fowl—continued to be sold and slaughtered in the retail live bird markets. After 1997, Hong Kong also established an elaborate system of blood tests, inspections, and quarantine rules to screen imported birds, as well as a surveillance system to test birds at the central slaughterhouse and in the live bird markets. However, Hong Kong can only control avian influenza viruses in its own domestic poultry. Hong Kong officials have no authority to monitor or regulate health and environmental conditions on Mainland China farms, nor are they able to control the avian influenza viruses in the millions of migratory wild birds in the area. Although the H5N1/97 virus was successfully eradicated from poultry, individual viruses containing its gene segments continued to circulate in birds in the region.

Avian Influenza in Hong Kong, 2001

For a time, Hong Kong's separation of terrestrial and aquatic poultry seemed to work. From 1999 to 2001, H5N1 viruses were intermittently isolated from geese and ducks at the central slaughterhouse, but no H5N1 viruses were found during routine surveillance in the live terrestrial poultry markets. Then, in April 2001, H5N1 viruses were found in three of eight retail markets; these viruses were isolated in fecal swabs from several apparently healthy chickens, silky chickens, pigeons, quail, and pheasants. This finding led to more intense scrutiny of the markets, and additional H5N1 isolates were found in cloacal swabs from dead chickens in 30 live bird markets. There were no symptoms of HPAI until mid-May, when three markets reported that the mortality rates in their poultry had increased greatly. On May 17, 2001, the Government of Hong Kong Special Administrative Region of China (SAR) reported an outbreak of highly pathogenic avian influenza type A (H5N1) virus to the OIE. The three affected live-bird markets were closed and all birds were destroyed. The following day all wholesale and retail markets selling chickens in Hong Kong were closed and the birds were culled. Beginning May 21 Hong Kong authorities depopulated approximately 1.2 million live birds as a precautionary measure. The cull covered 208 farms raising chickens, pigeons, and quail. Importation of live birds from Mainland China was stopped and retail markets for live poultry remained closed for four weeks. This outbreak is estimated to have cost $3.86 million including compensation to poultry vendors.

Although the cost of eradication was high, the surveillance system and quick response allowed Hong Kong to eliminate the H5N1/2001 viruses before illness became widespread in poultry. These viruses were found to be reassortants that contained gene segments from various influenza viruses of waterfowl. One of the parental viruses was, once again, a H5N1 Gs/Gd-like virus. This time, waterfowl viruses had been able to infect terrestrial poultry by reassorting with other waterfowl viruses. At least five different H5N1 genotypes were isolated during the 2001 outbreak. Although all five were highly pathogenic for chickens after experimental infection, only one was associated with the increased mortality rates in the three markets. This genotype had a mutation in the neuraminidase gene that increased its ability to spread in terrestrial poultry. The genetic analysis also suggested that the quick response to the outbreak might have prevented human disease. None of the H5N1/2001 viruses had the same genotype as the H5N1/97 virus and no human cases were reported in 2001. However, some of the viruses that had contributed gene segments to the H5N1/97 virus were still circulating in quail in the live bird markets. Given time, these viruses might have reassorted with the H5N1/2001 virus and produced another genotype that could infect humans. After the 2001 outbreak, Hong Kong authorities prohibited selling live quail where other poultry were sold in live bird markets.

The exclusion of waterfowl from Hong Kong's retail live bird markets, together with the screening of imported poultry, were successful in keeping H5N1/97-like viruses out of terrestrial poultry from 1998 until 2001. But the reassortant viruses found in 2001 seemed to be more difficult to exclude, perhaps due to their wider host range and/or more efficient transmission among birds. To interrupt the amplification of any viruses that might enter the retail markets, a once-a-month "rest-day" was introduced. On these rest days, the live bird markets are completely emptied of poultry, any remaining poultry are slaughtered to be sold as chilled carcasses, and the markets are thoroughly cleaned before being restocked the following day.

Avian Influenza in Hong Kong, 2002— an Unusual Outbreak in Wild Waterfowl

Late in 2002, Hong Kong once again had an outbreak with H5N1 viruses—this time in wild birds. The first episode occurred in Penfold Park, a small nature park that contained a number of resident waterfowl

Waterfowl have the potential to incubate avian influenza.
Source: Clint May, ISU

including geese, ducks, and swans, as well as captive psittacine and passerine birds, free-ranging white pigeons, and feral egrets. Neurologic disease and unusual deaths were first reported in early December. Thirty-one waterfowl died, and the remaining ducks and geese were culled on December 10. The second outbreak occurred at Kowloon Park, located 12 km away. This park had an aviary with 35 species of captive free-flying birds, and a bird lake that housed 26 species of captive pinioned waterfowl and flamingos. In addition, wild herons were seen at the waterfowl ponds and five species of feral birds visited

regularly to scavenge grain from the feeding troughs. The first unusual deaths occurred at this park from December 14 to 17, and the first confirmed case of H5N1 avian influenza was reported on December 17.

Kowloon Park, like Penfold Park, was closed, drained, and disinfected. All of the remaining resident waterfowl were quarantined. Many of the birds from the open ponds, including geese, ducks, swans, and flamingos died during December; however, the terrestrial and feral birds at these parks seemed to be unaffected. At the same time, H5N1 viruses were found in dead chickens in live bird markets and on a local chicken farm. H5N1 viruses were also isolated from dead little egrets, gray herons and other wild migratory birds that overwinter in Hong Kong. More than one virus seemed to be responsible for these outbreaks; at least three different H5N1 viruses isolated in late 2002 were able to cause severe disease and death in experimentally infected ducks.

Epidemics of avian influenza are very unusual in wild birds. Before this outbreak, researchers had seen little or no evolutionary change in the avian influenza viruses isolated from wild waterfowl over the last 60 years. Therefore, they believed that these viruses were stable in their normal reservoir hosts. Earlier viruses found in Hong Kong, including the H5N1/97 virus, did not replicate well in ducks and were asymptomatic in this species. The repeated outbreaks of H5N1 viruses in Hong Kong in 1997, 2001, and 2002 suggested that H5N1 viruses had become widespread in the region, and that new pandemic or panzootic strains could emerge through reassortment. There were also other concerns about these viruses. H5N1 viruses isolated in the region in 2001 and 2002 were much more variable than the H5 viruses isolated in Hong Kong between 1979 and 1997. In addition, it was worrisome that some of the new H5N1 isolates could infect the brain as well as the respiratory tract in both birds and mammals. During this time, there were also hints that viruses pathogenic to humans might be circulating in Mainland China. In 2003, a H5N1 virus infected two members of a Hong Kong family who had traveled to China. The 5-year old son recovered, but his 33-year old father died. Another family member died of a respiratory illness while in China, but no testing was done there.

Avian Influenza in Southeast Asia and Europe, 2003-2005

In 2003, a new epidemic broke out. This time, it was widespread. From late 2003 to March 2004, HPAI (H5N1) viruses were reported among poultry, particularly chickens, in Cambodia, China, Indonesia, Japan, Laos, South Korea, Thailand, and Vietnam. More than 100 million birds died or were culled in an effort to stop the outbreak. In rare instances, this virus was able to infect humans; 35 cases were confirmed in Thailand and Vietnam, most apparently the result of direct contact with birds. Twenty-four of the human infections were fatal. In many parts of Southeast Asia, humans live in close contact with their animals, including poultry. This facilitates the spread of influenza viruses between species, and may have contributed to the human infections. At first, culling and other measures appeared to control this virus. By March 2004, the outbreak seemed to be contained in poultry and human infections were no longer being reported in most nations. However, beginning in June 2004, a number of countries once again began seeing the disease. This time, infected poultry were reported in Cambodia, China, Indonesia, Malaysia, Thailand, Vietnam, and the Democratic People's Republic of Korea (North Korea). Human infections were seen in Indonesia, Vietnam, Thailand, Cambodia, and China. In addition, fatal H5N1 infections were reported in zoo and domestic cats fed infected poultry, and H5N1 virus transmission to domestic cats was confirmed in laboratory studies. In some of the infected tigers, which lived in a zoo in Thailand, the virus seems to have spread horizontally. There were also reports of infected zoo birds in Indonesia and pigs in China. In April 2005, a H5N1 virus killed more than 6,000 migratory birds at isolated Qinghai Lake in central China. Mongolia also reported the death of 89 migratory birds at two lakes in August 2005. These various reports were worrisome, as they suggested that the H5N1 viruses were adapting to multiple mammalian and avian hosts. As of November 2005, more than 150 million poultry had been culled or died in this outbreak, which was not yet under control. The U.S. Centers for Disease Control and Prevention (CDC) warned that the H5N1 virus now seemed to have become endemic among birds in Asia.

In 2005, H5N1 viruses spread beyond Southeast Asia. They were first reported in Russia and Kazakhstan. Authorities in these countries hoped to confine the virus to Asia by intensive eradication efforts. But within a few weeks, a H5N1 virus passed the Ural mountains, the boundary between Europe and Asia, and appeared in Turkey and Romania, prompting mass culls and fears of a worldwide panzootic. In Croatia, a H5 virus was found in dead wild swans at a fish pond. As a result, Croatia began to cull poultry in villages near the pond, and stopped all bird and poultry exports. In Germany, up to 25 wild geese and ducks were found dead at a pond in October 2005, and avian influenza virus was isolated from some of these birds. Cases of H5N1 HPAI were also reported in the Aegean Sea islands in Greece. How the H5N1 virus entered Europe is unknown, but there are suspicions that migrating wild birds might be carrying the virus into new regions. Some nations in the European Union mandated or recommended that poultry flocks, particularly those located near wetlands, be kept indoors to reduce the possibility of virus transmission from this source. In October 2005, the United Kingdom reported that the H5N1 virus had been found in mesias (a type of bird) that died in quarantine during the import process. Partly as a result of this finding, the European Commission banned the importation of wild birds into the E.U., with some exceptions allowed under special circumstances or quarantine conditions.

The specific origins and parent viruses of the currently circulating H5N1 viruses remain to be determined, but circumstantial evidence suggests that southern China may be the reservoir. Although they have not been fully characterized yet, these viruses seem to be related to H5N1 viruses found in Hong Kong from 1997 to 2002. Isolates from South Korea resemble the virus found in Penfold Park in 2002. The current H5N1 viruses also share some characteristics with one of the genotypes found during the 2001 outbreak. There is also some evidence that the H5N1 viruses may be evolving as the outbreak continues. Genetic differences have been reported between the South Korean viruses, which did not infect humans, and viruses that infected humans in Vietnam and Thailand. Isolates from South Korea, which acted very quickly to contain its outbreak, are genetically homogeneous; the H5N1 viruses found in some Southeast Asian countries with prolonged outbreaks are heterogeneous.

Fears of a Human Pandemic

One of the major concerns in the Southeast Asian outbreak has been the ability of the virus to infect humans. Between December 2003 and November 29, 2005, 133 human cases and 68 deaths were confirmed in Thailand, Vietnam, Cambodia, Indonesia, and China. Although a few of these cases may have been due to limited person-to-person transmission, the vast majority seemed to be caused by direct contact with poultry. However, authorities fear that the current viruses could recombine with a human influenza virus and produce an isolate that is more easily transmitted from person to person. An avian virus could also adapt to humans without reassortment, if it developed certain mutations. Fears of a new human pandemic are fueled, in part, by the recent discovery that the H1N1 virus responsible for the deadly 1918 pandemic was probably an avian influenza virus that became adapted to humans. The H5N1 viruses isolated from humans in the current epidemic share certain genetic features with the H1N1/1918 virus. In addition, the human population does not have immunity to H5N1; the currently circulating human influenza viruses are H1N1, H1N2 and H3N2.

As a result of this epidemic, countries are establishing plans to protect their populations in the event of an avian influenza pandemic in humans. Some countries have stockpiled antiviral drugs. A human H5N1 vaccine is also in development. Two events - reports of sustained human-to-human transmission, or genetic reassortment with human influenza viruses - may signal that the H5N1 virus is adapting to humans. As of November 2005, neither event had been reported.

Highly Pathogenic Avian Influenza and the U.S.

Highly pathogenic avian influenza is a foreign animal disease in the U.S. Although outbreaks of LPAI are relatively common, only three or four outbreaks of HPAI have been recorded in the U.S. since 1900. The first, in 1924-1925, was associated with live bird markets. This virus, which seemed to be disseminated mainly through the movement of poultry, spread to nine eastern states before being eradicated. HPAI was seen again in 1929; it may have been caused by the same virus or it may have been a new introduction. This disease was not reported again until the autumn of 1983, when a H5N2 virus caused an extensive epidemic in Pennsylvania and surrounding states. This virus, which was highly virulent in chickens, turkeys, and guinea fowl, was very similar to a LPAI virus that had been circulating in the area for 6 months. As a result, some birds had immunity to the HPAI virus, which complicated diagnosis and probably helped the virus spread further. Control and eradication of this epidemic, which was not completed until 1984, cost over $63 million in federal funds and an additional $350 million in increased consumer costs. Over 17 million birds died or were slaughtered. There was no evidence of transmission to humans. HPAI was not reported again until February 2004, when a virus was isolated from a south-central Texas broiler chicken flock This virus, which also had the subtype H5N2, caused symptoms consistent with LPAI in the Texas flock, and was not virulent for experimentally infected chickens. However, some of its genetic characteristics suggested that it was a HPAI virus. Researchers also found that further changes in its hemagglutinin gene could increase the mortality rate. As a result, this virus was designated as a HPAI virus, and the USDA and state of Texas culled the approximately 6,600 birds in the flock. Surveillance on all flocks within 10 miles of the affected farm revealed no additional cases. No zoonotic infections were reported.

Like other countries, the U.S. is concerned about the possibility that the H5N1 strains from Southeast Asia could enter domestic poultry flocks or wild birds. APHIS has re-examined its HPAI prevention and eradication plans in light of that epidemic. All imported birds, including pet birds of U.S. origin, must now be quarantined and tested for the avian influenza virus before they enter the country. In addition, APHIS has placed trade restrictions on the importation of poultry or poultry products from countries that have reported cases of HPAI. Poultry or poultry products from East and Southeast Asia must be processed or cooked before importation to destroy any influenza viruses. APHIS has also alerted the U.S. Department of Homeland Security to be particularly vigilant in its agricultural inspections of passengers and cargo from Asia, and has increased its surveillance of domestic markets for illegally imported poultry products. In addition, the USDA is working with the World Organization for Animal Health (OIE), the United Nations' Food and Agriculture Organization (FAO), and World Health Organization (WHO) to help affected countries and their neighbors with disease prevention, management, and eradication to reduce the global threat from this virus.

Sources of Information

Acha PN, Szyfres B (Pan American Health Organization [PAHO]). Influenza. In: Zoonoses and Communicable Diseases Common to Man and Animals. Volume 2. Chlamydioses, rickettsioses and viroses. 3rd ed. Washington DC: PAHO; 2003. Scientific and Technical Publication No. 580. p. 155-172.

Aiello SE, Mays A, editors. Influenza (Fowl plague). In: The Merck Veterinary Manual. 8th ed. Whitehouse Station, NJ: Merck and Co; 1998. p. 1983.

Alexander DY. A review of avian influenza [monograph online]. Available at: http://www.esvv.unizh.ch/gent_abstracts/Alexander.html. Accessed 30 Aug 2004.

BBC News. At-a-glance: Europe on bird flu alert. October 25, 2005. Available at: http://news.bbc.co.uk/1/hi/world/europe/4338490.stm. Accessed 2 Nov 2005.

BBC News. Lethal bird flu found in Croatia. October 26, 2005. Available at: http://news.bbc.co.uk/1/hi/world/europe/4378268.stm. Accessed 2 Nov 2005.

BBC News. EU bans imports of exotic birds. October 25, 2005. Available at: http://news.bbc.co.uk/1/hi/world/europe/4373584.stm. Accessed 2 Nov 2005.

Beard CW. Avian influenza. In: Buisch W, Hyde J, Mebus C, editors. Foreign Animal Diseases.7th ed. U.S. Richmond, Virginia: U.S. Animal Health Association; 1998. p. 71-80. Available at: http://www.vet.uga.edu/vpp/gray_book/FAD/index.htm. Accessed 15 Oct 2005.

Center for Infectious Disease Research and Policy (CIDRAP), University of Minnesota. Laboratory-confirmed human cases of H5N1 avian influenza, December 2003 to present (Sept 19, 2005). Available at: http://www.cidrap.umn.edu/cidrap/content/influenza/avianflu/case-count/avflucount.html. Accessed 7 Oct 2005.

Chen H, Deng G, Li Z, Tian G, Li Y, Jiao P, Zhang L, Liu Z, Webster RG, Yu K. The evolution of H5N1 influenza viruses in ducks in southern China. Proc Natl Acad Sci USA. 2004;101:-10452-10457.

Department for Environment, Food and Rural Affairs (DEFRA), United Kingdom. Epidemiology report published on H5N1 in Essex quarantine. New release 528/05. November 15, 2005. Available at: http://www.defra.gov.uk/news/2005/051115b.htm. Accessed 20 Nov 2005.

Enserink M, Kaiser J. Avian flu finds new mammal hosts. Science. 2004;305:1385.

Enserink M. 'Pandemic vaccine' appears to protect only at high doses. Science 2005;309(5737): 996.

European Commission. Health and Consumer Protecion Directorate-General. Scientific Committee on Animal Health and Animal Welfare. Directorate C - Scientific Health OpinionsUnit C3 - Management of scientific committees II. The definition of avian influenza & The use of vaccination against avian influenza. Adopted 27 June 2000. Available at: http://europa.eu.int/comm/food/fs/sc/scah/out45-final_en.pdf. Accessed 2 Nov 2005.

Fenner F, Bachmann PA, Gibbs EPJ, Murphy FA, Studdert MJ, White DO. Orthomyxoviridae. In: Veterinary Virology. San Diego, CA: Academic Press Inc.; 1987. p. 473-484.

Fouchier RAM, Schneeberger PM, Rozendaal FW, Broekman JM, Kemink SAG, Munster V, Kuiken T, Rimmelzwaan GF, Schutten M, van Doornum GJJ, Koch G, Bosman A, Koopmans M, Osterhaus ADME. Avian influenza A virus (H7N7) associated with human conjunctivitis and a fatal case of acute respiratory distress syndrome. Proc Natl Acad Sci U S A. 2004;101:1356–1361.

Guan Y, Peiris JS, Lipatov AS, Ellis TM, Dyrting KC, Krauss S, Zhang LJ, Webster RG, Shortridge KF.Emergence of multiple genotypes of H5N1 avian influenza viruses in Hong Kong SAR. Proc Natl Acad Sci U S A. 2002 Jun 25;99(13):8950-5.

Harper SA, Fukuda K, Uyeki TM, Cox NJ, Bridges CB. Prevention and control of influenza. Recommendations of the advisory committee on immunization practices (ACIP) Morb Mortal Wkly Rep. 2004;53(RR-6):1-40.

Hinshaw VS, Bean WJ, Webster RG, Rehg JE, Fiorelli P, Early G, Geraci JR, St Aubin DJ. Are seals frequently infected with avian influenza viruses? J Virol. 1984;51(3):863-5.

http://www.aphis.usda.gov/vs/ceah/cei/ai_hongkong0501.htm.* Accessed 2003.

International Society for Infectious Diseases. Promed-Mail. Available at: http://www.promedmail.org. Accessed 2003.

Kaleta EF, Honicke A. A retrospective description of a highly pathogenic avian influenza A virus (H7N1/Carduelis/Germany/72) in a free-living siskin (Carduelis spinus Linnaeus, 1758) and its accidental transmission to yellow canaries (Serinus canaria Linnaeus, 1758).Dtsch Tierarztl Wochenschr. 2005 Jan;112(1):17-9.

Kuiken T, Rimmelzwaan G, van Riel D, van Amerongen G, Baars M, Fouchier R, Osterhaus A. Avian H5N1 influenza in cats. Science [serial online]. 2004; 10.1126/science.1102287. Available at: http://www.sciencemag.org/cgi/rapidpdf/1102287v1.pdf. Accessed 3 Sept 2004.

Lee CW, Suarez DL, Tumpey TM, Sung HW, Kwon YK, Lee YJ, Choi JG, Joh SJ, Kim MC, Lee EK, Park JM, Lu X, Katz JM, Spackman E, Swayne DE, Kim JH. Characterization of highly pathogenic H5N1 avian influenza A viruses isolated from South Korea. J Virol. 2005 Mar;79(6):3692-702.

Lee CW, Swayne DE, Linares JA, Senne DA, Suarez DL. H5N2 avian influenza outbreak in Texas in 2004: the first highly pathogenic strain in the United States in 20 years? J Virol. 2005 Sep;79(17):11412-21.

Normile D. Potentially more lethal variant hits migratory birds in China. Science. 2005;309(5732):231.

Perkins LE, Swayne DE. Varied pathogenicity of a Hong Kong-origin H5N1 avian influenza virus in four passerine species and budgerigars.Vet Pathol. 2003 Jan;40(1):14-24.

Poultry Health Services Ltd. Highly pathogenic avian influenza summary fact sheet. Available at: http://www.poultry-health.com/fora/fowlplag.htm. Accessed 2003.

Reid AH, Taubenberger JK. The origin of the 1918 pandemic influenza virus: a continuing enigma. J Gen Virol. 2003;84:2285-92.

Sturm-Ramirez KM, Ellis T, Bousfield B, Bissett L, Dyrting K, Rehg JE, Poon L, Guan Y, Peiris M, Webster RG.Reemerging H5N1 influenza viruses in Hong Kong in 2002 are highly pathogenic to ducks. J Virol. 2004 May;78(9):4892-901.

Taubenberger JK, Reid AH, Lourens RM, Wang R, Jin G, Fanning TG. Characterization of the 1918 influenza virus polymerase genes. Nature. 2005 Oct 6;437(7060):889-93.

Thanawongnuwech R, Amonsin A, Tantilertcharoen R, Damrongwatanapokin S, Theamboonlers A, Payungporn S, Nanthapornphiphat K, Ratanamungklanon S, Tunak E, Songserm T, Vivatthanavanich V, Lekdumrongsak T, Kesdangsakonwut S, Tunhikorn S, Poovorawan Y. Probable tiger-to-tiger transmission of avian influenza H5N1. Emerg Infect Dis. 2005 May;11(5):699-701.

U.S. Centers for Disease Control and Prevention [CDC]. Avian flu [online]. CDC. Available at: http://www.cdc.gov/flu/avian/index.htm. Accessed 9 Nov 2005.

U.S. Centers for Disease Control and Prevention (CDC). Avian influenza outbreaks in North America. October 17, 2005. Available at: http://www.cdc.gov/flu/avian/outbreaks/us.htm. Accessed 3 Nov 2005.

U.S. Department of Agriculture (USDA), Animal and Plant Health Inspection Service (APHIS). Avian Influenza fact sheet. Release No. 0458.05. October 31, 2005. Available at: http://www.usda.gov/wps/portal/!ut/p/_s.7_0_A/7_0_1OB/.cmd/ad/.ar/sa.retrievecontent/.c/6_2_1UH/.ce/7_2_5JM/.p/5_2_4TQ/.d/0/_th/J_2_9D/_s.7_0_A/7_0_1OB?PC_7_2_5JM_contentid=2005/10/0458.xml&PC_7_2_5JM_navtype=RT&PC_7_2_5JM_parentnav=AI_FACTSHEETS&PC_7_2_5JM_navid=AI_FACTSHT#7_2_5JM. Accessed 2 Nov 2005.

U.S. Department of Agriculture (USDA), Animal and Plant Health Inspection Service (APHIS), Veterinary Services (VS). Safeguarding the United States from highly-pathogenic avian influenza (HPAI): USDA actions, plans, and capabilities for addressing the bird flu threat. October 2005. Available at: http://www.aphis.usda.gov/lpa/pubs/fsheet_faq_notice/fs_ahhpaiplan.html. Accessed 2 Nov 2005.

U.S. Department of State. Bureau of International Information Programs (USINFO.STATE.GOV). Highly contagious bird flu strain found in Texas. Available at: http://usinfo.state.gov/gi/Archive/2004/Feb/24-801538.html. Accessed 18 Oct 2005.

Webster RG. Influenza: An emerging disease. Emerg Infect Dis. 1998 Jul-Sep;4(3):436-41.

World Health Organization (WHO). Avian influenza fact sheet WHO; 2004 Jan. Available at: http://www.who.int/csr/don/2004_01_15/en/. Accessed 30 Aug 2005.

World Health Organization (WHO). Cumulative number of confirmed human cases of avian influenza A/(H5N1) reported to WHO. 29 November 2005. Available at: http://www.who.int/csr/disease/avian_influenza/country/cases_table_2005_11_29/en/index.html. Accessed 30 Nov 2005.

World Health Organization (WHO).Geographical spread of H5N1 avian influenza in birds - update 28. Available at: http://www.who.int/csr/don/2005_08_18/en/. Accessed 5 Oct 2005.

World Organization for Animal Health (OIE). Highly pathogenic avian influenza in Russia: follow-up report No. 2. OIE Disease Information. Vol. 18 - No. 3426. August 2005. Available at: http://www.oie.int/eng/info/hebdo/AIS_56.HTM. Accessed 6 Oct 2005.

World Organization for Animal Health (OIE). Highly pathogenic avian influenza. In: Manual of diagnostic tests and vaccines for terrestrial animals. OIE; 2004. Available at: http://www.oie.int/eng/normes/mmanual/A_summry.htm. Accessed 23 Oct 2005.

defunct link as of 2005

Bovine Spongiform Encephalopathy in the United Kingdom, 1986-2005

An epidemic of bovine spongiform encephalopathy (BSE) was first recognized in the United Kingdom in 1986. From 1986 to February 2003, over 179,900 cattle on more than 35,740 U.K. farms were affected. The epidemic peaked in January 1993 at almost 1,000 new cases per week. BSE also spread to other European countries that had imported cattle from the U.K., and eventually a small number of cases were recognized in North America. The BSE outbreak may have resulted from the feeding of scrapie-containing sheep meat-and-bone meal to cattle or it may have arisen as a rare spontaneous formation of a spongiform encephalopathy in a cow that then spread to other cattle through contaminated meat and bone meal. There is strong evidence and general agreement that the outbreak was amplified by feeding rendered bovine meat-and-bone meal to young calves. Most countries have now banned this practice and, as a result, the BSE epidemic has been waning for the last decade. A parallel outbreak of new-variant Creutzfeldt-Jakob disease (vCJD) in humans is most likely a result of the consumption of beef products contaminated by central nervous system tissue from cattle with BSE. As of June 2005,177 cases of vCJD had been reported, mainly in the United Kingdom. Deaths due to vCJD peaked in 2000 and have since been declining.

A cow in the U.K. displaying symptoms of bovine spongiform encephalopathy.
Source: USDA APHIS

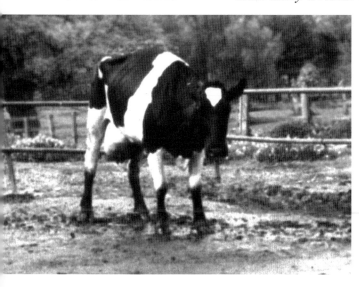

BSE developed into an epidemic as a consequence of an intensive farming practice—the recycling of animal protein in ruminant feed. The question of how to handle the BSE agent, a known hazard to cattle and potential hazard to humans, is key to the BSE story. The government took measures to address both hazards, but they were not always timely or adequately implemented and enforced because the basic biology of BSE was unknown and it was believed that BSE was not a threat to human life.

What are BSE and vCJD?

BSE is a progressive neurological disorder of cattle that results from infection by an unconventional transmissible agent. The causative agent of BSE and other transmissible spongiform encephalopathies (TSEs) is yet to be fully characterized. The BSE agent is smaller than most viral particles and is highly resistant to heat, ultraviolet light, ionizing radiation, and common disinfectants that normally inactivate viruses or bacteria. It causes no detectable immune or inflammatory response in the host and has not been observed microscopically. The incubation period for BSE ranges from two to eight years and clinical disease usually occurs in older animals. Most cases in the United Kingdom were seen in dairy cows between three and six years of age. Affected animals may display changes in temperament such as nervousness or aggression, abnormal posture, incoordination and difficulty in rising, decreased milk production, or loss of body condition despite continued appetite. Following the onset of clinical signs, the animal's condition deteriorates until it dies or is destroyed. This usually takes from two weeks to six months. There is no treatment.

Creutzfeldt-Jakob disease (CJD) is a rare and fatal human neurodegenerative disease of unknown cause. Patients with the conventional form are usually between 50 and 75 years of age. The new variant form (vCJD) in the United Kingdom mainly affects younger people; the median age at death is 28 years.

The first cases of BSE

Individual cattle were probably first infected by BSE in the 1970s. If they lived long enough to develop signs of disease, these were not reported to or investigated by the Central Veterinary Laboratory (CVL) of the State Veterinary Service (SVS). The first clinical cases were reported in 1984, although it was two years before the nature of the disease was actually recognized.

On December 22, 1984, Peter Stent of Pitsham Farm in Sussex called Dr. David Bee, a private veterinarian, to examine Cow 133. The cow had an arched back and had lost weight. Dr. Bee visited the farm several times over the following months, and continued to see animals showing unusual symptoms. Cow 133 developed a head tremor and incoordination before dying on February 11, 1985. By the end of April, five more cows on the farm had died. Dr. Bee requested assistance from Dr. J. M. Watkin-Jones, a veterinarian at the Winchester Veterinary Investigation Center (VIC) of the Veterinary Investigation Service. A number of samples of body tissue were submitted to the CVL for pathological analysis. Various possible ailments were identified, but despite a wide range of tests there was no definite diagnosis. The CVL suggested that Mr. Stent submit a live affected cow for

An epidemic of BSE was first recognized in the United Kingdom in 1986. The epidemic peaked in January 1993 at almost 1,000 cases per week. A parallel outbreak of new-variant Creutzfeldt-Jakob disease (vCJD) in humans is most likely a result of the consumption of beef products contaminated by central nervous system from cattle with BSE.

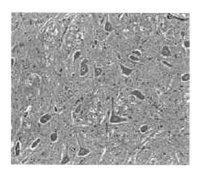

Normal bovine brain tissue

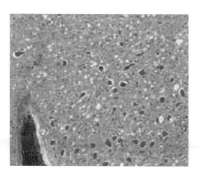

The spongiform lesions of BSE
Source: USDA APHIS

slaughter and post-mortem. Cow 142 was sent live to the CVL in September for euthanasia and a post-mortem examination. The pathologist on duty examined the tissues and concluded that the problem was associated with fungal contamination of feed and mycotoxin production. An April 1985 laboratory report stated that a fungal toxin called citrinin had been found in the feed at the farm. New cases ceased to develop on the farm and the veterinarians assumed that the problem had run its course (from www.bseinquiry.gov.uk/report/volume3/chapterd.htm).

The mysterious disease soon reappeared on other farms. At the end of 1986, the Pathology Department of the CVL considered four more cases of unusual neurologic disease in cattle from farms in Kent and Bristol. They identified these cases as a probable transmissible spongiform encephalopathy in cattle and named the new disease bovine spongiform encephalopathy. By the end of 1987, the CVL Epidemiology Department concluded that the cause of the reported cases of BSE was the consumption of meat-and-bone meal (MBM), which was made from animal carcasses and incorporated into cattle feed. At first it was thought that cattle were becoming infected from scrapie-contaminated sheep tissues and that the MBM had become infectious because rendering methods that had previously inactivated the conventional scrapie agent were changed. However, the cases of BSE identified between 1986 and 1988 were not index cases, and they were not the result of the transmission of scrapie. They were the consequences of recycling BSE-infected cattle into MBM. In addition, the theory that BSE resulted from changes in rendering methods is probably not correct because rendering methods have never been capable of completely inactivating TSEs. Although the origin of the disease will probably never be known, BSE probably originated from a novel source early in the 1970s, possibly a cow or other animal that developed the disease spontaneously. The disease did not become apparent until the agent had been disseminated to large numbers of cattle via MBM and, after a long incubation period, these cattle began developing clinical signs.

Precautions taken

In June 1988, the Southwood Working Party, set up to provide advice on the implications of BSE, recommended that cattle showing signs of BSE be destroyed and that compensation be paid to farmers. In February 1989, the Southwood Working Party submitted a report to the government that concluded that the risk of transmission of BSE to humans appeared remote and that 'it was most unlikely that BSE would have any implications for human health.' This assessment of risk was made assuming that BSE was probably derived from scrapie and could be expected to behave like scrapie. The Southwood Report never underwent a scientific review by experts in the field. Precautionary measures were put in place that went beyond those recommended by the Working Party and an expert committee was set up to advise BSE research.

Once MBM was identified as the probable vector of BSE in 1988, the government implemented a ban on incorporating ruminant protein in ruminant feed. This ban reduced the escalating rate of infection. After BSE was experimentally transmitted to a pig in 1990, new measures to protect pigs and poultry from BSE were introduced. However, the measures were unenforceable and widely disregarded. It was later discovered that a cow could become infected with the BSE agent by eating an amount of infectious tissue as small as a peppercorn. Cross-contamination in feedmills caused thousands of cattle to become infected, but because of the long incubation period this was not apparent until later. In 1994, because of the continuing infection, regulations were revised and a rigorous enforcement campaign was initiated. After March 1996, the incorporation of all animal protein in animal feed was banned. The BSE epidemic in the United Kingdom peaked in 1993 and, as a result of these control measures, has subsided.

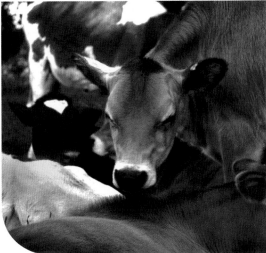

As of 2005, there is no diagnostic test to detect the BSE agent in living animals.
Source: Travis Engelhaupt, ISU

Recognition of the potential risks to humans

In June 1989, specified bovine offal (SBO) was banned from use in human food as a precaution. Specified bovine offal includes the brain, spinal cord, spleen, thymus, tonsils, and intestines of cattle. At the time of the ban, some questioned whether all of the spinal cord could be removed during the abattoir process. Questions were also raised about the process of mechanical recovery of scraps left attached to the vertebral column for use in human food (mechanically recovered meat). Instances of failure to remove all of the spinal cord from the carcass were discovered and in December 1995, the extraction of mechanically recovered meat from the spinal column of cattle was banned. Mechanically recovered meat can include dorsal root ganglia that have been demonstrated to be infectious in the late stages of incubation.

In May 1990, a domestic cat was diagnosed as suffering from a 'scrapie-like' spongiform encephalopathy. This generated widespread public and media concern that BSE had been transmitted to the cat and might also be transmissible to humans. As time passed, the increasing knowledge about BSE made the theory that it would behave like scrapie less and less viable. The public was not informed of any change in the perceived likelihood that BSE might be transmissible to humans and in fact was repeatedly reassured that it was safe to eat beef. There was, nevertheless, some recognition that the pathways by which bovine products or by-products might come into contact with humans or other animals needed to be examined. Known or suspected pathways included meat, vaccines, cosmetics, surgical instruments, bovine or human tissues, agricultural fertilizer, and agricultural waste. However, no coordinated consideration was implemented until March 1996.

The first human cases

Scientists suspected that if BSE were to spread to humans it would resemble Creutzfeldt-Jakob disease. In 1991, surveillance for atypical cases or changing patterns of CJD was put in place. Three dairy farmers who had had BSE in their herds were diagnosed with CJD in August 1992, July 1993, and December 1994. The fourth annual report of the CJD Surveillance Unit (CJDSU), issued in August 1995, noted the apparently high incidence of CJD in farmers. The Spongiform Encephalopathy Advisory Committee (SEAC) released a press release about suspected CJD in a cattle farmer in October 1995.

In May 1995, Stephen Churchill, age 18, died. He was later confirmed as the first known victim of vCJD. His was one of three vCJD deaths in 1995. The CJDSU identified its second suspect vCJD death in a remarkably young patient in August 1995. A third individual died in November 1995. Both cases were later confirmed as vCJD. The CJDSU announced the emergence of vCJD and on March 16, 1996, the SEAC announced that the most likely explanation for the cases of a new variant of CJD in young people was exposure to BSE. This has since been compellingly supported by scientific evidence. A policy of banning consumption of cattle over 30 months of age was introduced. However, the incubation period for transmissible spongiform encephalopathies is long and, not surprisingly, cases of vCJD continue to be diagnosed. Annual vCJD-related deaths in the U.K. rose gradually to a high of 28 in 2000, and tapered to nine in 2004. Three deaths were reported from January 1, 2005 to October 8, 2005, bringing the total number of deaths in the U.K. to 151. As of June 2005, 177 cases of vCJD had been reported worldwide, including one from the U.S. in 2002. Nearly all of these people had lived in the U.K. during multiple years between 1980 and 1996 and had been exposed to BSE there.

BSE outside the United Kingdom

When the BSE epidemic became evident, the European Union prohibited the export from the U.K. of live bovine animals, their semen and embryos, mammalian-derived MBM, or the meat of bovine animals slaughtered in the U.K. that is liable to enter the animal feed or human food chain. The export of materials destined for use in medicinal products, cosmetics, or pharmaceuticals was also banned. Despite these measures, BSE spread to countries outside the U.K. Eighteen European countries have reported at least one case of BSE in indigenous cattle. Portugal had the highest incidence rate; in 2001, it reported more than 100 indigenous cases per million cattle aged over 24 months. Significant numbers of cases were also reported from the Republic of Ireland, with 62 BSE cases per million (cpm), Switzerland (49 cpm), Belgium (28 cpm), Spain (24 cpm), Germany (20 cpm), France (20 cpm), Slovakia (18 cpm), Italy (14 cpm), and the Netherlands (10 cpm). Denmark, Slovenia, Greece, the Czech Republic, Finland, Japan, and Austria reported between one and seven BSE cases per million. Other countries likely to have been affected by BSE include Albania, Bulgaria, Croatia, Cyprus Republic, Estonia, Hungary, Latvia, Lithuania, Luxembourg, Poland, Romania, San Marino Republic, Slovic Republic, and Turkey. Japan reported its first case in indigenous cattle in 2001 and Israel in 2002. Infections were also seen in imported cattle in Oman, Liechtenstein, and the Falkland Islands; however, eradication efforts centered on such imported animals may prevent BSE from becoming established in a country.

Canada has found BSE in imported cattle and, more recently, in three indigenous cattle. The first indigenous case was confirmed in May, 2003, and the remaining two cases in January, 2005. The three animals were, respectively, a downer Angus beef cow with neurologic signs, an 8-year old downer dairy cow, and a 6-year old Charolais beef cow. All three animals came from the province of Alberta. Two animals appear to have been exposed to BSE in MDM before Canada imposed a ban on this product in ruminant feed in 1997. The third may have been exposed in feed produced shortly after the ban, but the actual source is unknown. Investigations revealed no other BSE cases in the birth cohorts or recently born offspring of any of these animals. Canada is considered to be an OIE minimal risk country for BSE, based on its surveillance, prevention and control measures, and the incidence of disease.

BSE and the United States

In 1989, to prevent BSE from entering the United States, restrictions were placed on the importation of live ruminants and certain ruminant products from countries where BSE was known to exist. These restrictions were later extended to include the importation of ruminants and certain ruminant products from all European countries. On August 4, 1997, the Food and Drug Administration (FDA) established regulations that prohibit the feeding of most mammalian proteins to ruminants. Active surveillance efforts by the USDA Animal and Plant Health Inspection Service (APHIS) were instituted in May 1990.

As a result of this surveillance, BSE was found in a Holstein dairy cow in Washington state in December 2003. The cow had been imported from Canada in September 2001, along with 81 others. Samples were taken from 255 animals located on farms in the U.S. where cows from the index herd in Canada were being raised. All tested negative to BSE.

In response to this case, the USDA banned the use of certain bovine tissues in human foods and made extensive changes in slaughter and processing facilities to reduce the risks to human health. In addition, APHIS undertook an intensified testing program to determine whether BSE currently exists in U.S. cattle and at what level. This program, which began in June 2004, will test as many high-risk animals as possible over a 12- to 18-month period, as a one-time 'snapshot' of the BSE picture in the U.S. Most of the samples are being taken from high-risk animals such as downer cattle, cattle with neurological disease, emaciated or injured cattle, and dead cattle. A limited number of older, normal cattle are also being randomly tested. The carcasses of the tested animals are not allowed to enter the food chain until testing is negative. The USDA estimates that this surveillance can detect one infected animal in 10 million if 201,000 cattle are tested, given the assumption that all positives are in the high-risk population.

As of October 2005, the intensified surveillance has found one case of BSE in an indigenous animal. A 12 year old Brahma cross cow from Texas was sold in a livestock sale and transported to a packing plant. The animal, which was dead on arrival, was sent on to a pet food plant, where it was sampled for BSE. The carcass was incinerated and was not used in pet food. The test results on this animal were initially conflicting, but in June 2005, a sample sent to a BSE reference laboratory in the U.K. was determined to be positive. APHIS, the FDA, the Texas Animal Health Commission and the Texas Feed and Fertilizer Control Service conducted a joint investigation to determine the source of the infection and test the infected cow's cohorts and offspring. The infected animal was traced to the ranch in Texas where it had been born and raised. All adult animals that left this farm after 1990, and the two calves born to the infected cow within 2 years of its death were traced. Most of these animals had been slaughtered, died or were presumed to be dead, although a few animals were untraceable. One surviving animal was tested and found to be negative, and another was determined to be of no interest due to its age. As the BSE-infected cow had been born before the USDA implemented the ban on MBM in ruminant feeds in 1997, it appears to have been infected from that source.

As of October 8, 2005, the surveillance program has tested more than 484,000 cattle, with no additional positive animals found. However, because of these two BSE cases, a number of countries have banned the importation of a variety of ruminant products or live animals from the U.S. These bans vary greatly. While some nations now prohibit the importation of all U.S. beef, others have placed only temporary or limited bans, such as a ban on beef products from Texas and Washington states. Some countries allow certain products from animals of a specified age or under specific conditions.

Sources of Information

Canadian Food Inspection Agency. Animal Health and Production Division. Bovine spongiform encephalopathy (BSE) in North America. Available at: http://www.inspection.gc.ca/english/anima/heasan/disemala/bseesb/bseesbindexe.shtml. Accessed 21 Sept 2005.

Department for Environment, Food and Rural Affairs (DEFRA), United Kingdom. Bovine spongiform encephalopathy. Available at: http://www.defra.gov.uk/animalh/bse/. Accessed 2003.

Department of Health, United Kingdom. Monthly Creutzfeldt-Jakob disease statistics. April 7, 2003. Available at: http://www.doh.gov.U.K./cjd/stats/apr03.htm *. Accessed 2003.

Department of Health and Human Services, U.S. Food and Drug Administration (FDA). Report on Food & Drug Administration, Dallas District, investigation of bovine spongiform encephalopathy event in Texas 2005. Aug 30, 2005. Available at: http://www.fda.gov/cvm/texasfeedrpt.htm. Accessed 21 Sept 2005.

Lord Phillips, chair. The BSE inquiry: The report. A report to the Minister of Agriculture, Fisheries and Food, the Secretary of State for Health and the Secretaries of State for Scotland, Wales and Northern Ireland. London: Her Majesty's Stationery Office; 2000. Report no HC 887-1. Crown copyright. Available at: http://www.bseinquiry.gov.uk/report/. Accessed 2003.[Information from the sections titled "The first cases of BSE," "Precautions Taken," and "The First Human Cases" is from this report]

The National Creutzfeldt-Jakob Disease Surveillance Unit, United Kingdom. CJD statistics. Available at: http://www.cjd.ed.ac.uk/figures.htm. Accessed 21 Sept 2005.

US Centers for Disease Control and Prevention (CDC). BSD and CJD information and resources. Available at: http://www.cdc.gov/ncidod/diseases/cjd/cjd.htm. Accessed 2003.

US Centers for Disease Control and Prevention (CDC). New variant CJD fact sheet. Available at: http://www.cdc.gov/ncidod/diseases/cjd/cjd_fact_sheet.htm. Accessed 2003. [Current vCJD information is now available at http://www.cdc.gov/ncidod/dvrd/vcjd/]

US Centers for Disease Control and Prevention (CDC). Update 2002: Bovine spongiform encephalopathy and variant Creutzfeldt-Jakob disease. Available at: http://www.cdc.gov/ncidod/diseases/cjd/bse_cjd.htm.* Accessed 2003.

U.S. Centers for Disease Control and Prevention (CDC). Questions and answers regarding bovine spongiform encephalopathy (BSE) and variant Creutzfeldt-Jakob disease (vCJD). June 29, 2005. Available at: http://www.cdc.gov/ncidod/dvrd/vcjd/qa.htm. Accessed 19 Sept 2005.

United States Department of Agriculture (USDA), Animal and Plant Health Inspection Service (APHIS)Bovine spongiform encephalopathy. Available at: http://www.aphis.usda.gov/lpa/issues/bse/bse.html. Accessed 2003.

USDA Animal and Plant Health Inspection Service (APHIS). Bovine spongiform encephalopathy (BSE) surveillance, March 2003. Available at: http://www.aphis.usda.gov/lpa/issues/bse/bse-surveillance.html. Accessed 2003.

USDA Animal and Plant Health Inspection Service (APHIS). BSE testing page. Frequently asked questions. Available at: http://www.aphis.usda.gov/lpa/issues/bse_testing/faq.html. Accessed 21 Sept. 2005.

USDA Animal and Plant Health Inspection Service (APHIS). BSE trade ban status as of 08/04/05. Available at: http://www.aphis.usda.gov/lpa/issues/bse/trade/bse_trade_ban_status.html. Accessed 20 Sept 2005.

USDA Animal and Plant Health Inspection Service (APHIS). Press release: Investigation results of Texas cow that tested positive for bovine spongiform encephalopathy (BSE) Aug. 30, 2005. Release no. 0336.05. Available at: http://www.usda.gov/wps/portal/!ut/p/_s.7_0_A/7_0_1OB/.cmd/ad/.ar/sa.retrievecontent/.c/6_2_1UH/.ce/7_2_5JM/.p/5_2_4TQ/.d/1/_th/J_2_9D/_s.7_0_A/7_0_1OB?PC_7_2_5JM_contentid=2005/08/0336.xml&PC_7_2_5JM_navtype=RT&PC_7_2_5JM_parentnav=LATEST_RELEASES&PC_7_2_5JM_navid=NEWS_RELEASE#7_2_5JM. Accessed 21 Sept 2005.

USDA Animal and Plant Health Inspection Service (APHIS). Statistics from the nationwide BSE surveillance program. Available at: http://www.aphis.usda.gov/oa/bse/bsesurvey.html#charts. * Accessed 2003.

Originally reviewed by:
Dr. Harley Moon, F.K. Ramsey Distinguished Professor,
Iowa State University, College of Veterinary Medicine

*defunct link as of 2004, 2005

Canine Influenza, 2004-2005

Viruses rarely jump from one species into another. When they do, the outbreak tends to be brief; typically, the virus is poorly adapted to the new host and cannot be transmitted efficiently in the new species. Two characteristics of influenza viruses – their high mutation rate and their ability to recombine with each other – help them adapt to new species. Although most cross-species infections by these viruses are self-limited, there are records of a few permanent jumps. One is currently occurring in dogs, which have acquired an equine influenza virus from horses.

In January 2004, 22 racing greyhounds at a Florida racetrack became ill with an unknown respiratory disease. Fourteen of the dogs developed a fever, followed by a persistent cough that lasted for 10 to 14 days. These dogs recovered. Eight other dogs died suddenly with evidence of hemorrhages in the respiratory tract. At necropsy, the fatal cases had signs of severe hemorrhagic pneumonia. Using lung tissue samples from the dead dogs, researchers discovered an influenza A virus that was very similar to a H3N8 equine influenza virus circulating in horses. All of the genes in the canine virus were of equine origin, suggesting that the virus had been transmitted whole from horses into dogs. Serology using paired acute and convalescent sera demonstrated that the recovered dogs had also been infected by this virus. Some asymptomatic dogs that had been exposed during the outbreak also seroconverted. In addition, it became apparent that the canine influenza virus had been circulating among greyhounds in Florida for several years. Some Florida racetracks had experienced outbreaks of an unknown respiratory disease from 1999 to 2003; seropositive dogs were found at these tracks. Antibodies to the virus were not found in canine serum samples from 1996 to 1998. The same virus, or a very similar one, was also found in preserved lung tissues from a greyhound that died of an unknown respiratory disease in 2003. At first, the canine influenza virus did not seem to be a threat to other breeds of dogs. Experimentally infected beagles developed a fever, but no respiratory signs.

In 2004 and 2005, canine influenza continued to be reported in greyhounds. Between June and August 2004, outbreaks of respiratory disease were seen at 14 greyhound racetracks in Alabama, Arkansas, Florida, Kansas, Texas, and West Virginia. Some of these outbreaks were linked to the canine influenza virus and others were not investigated. From January to May 2005, more episodes were seen. The disease affected greyhounds at 20 tracks in Arkansas, Arizona, Colorado, Florida, Iowa, Kansas, Massachusetts, Rhode Island, Texas, and West Virginia. The evidence that the new virus was circulating widely in racing greyhounds made researchers suspect that it might become a threat to other breeds of dogs. Serology on dogs with respiratory disease in shelters and veterinary clinics in Florida and New York revealed evidence of the virus in pets and prompted state officials to issue a warning to the public. Recently, cases of canine influenza were identified in pets in other states including California and Washington. It now appears that this virus may be an unrecognized cause of respiratory disease in dogs throughout the U.S.

What are influenza viruses and how do they jump from species to species?

Influenza is caused by influenza viruses, members of the Orthomyxo-virus family: There are three genera of these viruses: influenzavirus A, influenzavirus B and influenzavirus C. The influenza B and C viruses mainly infect humans, while the influenza A viruses also infect other mammals and birds. Influenza A viruses are classified into subtypes based on two proteins, the hemagglutinin ('H') and neuraminidase ('N'). There are at least 16 different hemagglutinin antigens (H1 to H16) and 9 neuraminidase antigens (N1 to N9). Antibodies to the hemagglutinin and neuraminidase proteins are important in immunity to these viruses. The H and N proteins also help the virus attach to cells and aid in releasing newly formed viruses from a cell; therefore, these proteins help determine the species specificity of each influenza virus. However, these proteins are not the only ones important in adapting the virus to a species; internal virus proteins must also have a good 'fit' with the cell if the virus is to efficiently replicate and spread. Wild birds, particularly waterfowl, are the reservoirs for the influenza A viruses; these birds carry all of the subtypes but rarely become ill themselves. The avian influenza viruses are sometimes transmitted to poultry, which may cause outbreaks of avian influenza in these birds. Some influenza viruses have become adapted to mammals. They include the equine influenza viruses, swine influenza viruses, and human influenza viruses. The equine, swine, and human viruses are now well adapted to their host species and are not easily transmitted to other species of mammals or birds.

Although jumps from one species to another are rare, they are aided by the influenza virus' tendency to change. Influenza viruses quickly accumulate small mutations, a process called 'antigenic drift.' In addition, they can exchange proteins with other influenza viruses, an ability facilitated by their segmented genome. If two influenza viruses infect a cell simultaneously, the segments may mix when new virus particles are assembled. An influenza virus can 'reassort' with any other influenza virus, regardless of its origin. For example, if a cell is infected by a swine and a human influenza virus, the new viruses budding from that cell might contain some pieces from the swine influenza virus and other pieces from the human influenza virus—a process that could make the swine virus better able to infect human cells. Reassortment is particularly common in pigs, which have receptors for the human, swine and avian influenza viruses. Sometimes, an influenza virus can also jump 'whole'

Between June and August 2004, outbreaks of respiratory disease were seen at 14 greyhound racetracks in Alabama, Arkansas, Florida, Kansas, Texas, and West Virginia. Some of these outbreaks were linked to the canine influenza virus and others were not investigated.

from one species to another. Such jumps have been seen when avian influenza viruses infected people, cats, mink, seals, horses and other animals, and swine influenza viruses infected humans and turkeys. Usually, the virus is poorly adapted to the new species, can't be transmitted efficiently, and quickly dies out. Occasionally, a virus is able to replicate and spread well in the new hosts, and a permanent jump is made. Such permanent jumps were seen in 1918, when pigs acquired their first influenza viruses, and in China in 1989, when horses were infected by a new kind of equine influenza virus. Until recently, no influenza viruses circulated in dogs or cats.

Where did the canine influenza virus come from?

An analysis of the canine influenza virus isolated from greyhound lung tissue has demonstrated that this virus is most closely related the H3N8 "Florida lineage" equine influenza virus that emerged in the early 1990s. There are four amino acid differences between the hemagglutinin proteins in the equine and canine viruses; these changes were probably important in adapting the virus to dogs. Although it's remotely possible that this virus was repeatedly introduced into dogs from some other species, the evidence suggests that a single virus was transmitted whole from horses to dogs, as a one-time event. Transmission between dogs probably occurs via aerosols, similarly to other influenza viruses. However, canine influenza viruses have, so far, proven impossible to isolate from naturally infected, live animals, possibly because virus isolation has always been attempted relatively late in the infection, after the symptoms have appeared.

What can we expect from the canine influenza virus?

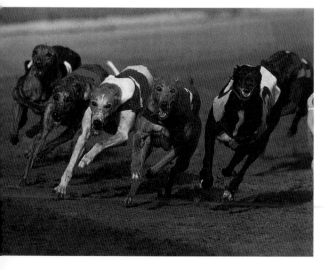

Canine influenza was first identified in racing greyhounds.
Source: www.gettyimages.com

Canine influenza is an emerging disease in dogs. Dogs are not expected to have any naturally-acquired or vaccine-induced immunity to this virus, and some experts warn that the canine population may be facing a pandemic similar to the influenza pandemics that swept through humans in 1918, 1957 and 1968, or swine in 1918. Although early reports suggested that canine influenza was limited to greyhounds, all dogs regardless of breed or age are now considered to be susceptible. In kennels, the infection rate may reach 100% and symptoms may be seen in 75% of the dogs infected. Most dogs are expected to develop the less severe form of the disease, and recover. In this form, the major symptom is a cough that may persist for up to 3 weeks, in spite of treatment. Occasionally, the cough is accompanied by a fever and/ or a nasal discharge that responds to antibiotics. A few dogs develop a more severe form with pneumonia and possibly pulmonary hemorrhages. In dogs with severe disease, the overall mortality rate is thought to be 1-5%. However, as experience with this virus grows, these numbers may be adjusted up or down; some sources suggest that the mortality rate may be as high as 10%, while others expect a high prevalence of mild, self-limiting or asymptomatic infections and suggest that the overall mortality rate in pets will be less than 1%. A vaccine for dogs, based on the equine influenza vaccine, is in development and may be available soon.

Once some dogs develop either naturally-acquired or vaccine-induced immunity to this virus, any epidemic or pandemic will probably subside. However, all influenza viruses constantly acquire small changes and periodic outbreaks may continue, similar to the yearly flu epidemics in humans or outbreaks of equine influenza in horses.

Are there any public health concerns about this virus?

There is currently no evidence that any other species, including humans, can be infected by the canine influenza virus. However, some experts are concerned that, due to their close associations with humans, dogs might become a source of novel influenza virus transmission to humans. As a precaution, physicians, veterinarians and others have been asked to report any cases of human influenza that seem to be linked to exposure to canine influenza.

Sources of Information

Acha PN, Szyfres B (Pan American Health Organization [PAHO]). Zoonoses and Communicable Diseases Common to Man and Animals. Volume 2. Chlamydiosis, rickettsioses and viroses. 3rd ed. Washington DC: PAHO; 2003. Scientific and Technical Publication No. 580. Influenza; p. 155-172.

Associated Press. Dog flu arrives in Oregon. October 1, 2005. Available at: http://www.kgw.com/sharedcontent/APStories/stories/D8CVD5E01.html. Accessed 3 Oct. 2005

Canine influenza virus emerges in Florida [online]. J Am Vet Med Assoc News Express. Sept. 22, 2005. Available at: http://www.avma.org/onlnews/javma/oct05/x051015b.asp. Accessed 27 Sept 2005.

Carey, S. UF researchers: equine influenza virus likely cause of Jacksonville greyhound deaths [online]. News Releases, University of Florida College of Veterinary Medicine. Available at: http://www.vetmed.ufl.edu/pr/nw_story/greyhds.htm. Accessed 27 Sept 2005.

Centers for Disease Control and Prevention [CDC]. Avian flu [online]. CDC. Available at: http://www.cdc.gov/flu/avian/index.htm. Accessed 24 Aug 2004

Cornell University College of Veterinary Medicine. Canine influenza virus detected [online]. Animal Health Diagnostic Center Announcements. Sept 21, 2005. Available at: http://www.diaglab.vet.cornell.edu/news.asp. Accessed 27 Sept 2005.

Cornell University College of Veterinary Medicine. Samples for detecting the presence of canine influenza virus [online]. Animal Health Diagnostic Center Announcements. Sept 21, 2005. Available at: http://www.diaglab.vet.cornell.edu/news.asp. Accessed 27 Sept 2005.

Crawford PC, Dubovi EJ, Castleman WL, Stephenson I, Gibbs EPJ, Chen L, Smith C, Hill RC, Ferro P, Pompey J, Bright RA, Medina M-J, Johnson CM, Olsen CW, Cox NJ, Klimov AI, Katz JM, Donis RO. Transmission of equine influenza virus to dogs. Science. 2005 Sep 26; [Epub ahead of print]. Available at: http://www.sciencemag.org/cgi/rapidpdf/1117950v1. Accessed 27 Sept 2005.

Daly JM, Mumford JA. Influenza infections [online]. In: Lekeux P, editor. Equine respiratory diseases. Ithaca NY: International Veterinary Information Service [IVIS]; 2001. Available at: http://www.ivis.org/special_books/Lekeux/toc.asp. Accessed 10 May 2004.

Enserink M, Kaiser J. Avian flu finds new mammal hosts. Science. 2004;305:1385.

Enserink M. Flu virus jumps from horses to dogs [monograph online]. Science Now. 26 September 2005. Available at: http://sciencenow.sciencemag.org/cgi/content/full/2005/926/2. Accessed 27 Sept 2005.

Fenner F, Bachmann PA, Gibbs EPJ, Murphy FA, Studdert MJ, White DO. Veterinary virology. San Diego, CA: Academic Press Inc.; 1987. Orthomyxoviridae; p. 473-484.

Heinen P. Swine influenza: a zoonosis. Vet Sci Tomorrow [serial online]. 2003 Sept 15. Available at: http://www.vetsite.org/publish/articles/000041/print.html. Accessed 26 Aug 2004.

Hinshaw VS, Bean WJ, Webster RG, Rehg JE, Fiorelli P, Early G, Geraci JR, St Aubin DJ. Are seals frequently infected with avian influenza viruses? J Virol. 1984;51(3):863-5.

Influenza, canine - USA (multistate). PromedMail Oct 2, 2005. Archive Number 20051002.2883. Available at: http://www.promedmail.org. Accessed 3 Oct 2005.

Kuiken T, Rimmelzwaan G, van Riel D, van Amerongen G, Baars M, Fouchier R, Osterhaus A. Avian H5N1 influenza in cats. Science [serial online]. 2004; 10.1126/science.1102287. Available at: http://www.sciencemag.org/cgi/rapidpdf/1102287v1.pdf. Accessed 3 Sept 2004.

Lamb S., McElroy T. Bronson alerts public to newly emerging canine flu. Florida Department of Agriculture and Consumer Services, Department Press Release. Sept. 20, 2005. Available at: http://doacs.state.fl.us/press/2005/09202005.html. Accessed 27 Sept 2005.

Reid AH, Taubenberger JK. The origin of the 1918 pandemic influenza virus: a continuing enigma. J Gen Virol. 2003;84:2285-92.

U.S. Centers for Disease Control and Prevention (CDC). Media briefing on canine influenza. September 26, 2005. Available at: http://www.cdc.gov/od/oc/media/transcripts/t050926.htm. Accessed 3 Oct. 2005.

Vet Association: Canine Flu Found In Southern California. NBC4.TV. Sept 30, 2005. Available at: http://www.nbc4.tv/health/5044261/detail.html. Accessed 3 Oct. 2005.

Classical Swine Fever in Great Britain, 2000

This is an example of how the British veterinary infrastructure was able to trace, control, and eradicate an outbreak of classical swine fever before the disease became widespread. Classical swine fever is an exotic disease that has been eradicated from a number of developed countries; however, it still exists in some parts of the world and could be re-introduced at any time in infected animals or animal products.

On August 4, 2000, a suspected case of classical swine fever (CSF) in a pig herd was reported to the British Ministry of Agriculture, Fisheries, and Food (MAFF) Animal Health Divisional Office at Bury St Edmunds, Suffolk. The herd consisted of 3,500 weaned pigs in seven houses. The pigs had been ill since July 11, when weaned pigs had been introduced from a breeding/multiplier unit. The infection had spread to four houses and as of August 4, a total of 1,110 pigs were ill and about 200 had died. A MAFF veterinary officer visited the premises the same day and, after examining the pigs on site, placed the holding under official movement restrictions and took blood samples to test the pigs for classical and African swine fever. On August 7, two cases of suspected classical swine fever were reported on other farms. One case was in a herd of rearing pigs. The second was in a breeding herd that had supplied weaned pigs to the other two infected farms. Both herds were immediately placed under quarantine and blood samples were sent for laboratory examination.

An outbreak of classical swine fever was declared on August 8, 2000. National and local crisis centers were established to deal with the outbreak. Three-kilometer protection and 10-kilometer surveillance zones were established around the infected premises and the movement of all pigs within the zones was prohibited. The remaining 3,300 pigs on the first identified farm were killed on August 10 and their carcasses destroyed by rendering. The premises were cleaned and disinfected on August 11. The other two farms were also depopulated. The movements of pigs, feedstuffs, vehicles, and people onto and off the premises were traced to identify possible sources of the virus and limit the spread of infection.

During the next few months, classical swine fever was found on several more farms. Before the first farm had been placed under quarantine, it had sent infected pigs to four other premises. The disease also spread to two contiguous outdoor pig farms. From one of those, classical swine fever spread to another contiguous holding and then, through the movement of pigs, to two additional premises. Two more outbreaks occurred in pig units owned by haulage operators. A total of 16 infected sites were confirmed in Great Britain between August 4 and November 3. However, by December the outbreak had been contained. All controls relating to the 16 infected premises were lifted on December 30, 2000.

What is classical swine fever?

Classical swine fever, also known as hog cholera, is a contagious febrile disease of pigs. This disease is caused by infection with the classical swine fever virus, a member of the Pestivirus genus of the Flaviviridae family of RNA viruses. Pigs can become infected by ingestion, inhalation, genital (semen) infection, or wound contamination. Classical swine fever is most easily spread by contact with infected pigs or the feeding of inadequately cooked garbage (swill). Spread of the virus by fomites or by biting insects is also possible. The clinical signs include lethargy, yellow diarrhea, conjunctivitis, incoordination, fever, and excessive thirst. Additional signs include skin lesions ranging from cyanotic patches on the ears and abdomen to raised, scabby lesions mainly on the legs. Classical swine fever strongly resembles African swine fever and must be distinguished from it by laboratory tests.

Tracing the virus' footsteps

The source of the outbreak appears to have been the breeding farm identified on August 7. The epidemiological inquiry found that the CSF virus probably entered the breeding unit on May 1 then spread to the index farm and hered rearing of pigs by the movement of infected pigs.

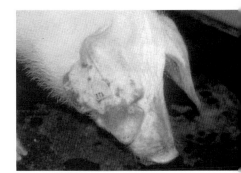

A purplish discoloration of the skin can sometimes be seen in pigs with classical swine fever as well as some other diseases.
Source: USDA APHIS

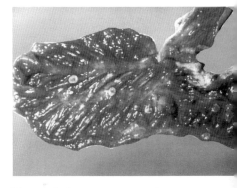

'Button' ulcers are sometimes found in the lining of the intestine at necropsy.
Source: USDA APHIS

> *Classical swine fever is most easily spread by contact with infected pigs or the feeding of inadequately cooked garbage (swill). Spread of the virus by fomites or by biting insects is also possible.*

These three farms were all owned by or contracted to the U.K.'s largest outdoor pig rearing company. The company's pigs were born on breeding units and remained there for approximately three to four weeks before being moved to rearing premises where they remained for a further six to eight weeks. From the rearing units, the pigs moved to finishing units where they remained for 10 weeks before being slaughtered. This method of swine production was designed to reduce the transmission of enzootic diseases by early weaning of pigs from the breeding farm to a series of remote locations. Disease transmission from older finishing pigs to young growing pigs is avoided by having a series of separate finishing farms.

All rearing and finishing premises that had received pigs born after May 1 at the breeding unit were traced, tested for classical swine fever, and placed under official movement restrictions. All the pigs on premises that had received pigs born after June 1 were treated as "dangerous contacts" and were destroyed. The other 47 breeding herds owned by or contracted to the production company were traced, placed under quarantine, clinically inspected by a MAFF veterinary officer, and sampled for evidence of CSF. The government traced the movements of the transporter who took weaned pigs from the breeding premises. All the premises that the transporter visited were tested and placed under official movement restrictions.

The origin of the virus and its route of introduction were not established with complete certainty. However, the evidence strongly suggests that infection did not come through the introduction of infected pigs, contact with feral pigs, contaminated vehicles or personnel, discharges of effluent, or contaminated vaccines or biological products. It appears more likely that the infection was introduced in contaminated pig meat in food discarded by people; a public footpath runs adjacent to the outdoor paddocks containing dry sows on the breeding farm. Genetic typing showed that the outbreak was caused by a virus strain that is not currently present in Europe. This strain is in the same genetic group that was isolated during a classical swine fever outbreak in Belgium, Italy, the Netherlands, and Spain in 1997–98.

Sources of Information

Department for Environment, Food and Rural Affairs (DEFRA), United Kingdom. Disease factsheet: Classical swine fever. Available at: http://www.defra.gov.uk/animalh/diseases/notifiable/disease/classicalsf.htm. Accessed 2003.

http://www.aphis.usda.gov/vs/ceah/cei/csf_uk0800e.htm.* Accessed 2003.

PigHealth.com. Classical swine fever. Available at: http://www.pighealth.com/csf.htm. Accessed 2003.

ThePigSite.com. Available at: http://www.thepigsite.com. Accessed 2003.

World Organization for Animal Health (OIE). OIE disease information, 20 August 2004, Vol. 17 - No. 34. Available at: http://www.oie.int/eng/info/hebdo/AIS_31.HTM. Accessed 2003.

Reviewed by:

John Carr, Assistant Professor, ISU, College of Veterinary Medicine

defunct link as of 2005

This is example of how foot and mouth disease can spread in a country with a veterinary infrastructure similar to that of the United States and how the international community reacted to an outbreak in the U.K. Outbreaks of foot and mouth disease cause major economic and trading difficulties for infected countries. Because the disease can spread on fomites as well as between animals, it can sweep through a country rapidly in spite of control measures.

How it began

On February 19, 2001, a veterinary inspector from the State Veterinary Service of the Ministry of Agriculture, Fisheries and Food (MAFF), undertaking routine inspections at an abattoir at Little Warley near Brentwood, Essex, saw vesicular lesions on 27 sows and one boar. Vesicles (skin blisters) are a characteristic symptom of foot and mouth disease (FMD). Vesicles caused by FMD are clinically indistinguishable from those caused by other vesicular diseases such as vesicular stomatitis, swine vesicular disease, or vesicular exanthema of swine. In this case, laboratory tests confirmed the disease to be foot and mouth disease. On February 20, MAFF announced an immediate "stop movement" of all susceptible livestock in the United Kingdom, including the movement of animals to abattoirs, sale markets, and pastures.

Efforts to trace the disease back to the infected farm and suppress the outbreak began immediately. The infected pigs had arrived at the abattoir on February 16 from farms in Buckinghamshire and the Isle of Wight. The pigs were traced back to a farm at Heddon-on-the-wall, Northumberland. By the time the outbreak was discovered, foot and mouth disease had spread to a cluster of holdings in the County of Essex through the movement of pigs and people and local airborne spread. Infected sheep from the farm at Heddon-on-the-wall had also been moved to the Longtown market near Carlisle. These sheep infected thousands of additional sheep and cattle holdings in other parts of Great Britain, initially through the movement of sheep through markets and subsequently by local spread around infected holdings.

What is foot and mouth disease?

Foot and mouth disease is a highly infectious viral disease that can affect all cloven-hoofed animals including cattle, swine, deer, goats, and sheep. More rarely, it affects hedgehogs, rats, elephants, giraffes, and antelopes. The FMD virus is spread in aerosols and on fomites such as manure-contaminated tires, boots, and clothing. The disease is characterized by fever and vesicles, which progress to erosions in the mouth, nares, muzzle, feet, or teats. In cattle, oral lesions are common, with vesicles on the tongue, dental pad, gums, soft palate, nostrils, or muzzle. Hoof lesions can be found in the area of the coronary band and interdigital space. The erosions are quite painful and affected animals are lame, refuse to eat, and may lose weight. The mouth lesions can cause profuse salivation. Sheep and goats show very mild, if any, signs. Animals generally recover in about two weeks but secondary infections may lead to a longer recovery time.

How it entered the U.K.

Seven immunogically different serotypes of the FMD virus are known to exist. The virus in the U.K. was identified as serotype "O" Pan-Asian. This strain was first recognized in India in 1990 and has since spread to a number of countries around the world. It is identical to the virus found in recent outbreaks in Africa, including one in South Africa where the virus was traced to pig swill—waste food from human tables—sold illegally from an Asian boat.

The source of the 2001 epizootic in the U.K. is also thought to have been pig swill. The feeding of pig swill is a practice that has been going on for generations. Today, pig swill comes from restaurants, schools, and anywhere humans eat and waste food on a large scale. In recent years, the feeding of pig swill has declined because it is thought to be inefficient and outmoded. In 1998, a government panel of agricultural experts advised that it be banned; however, the advice was rejected by ministers who did not want to impose new costs on hard-pressed farmers. Only about one percent of producers in the U.K. were using pig swill at the time of the outbreak. Farmers are supposed to treat the swill by heating it to 100 degrees centigrade to kill potential pathogens. MAFF officials suspect that the infectious swill originated as waste food from a ship or international restaurant that was not properly heat-treated.

The spread

By March 2, foot and mouth disease had spread to 40 locations, with many linked to infected markets. A total of 25,000 animals had been destroyed and incinerated on-farm. An outbreak was also confirmed in County Armagh in Northern Ireland. (The term "outbreak" used here refers to infections at a farm or abattoir that was previously uninfected.) On March 9, there were cases in 127 locations. The MAFF sent information to farmers and veterinarians on how to avoid spreading FMD and how to report suspected outbreaks. It also publicized the details of the clinical signs of FMD in sheep, as the symptoms in this species can be subtle.

At the start of the outbreak, MAFF veterinarians who had been on infected premises were required not to have contact with uninfected, susceptible animals for five days. A shortage of "clean" unexposed veterinarians quickly developed. Private practice veterinarians and foreign government veterinarians were enlisted to help with the outbreak. The U.S.

sent the first group of 20 veterinarians the week of March 5. One month after the start of the outbreak, MAFF decreased the time required to become "clean" from five to three days to enable more veterinarians to investigate potentially infected premises. Eventually the time required to become "clean" decreased to 24 hours to visit a highly suspect farm. Veterinary teams for infected premises, surveillance, and trace back from sale markets were established to better utilize personnel.

The control measures implemented by MAFF resulted in a number of difficulties. Because of the restriction of animal movement, cows could not cross roads for milking or be moved to fresh grazing pastures. Pregnant ewes were prevented from moving to shelter for lambing. There was a public outcry to allow some animal movement for welfare reasons. To reduce the transmission of virus by humans, footpaths in the countryside were closed and the public was strongly discouraged from going anywhere near livestock farms. Carcass disposal also became a problem. The MAFF initially planned to render the carcasses of destroyed livestock rather than incinerate them on-farm. However, the large number of carcasses resulted in a lack of sealed trucks for hauling carcasses to rendering plants, delays in burial, and shortages of material for incineration. The National Farmers Union (NFU) protested the delay of several days in destroying infected animals and burning carcasses. About one month after the start of the outbreak the military became involved to coordinate the disposal of carcasses.

In spite of control measures, the epidemic continued to spread and cases began to appear outside the U.K. On March 13, FMD was confirmed at La Baroche-Gondouin in northwestern France. The infected farm was already in a movement control zone, put in place around a sheep farm that had imported sheep from the U.K. two weeks earlier. The sheep had been preventively slaughtered at that time. Six cattle on the farm showed symptoms of FMD, and the entire herd of 114 cattle was destroyed. On March 15, the MAFF made the decision to "ring depopulate" in the U.K. A ring was defined as three kilometers around an infected premises. A total of 251 farms were infected on March 15 and about a million healthy animals were scheduled to be killed. The media called it "the mass cull." On March 20, FMD was found in the Republic of Ireland; typical FMD lesions were detected in sheep on a farm only four miles away from the single outbreak which occurred in Northern Ireland. The farm was within the surveillance zone established after this earlier incident. The source of the Republic of Ireland outbreak was believed to be sheep imported via N. Ireland from mainland U.K.

On March 21, FMD was confirmed in four cows on a farm in the Netherlands. Temporary restrictions were imposed throughout the country on the movement of cattle, poultry, transport vehicles for cattle and

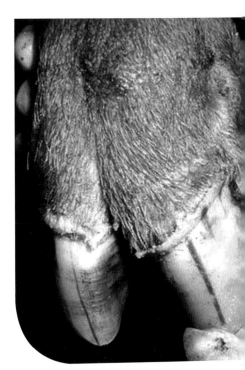

Animals with foot and mouth disease develop vesicles and erosions on the mouth, muzzle, feet, or teats. These lesions are indistinguishable from the lesions found in other vesicular diseases such as swine vesicular disease, vesicular stomatitis, or vesicular exanthema of swine.
Source: USDA

poultry, and the semen, ova, and embryos of ungulates. All animals on the affected farm were immediately culled. The animals on the six farms within a one-kilometer radius of the infected holding were also destroyed. Animals were either buried on the farm or burned. All farms within a radius of three kilometers of the affected farm were inspected for signs of FMD. The FMD virus is believed to have reached the Netherlands via a shipment of veal calves from the Republic of Ireland. The calves were rested in an animal holding near Barouche Gondouin, France for 12 hours, where they were apparently infected by sheep coming from the U.K. On March 23, to fight the spread of FMD, European Union veterinarians in Brussels agreed to limited emergency vaccination in the Netherlands around infected farms and animals awaiting slaughter. This overturned the 15-year E.U. policy of prohibiting vaccination for FMD.

On March 30, there were 60 new outbreaks in the U.K., the highest daily total of the epidemic so far, with a total of 839 outbreaks to that date. The farming and tourism industries had by this point been devastated, and even politics was affected. On April 2, Prime Minister Tony Blair announced that the general election scheduled for May 3 would be delayed until June 7 because of the FMD crisis. However, the severe control measures eventually succeeded in controlling the epidemic. By June 12 the spread had slowed; only four new locations were affected that day, bringing the total number of new outbreaks to 1,736. By this time, over 3,281,000 animals had been slaughtered, and 8,334 premises had been affected.

The international reaction

The U.K. was required to notify the World Organization for Animal Health (OIE) of the outbreak within 24 hours of the first case. On the following day, February 21, the European Commission banned the export of live animals, germplasm, fresh meat, meat products, milk and milk products, hides, and skins of FMD susceptible species from all of the U.K.

The U.S./USDA response

Immediately after FMD was confirmed in the U.K., the USDA stepped up its efforts to guard against FMD. The importation of swine, ruminants, any fresh swine or ruminant meat (chilled or frozen), and other products of swine and ruminant origin from the European Union was temporarily prohibited. Travelers were prevented from carrying into the U.S. any agricultural products, particularly animal products from the European Union that could spread the disease. Security was tightened at ports of entry and airports to ensure that passengers, luggage, and cargo were checked as appropriate. The USDA also heightened the alert and coordination with state agriculture officials and other USDA officials stationed around the globe to monitor the situation, and developed a public education campaign that included additional signs in airports, public service announcements, an information hotline, website, and other tools to inform the public about the issue. In addition, the U.S. sent a team of experts to the European Union to monitor, evaluate, and assist in containment efforts.

As the FMD outbreak grew in the U.K., the USDA also established an emergency operations center to coordinate communication, answer technical questions, and provide consumer and traveler information about FMD and other related issues. In addition, the USDA reviewed its current Animal and Plant Health Inspection Service programs and staffing to ensure appropriate resources were available to prevent the entry of FMD into the United States, both short and long-term. Federal and state emergency operations plans were also reviewed to ensure that appropriate response mechanisms were in place to act quickly if FMD were ever to enter the United States.

Final statistics

The last case of this outbreak was reported on September 30, 2001, bringing the total number of confirmed cases in the U.K. to 2,030. Many more animals had been killed to prevent the spread of the disease. According to official U.K. government figures, 4,068,000 animals were culled between the first case on February 20, 2001 and the last case on September 30, 2001. Unofficial figures from the Meat and Livestock Commission put the number of animals slaughtered at more than 10 million. Those figures include animals slaughtered for welfare reasons such as dwindling feed and space, animals killed because there was no market for them, and animals killed with their mothers and only counted as one animal. On January 22, 2002, the OIE declared that the U.K. had regained its previously recognized FMD-free status without vaccination, clearing the way for international export trade in animals and animal products.

Sources of Information

Department for Environment, Food and Rural Affairs (DEFRA), U.K. Foot and mouth disease. Available at: http://www.defra.gov.uk/footandmouth/. Accessed 2003.

http://www.aphis.usda.gov:80/oa/fmd/informwp.html. * Accessed 2003.

International Society for Infectious Diseases. Promed-Mail. Available at: http://www.promedmail. org. Accessed 2003.

PigHealth.com. Available at: http://www.pighealth.com. Accessed 2003.Reviewed by:

Dr. Larry Ludemann, USDA APHIS, VS, Center for Veterinary Biologics, and a veterinarian assigned to assist with the outbreak in the U.K. in spring 2001.

*defunct link as of 2004

Foot and Mouth Disease in Uruguay, 2001

Foot and mouth disease (FMD) also occurred in Uruguay at the same time as the epidemic in the U.K. Although these two countries are approximately the same size, their livestock composition is quite different. Uruguay has nearly seven times as many cattle as the U.K. (10.6 million compared to 1.6 million) but fewer sheep and pigs. Faced with a similar number of FMD-infected farms, the two countries' approach to this disease was drastically different. The U.K. used a stamping-out policy with no vaccination, while Uruguay culled few animals and concentrated its efforts on a massive vaccination campaign. In the U.K., more than 6 million animals were killed. In Uruguay, a little over 6,900 animals were killed, and over 24 million doses of vaccine were used. The two outbreaks lasted about the same time, but the overall cost to control the epidemic was far less in Uruguay. The FMD outbreak in the U.K. is estimated to have cost approximately $5 billion to agriculture and the food chain and an additional $5 billion from loss of tourism. The cost of the outbreak in Uruguay was $243.6 million, with much of this due to the loss of export markets. This outbreak illustrates how vaccination can be effective in controlling and eradicating FMD.

In 1987, the countries of South America established the Hemispheric Plan for the Eradication of Foot and Mouth Disease (PHEFA). Under this plan, comprehensive vaccination with modern, improved vaccines is the backbone of eradication efforts, but depopulation is also conducted if the disease threatens a disease-free region. The adoption of PHEFA led to a decrease in the number of FMD outbreaks reported in South America from 955 in 1990 to 130 in 1999. The adoption of PHEFA also strengthened veterinary systems overall and promoted private sector cooperation in control and eradication activities, resulting in an overall improvement in national animal health programs and services in nearly all countries.

Livestock breeding is the major agricultural activity in Uruguay, and a significant contributor to its economy. In 2001, Uruguay had 10.6 million cattle, 12.1 million sheep, 480,000 horses, and 270,000 pigs. Livestock production represents more than 65 percent of all Uruguayan exports. The presence of FMD, however, places significant restrictions on trade. In the 1990s, the European Union decided to stop general vaccination for FMD, prompting South American meat-exporting countries to discontinue vaccination if possible and acquire a more favorable trade status. In 1994, Uruguay was recognized by the OIE as "FMD free where vaccination is practiced." In the same year, it discontinued vaccination, in the hope of obtaining the status of "FMD free without vaccination," a goal it achieved in 1996. Also hoping to achieve the coveted "FMD free without vaccination" status, Argentina and Paraguay stopped vaccinating in 1999, as did portions of Brazil in 2000. However, Ecuador, Peru, Bolivia, Colombia, Venezuela and parts of Brazil continued to report FMD outbreaks through the 1990s and continued to vaccinate.

As a result of discontinuing vaccination, Uruguay, Argentina, Paraguay and parts of Brazil were at great risk for FMD. Their increased susceptibility was due to the progressive loss of immunity in large cattle populations over a short period of time, the continual danger of the spread of FMD from the remaining endemic areas, and the movement of large numbers of now-susceptible young livestock to fattening areas. Because they were free of FMD, these countries devoted fewer people and resources to the eradication project. Some people believe that the decreased resources contributed to the failure of surveillance and communication systems between countries. Education and training of public and private individuals also decreased, and political and commercial interests became more important than sanitary requirements. In a few years, the entire veterinary infrastructure promoted by PHEFA was weakened, and FMD invaded the southern region of South America, including Uruguay.

The re-introduction of FMD into the region

In 2000, Argentina, Brazil and Uruguay reported outbreaks of foot and mouth disease with both the type O and the type A viruses. FMD types A and type O were reported in Argentina, where 124 premises were eventually involved. Twenty-two facilities were affected in Brazil, with 12 confirmed as type O, and three farms were infected in an adjacent part of Uruguay. All three countries conducted depopulation ('stamping-out') campaigns and, by the end of 2000, believed the viruses to be eradicated. However, in February 2001, Argentina reported the first cases of a massive FMD outbreak that would eventually affect all three countries. This virus, a type A, spread rapidly and explosively through the central and eastern part of Argentina, although a special control region prevented the epidemic from extending into the south. Despite extensive depopulation efforts, the disease had affected over 2,000 premises by the end of 2001 and was still out of control in Argentina. Brazil reported its first outbreak with this virus in May 2001, in the state of Rio Grande do Sul. The affected herd and contact animals were immediately culled, and a vaccination campaign was initiated that prevented the virus from spreading outside this state. Ultimately, Brazil would report 37 outbreaks of FMD in Rio Grande do Sul in 2001.

On April 23, 2001, FMD type A appeared in Uruguay, from Argentina. The first infected farm was reported in Palmitas, Soriano Department (state). Palmitas is approximately 70 km from Uruguay's border with Argentina, the Uruguay River. Thirty-nine of the 430 cattle on the affected farm had signs of FMD. Lesions were not seen on the farm's 640 sheep. The affected and exposed animals were killed the following day. On April 26, FMD was found on a neighboring farm, which had a mixed population of cattle, sheep and pigs. At the same time, several FMD outbreaks occurred in the adjacent Colonia Department, 25 km from the Uruguay River and 40 km from the first cases. The zone where the outbreak first occurred is economically integrated with the adjacent region of Argentina, which was experiencing FMD outbreaks, and the virus is assumed to have spread from this region via fomites or people.

Quarantines were immediately placed on both affected departments and, the following day, the remaining affected and exposed animals were destroyed and buried. In total, 5,093 cattle, 1,511 sheep, and 333 pigs were culled. Three days later, the government was forced to suspend the stamping-out procedure because of strong resistance by local farmers and the discovery that the disease had spread to other areas of the country. Authorities learned that, a few days before the first cases were recognized, cattle had been sold at auction and delivered to other parts of Uruguay. The movement of people, agricultural equipment and machinery, and milk and beef trucks are also thought to have contributed to the spread of the virus. On April 26, Uruguay began ring vaccination of cattle within a 10 km radius of the affected farms. Beginning on April 27, all movement and trade of animals were prohibited throughout the country. On April 30, vaccination was extended to form a protective barrier to prevent the virus from entering uninfected states or neighboring countries.

The vaccination program

On May 5, Uruguayan authorities initiated a massive vaccination program for all cattle. The Uruguayan veterinary services established a vaccination timetable, scheduling routes, dates, and times. The vaccine was provided to farmers free of charge, and the farmers were responsible for vaccinating their animals within a given time period. Animals in areas adjacent to the state of Rio Grande do Sul were vaccinated first in order to protect Brazilian livestock. Vaccination proceeded from north to south and from east to west, and was completed on June 7; movement and transit restrictions were then relaxed. In total, nearly 11 million cattle were vaccinated. Government-administered serological tests at the completion of the vaccination program suggested that compliance had been 99 percent. Uruguay's 12 million sheep, which share pastures with the cattle, were not vaccinated; however, this did not seem to hamper the eradication of the virus. The approximately 270,000 pigs were also left unvaccinated, as the vaccine used was not thought to be effective in this species. At the height of the epidemic, 40-60 new infected farms were being found each day; however, by the end of the first round of vaccination, there were fewer than 10 new foci per day.

From June 15 to July 22, Uruguay conducted a re-vaccination program. A total of 24 million doses of FMD oil-adjuvanted vaccines were distributed during these two vaccination rounds. In November 2001, an additional 4.5

million young cattle that had been born since 2000 were vaccinated or re-vaccinated, and each animal was identified by an ear-tag tracking system. This revaccination effort boosted immunity in the cattle population to the optimum levels, and decreased the risk that vaccinated animals might become carriers. A few days after the completion of the second round of vaccination, only a few sporadic cases were being found. The last case of FMD was found on a dairy farm on August 21. By October, Uruguay was again classified as "free of FMD, with vaccination." Re-vaccination of all cattle was carried out again in February 2002 and May 2002.

There have been some concerns about the use of vaccines in eradication efforts. Some FMD outbreaks in the past were linked to incompletely inactivated, older vaccines. Although newer vaccines use better inactivation methods, there are still fears that this could occur. It may also be possible for animals to become FMD carriers, even when vaccinated. In this South American epidemic, there were no documented cases of vaccinated animals causing new outbreaks.

The cost of the outbreak

From April 23 to August 21, 2001, a total of 2,057 farms or facilities in Uruguay were affected by FMD, a number similar to the farms affected by the epidemic in the U.K. However, Uruguay was able to eradicate its extensive outbreak solely by restrictions on livestock movement and the vaccination of cattle, in spite of having a large and fully susceptible sheep population in close contact with the cattle. The total direct cost of eradication was estimated at $13.6 million. Vaccine purchases accounted for $7.5 million, with the remainder used for compensation payments to farmers, cleaning and disinfection, and operating expenses. The $13.6 million does not include some expenses incurred by the Army, which collaborated by controlling illegal livestock movements in border areas and providing other support. Argentina and Brazil also managed to control their epidemics, in part by vaccination.

The loss of export markets and a pronounced decrease in livestock prices associated with the epidemic were costly for Uruguay. The estimated losses as a result of the closing of external markets to Uruguayan farmers exceeded $200 million. Financial losses to meat and dairy producers, in particular, had a significant negative impact on the national economy. In addition, movement restrictions on the entire livestock sector affected many workers and associated industries such as packing plants. Losses associated with closed packing plants, as well as the return of 380 containers of meat that were in transatlantic transit at the time of the outbreak, added approximately $30 million in costs. In total, the epidemic cost Uruguay approximately $243.6 million, a much smaller figure than the approximately $10 billion in losses to agriculture, the food chain and tourism during the outbreak in the U.K. In addition,

> *Uruguayan authorities initiated a massive vaccination program for all cattle. The Uruguayan veterinary services established a vaccination timetable, scheduling routes, dates, and times. The vaccine was provided to farmers free of charge, and the farmers were responsible for vaccinating their animals within a given time period.*

> *Uruguay was able to eradicate its extensive outbreak solely by restrictions on livestock movement and the vaccination of cattle, in spite of having a large and fully susceptible sheep population in close contact with the cattle.*

approximately 6,900 animals were culled in Uruguay compared with the more than 6 million animals killed in the U.K.

Sources of Information

Barteling SJ. Development and performance of inactivated vaccines against foot and mouth disease. Rev Sci Tech. 2002; 21(3):577-588.

Casas Olascoaga R. (Direct Advisor of the Minister of Livestock, Agriculture and Fish. Uruguay). Foot-and-mouth disease in 2000-2001 period. In: International Conference on Control and Prevention of Foot-and-mouth disease; 2-13 Dec 2001; Brussels. Available at: http://bvs.panaftosa.org.br/textoc/FMD%20Uruguay%20(Casas).doc. Accessed 15 Sept 2005.

Correa Melo E, Saraiva V, Astudillo V. Review of the status of foot and mouth disease in countries of South America and approaches to control and eradication. Rev Sci Tech. 2002; 21(3):429-436

Sutmoller P, Barteling S, Casas Olascoaga R, Sumption KJ. Control and eradication of foot-and-mouth disease. Virus Res. 2003; 91: 101-144.

Sutmoller P,* Casas Olascoaga R. The successful control and eradication of foot and mouth disease epidemics in South America in 2001. Evidence for the Temporary Committee on Foot-and-Mouth Disease of the European Parliament; September 2, 2002. Presented by Paul Sutmoller. Available at: http://www.humanitarian.net/biodefense/papers/sutmoeller_en.pdf. Accessed 2003.

Thompson D, Muriel P, Russell D, Osborne P, Bromley A, Rowland M, Creigh-Tyte S, Brown C. Economic costs of the foot and mouth disease outbreak in the UK in 2001. Rev Sci Tech. 2002; 21(3):675.

Thomson G. Foot and mouth disease: Facing the new dilemmas. Rev Sci Tech. 2002;21(3): 425-8.

United States Department of Agriculture (USDA), Animal and Plant Health Inspection Service (APHIS). Report on the foot and mouth disease situation in Uruguay. 20th September 2002. Available at: https://web01.aphis.usda.gov/db/mtaddr.nsf/0/34e2047f2c384e8385256c4c0059a38d/$FILE/InformeF_.doc. Accessed 23 Sept 2005.

Monkeypox in the United States, 2003

Veterinarians work to prevent, diagnose and treat disease in a wide variety of species, but they also take on the role of gatekeeper to decrease the incidence of disease transmission between humans and animals. Veterinarians need to have a knowledge of zoonotic diseases, and should question animal owners about illness if a zoonosis is suspected in animals or people. The 2003 monkeypox outbreak demonstrates the importance of close cooperation between the medical, public health, and veterinary communities in addressing zoonotic diseases.

On June 7, 2003, public health officials from the Centers for Disease Control and Prevention (CDC) and the states of Wisconsin, Illinois, and Indiana reported the first outbreak of human monkeypox in the Western Hemisphere. Monkeypox is a rare, zoonotic viral disease that occurs primarily in the rain forest countries of Central and West Africa. The monkeypox virus is a member of the orthopox family of viruses. Other orthopoxviruses that can infect humans include variola (smallpox), vaccinia (the attenuated virus used in the smallpox vaccine), cowpox virus, buffalopox virus, and the newly described Cantagalo virus in Brazil. In humans, infection with the monkeypox virus results in a rash illness similar to, but less infectious than, smallpox. The incubation period is approximately 12 days. Monkeypox in humans is not usually fatal; depending on the outbreak, deaths typically occur in 1-10% of all cases.

Animal species known to be susceptible to monkeypox include non-human primates, rabbits, and some rodents.

How did monkeypox get to the United States?

Traceback investigations found that the source of the infection was a shipment of animals from Ghana imported into Texas on April 9. The shipment contained approximately 800 small mammals of nine different species, including six African rodents. The rodents included rope squirrels, tree squirrels, Gambian giant rats, brush-tailed porcupines, dormice, and striped mice. Some of these animals had reportedly become ill and died suddenly, soon after their arrival in the U.S. The CDC tested some of the surviving animals by PCR and virus isolation, and found that one Gambian giant rat, three dormice, and two rope squirrels were infected with the monkeypox virus.

Before the outbreak was detected, the monkeypox virus had spread into several states in these animals and in prairie dogs. Some of the imported animals were shipped from Texas to an Iowa distributor and then to a distributor in Illinois. In Illinois, the Gambian rats and dormice were kept in close proximity to prairie dogs, which became infected. The prairie dogs were then sold to other dealers and individuals in several states, including a Milwaukee animal distributor who purchased prairie dogs and a Gambian giant rat that was ill at the time. In May, some of these prairie dogs were sold to two pet shops in the Milwaukee area. Others were sold or traded during a pet "swap meet" (pets for sale or exchange) in northern Wisconsin. All of the exposed prairie dogs could not be traced during the investigation.

The first human case of monkeypox occurred in a child who had been bitten by an infected pet prairie dog. The child's mother and father also became infected through contact with this animal. Scientists at the Marshfield Clinic in Marshfield, Wisconsin recovered the first viral isolates from one of the patients and a prairie dog. Using electron microscopy, they found a poxvirus in the skin of the human patient and the lymph node of the prairie dog. The CDC conducted further laboratory testing including PCR, serology, immunohistochemistry, and gene sequencing that confirmed these results and demonstrated that the poxvirus was the monkeypox virus. The CDC advised physicians, veterinarians, and the public to report instances of rash illness associated with exposure to prairie dogs, Gambian rats, or other animals to local and state public health authorities. In total, 37 laboratory-confirmed and 35 suspected human cases were reported in Illinois, Indiana, Kansas, Missouri, Wisconsin and Ohio. In most patients, the disease took the form of fever and vesicular skin eruptions. Two patients, both

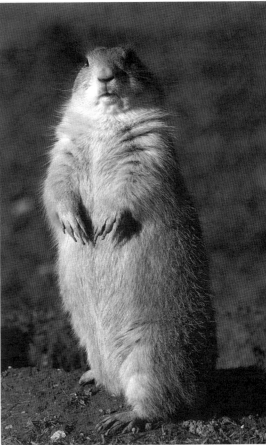

Prairie dogs housed in close proximity to imported Gambian rats and dormice became infected with monkeypox virus.
Source: www.gettyimages.com

children, had serious illnesses including one case of encephalitis. However, this outbreak was unusual in that no human deaths were reported. Distinct monkeypox isolates are found in West Africa and the Congo basin, with the Congo strains more virulent for primates. The strain that entered the U.S. was a West African virus, a factor that seems to account for the mildness of the outbreak.

All of the human patients reported direct or close contact with sick prairie dogs. Cases of monkeypox were also reported in animals. In prairie dogs, the illness included fever, cough, conjunctivitis, and lymphadenopathy, followed by a nodular rash. Some prairie dogs died and others apparently recovered. Preliminary information suggests that the Gambian giant rat under investigation experienced a much milder illness with no respiratory signs and possibly limited dermatologic involvement. Veterinarians who suspected monkeypox in an animal were asked to contact the state health department for information on specimen submission, and not to perform necropsies or biopsies because of the risk of infection. The CDC recommended that all animals with suspected monkeypox be humanely euthanized to prevent further spread of the disease and the carcass be incinerated. If the animal was associated with a human case, it was to be tested to confirm the disease. In addition, the CDC recommended that all rodents from the April 9 shipment, and any prairie dogs on the premises at the same time as these African rodents, be euthanized. Other mammals that had been in contact with these animals were placed under quarantine for 6 weeks.

On June 25, 2003, the CDC issued updated interim guidelines on the use of the smallpox vaccine, the antiviral drug cidofovir and vaccine immune globulin. The CDC recommended that people who had close or intimate contact with a confirmed case be vaccinated with the smallpox vaccine. These people could be vaccinated up to 14 days after exposure. Seven people including three veterinarians, two laboratory workers, and two health-care workers received pre-exposure prophylaxis. Another 23 people were vaccinated after exposure. The CDC also issued recommendations to medical workers on preventing transmission. Limited person-to-person transmission has been reported in monkeypox outbreaks in Africa, and health care personnel attending hospitalized patients were advised to follow standard precautions for guarding against airborne or contact illness. No cases of human-to-human transmission were confirmed in the outbreak in the U.S. Veterinarians examining or treating sick rodents, rabbits, and exotic pets like prairie dogs and Gambian rats were advised to use personal protective equipment such as gloves, surgical masks or N-95 respirators, and gowns.

Table 3: Monkeypox: Report of Cases in the United States

Data reported to CDC as of July 30, 2003. This is the final report.

State	Cases Under Investigation	Lab-Confirmed Cases
Illinois	13	9
Indiana	16	7
Kansas	1	1
Missouri	2	2
Ohio	1	0
Wisconsin	39	18
Total	72	37

On June 11, 2003, the CDC and the FDA issued a joint order announcing an immediate embargo on the importation of all rodents from Africa, due to the potential for these rodents to spread the monkeypox virus to other animal species and to humans. The joint order also banned within the U.S. any sale, offering for distribution, transport, or release into the environment, of prairie s and six genera of African rodents implicated in the monkeypox outbreak. On November 3, 2003, the joint order was replaced by an interim final rule in which the CDC restricts importation of these animals and the FDA restricts domestic interstate and intrastate movement, with exemption procedures to accommodate special circumstances. The last human case of monkeypox in the U.S. was acquired on June 20, 2003.

Sources of Information

Chen N, Li G, Liszewski MK, Atkinson JP, Jahrling PB, Feng Z, Schriewer J, Buck C, Wang C, Lefkowitz EJ, Esposito JJ, Harms T, Damon IK, Roper RL, Upton C, Buller RM. Virulence differences between monkeypox virus isolates from West Africa and the Congo basin. Virology. 2005;340(1):46-63.

Guarner J, Johnson BJ, Paddock CD, Shieh W-J, Goldsmith CS, Reynolds MG, et al. Monkeypox transmission and pathogenesis in prairie dogs. Emerg Infect Dis. 2004 Mar;10(3):426-31. Available at: http://www.cdc.gov/ncidod/EID/vol10no3/03-0878.htm. Accessed 20 Sept 2005.

Update: Multistate outbreak of monkeypox —Illinois, Indiana, Kansas, Missouri, Ohio, and Wisconsin, 2003. Morb Mortal Wkly Rep. 2003 June 13; 52(23):537-40.

Update: Multistate outbreak of monkeypox—Illinois, Indiana, Kansas, Missouri, Ohio, and Wisconsin, 2003. Morb Mortal Wkly Rep. 2003 June 20;52(24):561-4.Update: Multistate outbreak of monkeypox—Illinois, Indiana, Kansas, Missouri, Ohio, and Wisconsin, 2003. Morb Mortal Wkly Rep. 2003 July 11;52(27):642-646.

U.S. Centers for Disease Control and Prevention(CDC). Monkeypox infections in animals: Updated interim guidance for veterinarians. July 31, 2003. Available at: http://www.cdc.gov/ncidod/monkeypox/animalguidance.htm. Accessed 2003.

U.S. Centers for Disease Control and Prevention(CDC). Monkeypox report of cases in the United States. July 30, 2003. Available at: http://www.cdc.gov/od/oc/media/mpv/cases.htm. Accessed 2003.

U.S. Centers for Disease Control and Prevention(CDC). Monkeypox report of cases in the United States Final count, as of July 30, 2003. Available at: http://www.cdc.gov/od/oc/media/mpv/cases.htm. Accessed 2 Oct 2005.

U.S. Centers for Disease Control and Prevention(CDC). Public health investigation uncovers first outbreak of human monkeypox infection in Western Hemisphere. CDC Press Release. June 7, 2003. Available at: http://www.cdc.gov/od/oc/media/pressrel/r030607.htm. Accessed 2003.

U.S. Centers for Disease Control and Prevention(CDC). Questions and answers about monkeypox. November 4, 2003. Available at: http://www.cdc.gov/ncidod/monkeypox/qa.htm. Accessed 2003.

Nipah Virus in Malaysia, 1999-2000, and Bangladesh, 2001-2004

The Nipah virus is an example of an emerging viral pathogen. This virus is a previously unknown member of the family Paramyxoviridae that has been identified primarily in humans, pigs, and fruit bats. It was first recognized during an outbreak of respiratory and neurologic disease in pigs. More than 200 people who had contact with infected pigs developed encephalitis, which was often fatal. The virus later reappeared briefly in Malaysia, and several times in Bangladesh. Two elements that can be significant in the emergence of a viral epidemic or epizootic are the agent's pathogenicity to the host and its capacity to establish itself in new hosts. The Nipah virus, which appears to exist naturally in fruit bats, became established in pigs in Malaysia and was lethal to humans. Enormous numbers of pigs contracted the disease, which became so widespread that for public health protection, half of Malaysia's commercial pig population had to be destroyed. In Bangladesh, where pigs are uncommon, clusters of encephalitis were seen periodically in humans between 2001 and 2004, but these outbreaks were self-limiting and unrelated to exposure to livestock.

From late 1998 through the first half of 1999, a new pig disease characterized by pronounced respiratory and neurologic signs, sometimes with sudden death in sows and boars, began to spread among pig farms in Malaysia. It was not initially identified as a new syndrome because the morbidity and mortality rates were not high and the symptoms were not markedly different from other known diseases including Japanese encephalitis, a mosquito-borne disease prevalent in most countries in Asia. But when measures to control Japanese encephalitis did not prevent an increased incidence of viral encephalitis in pig farm workers, attention was again focused on the mysterious pig disease. In March 1999, Malaysian researchers isolated an unknown virus, which was identified by the U.S. Centers for Disease Control and Prevention (CDC) as a previously unknown paramyxovirus. The virus was termed the Nipah virus and the syndrome in pigs became known as the Porcine Respiratory and Encephalitis Syndrome, Porcine Respiratory and Neurologic Syndrome, or simply Barking Pig Syndrome after the loud cough seen in infected pigs.

By the time the virus was identified, pigs on many farms in peninsular Malaysia were already showing signs of the disease. Transmission between farms was attributed to the movement of pigs, as well as the sharing of boar semen and possibly the movement of dogs and cats. The Nipah virus spread rapidly among pigs on the infected farms, probably by

EM of the Nipah Virus
Source: Dept. of Veterinary Sciences,
Malaysian Government

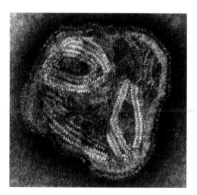

direct contact with infected pigs' excretions and secretions such as urine, saliva, or pharyngeal and bronchial secretions. Pigs in Malaysia are typically kept in close confinement, which can encourage the spread of pathogens between animals.

What is the Nipah virus?

The Nipah virus is a previously unrecognized paramyxovirus that appears to be related to another emerging virus, the Hendra virus in Australia. The Nipah virus can infect pigs, humans, dogs, and goats. Antibodies to the virus have also been reported in cats and horses, and viral antigens were found in one case of meningitis in a horse. Sheep may also be affected. In pigs, the Nipah virus causes rapid and labored breathing, an explosive and non-productive cough, neurologic changes including lethargy or aggressive behavior, and sudden death. The Nipah virus spreads readily from infected swine to other species. In pigs, the virus is found in high concentrations in the epithelial cells of the airways, facilitating its airborne spread.

In Malaysia, most human cases seemed to occur after close direct contact with the excretions or secretions from an infected pig. No cases of human-to-human transmission were documented during this epidemic; however, researchers suspect that person-to-person transmission occurred during more recent outbreaks in Bangladesh. In humans, the Nipah virus localizes in the brain after it circulates in the blood. The most common signs of infection are fever, severe headache, myalgia, encephalitis, or meningitis. Approximately half of all human cases seen to date have been fatal.

Where did the virus come from?

Fruit bats (flying foxes) are thought to be the natural hosts for the Nipah virus. Environmental circumstances could have led to the emergence of the virus from this species into pigs. There is greater contact between humans and their domestic animals and bats as intensive farming practices encroach into previously undisturbed natural habitats. The concentration of pigs and fruit trees on the same farms can lead to increased contact between fruit bats and pigs. Biologists have also noted that flying foxes are increasingly seen in urban areas. When a virus exists in a ubiquitous wild animal reservoir, such as bats, its emergence into humans and domestic animals can be difficult to prevent. Recently, researchers have found that at least two major strains of the Nipah virus circulated in pigs during the 1998 epidemic. A strain isolated from the initial outbreak in the northern regions differs significantly from a strain isolated four months later in the south. These results suggest that the Nipah epidemic in Malaysia was not due to a single transmission of the virus from fruit bats into pigs. Instead,

> *The Nipah virus, which appears to exist naturally in fruit bats, became established in pigs and was lethal to humans.*

it now seems that the virus may have emerged at least twice over the course of this outbreak.

Advances in microbiological techniques can also contribute to the recognition of emerging diseases. The discovery of the Nipah virus was facilitated by increased technical abilities, as well as by the discovery of a related virus, the Hendra virus, in Australia in 1994. Like the Nipah virus, the Hendra virus appears to be found in fruit bats in nature and was only discovered when it emerged into other species and caused disease.

Control measures

The Nipah virus is a biosafety level 4 agent because it causes death in people and there is no treatment or vaccine. At the time of the outbreak, there were no biosafety level 4 laboratories in Malaysia. Researchers from both the U.S. CDC and the Australian Commonwealth Scientific and Industrial Research Organization (CSIRO) helped the Malaysian government to isolate the virus, develop diagnostic tests, conduct transmission studies, and implement an eradication program.

The primary measure used to control the Nipah virus outbreak was the culling of pigs. Between the end of February and the end of April 1999, over 900,000 pigs from almost 900 farms were destroyed. The depopulation of infected pigs successfully controlled the human epidemic. The culling program was stopped after all known and suspected infected herds were destroyed. An ELISA test was developed to identify infected farms and a national swine testing and surveillance program was begun at the end of April 1999. The program required that each farm be sampled twice, with a minimum interval of three weeks between sampling. In the following three months, 889 farms were tested and 50 farms were found to be positive. The positive farms were considered infected and 172,750 pigs were destroyed. The government then developed a control program to provide continued monitoring of all pigs prior to slaughter. An educational program for farmers was also implemented.

Before the outbreak, pigs were second only to poultry in the Malaysian livestock industry. The Nipah outbreak resulted in the reduction of the Malaysian swine population from 2.4 million to 1.32 million pigs. The total number of farms decreased from 1,885 to 829. The outbreak also caused dramatic changes in the pig farming industry. In one state, Negeri Sembilan, pig farming is completely prohibited. In other areas, pig farming is now only allowed in an identified Pig Farming Area. The restocking of farms that had been depopulated is subject to government approval. After the outbreak, farmers were encouraged to undertake other agriculture and livestock activities.

Continued threats from the virus in Malaysia, Bangladesh and other countries

The presence of the Nipah virus in native wildlife populations poses a continuing threat to the pig and human populations in Malaysia. The Nipah virus may have reemerged in June and July 2000 when neutralizing antibodies were found in pigs on some farms in Peninsular Malaysia. A total of 1,700 pigs were destroyed in two farms in the state of Perak. In July 2000, IgG antibodies to the Nipah virus were also found in pigs on some farms in Sarawak. Four pig workers in Sarawak also had antibodies. Approximately 6,000 pigs were destroyed to control this outbreak.

More recently, a series of Nipah virus outbreaks unrelated to pigs have been reported in Bangladesh. In April and May 2001, several people in Chandpur village, Meherpur District developed an unknown neurologic disease with fever. The first case occurred in a 33 year old farmer who became ill on April 20 and died 6 days later. The farmer's wife, son, brother, and sister also developed the disease. In total, 13 cases and 9 deaths occurred in eight households. Japanese encephalitis, dengue fever, and malaria were ruled out. No samples were taken from the nine patients who died, but a later investigation revealed Nipah virus antibodies in the four surviving patients. From January 11 to 28, 2003, a cluster of similar cases appeared in villages in Naogaon District, approximately 150 km from the first outbreak. Twelve people in eight households were affected. Eight patients died, usually within a few days of the disease onset; no diagnostic samples were available from these cases. The four survivors of this outbreak also had Nipah virus antibodies.

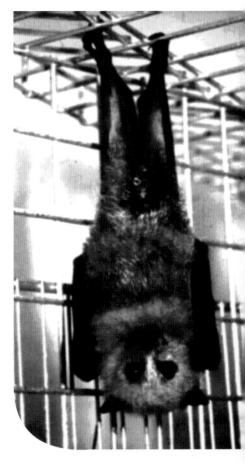

Fruit bats are thought to be the natural hosts for both the Nipah virus in Malaysia and the Hendra virus in Australia.
Source: Ministry of Agriculture, Malaysia

No obvious zoonotic source was found in either of these two outbreaks. No clusters of illness were seen in pigs, which are uncommon in Bangladesh, or in any other species. Serum samples collected from 2 pigs and 31 bats in Meherpur were all negative for Nipah virus antibodies. In Naogaon, 50 animals including 10 birds, 4 pigs, 4 dogs, 2 shrews, 5 rodents, and 25 bats were tested by serology. Antibodies to the Nipah virus were found only in two flying foxes. Although case control studies did suggest that patients were more likely than controls to have been in contact with a sick cow, no cows were available for testing and this association may be due to chance. It also appears that the virus might have been spread, in part, by person-to-person transmission. There were several clusters of cases within households, with family members becoming ill over a short period. In addition, people in Meherpur were more likely to be infected if they lived with or cared for patients, particularly if they had contact with secretions such as saliva or urine.

From January through April 2004, two new clusters of fatal encephalitis were seen in Bangladesh. The first occurred in Manikganj, Rajbari Jaipurhat, Naogaon and Faridpur provinces from early January through

February. As of February 26, 22 cases and 17 deaths were attributed to the Nipah virus, with an additional 51 cases still under investigation. Another cluster of cases was reported in April in Faridpur district. As of April 20, 30 cases and 18 deaths had been seen. In both outbreaks, CDC laboratories confirmed that the Nipah virus was the cause of disease in a number of the cases.

Health officials continue to be on the lookout for the Nipah virus or similar viruses, which could re-emerge in Bangladesh, Malaysia, or other countries. Although henipavirus (Nipah and Hendra) outbreaks have been reported only in Australia, Malaysia, and Bangladesh, their actual range could be considerably broader. Flying foxes, the natural hosts for these viruses, can be found from the east coast of Africa across south and Southeast Asia, east to the Philippines and Pacific islands, and south to Australia. Recently, the Nipah virus was isolated from Lyle's bats in Cambodia.

Sources of Information

AbuBakar S, Chang LY, Ali AR, Sharifah SH, Yusoff K, Zamrod Z. Isolation and molecular identification of Nipah virus from pigs. Emerg Infect Dis. 2004 Dec;10:2228-30.

Hooper PT. New fruit bat viruses affecting horses, pigs and humans. In: Brown C, Bolin C, editors. Emerging Diseases of Animals. Washington, DC: ASM Press; 2000. pp. 85–100.

Hsu VP, Hossain MJ, Parashar UD, Ali MM, Ksiazek TG, Kuzmin I, Niezgoda M, Rupprecht C, Bresee J, Breiman RF. Nipah virus encephalitis reemergence, Bangladesh. Emerg Infect Dis. 2004 Dec;10:2082-7.

Mohd Nor MN, Gan CH, Ong BL. Nipah virus infection of pigs in peninsular Malaysia. Rev Sci Tech. 2000 April; 19 (1):160.

Reynes JM, Counor D, Ong S, Faure C, Seng V, Molia S, Walston J, Georges-Courbot MC, Deubel V, Sarthou JL. Nipah virus in Lyle's flying foxes, Cambodia. Emerg Infect Dis. 2005 Jul;11:1042-7.

United States Department of Agriculture (USDA), Animal and Plant Health Inspection Service (APHIS), Center for Emerging Issues. Available at: http:// www.aphis.usda.gov:80/vs/ceah/cei/nipahupd.htm.* Accessed 2003.

World Health Organization (WHO). Nipah-like virus in Bangladesh. 12 February 2004. Available at: http://www.who.int/csr/don/2004_02_12/en/index.html. Accessed 14 Sept 2005.

World Health Organization (WHO). Nipah-like virus in Bangladesh – update 26 February 2004. Available at: http://www.who.int/csr/don/2004_02_26/en/index.html. Accessed 14 Sept 2005.

World Health Organization (WHO). Nipah virus in Bangladesh. 20 April 2004. Available at: http:// www.who.int/csr/don/2004_04_20/en/index.html. Accessed 14 Sept 2005.

Originally reviewed by:

Jasbir Singh, Department of Veterinary Sciences, Malaysian government and former ISU graduate student

defunct link as of 2005

Screwworm–New World

(*Cochliomyia hominivorax*) in the United States, 2000

This is an example of how prompt actions taken by veterinary practitioners prevented the introduction and spread of screwworm myiasis, a devastating disease. Screwworms were once endemic throughout the southern United States, but were eradicated by a program that involved the release of sterile male flies. The New World screwworm still exists in parts of the Caribbean and South America and could be re-introduced to the U.S. at any time.

On February 27, 2000, a shipment of 17 horses from Argentina arrived at a quarantine facility in Miami, Florida. Two days later, 16 of the 17 horses were released from quarantine. On March 1, the one remaining horse, a four-year-old chestnut thoroughbred gelding, was also released. The next day, a private practitioner performed a physical examination on this horse and found minor discharge from the prepuce, no swelling, and a bad odor—and, on closer examination, a number of insect larvae in the penis. The practitioner collected 50-100 larvae from the distal penis of the horse and contacted federal authorities. On March 3, a USDA APHIS foreign animal disease diagnostician (FADD) submitted samples of larvae from the horse to the USDA National Veterinary Services Laboratories (NVSL) in Ames, Iowa, and appropriately treated the horse and premises. On March 4, the NVSL confirmed that the samples from the horse were screwworm larvae in the third instar stage. The horse received a second treatment on March 6 and remained in quarantine until its wound was completely healed. It was released from quarantine on March 15, after being examined by a federal veterinarian. The other 16 horses in the February 27 shipment were traced and each horse was examined twice by a FADD, at three to five day intervals. No evidence of disease was found in any of these horses. APHIS Veterinary Services began intensive screwworm surveillance in Florida and sentinel animals were placed in the West Palm Beach area from March 10 to April 17. Screwworms were not found.

Another screwworm incident occurred in December 2000 in Dade County, Florida, in a pet cat that had traveled with a U.S. military employee from the Guantanamo Bay military base in Cuba to the U.S. In Cuba, a veterinarian had treated an abscess on the foot of the cat with ivermectin for five consecutive days before departure. Throughout the treatment, the veterinarian removed several dead larvae from the wound, which was healing over. When the owner arrived in Florida, he took the cat to a private practitioner, who removed one larva from the partially healed abscess. The practitioner shipped the larva to the NVSL where the diagnostician identified a mature *Cochliomyia hominivorax* larva in the third instar stage. The cat was treated and the disease did not spread.

What are screwworms?

Screwworm myiasis is a devastating parasitic disease that has long been a leading cause of livestock losses in tropical areas of the Western Hemisphere. The larvae of the New World screwworm fly, *Cochliomyia hominivorax*, feed on the open wounds of warm-blooded animals, including humans. Unlike ordinary maggots that subsist on debris and dead tissue, screwworm larvae attack living flesh, causing debilitation and sometimes even death. Wounds prone to screwworm infestation include those caused by feeding ticks, the bites of vampire bats, castra-

> *Screwworms have been eradicated from the United States and most of Central America by the release of sterile male screwworm flies. These flies mate with screwworm females and prevent them from laying viable eggs.*

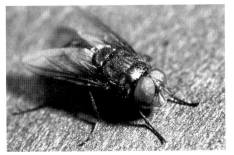

An adult Screwworm fly
Source: USDA APHIS

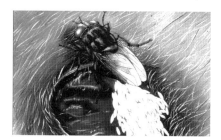

The screwworm fly lays her eggs at the edge of a wound on a warm-blooded animal.

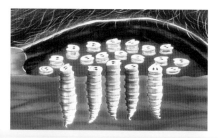

Larvae develop in the wound, feeding on the flesh, and then drop out of the wound onto the ground.

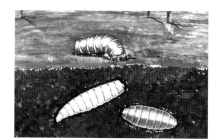

Mature larvae burrow into the ground where they pupate.

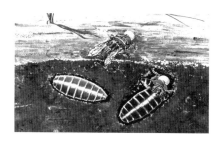

Adult flies emerge from the pupal stage to mate and begin the cycle again.
Source: USDA APHIS

tion, dehorning, branding, shearing, wire cuts, sore mouth in sheep, and shedding of the velvet in deer. The navels of newborn mammals are also common sites of infestation.

New World screwworms were once found throughout the tropical and subtropical regions of North, Central, and South America, but have been eradicated from many countries by a series of cooperative programs involving the release of sterile male flies. This approach, conducted and sustained by the USDA APHIS, has systematically eliminated screwworms from the U.S., Mexico and most of Central America over the last five decades. In late 1998, the USDA and Panama began the final phase of the Screwworm Eradication Program in that southernmost Central American country. Because there is no screwworm control plan for South America, sterile fly releases across eastern Panama will continue to be necessary even after Panama becomes screwworm-free. The sterile flies will create and maintain a biological barrier in Panama's Darien Gap, halting the pest's northward migration at the Panama-Colombia border. In addition to South America, screwworm is endemic on a few islands in the Caribbean, including Hispanola, Cuba and Jamaica.

Sources of Information

Emergency reports submitted to the OIE by the USDA in 2000. Accessed 2003.

Personal communication, Dr. James Mertins, USDA, APHIS, NVSL, Ames, Iowa 50010

Thomas TM. (US Army Veterinary Corps). Screwworm containment in Panama during final military withdrawal. Available at: http://www.aphis.usda.gov:80/vs/training/ss_2000/pdf/pan-can-shutdown.pdf. Accessed 2003.

United States Department of Agriculture (USDA), Animal and Plant Health Inspection Service (APHIS). Factsheet: Screwworm. Available at: http://www.aphis.usda.gov/lpa/pubs/fsheet_faq_notice/fs_ahscrewworm.html. Accessed 2003.

World Organization for Animal Health (OIE). Available at: http://www.oie.int. Accessed 2003.

Reviewed by:
Dr. James Mertins, USDA, APHIS, NVSL, Ames, Iowa 50010

defunct link as of 2004

West Nile Virus in the United States, 1999–2005

The outbreak of West Nile fever in New York in 1999 illustrates how a mosquito-borne disease that affects both humans and animals can spread. The West Nile virus had never before been reported in this hemisphere. The outbreak provides lessons about detecting and responding to a new disease, including the importance of local disease surveillance and response systems, communication among public health agencies, and links between public and animal health agencies. Veterinarians played an important role in the initial diagnosis of this outbreak. West Nile is now considered an endemic disease in the U.S.

In early August 1999, Tracy McNamara, DVM, head of the department of pathology at the Bronx Zoo, became concerned when she heard that a large number of crows had been dying around the zoo. By late August, 40 crows had died. Then birds at the zoo began to die. Over the Labor Day weekend, the zoo lost a Guanay Cormorant, three Chilean flamingos, a pheasant, and a bald eagle. Because these deaths followed those of the crows, experts strongly doubted that the disease originated in the zoo. Necropsies of the birds revealed streaking in the heart and brain hemorrhages. Eastern equine encephalitis was suspected but McNamara was skeptical because the emus in her care, which are very susceptible to eastern equine encephalitis virus, were thriving. "It was becoming more and more suggestive that this was not a regular bird disease," McNamara said. When two more flamingos died on September 9, she sent samples to the USDA's National Veterinary Services Laboratories (NVSL) in Ames, Iowa. The NVSL ruled out avian influenza and Newcastle disease viruses. The Centers for Disease Control and Prevention (CDC) was also sent samples, as were doctors at an Army laboratory in Fort Detrick, Maryland.

Meanwhile, on August 23, 1999, an infectious disease physician from a hospital in northern Queens contacted the New York City Department of Health (NYCDOH) to report two patients with encephalitis. On investigation, NYCDOH initially identified a cluster of six patients with encephalitis, five of whom had profound muscle weakness. Testing of these initial cases was positive for St. Louis encephalitis virus on September 3 at the CDC. Eight of the earliest case-patients were residents of a 2 x 2-mile area in northern Queens. On the basis of these findings, aerial and ground applications of mosquito adulticides and larvacides were instituted in northern Queens and South Bronx on September 3.

What happened next?

In Ames, Iowa, the NVSL isolated a virus from the birds' tissues and, after ruling out several viral agents that cause encephalitis in birds, performed an electron microscopy examination. Forty nanometer virus particles with the morphology of togaviruses or flaviviruses were observed. On September 20, the NVSL forwarded the virus cultures to the CDC for identification and characterization. Testing at the CDC on September 23 indicated that the isolate was closely related to the West Nile virus (WNV), which had never been isolated in the western hemisphere. CDC experts also detected flavivirus antigens in one of the human autopsy specimens by immunohistochemistry and found a West Nile-like virus genomic sequence in a human brain specimen from an encephalitis case; this sequence was identical to that derived from the bird tissues. Concurrently, specimens of brain tissue from three human encephalitis cases, forwarded by the New York State Department of Health to the University of California, Irvine, were reported as positive for the West Nile-like virus sequence by genomic analysis.

By September 28, a total of 17 confirmed and 20 probable human cases and four deaths had been reported in New York City and the surrounding counties. The four deaths occurred among persons over 68 years of age. The onset dates ranged from August 5 to September 16. The median age of the patients was 71 years (range 15-87 years), with the most severe clinical cases and all fatalities occurring among older persons. In October 1999, the NVSL first isolated the West Nile virus from the brain tissue of a Long Island horse that had clinical encephalitis. WNV was also isolated at NVSL from two additional encephalitic horses in 1999 and WNV antibodies were identified in ill horses in Suffolk and Essex counties, New York. Retrospective classification of likely West Nile cases occurring prior to October resulted in a total of 25 equine cases.

What is the West Nile virus?

The West Nile virus is a flavivirus belonging taxonomically to the Japanese encephalitis subgroup. This subgroup also includes the St. Louis encephalitis virus, Kunjin virus, Murray Valley encephalitis virus, and others. The West Nile virus was first isolated in the West Nile province of Uganda in 1937. It is a mosquito-transmitted virus that, in endemic regions, cycles between birds and mosquitoes. Many infected birds are asymptomatic, but high mortality rates have been seen in some species—particularly crows, ravens, and jays. When environmental conditions favor high viral amplification, mosquitoes can also spread the virus to mammals. In the northern United States, the West Nile virus has been most closely associated with *Culex pipiens*, a mosquito species that breeds in standing water, especially water polluted with organic matter. It has been thought that these mosquitoes "prefer" to bite birds, but if breeding sites are available near homes and domestic animal enclosures, *Culex pipiens* may bite people and domestic animals. *Culex pipiens* is most active at dawn and dusk. Another hypothesis suggests that other species of mosquitoes, not *Culex pipiens*, acts as a "bridge," biting both birds and mammals. Some recent evidence indicates that *Culex salinarius* is responsible for WNV transmission to people. *C. salinarius* is found in fresh and saltwater marshes, lakes, ponds, and seepage areas, as well as in the many types of artificial containers found around human residences and businesses. This species is active from sunset to sunrise. Like the St. Louis encephalitis virus, the West Nile virus is not transmitted from person to person or from birds to people.

Among mammals, symptomatic infections mainly seem to occur in humans and horses. In humans, many cases of West Nile fever are mild and flu-like; however, in more severe cases, there may be signs of encephalitis, meningoencephalitis or meningitis. Horses develop symptoms of encephalitis, often without a fever. The first recorded epidemics of West Nile fever occurred in Israel during 1950-1954 and in 1957. The largest recorded epidemic occurred in South Africa in 1974. Epidemics were also reported in Europe in the Rhone delta of France in 1962 and in Romania in 1996. The West Nile virus had never been recognized in the United States or any other area of the Western Hemisphere prior to 1999.

The response to the outbreak

Vector control measures had been initiated in northern Queens and the South Bronx on September 3. These measures were followed by a citywide pesticide application, after a laboratory confirmed a case of West Nile encephalitis in a Brooklyn resident with no travel history to Queens and two additional cases in the South Bronx. Surveillance of wild birds and sentinel chickens was instituted to assess WNV distribution in the region. Emergency telephone hotlines were established in New York City on September 3 and in Westchester County on September 21 to address public inquiries about the encephalitis outbreak and pesticide application. Approximately 300,000 cans of DEET-based mosquito repellant were distributed citywide through local firehouses, and 750,000 public health leaflets were distributed with information about personal protection against mosquito bites. Recurring public messages were announced on radio, television, web sites, and in newspapers, urging personal protection against mosquito bites. Recommended actions included limiting outdoor activity during the peak hours of mosquito activity, wearing long-sleeved shirts and long pants, using DEET-based insect repellents, and eliminating any potential mosquito breeding niches. Spraying schedules were also publicized and people were advised to remain indoors during spraying to reduce pesticide exposure.

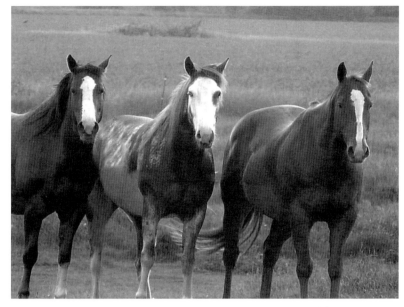

Horses are highly susceptible to the West Nile virus.
Source: Clint May, ISU

By the end of 1999, the West Nile virus had been identified in a limited area of the northeastern United States in wild birds, mosquitoes, humans, and horses. Naturally occurring virus had been found in birds and mosquitoes in parts of Connecticut, New York, New Jersey, and in one county in Maryland. Clinical illness in humans and horses occurred during a period from early August through late October and was limited to New York. WNV activity ended for the season because of various factors, including climate and vector control activities. In all, 62 human cases, with seven deaths, were recognized in 1999. Twenty-five cases of West Nile encephalitis were also identified in horses, all in Suffolk and Nassau Counties on Long Island, New York. Because horses are known not to play a role in the transmission of WNV, quarantines were never placed on any non-clinically ill horses in the outbreak area. However, the movement of horses was restricted, particularly the export of horses from affected areas to the European Union and the shipment of any horses to the E.U. via Kennedy airport.

In genetic sequencing studies, the West Nile virus isolates from the New York outbreak showed strong similarities to isolates from Israel, suggesting that this region may have been the origin of the virus. How the West Nile virus was introduced into the United States is unknown, but speculation has centered on infected humans, mosquitoes, or birds being transported by aircraft. Several other speculated routes of entry also exist.

The continuing spread of the West Nile virus

In 2000, 21 human cases of West Nile encephalitis were reported. Two elderly patients, an 82-year-old man in New Jersey and an 87-year-old woman in New York, died of the disease. Sixty confirmed equine cases were confirmed in seven states; 37 horses survived and 23 (38%) died or were euthanized. Six wild mammals were classified as WNV-positive and 4,323 infected birds were documented in 12 states plus the District of Columbia. A total of 143 counties in 12 eastern states and the District of Columbia had confirmed findings of WNV in a mosquito, bird, or mammal.

In 2001, the virus spread through bird migration south to Florida, west to Iowa, and north to Canada. There were 66 human cases in 10 states, including nine deaths. As before, most of the cases occurred in older patients; the median age was 68 and the range was 9 to 90 years. A total of 733 equine cases were reported from 127 counties in 19 states, a 12-fold increase from 2000. More than 7,000 WNV-positive wild birds were found in 328 counties in 27 states and the District of Columbia. In 66 percent of the counties, dead crows were the first indication of West Nile virus activity. Positive birds were collected from April to December 2001. West Nile virus did not affect any commercial poultry.

From 2002 to 2005, the virus continued to spread across North and South America. By the end of the 2002 mosquito season, the West Nile virus was found throughout the Midwest and was spreading into the western states. In 2003, this virus was first reported from some countries in South America. By 2005, it was found in all U.S. states except Alaska and Hawaii. The first West Nile virus vaccine for horses was licensed in 2002 and a second vaccine was licensed in 2003. As a result, the number of West Nile virus cases in horses decreased from more than 15,000 in 2002, to approximately 1400 in 2004. Reported human infections also declined from over 9800 cases and 264 deaths in 2003, to approximately 2500 cases and 100 deaths in 2004. As of Sept 13, 1299 cases and 29 fatalities had been reported in 2005. The reasons for the declining case rate in humans are unknown but may include weather patterns, mosquito control programs, public education, or other factors.

Sources of Information

Batieha A, Saliba EK, Graham R, Mohareb E, Hijazi Y, Wijeyaratne P. Seroprevalence of West Nile, Rift Valley, and sandfly arboviruses in Hashimiah, Jordan. Emerg Infect Dis. 2000 Jul-Aug;6(4):358-62.

Canadian Food Inspection Agency. West Nile virus. Available at: http://www.inspection.gc.ca/english/anima/heasan/disemala/wnvvno/wnvfse.shtml. Accessed 12 Sept 2005.

Cornell University. Environmental risk analysis program. West Nile virus. Available at: http://www.cfe.cornell.edu/erap/wnv/. Accessed 2003.

International Society for Infectious Diseases. NVSL first to… ProMED Mail, Tue, 28 Sep 1999 11:30:16 -0500, from Beverly J. Schmitt of the USDA APHIS National Veterinary Services Laboratories. Archive Number 19990928.1739. Available at: http://www.promedmail.org. Accessed 2003.

Lvov DK, Butenko AM, Gromashevsky VL, et al.. Isolation of two strains of West Nile virus during an outbreak in southern Russia, 1999. Emerg Infect Dis. 2000 Jul-Aug;6(4):373-6.

Ostlund EN, Andresen JE, Andresen M. West Nile encephalitis. Vet Clin N Am Equine Pract. 2000;16:427-41.

Rappole JH, Derrickson SR, Hubalek Z. Migratory birds and spread of West Nile virus in the Western Hemisphere. Emerg Infect Dis. 2000 Jul-Aug;6(4):319-28.

Shieh WJ, Guarner J, Layton M, Fine A, Miller J, Nash D, Campbell GL, Roehrig JT, Gubler DJ, Zaki SR. The role of pathology in an investigation of an outbreak of West Nile encephalitis in New York, 1999. Emerg Infect Dis. 2000 Jul-Aug;6(4):370-2.

Steinhauer J. African virus may be culprit in mosquito-borne illnesses in New York region. New York Times; Sunday, 26 September 1999 Available at: http://www.nytimes.com/library/national/regional/092599ny-encephalitis.html. Accessed 2003.

U.S. Centers for Disease Control and Prevention (CDC). 2003 West Nile virus activity in the United States. April 15 2003. Available at: http://www.cdc.gov/ncidod/dvbid/westnile/surv&controlCaseCount03_detailed.htm. Accessed 2003.

U.S. Centers for Disease Control and Prevention (CDC). 2004 West Nile virus activity in the United States. Available at: http://www.cdc.gov/ncidod/dvbid/westnile/surv&controlCaseCount04_detailed.htm. Accessed 13 Sept 2005.

U.S. Centers for Disease Control and Prevention (CDC). 2005 West Nile virus activity in the United States. Available at: http://www.cdc.gov/ncidod/dvbid/westnile/surv&controlCaseCount05_detailed.htm. Accessed 13 Sept 2005.

United States Department of Agriculture (USDA) Animal and Plant Health Inspection Service (APHIS). Update on the current status of West Nile virus. Equine cases of West Nile virus illness in 2002: 1 January through 31 December. Available at: http://www.aphis.usda.gov/lpa/issues/wnv/wnvstats.html.* Accessed 2003.

USDA Animal and Plant Health Inspection Service (APHIS). West Nile virus. Available at: http://www.aphis.usda.gov/lpa/issues/issues_archive/wnv/wnv.html. Accessed 2003.

US General Accounting Office. West Nile virus outbreak, lessons for public health preparedness. Report to Congressional requesters. Washington: September 2000. . Report nr HEHS-00-180. Available at: http://www.gao.gov/new.items/he00180.pdf. Accessed 2003.

United States Geological Survey (USGS). USGS West Nile virus maps – 2002-2005. Available at: http://westnilemaps.usgs.gov/index.html. Accessed 13 Sept 2005.

West Nile virus activity—United States, 2001. Morb Mortal Wkly Rep. June 14, 2002 / 51(23);497-501. Available at: http://www.cdc.gov/mmwr/preview/mmwrhtml/mm5123a1.htm. Accessed 2003.

Originally reviewed by:

Beverly J. Schmitt and Eileen Ostlund of the USDA APHIS NVSL in Ames, Iowa 50010

defunct link as of 2005

Section 2
• Fact Sheets for Emerging and Exotic Diseases of Animals •

Anna Rovid Spickler, DVM, PhD

This section contains brief fact sheets on a number of animal diseases that are exotic to the United States as well as some additional OIE listed diseases and other important infectious diseases. Veterinarians are obligated to report the suspected occurrence of these diseases to appropriate state or federal authorities. Although these fact sheets contain information on diagnosis, veterinarians should not attempt to collect and submit samples from suspected foreign animal diseases directly to the national disease laboratories. Instead, veterinarians who suspect an exotic disease should immediately contact their state veterinarian or APHIS Area Veterinarian in Charge for help. It is important to note that reportable diseases vary from state to state and the lists of these diseases may change. As a practicing veterinarian, you need to be familiar with the current list of reportable diseases for your area rather than rely upon the general information in these fact sheets.

These fact sheets were developed beginning in the fall of 2000 by Anna Rovid Spickler, DVM, PhD and Kris August, DVM under the guidance of James A. Roth, DVM, PhD. The fact sheets were originally developed for use in the Emerging and Exotic Diseases of Animals Internet course. Dr. Spickler updated and revised all the fact sheets in 2002-2003. She developed additional fact sheets and updated others in 2004-2006. Members of the Center for Food Security and Public Health (CFSPH) staff have also worked to update and maintain this resource. Glenda Dvorak, DVM, MS, MPH manages the fact sheets for the CFSPH website and ensures that they are as up to date as possible. Other members of the CFSPH team who have helped with the fact sheets include: Danelle Bickett-Weddle, DVM, MPH, Susan Brockus, DVM, MPH, Dipa Brahmb-hatt, DVM, MPH, Bryan Buss, DVM, MPH, Kristine Edwards, DVM, MPH, Stacy Holzbauer, DVM, MPH, LeMac Morris, DVM, MPH, Vicky Olson, DVM, MPH, Ann Peters Garvey, DVM, MPH, Alex Ramirez, DVM, MPH, Jamie Snow, DVM, MPH, Katie Steneroden, DVM, MPH, Jared Taylor, DVM, MPH, Ingrid Trevino, DVM, MPH, Gayle Brown, DVM, PhD, and Jane Galyon, MS. Dr. Alfonso Torres, Cornell University, reviewed a number of the fact sheets for an APHIS project and his comments and suggestions were incorporated. Dr. Steven Sorden, DVM, PhD reviewed and also improved a number of the fact sheets. Comments and suggestions on these fact sheets are always encouraged. As new information becomes available, the fact sheets are updated and can be found at www.cfsph.iastate.edu/DiseaseInfo

Section 2-Fact Sheets for Emerging and Exotic Diseases of Animals
Section 3-Images of Emerging and Exotic Diseases of Animals

African Horse Sickness

Perdesiekte, Pestis Equorum,
La Peste Equina, Peste Equina Africana

Importance

African horse sickness is a serious viral disease of horses spread by midges. Mortality can be as high as 95% in some forms of this disease. Asymptomatic or mild infections may occur in zebras, African donkeys, and horses previously infected by another serotype of the virus. Potential arthropod vectors may exist in the United States.

Etiology

African horse sickness is caused by the African horse sickness virus, an arthropod–borne orbivirus in the family Reoviridae. There are nine serotypes of the virus.

Species affected

African horse sickness can affect horses, donkeys, mules, zebras, and camels. Zebras may be asymptomatic carriers in Africa, and horses and mules may be accidental hosts. Dogs are susceptible to experimental infections. African elephants have been found to carry antibodies to the African horse sickness virus, but there is no evidence of virus replication in this species.

Geographic distribution

African horse sickness is endemic in sub–Saharan central and east Africa. This disease often spreads to southern Africa and occasionally to northern Africa. Outbreaks have been seen in Egypt and other parts of the Middle East, as well as in Spain.

Transmission

African horse sickness is not contagious. The causative virus is transmitted by midges of the genus *Culicoides*. Field vectors include *Culicoides imicola* and *C. bolitinos*; *Culicoides imicola* appears to be the most important vector. Potential *Culicoides* vectors may exist in the United States.

Transmission by insects other than midges is thought to be a minor source of infection. Mosquitoes have been implicated as biological vectors, and biting flies in the genera *Stomoxys* and *Tabanus* may be able to transmit the virus mechanically.

Incubation period

In experimental infections, the incubation period can range from 2 to 14 days; most often, clinical signs appear 5 to 7 days after infection. In natural infections, the incubation period appears to be approximately 7 to 14 days.

Clinical signs

Four different forms of African horse sickness may be seen: the peracute or pulmonary form, the subacute edematous or cardiac form, the acute or mixed form, and horsesickness fever.

The peracute or pulmonary form

This form of African horse sickness usually begins with an acute fever, followed by the sudden onset of severe respiratory distress. Infected animals often stand with forelegs spread, head extended, and nostrils fully dilated. Other clinical signs may include tachypnea, forced expiration, profuse sweating, spasmodic coughing, and a frothy serofibrinous nasal exudate. Dyspnea usually progresses rapidly, and the animal often dies within a few hours after the respiratory signs appear.

The subacute edematous or cardiac form

The cardiac form of African horse sickness usually begins with a fever that lasts for 3 to 6 days. Shortly before the fever starts to subside, edematous swellings appear in the supraorbital fossae and eyelids. These swellings later spread to involve the cheeks, lips, tongue, intermandibular space, laryngeal region, and sometimes the neck, shoulders, and chest. However, it is important to note that no edema of the lower legs is observed. Other clinical signs, usu-ally seen in the terminal stages of the disease, can include severe depression, colic, and petechiae under the ventral surface of the tongue and in the conjunctivae. Death often occurs from cardiac failure. If the animal recovers, the swellings gradually subside over the next 3 to 8 days.

The acute or mixed form

In this form of African horse sickness, symptoms of both the pulmonary and cardiac forms are seen. In most cases, the cardiac form is subclinical and is followed by severe respiratory distress. Occasionally, mild respiratory signs may be followed by edema and death from cardiac failure. The mixed form of African horse sickness is rarely diagnosed clinically, but is often seen at necropsy in horses and mules.

Horsesickness fever

In horsesickness fever, the clinical signs are mild. The characteristic fever usually lasts for 3 to 8 days; morning remissions and afternoon exacerbations are often seen. Other symptoms are generally mild and may include mild anorexia or depression, congested mucous membranes, and an increased heart rate. This form of the disease is rarely fatal.

Post mortem lesions

In the pulmonary form of African horse sickness, the typical lesions are edema of the lungs and hydrothorax. In the most acute cases, frothy fluid flows from the nostrils and the cut surface of the lungs, which are mottled red, noncollapsed, and heavy. In more prolonged cases, there may be extensive interstitial and subpleural edema, and hyperemia may be less apparent. Occasionally, extensive fluid accumulation may be noted in the thoracic cavity (hydrothorax), with near normal appearance of the lungs. The lymph nodes, particularly the nodes in the thoracic and abdominal cavities, are usually enlarged and edematous. Less often, there may be subcapsular hemorrhages in the spleen, congestion in the renal cortex or gastric fundus, and edematous infiltration around the aorta and trachea. Hyperemia and petechial hemorrhages may be apparent in the small and large intestines, and the pericardium may contain petechiae.

In the cardiac form, a yellow gelatinous infiltrate can be seen in the subcutaneous and intermuscular fascia of the head, neck, and shoulders, and occasionally the brisket, ventral abdomen and rump. Hydropericardium is common. The epicardium and endocardium often contain petechial and ecchymotic hemorrhages. Lesions may also be found in the gastrointestinal tract, resembling the pulmonary form. In addition, prominent submucosal edema may be noted in the cecum, large colon, and rectum. In the cardiac form, the lungs are usually normal or slightly engorged, and the thoracic cavity rarely contains excess fluid.

In the mixed form, the post–mortem lesions are a mixture of typical findings from both the cardiac and pulmonary forms.

Morbidity and mortality

Morbidity and mortality vary with the species of animal and previous immunity. Horses are particularly susceptible to this disease. In this species, the mortality rate varies from 50% to 95%, depending on the form of the disease. In the cardiac form, mortality is usually 50% to 70% and, in the mixed form, greater than 80%. The pulmonary form is almost always fatal, but horsesickness fever rarely results in death. In other species of Equidae, African horse sickness is generally less severe. In mules, the mortality rate is approximately 50%, and in European and Asian donkeys, 5% to 10%. Death is rare in African donkeys and zebra.

Animals that recover from African horse sickness develop good immunity to the infecting serotype, and partial immunity to other serotypes. A live attenuated vaccine is available in endemic countries. However, this vaccine is not safe for use in AHS–free countries. A killed vaccine was produced only against serotype 4.

Diagnosis

Clinical

African horse sickness should be suspected in animals with typical symptoms of the cardiac, pulmonary, or mixed forms of the disease. The supraorbital swellings are particularly characteristic of this disease. The horsesickness form can be difficult to diagnose.

Differential diagnosis

The differential diagnosis includes anthrax, equine viral arteritis, equine infectious anemia, Hendra virus infection, purpura hemorrhagica, and equine piroplasmosis. In Africa, equine encephalosis virus (another orbivirus transmitted by *Culicoides*) causes a syndrome resembling horsesickness fever.

Laboratory tests

African horse sickness can be diagnosed by isolating the virus or detecting its nucleic acids or antigens. More than one test should be used to diagnose an outbreak. Virus isolation is particularly important when outbreaks are seen outside endemic areas. Suitable cultures for inoculation include baby hamster kidney (BHK–21), monkey stable (MS) or African green monkey kidney (Vero) cells. Isolation is also possible in embryonic eggs or newborn mice. The virus isolate should be serotyped by virus neutralization or other methods.

Viral antigens can be detected by enzyme–linked immunosorbent assays (ELISAs). A reverse–transcription polymerase chain reaction (RT–PCR) technique is used to detect viral RNA.

African horse sickness may also be diagnosed by serology. Antibodies can be detected within 8 to 12 days after infection and may persist for 1 to 4 years. The African horse sickness virus does not cross–react with other known orbiviruses. Available serologic tests include complement fixation, ELISAs, immunoblotting, and virus neutralization. The indirect ELISA and complement fixation tests are the prescribed tests for international trade. The virus neutralization test is used for serotyping. Immunodiffusion and hemagglutination inhibition tests have also been described.

Samples to collect

Before collecting or sending any samples from animals with a suspected foreign animal disease, the proper authorities should be contacted. Samples should only be sent under secure conditions and to authorized laboratories to prevent the spread of the disease.

In live animals, uncoagulated blood samples should be taken for virus isolation. Success is most likely if these samples are collected early during the febrile stage. Necropsy samples for virus isolation should include small (2–4 g) samples of the spleen, lung, and lymph nodes. The samples for virus isolation should be stored and transported at 4°C. Serum should also be taken for serology.

Recommended actions if
African horse sickness is suspected

Notification of authorities

African horse sickness should be reported immediately to state or federal authorities upon diagnosis or suspicion of the disease.

Federal: Area Veterinarians in Charge (AVICs):
http://www.aphis.usda.gov/vs/area_offices.htm

State Veterinarians:
http://www.aphis.usda.gov/vs/sregs/official.html

Quarantine and disinfection

Horses cannot enter the U.S. from an African horse sickness endemic country unless they have been in a AHS–free country or area of the world for at least 60 days. Upon entering the U.S., horses are then subject to the regular 3 or 7 day quarantine period at the point of entry.

If African horse sickness is detected in a country where it is not endemic, a strict quarantine zone should be established. All Equidae should be sprayed with insect repellants and, at a minimum, stabled from dusk to dawn. If possible, animals should be stabled in insect–proof housing. Each susceptible animal should have its temperature taken regularly (optimally, twice daily). Those animals that develop a fever should be kept in insect–free stables until the cause of the fever has been established. These control measures should be implemented upon suspicion of the disease. Vaccination should be considered once the diagnosis has been confirmed.

The African horse sickness virus can be inactivated in the laboratory by formalin, β-propriolactone, acetylethyleneimine derivatives, or radiation. It is also destroyed at a pH less than 6, or pH 12 or greater.

Public health

Humans are not natural hosts for the African horse sickness virus, and no cases have been seen after contact with field strains. However, a neurotropic vaccine strain, adapted to mice, can cause encephalitis and retinitis in humans.

For more information

World Organization for Animal Health (OIE)
http://www.oie.int

OIE Manual of Standards
http://www.oie.int/eng/normes/mmanual/a_summry.htm

OIE International Animal Health Code
http://www.oie.int/eng/normes/mcode/A_summry.htm

USAHA Foreign Animal Diseases Book
http://www.vet.uga.edu/vpp/gray_book/FAD/

References

"African Horse Sickness." In *Manual of Standards for Diagnostic Tests and Vaccines*. Paris: World Organization for Animal Health, 2000, pp. 178–188.

"African Horse Sickness." In *The Merck Veterinary Manual*, 8th ed. Edited by S.E. Aiello and A. Mays. Whitehouse Station, NJ: Merck and Co., 1998, pp. 496–497.

Erasmus, B.J. "African Horse Sickness." In *Foreign Animal Diseases*. Richmond, VA: United States Animal Health Association, 1998, pp. 41–51.

African Swine Fever

Pesti Porcine Africaine, Fiebre Porcina Africana, Maladie de Montgomery

Importance

African swine fever is a serious viral disease of pigs, endemic in Africa. Isolates vary in virulence from highly pathogenic strains that cause near 100% mortality to low–virulence isolates that can be difficult to diagnose. Disease outbreaks have occurred in numerous countries and the cost of eradication has been significant. During outbreaks in Malta and the Dominican Republic, the swine herds of these countries were completely depopulated.

Etiology

African swine fever results from infection by the African swine fever virus (ASFV). Formerly classified as a member of the family Iridoviridae, this virus is currently the only member of the family Asfarviridae. The ASF virus is the only DNA virus that is transmitted by arthropods. The virulence of virus isolates varies.

Species affected

African swine fever affects domestic pigs and wild pigs, including the warthog, bush pig, and giant forest hog in Africa. Symptomatic infections occur in domestic pigs and feral pigs;

infections are generally asymptomatic in warthogs, bush pigs, and giant forest hogs.

Geographic distribution

African swine fever is endemic in most of sub–Saharan Africa; the highest incidence of disease is seen from the equator to the northern Transvaal. This disease is also found in feral pigs in Sardinia, Italy.

Transmission

African swine fever can be transmitted by direct contact with infected animals, indirect contact on fomites, and by tick vectors. Transmission during direct contact is usually by oronasal spread. African swine fever virus can be found in all tissues and body fluids, but particularly high levels are found in the blood. Massive environmental contamination may result if blood is shed during necropsies or pig fights, or if a pig develops bloody diarrhea. The virus can also spread on fomites, including vehicles, feed, and equipment. There is evidence that some pigs may become carriers.

African swine fever often spreads to new areas when pigs are fed uncooked scraps that contain ASFV–infected pork. In one outbreak, pigs became infected after being fed the intestines of guinea fowl that had eaten infected ticks. The African swine fever virus is highly resistant to environmental conditions. It can survive for 15 weeks in chilled meat, a year and a half in blood stored at 4°C, 11 days in feces at room temperature, and at least a month in contaminated pig pens. The virus will also remain infectious for 150 days in boned meat stored at 39°F, 140 days in salted dried hams, and several years in frozen carcasses.

African swine fever is also spread through the bite of infected *Ornithodoros* spp.soft ticks. In tick populations, transstadial, transovarial, and sexual transmission occur. In Africa, this disease is thought to cycle between newborn warthogs and the soft ticks that live in their burrows. Infected soft tick colonies can maintain the ASF virus for years.

Incubation period

The incubation period is 5 to 15 days.

Clinical signs

African swine fever can be a peracute, acute, subacute, or chronic disease. More virulent isolates cause a high fever, moderate anorexia, leukopenia, recumbency, and skin reddening that is most apparent in white pigs. Some pigs develop cyanotic skin blotching on the ears, tail, lower legs, or hams. Diarrhea and abortions are sometimes seen, but most pigs infected with acute African swine fever remain in good condition. In infections with highly virulent isolates, progressive anorexia and depression develop and are usually followed by death within 7 to 10 days. The death rate is generally lower in animals infected with moderately virulent isolates, but may still be very high in very young animals.

Animals infected with isolates of low virulence may seroconvert without symptoms, abort, or develop chronic African swine fever. The symptoms of chronic disease are a low fever, which may recur, and sometimes pneumonia or painless swelling of the joints, particularly the carpal and tarsal joints. Reddened foci may appear on the skin and become raised and necrotic. In some cases, the only clinical signs may be emaciation and stunting. Chronic African swine fever can be fatal.

Post mortem lesions

The most consistent and characteristic lesions occur in the spleen and lymph nodes. In animals infected with highly virulent isolates, the spleen is usually very large, friable, and dark red to black. In pigs infected with moderately virulent isolates, the spleen is also enlarged, but not friable, and the color is closer to normal. The lymph nodes are often swollen and hemorrhagic and may look like blood clots; the nodes most often affected are the gastrohepatic, renal, and mesenteric lymph nodes. Edema may

also be seen in other lymph nodes, and the tonsils are often swollen and reddened.

Less consistent clinical signs include hemorrhages, petechiae, and ecchymoses in other organs. Petechiae may be present on any organ, but most are located on the renal cortex, bladder, lungs, and heart. Ecchymoses and "paint–brush" hemorrhages are often found on the serosa of the stomach and intestines. Edema may be seen in the lungs and gall bladder, and the pleural, pericardial, and peritoneal cavities may contain excess fluid. In some pigs, dark red or purple areas may be found on the skin of the ears, feet, and tail. Aborted fetuses may be anasarcous, have a mottled liver, and have petechiae in the placenta, skin, and myocardium.

In animals with chronic African swine fever, the most common post–mortem lesions are focal areas of skin necrosis, consolidated lobules in the lung, fibrinous pericarditis, generalized lymphadenopathy, and swollen joints.

Morbidity and mortality

In domestic pigs, morbidity approaches 100% in herds that have not been previously exposed to the virus. Mortality varies with the virulence of the isolate, and can range from 0% to 100%. Low virulence isolates are more likely to be fatal in pigs with a concurrent disease, pregnant animals, and young animals. Mild or asymptomatic disease is usually seen in warthogs and bush pigs.

No treatment or vaccine exists for this disease.

Diagnosis

Clinical

African swine fever should be suspected in pigs with a fever, when the necropsy findings include a very large, friable, dark red to black spleen and greatly enlarged and hemorrhagic gastrohepatic and renal lymph nodes.

Differential diagnosis

The differential diagnosis includes hog cholera (classical swine fever), porcine dermatitis and nephropathy syndrome, erysipelas, salmonellosis, eperythrozoonosis, actinobacillosis, Glasser's disease (*Haemophilus parasuis* infection), Aujeszky's disease, thrombocytopenic purpura, warfarin poisoning, and heavy metal toxicity.

Laboratory tests

In areas where African swine fever is not endemic, this disease should be diagnosed by virus isolation and the detection of viral antigens. Blood and tissue samples from suspect pigs are inoculated into pig leukocyte or bone marrow cultures for virus isolation. African swine fever virus induces hemadsorption of pig erythrocytes to the surface of infected cells. The virus can also be detected with peripheral blood leukocytes from infected pigs in a hemadsorption "autorosette" test.

African swine fever virus antigens can be found in tissue smears or cryostat sections by the fluorescent antibody test (FAT). Nucleic acids can be detected by a polymerase chain reaction (PCR) assay. PCR is particularly useful in putrefied samples that cannot be used for virus isolation and antigen detection.

Serology is carried out simultaneously with virus isolation. Antibodies to ASFV persist for long periods of time after infection. Serology may also be used for diagnosis in endemic areas. Available serologic tests include the enzyme–linked immunosorbent assay (ELISA), immunoblotting, indirect fluorescent antibody (IFA), and counter immunoelectrophoresis (immunoelectro–osmophoresis) tests. The ELISA is prescribed for international trade.

Samples to collect

Before collecting or sending any samples from animals with a suspected foreign animal disease, the proper authorities should be contacted. Samples should only be sent under secure conditions and to authorized laboratories to prevent the spread of the disease.

For virus isolation from live animals, blood should be collected into an anticoagulant. At necropsy, samples of the spleen, lung, liver, kidney, and tonsils, as well as the submandibular, inguinal, and gastrohepatic lymph nodes should be collected aseptically. Samples of the bone marrow should be sent if significant postmortem changes are seen. ASFV is not found in aborted fetuses; in cases of abortion, a blood sample should be collected from the dam. Samples for virus isolation should be transported cold on wet ice or frozen gel packs.

Samples of the same tissues, the brain, and any other grossly abnormal tissues should be submitted for histology. Serum and/or tissue fluids should be submitted for serology

Recommended actions if African swine fever is suspected

Notification of authorities

African swine fever should be reported to state or federal authorities immediately upon diagnosis or suspicion of the disease.
Federal: Area Veterinarians in Charge (AVICs):
http://www.aphis.usda.gov/vs/area_offices.htm
State Veterinarians:
http://www.aphis.usda.gov/vs/sregs/official.html

Quarantine and disinfection

To prevent introduction of the African swine fever virus into areas free of the disease, all garbage fed to pigs should be cooked. Unprocessed meat must be heated to at least 70°C for 30 minutes to inactivate the virus; 30 minutes at 60°C is sufficient for serum and bodily fluids.

African swine fever is a contagious disease. Eradication is by slaughter of infected and in–contact animals, and disposal of carcasses, often by burying, rendering or burning. Strict quarantine must be imposed, and potential tick vectors should be controlled with acaricides. In cases of ASF outbreaks, there must be a detailed entomological investigation for the possibility of soft tick vectors and their role as long term carriers. In the outbreaks in the Americas, the *Ornithodoros* ticks never became chronically infected. But in Spain, Portugal and Africa, infected soft ticks can carry the ASFV for many years. Many common disinfectants are ineffective; care should be taken to use a disinfectant specifically approved for African swine fever. Sodium hypochlorite and some iodine and quaternary ammonium compounds are effective.

Public health

Humans are not susceptible to African swine fever virus.

For more information

World Organization for Animal Health (OIE)
http://www.oie.int
OIE Manual of Standards
http://www.oie.int/eng/normes/mmanual/a_summry.htm
OIE International Animal Health Code
http://www.oie.int/eng/normes/mcode/A_summry.htm
USAHA Foreign Animal Diseases Book
http://www.vet.uga.edu/vpp/gray_book/FAD/

References

"African Swine Fever." *Animal Health Australia*. The National Animal Health Information System (NAHIS). 18 Oct 2001. http//www.brs.gov.au/usr–bin/aphb/ahsq?dislist=alpha.

"African Swine Fever." In *Manual of Standards for Diagnostic Tests and Vaccines*. Paris: World Organization for Animal Health, 2000, pp. 189–198.

"African Swine Fever." In *The Merck Veterinary Manual*, 8th ed. Edited by S.E. Aiello and A. Mays. Whitehouse Station, NJ: Merck and Co., 1998, pp. 504–506.

Mebus, C.A. "African Swine Fever." In *Foreign Animal Diseases*. Richmond, VA: United States Animal Health Association, 1998, pp. 52–61.

Shirai J, T. Kanno, Y. Tsuchiya, S. Mitsubayashi, and R. Seki. "Effects of chlorine, iodine, and quaternary ammonium compound disinfectants on several exotic disease viruses." *J Vet Med Sci* 62, no. 1 (2000): 85–92.

Akabane

Congenital Arthrogryposis-Hydranencephaly Syndrome, A-H Syndrome, Akabane Disease, Congenital Bovine Epizootic A-H Syndrome, Acorn Calves, Silly Calves, Curly Lamb Disease, Curly Calf Disease, Dummy Calf Disease

Importance

Akabane is a viral disease that may cause serious economic losses in ruminants. Inapparent infections in adults can lead months later to abortions, stillbirths, premature births, and severe congenital defects in newborns. Most affected neonates die or must be euthanized. There is no treatment for this disease.

Etiology

Akabane is caused by Akabane virus, an arbovirus in the Simbu group of the family Bunyaviridae. Several closely related viruses—Aino, Peaton, Tinaroo, and Douglas viruses—can also produce fetal defects. Cache Valley virus causes a similar syndrome in ruminants in the United States.

Species affected

Symptomatic infections are seen only in cattle, sheep, and goats. Wild ruminants can be infected with Akabane virus; congenital defects may occur in these species but have not been reported. Antibodies to the virus have also been found in horses, buffalo, deer, camels, and dogs.

Geographic distribution

Akabane is common in the tropics and subtropics between latitude 35°N and 35°S. This disease is endemic in the northern half of Australia; occasional outbreaks occur in southern Australia when conditions are favorable for the virus to spread. Akabane disease has also been seen in Japan, Cyprus, Korea, Zimbabwe, Israel and other countries in the Middle East, and South Africa. Serological evidence of the virus has been found throughout Africa, Asia, and Australia.

Transmission

The vector for Akabane is not proven, but epidemiological evidence suggests that the virus is spread by mosquitoes and gnats. Akabane virus has been isolated from *Aedes vexans, Culex triteeniorhynchus*, and *Culicoides oxystoma* in Japan, *Anopheles funestus* in Kenya, and *Culicoides milnei* and *Culicoides imicola* in Africa. In Australia, the virus has been isolated from *Culicoides brevitarsis* and *Culicoides wadei* gnats; the main vector appears to be *C. brevitarsis*. Akabane virus is not transmitted by contact, infected tissues, exudates, or fomites. Ruminants do not appear to become long–term carriers of this virus.

Incubation period

In adults, the infection is asymptomatic, but viremia usually occurs 1 to 6 days after infection and lasts for 1 to 9 days. The symptoms of fetal infection are not seen until much later or at term.

Clinical signs

Infections in non–pregnant animals are asymptomatic. In pregnant ruminants, abortions, stillbirths, premature births, and dystocia may be seen.

Congenital abnormalities are a hallmark of this disease. Calves that were infected late in the first trimester are usually bright and alert, but cannot stand. Although some can rise with assistance, they are incoordinated, ataxic, and may be paralyzed in one or more limbs. Muscle atrophy, limb rotation, exophthalmos, excessive lacrimation, and abnormal vocalization have also been seen.

Calves infected during the second trimester usually have arthrogryposis at birth; most cannot stand. The joints are rigid and fixed in flexion (or, less often, in extension) and the muscles are usually severely atrophied. Torticollis, scoliosis, and kyphosis may also be seen. Some newborns may have both arthrogryposis and neurologic abnormalities.

"Dummy" calves are animals that were infected late in pregnancy. These animals can usually stand and walk, but have behavioral abnormalities that may include a slow or absent suckle reflex, depression, dullness, periodic hyperexcitability, deafness, nystagmus, incoordination, or blindness. Skull deformities are common.

Most affected neonates die or must be euthanized soon after being born. Animals with mild symptoms may gradually become more mobile, but most die by six months.

Post mortem lesions

Fetuses or newborns may have arthrogryposis, hydranencephaly, or both syndromes. In animals with arthrogryposis, most of the affected joints are ankylosed and cannot be straightened. Central nervous system (CNS) lesions may include hydranencephaly, hydrocephalus, agenesis of the brain, microencephaly, porencephaly, or cerebellar cavitation. Gelatinous softenings and fluid–filled cysts are sometimes found in the cerebral hemispheres and, less often, in the midbrain and cerebellum. Fibrinous leptomeningitis, fibrinous ependymitis, and spinal cord agenesis or hypoplasia have also been seen. Other abnormalities may include torticollis, scoliosis, brachygnathism, cataracts, ophthalmia, presternal steatosis, hypoplasia of the skeletal muscles and lungs, fibrinous polyarticular synovitis, and fibrinous omphalitis. Shallow erosions are sometimes found around the muzzle and nares and between the digits.

Morbidity and mortality

Most animals in endemic areas are immune to the virus by sexual maturity. Outbreaks usually occur at the limits of the virus' geographic range, when the virus is spread to susceptible animals by favorable environmental conditions. Pregnant animals that are moved into endemic areas are also at risk. Subsequent pregnancies are not affected, and vaccines are available in some countries.

The mortality rate is very high in affected newborns. Most animals die soon after birth or must be euthanized.

Diagnosis

Clinical

Akabane disease should be suspected during an outbreak of aborted, mummified, premature, or stillborn fetuses with arthrogryposis and hydranencephaly. No history of disease is expected in the dam.

Differential diagnosis

In the United States, Akabane disease in small ruminants must be differentiated from infection with Cache Valley virus. Bovine virus diarrhea, Border disease, Wesselsbron disease, and a variety of nutritional, genetic, and toxic diseases should also be considered.

Laboratory tests

Akabane disease is often diagnosed by serology. Antibodies can be found in serum samples from the fetus or the presuckle neonate, and sometimes in cerebrospinal fluid or other body fluids. The absence of antibodies in the fetus or newborn does not rule out this disease. In adults, serology is only useful in areas where the virus is nonendemic; lack of a maternal immune response rules out Akabane infection. Available serologic tests include microtiter neutralization, agar gel immunodiffusion, hemagglutination inhibition, and hemolysis inhibition assays. Low titers in unpaired serum samples may be due to cross–reactions.

Akabane virus can be isolated by inoculating tissues into suckling mice, 4–day old chick embryos, or a variety of cell lines. The virus is identified by immunofluorescence and virus neutralization. Virus isolation is rarely successful unless the fetus and placenta were aborted before the fetus developed an immune response. Akabane virus cannot be isolated from maternal tissues by the time the affected fetuses are born.

Immunofluorescent staining can also be used to detect virus antigens in the brain and muscle of aborted fetuses.

Samples to collect

Before collecting or sending any samples from animals with a suspected foreign animal disease, the proper authorities should be contacted. Samples should only be sent under secure conditions and to authorized laboratories to prevent the spread of the disease.

Samples of the placenta, as well as muscle, cerebrospinal fluid, and nervous tissue should be collected from the fetus for virus isolation. Serum samples should be taken from the dam, the fetus, or the neonate before it is allowed to suckle. Pieces of liver, spleen, kidney, heart, lung, lymph nodes, spinal cord, brain, and affected muscle should be placed in 10% buffered formalin for histopathology. The samples should be delivered (on ice) to a laboratory within 24 hours. If shipping will be delayed, the specimens should be quick–frozen and not allowed to thaw during delivery.

Recommended actions if Akabane disease is suspected

Notification of authorities

Akabane disease should be immediately reported to state or federal authorities.

Federal: Area Veterinarians in Charge (AVICs):
http://www.aphis.usda.gov/vs/area_offices.htm
State Veterinarians:
http://www.aphis.usda.gov/vs/sregs/official.html

Quarantine and disinfection

Akabane virus does not appear to be transmitted between animals except by arthropods. Care should be taken to prevent infection by potential vectors such as mosquitoes or gnats. If disinfection is necessary, enveloped viruses such as the Bunyaviridae are susceptible to most common viral disinfectants including hypochlorite (bleach), detergents, chlorhexidine, alcohol, phenols, and commercial disinfectants.

Public health

Human infections by Akabane virus have not been reported.

For more information

World Organization for Animal Health (OIE)
http://www.oie.int
OIE Manual of Standards
http://www.oie.int/eng/normes/mmanual/a_summry.htm
OIE International Animal Health Code
http://www.oie.int/eng/normes/mcode/A_summry.htm
USAHA Foreign Animal Diseases Book
http://www.vet.uga.edu/vpp/gray_book/FAD/

References

"Akabane." In *The Merck Veterinary Manual,* 8th ed. Edited by S.E. Aiello and A. Mays. Whitehouse Station, NJ: Merck and Co., 1998, pp. 451–452.

Charles, J.A. "Akabane Virus." *Veterinary Clinics of North America: Food Animal Practice* 10, no. 3 (1994): 525–546.

"Selection and Use of Disinfectants. Nebraska Cooperative Extension G00–1410–A." May 2001. University of Nebraska – Lincoln. 3 Oct 2001. http://ianrsearch.unl.edu/pubs/animaldisease/g1410.htm.

St. George, T.D. "Akabane." In *Foreign Animal Diseases*. Richmond, VA: United States Animal Health Association, 1998, pp. 62–70.

Amblyomma hebraeum

Bont Tick, Southern Africa Bont Tick

Importance

Amblyomma hebraeum is a hard tick that infests livestock and wildlife. This tick can leave large wounds that may become infected by bacteria or infested by screwworms. It can also transmit heartwater (infection by *Ehrlichia*—formerly *Cowdria*—*ruminantium*) to ruminants. Its larvae transmit tick typhus (infection by *Rickettsia conorii*) to humans.

Species affected

Immature ticks feed on small mammals, ground–feeding birds, and reptiles. Adult ticks can be found on livestock and wildlife including antelope.

Geographic distribution

A. hebraeum is found in the tropics and subtropics. It prefers moderately humid, warm savannas. This tick is endemic in South Africa, Zimbabwe, Botswana, Namibia, Malawi, Mozambique, and Angola.

Life cycle

Amblyomma hebraeum is a three–host tick. Immature ticks feed on small mammals, ground–feeding birds, reptiles and all domestic ruminant species. Adult ticks can be found on livestock and wildlife including antelope. Adults can usually be found on the relatively hairless parts of the body. Most are found on the ventral body surface, the perineum, axillae and under the tail.

Identification

A. hebraeum is a member of the family Ixodidae (hard ticks). Hard ticks have a dorsal shield (scutum) and their mouthparts (capitulum) protrude forward when they are seen from above. Amblyomma ticks are large variegated ticks with long, strong mouthparts. The palps are long; the second segment is twice as long as it is wide. Eyes are present and the festoons are well developed. The males have no adanal shields, accessory shields, or subanal shield.

A. hebraeum males are 4.2–5.7 mm long, oval ticks. The capitulum is long, with a rectangular basis; the lateral margins are rounded and the posterolateral angles are rounded and slightly salient. Palpal segment 2 is approximately three times as long as palpal segment 3. The hypostomal dentition is 3.5/3.5. The scutum is smooth and convex, with fine black or brown spots and stripes on a pale greenish white background. The posteromedian stripe is narrow and is knobbed anteriorly; it rarely reaches the falciform stripe. The poster–accessory stripes are short and well separated from the third lateral spots. The festoons, with the exception of the external festoons, are pale. The scutal eyes are small, slightly convex, and circular. The ventral surface is dull greenish yellow, with distinct ventral plaques and festoons with dark brown scutes (obsolete on the external one). The spiracular plate is moderately large and triangular, with rounded angles. The legs are dark brown, moderately stout, and have apical yellow banding at the distal end of each segment. Coxa I has two unequal spurs, coxae II and III contain salient ridges, and coxa IV has a short stout spur. The tarsi are short and abruptly attenuated.

Unfed *A. hebraeum* females are 5 mm long; engorged females can be up as long as 20 mm. The dorsum is dark greenish–brown or black, punctate and striate. The capitulum is 2 mm long, with a rectangular basis, convex lateral margins, and slightly salient posterolateral angles. The palpi are slender; segment 2 is slightly curved and is approximately 2.5 times as long as segment 3. The hypostome is long and slightly spatulate. The dentition is 3.5/3.5. The scutum is ornate, with widespread pale coloration, and is slightly longer than wide. The cervical grooves are deep anteriorly, but become shallow and end in the posterior third of the scutum. The cervical stripe extends posteriorly to the limiting spots and is generally connected to a small frontal spot by a thin line. The scapulae are dark and the punctuations are fine; however, the punctuations are coarser and more crowded in the scapular field. The eyes are pale, circular, and bulging. The genital opening is level with the interspace between coxa II and coxa III. The legs are thinner than in the male and legs III and IV have pale stripes.

Recommended actions if *Amblyomma hebraeum* is suspected

Notification of authorities

Known or suspected *A. hebraeum* infestations should be immediately reported to state or federal authorities.

Federal: Area Veterinarians in Charge (AVICs):
http://www.aphis.usda.gov/vs/area_offices.htm
State Veterinarians:
http://www.aphis.usda.gov/vs/sregs/official.html

Control measures

Acaricides can eliminate these ticks from the animal, but do not prevent reinfestation. Three–host ticks spend at least 90% of their life cycle in the environment rather than on the host animal; ticks must be controlled in the environment to prevent their spread.

Public health

A. hebraeum larvae transmit tick typhus (infection by *Rickettsia conorii*) to humans.

For more information

World Organization for Animal Health (OIE)
http://www.oie.int
OIE International Animal Health Code
http://www.oie.int/eng/normes/mcode/A_summry.htm
USAHA Foreign Animal Diseases Book
http://www.vet.uga.edu/vpp/gray_book/FAD/
Identification of the Paralysis Tick *I. holocyclus* and Related Ticks
http://members.ozemail.com.au/~norbertf/identification.htm
Hard Ticks (photographs) from the University of Edinburgh
http://www.nhc.ed.ac.uk/collections/ticks/hard.htm#Amblyomma

References

"*Amblyomma* spp." In *The Merck Veterinary Manual*, 8th ed. Edited by S.E. Aiello and A. Mays. Whitehouse Station, NJ: Merck and Co., 1998, pp. 673–674.

Arthur, D.R. "Genus *Amblyomma*." In *Ticks and Disease*. New York: Pergamon Press, 1961, pp. 77–79.

"Disease Information." 2001 Merial. 3 December 2001. http//nz.merial.com/farmers/sheep/disease/haema.html.

"Identification of the Paralysis Tick *I. holocyclus* and Related Ticks." February 2001. New South Wales Department of Agriculture. 29 November 2001. http//members.ozemail.com.au/~norbertf/identification.htm>.

Amblyomma variegatum

Tropical Bont Tick, Tropical African Bont Tick

Importance

Amblyomma variegatum is a hard tick that feeds on a number of domestic animals including cattle, sheep, goats, horses, and dogs. Its bite is severe and painful and may result in septic wounds, abscesses, inflammation on the teats of cows, and significant damage to the skin. In some regions, the bites may become infested by screwworms. This tick can transmit heartwater (infection by *Ehrlichia*—formerly *Cowdria*—*ruminantium*) to ruminants. It also spreads acute bovine dermatophilosis and is a host for Crimean–Congo hemorrhagic fever virus, Dugbe virus, Thogoto virus, Bhanja virus, Jos virus, and yellow fever virus. Its larvae transmit tick typhus (infection by *Rickettsia conorii*) to humans.

Species affected

Immature ticks feed on small mammals, ground–feeding birds, reptiles, cattle, sheep, and goats. Adult ticks prefer cattle, but can also be found on sheep, goats, horses, camels, dogs, and some large wildlife including antelope.

Geographic distribution

A. variegatum is found in the tropics and subtropics. This tick is endemic in sub–Saharan savannas in many countries in Africa, as well as in southern Arabia, the Caribbean, and some islands in the Atlantic and Indian Oceans. An eradication program is in progress in the Caribbean.

Life cycle

A. variegatum is a three–host tick. Immature ticks feed on small mammals, ground–feeding birds, and reptiles, as well as cattle, sheep, and goats. Adult ticks prefer cattle, but can also be found on other livestock, dogs, and some wildlife. The adult ticks are usually found on the relatively hairless parts of the body. Most are located on the ventral body surface, the genitalia, and under the tail.

Identification

A. variegatum is a member of the family Ixodidae (hard ticks). Hard ticks have a dorsal shield (scutum) and their mouthparts (capitulum) protrude forward when they are seen from above. Amblyomma ticks are large ticks with long, strong mouthparts. The palps are long; the second segment is twice as long as it is wide. Eyes are present and the festoons are well developed. The males have no adanal shields, accessory shields, or subanal shield. Female *A. variegatum* are brown, but the males are brightly ornamented with orange. When they are engorged, the adult female ticks are about the size of a nutmeg.

Recommended actions if *Amblyomma variegatum* is suspected

Notification of authorities

Known or suspected *A.variegatum* infestations should be immediately reported to state or federal authorities.

Federal: Area Veterinarians in Charge (AVICs):
http://www.aphis.usda.gov/vs/area_offices.htm
State Veterinarians:
http://www.aphis.usda.gov/vs/sregs/official.html

Control measures

Acaricides can eliminate these ticks from the animal, but do not prevent reinfestation and must be repeated periodically. Three–host ticks spend at least 90% of their life cycle in the environment rather than on the host animal; ticks in the environment must also be controlled to prevent their spread.

Public health

A. variegatum can spread a number of exotic diseases to humans, including Crimean–Congo hemorrhagic fever virus, yellow fever virus, and tick typhus.

For more information

World Organization for Animal Health (OIE)
http://www.oie.int
OIE International Animal Health Code
http://www.oie.int/eng/normes/mcode/A_summry.htm
USAHA Foreign Animal Diseases Book
http://www.vet.uga.edu/vpp/gray_book/FAD/
Identification of the Paralysis Tick *I. holocyclus* and Related Ticks
http://members.ozemail.com.au/~norbertf/identification.htm
Hard Ticks (photographs) from the University of Edinburgh
http://www.nhc.ed.ac.uk/collections/ticks/hard.htm#Amblyomma

References

"*Amblyomma spp.*" In *The Merck Veterinary Manual*, 8th ed. Edited by S.E. Aiello and A. Mays. Whitehouse Station, NJ: Merck and Co., 1998, pp. 673–674.

"Identification of the paralysis tick *I. holocyclus* and related ticks." February 2001. New South Wales Department of Agriculture. 29 November 2001. http//members.ozemail.com.au/~norbertf/identification.htm.

Pegram, R.G., A. Rota, R. Onkelinx, D.D. Wilson, P. Bartlette, B.S. Nisbett, G. Swanston, P. Vanterpool, and J.J. de Castro. "Eradicating the tropical bont tick from the Caribbean." 30 November 2001. http//www.fao.org/ag/AGa/AGAP/WAR/warall/W2650T/W2650t06.htm.

Wilson, D.D. and R.A. Bram. "Foreign pests and vectors of arthropod–borne diseases." In *Foreign Animal Diseases*. Richmond, VA: United States Animal Health Association, 1998, pp. 225–239.

Anthrax

Charbon, Malignant Pustule, Malignant Carbuncle, Milzbrand, Splenic Fever, Woolsorter's Disease

Importance

Outbreaks of anthrax can have economic importance due to high mortality, especially among ruminants. Anthrax is a potentially fatal zoonotic disease. Spores can survive in the environment for many decades making eradication difficult. Historically, anthrax was the first disease of man and animals to be demonstrated to be caused by a microorganism. Much of the early research on bacteria and vaccines was done using anthrax.

Etiology

Anthrax is caused by *Bacillus anthracis*, a spore–forming, encapsulated, Gram–positive rod–shaped bacterium.

Species affected

Herbivores are the primary hosts of *Bacillus anthracis*. Other mammals, including humans, are more resistant and considered incidental hosts.

Geographic distribution

Anthrax has a world–wide distribution. Infection is common in some areas of Africa and Asia. Outbreaks occasionally occur in Europe, America, and Australasia.

Transmission

Transmission can occur through ingestion, inhalation or cutaneous routes. Animals are most commonly infected by ingestion of spores from contaminated soil. Human infection is frequently caused by exposure of open wounds on the skin to animal products such as meat, hides, or wool. Infection can also occur by inhalation of spores and possibly fly bites in some regions.

Incubation period

The incubation period varies from 1 to 20 days.

Clinical signs

The clinical signs in different species can vary due to susceptibility and route of infection. Many of the signs are due to toxin production by the bacteria. Ruminants are the most susceptible to infection and sudden death may occur without observation of other signs. The animal may appear healthy even a few hours before death. Signs prior to death include fever, disorientation, muscle tremors, dyspnea, congested mucous membranes, terminal convulsions, and collapse. Some animals may show signs up to 48 hours prior to death.

In horses, in addition to signs of septicemia, ingestion causes enteritis and colic, while cutaneous injection of spores by biting flies may cause edematous swellings. Death usually occurs in 1 to 3 days, but some animals can survive up to a week.

Pigs, dogs, and cats are more commonly affected with signs of fever, depression, anorexia, weakness, prostration, and death, or chronic infection with localized swelling, fever, enlarged lymph nodes, and possible death if the airway becomes obstructed. Ingestion is the most common route of infection in these species and the organism may localize in pharyngeal lymph nodes, or cause generalized bacteremia or acute gastroenteritis. Carnivores are generally more resistant and recovery is not uncommon.

Post mortem lesions

In ruminants, lesions consistent with generalized septicemia are seen including a rapidly decomposing bloated carcass with incomplete rigor mortis, poorly clotted dark blood coming from the anus, vulva, nostrils and mouth, multiple petechial hemorrhages, and an enlarged spleen with 'blackberry jam' consistency. These lesions can be similar to those caused by other infectious and toxic causes of acute death. Horses will have similar septicemic lesions and may also have edematous lesions especially of the throat and neck. In omnivores (pigs) and carnivores, findings of septicemia as described for ruminants may occur, but more often there is extensive edema and inflammation in the pharyngeal area. If the infection is in the gastrointestinal tract, severe inflammation, sometimes with hemorrhage and necrosis, may be seen in the stomach, intestines, and mesenteric lymph nodes, accompanied by peritonitis and excessive peritoneal fluid.

Morbidity and mortality

Mortality can be very high, especially in ruminants. In carnivores, mortality is relatively low.

Diagnosis

Clinical

Anthrax should be considered a possibility in cases of sudden death in herbivores with unclotted blood from nose, mouth, anus or vulva. In pigs and carnivores, localized edema especially in the neck area is suggestive of anthrax infection.

Differential diagnosis

In animals, differentials include blackleg, botulism, toxicosis (plants, heavy metals, snake bite), lightning strike, and peracute babesiosis.

Laboratory tests

Laboratory diagnostic tests include susceptibility to specific bacteriophages, sensitivity to penicillin (*B. anthracis* exhibits a characteristic 'string–of–pearls' formation when grown with penicillin), and animal inoculation (mice, guinea pigs) to satisfy Koch's postu-

lates. A thermoprecipitin test described by Ascoli in 1911 has been used to detect *B. anthracis* in decomposed carcasses.

Serological tests are rarely used for diagnosis in animals. In humans, the following tests have been used: agar gel immunodiffusion, indirect microhemagglutination, enzyme immunoassay which includes enzyme–linked immunosorbent assay, and electrophoretic immunotransblot.

Samples to collect

If anthrax is suspected, it is best not to perform a necropsy in order to prevent environmental contamination with spores. Anthrax is a zoonotic disease; samples should be collected and handled with all appropriate precautions. The collection and shipment of samples should conform to all state and federal regulations.

Due to poor clotting, a blood sample can be taken post mortem from a vein, such as the caudal vein. Blood smears should be made and the blood submitted for isolation of *B. anthracis*. The collection site should be covered with a disinfectant–soaked bandage to prevent leakage of contaminated blood.

Recommended actions if anthrax is suspected

Notification of authorities

State and/or federal veterinarians should be informed of any suspected anthrax case.

Federal: Area Veterinarians in Charge (AVICs):
http://www.aphis.usda.gov/vs/area_offices.htm
State Veterinarians:
http://www.aphis.usda.gov/vs/sregs/official.html

Quarantine and disinfection

Quarantine of the affected premises and disinfection are important. *B. anthracis* can be destroyed with 5-10% formaldehyde (15-30% formalin). Chlorine solutions must be very strong to eliminate anthrax spores. Vaccination of susceptible animals in surrounding areas may be necessary. Carcasses are best destroyed by burning. Burial has not been found to be sufficient as spores can survive for decades in the environment.

Public health

Veterinarians, animal handlers, laboratory personnel and industrial workers can all be exposed to anthrax through contact with infected tissues. Protection using latex gloves, face mask, and other protective clothing is recommended when handling specimens suspected to be infected with *B. anthracis*.

In humans, the cutaneous form is most common due to exposure to infected animals or animal products. The infective spores enter the skin through open wounds or abrasions. Within 3 to 5 days (up to 12 days) a small pimple appears which progresses to a typical anthrax eschar over another 2 to 3 days. This ulcerated dry black scab surrounded by vesicles and edema can vary in size from two to several centimeters. The lesion begins to heal in about 10 days taking 2 to 6 weeks to completely resolve. Cutaneous infections can occasionally lead to systemic bacteremia, septicemia and death if not treated. Pulmonary and intestinal forms, due to inhalation or ingestion of spores, begin with mild symptoms of slight fever, malaise and gastroenteritis for a few days then progress to severe illness with signs of fever, chills, prostration, shock, collapse and death within just a few hours. In humans, 10% to 20% of cutaneous cases may be potentially fatal without antibiotic treatment. Early treatment with antibiotics is important when signs suggestive of anthrax are seen in people with potential exposure to the disease. A vaccine is available for those with increased risk for exposure.

For more information

World Organization for Animal Health (OIE)
http://www.oie.int

OIE Manual of Standards
   http://www.oie.int/eng/normes/mmanual/a_summry.htm
OIE International Animal Health Code
   http://www.oie.int/eng/normes/mcode/A_summry.htm
USAHA Foreign Animal Diseases Book
   http://www.vet.uga.edu/vpp/gray_book/FAD/

References

"Anthrax." In *Manual of Standards for Diagnostic Tests and Vaccines.*
   Paris: World Organization for Animal Health, 2000, pp.
   233–244.
Turnbull, P.C.B. In *Zoonoses.* Edited by S.R. Palmer, E.J.L. Soulsby
   and D.I.H Simpson. New York: Oxford University Press,
   1998, pp. 3-16.

Aujeszky's Disease

Pseudorabies, Mad Itch

Importance

Aujeszky's disease is an economically significant disease of pigs. This viral infection causes central nervous system (CNS) signs and high mortality in young animals and respiratory illness in older pigs. The causative virus can also infect other species, resulting in a fatal CNS disease. An eradication program for Aujeszky's disease was established in 1989; as of May 2005 all U.S. states were free of this disease.

Etiology

Aujeszky's disease results from infection by pseudorabies virus, an alphaherpesvirus in the family Herpesviridae. This virus can become latent in the trigeminal ganglia in pigs.

Species affected

Pigs are the natural host for the pseudorabies virus and the only animal to become latently infected. However, the virus can infect nearly all mammals, including cattle, sheep, goats, cats, and dogs. It does not infect humans or many other primates, and infections in horses are rare.

Geographic distribution

Aujeszky's disease can be found in most of Europe, Mexico, Cuba, Brazil, Venezuela, New Zealand, Samoa, and Southeast Asia. A surveillance program is ongoing in the United States; as of May 2005, all states had achieved status V (free).

Transmission

The pseudorabies virus is transmitted by respiratory or fecal–oral routes. In pigs, the virus can be found in the tonsillar epithelium, milk, urine, and vaginal and preputial secretions for more than two weeks during acute infections. The virus can remain infectious for as long as seven hours in the air, if the relative humidity is at least 55%, and may travel up to three kilometers as an aerosol. Under favorable conditions, it can also survive for several days in contaminated bedding and water. Infected pigs can become latent carriers. The inactive virus is carried in the trigeminal ganglia and can become reactivated after stressors such as transport, crowding, corticosteroid injections, or farrowing.

Other animals usually become infected through contact with infected pigs. Sheep and cattle are generally thought to be dead–end hosts, but may occasionally excrete some virus. Infected rats, other wildlife, and dogs and cats may act as vectors.

Incubation period

The incubation period in pigs is one week.

Clinical signs

In pigs, the clinical signs depend on the age of the animal. Piglets less than a week old may die within hours with no symptoms, or may have fever, anorexia, weight loss, tremors, paddling, or other symptoms of CNS involvement. Mortality in this age group is very high. In slightly older pigs, the clinical signs can include fever, anorexia, vomiting, depression, respiratory symptoms, and CNS signs. Common CNS signs include incoordination, muscle twitching, somnolence, convulsions, paralysis, or a "goose–stepping" gait. In weaned pigs, Aujeszky's disease is mainly a respiratory illness. In this age group, the symptoms may include a fever, anorexia, weight loss, coughing, sneezing, conjunctivitis, and dyspnea. CNS signs are occasionally seen. In adults, the infection is usually mild or inapparent; respiratory symptoms predominate. Pregnant sows may reabsorb the infected fetuses or abort. Piglets born alive may be weak and trembling.

In cattle and sheep, Aujeszky's disease is almost always fatal within a few days. The first symptom is intense pruritis of a patch of skin, which usually leads to severe licking, rubbing, or gnawing. Self–mutilation is common. Animals become progressively weaker and eventually recumbent. Convulsions, bellowing, teeth grinding, pharyngeal paralysis, cardiac irregularities, and rapid, shallow breathing are common. The clinical signs are similar in dogs and cats. Profuse salivation may resemble rabies.

Post mortem lesions

In pigs, post–mortem lesions are often subtle or difficult to find. Many pigs have a serous or fibrinonecrotic rhinitis; this may be visible only if the head is split and the nasal cavity opened. Other lesions may include necrotic tonsillitis, pharyngitis, or placentitis, and secondary pneumonia. Pulmonary edema, congestion, or consolidation can sometimes be found. The pulmonary lymph nodes may contain petechial hemorrhages, and the liver may have necrotic foci. Often, there are no gross lesions.

Typically, nonsuppurative meningoencephalitis is found upon microscopic examination of the white and gray matter. The meninges are usually thickened from mononuclear cell infiltration. Mononuclear perivascular cuffing and neuronal necrosis may be seen. Additional findings can include necrotic tonsillitis, bronchitis, bronchiolitis, and alveolitis. There may be focal necrosis in the liver, spleen, adrenal glands, and lymph nodes.

In species other than pigs, the only lesions may be areas of edema, congestion, and hemorrhage in the spinal cord. These lesions are usually found in the portion of the spinal cord that innervates the area of pruritis. Microscopically, there is cellular infiltration and neuronal degeneration. CNS lesions similar to those found in pigs, but milder, are often found.

Morbidity and mortality

Aujeszky's disease is most common in pigs. In this species, mortality may be as low as 1% to 2% in grower and finisher pigs, up to 50% in nursery pigs, and as high as 100% in animals less than a week old. Sporadic cases are seen in other species in close contact with pigs. In these species, the disease is always fatal.

A vaccine is available, but there is no specific treatment for infections.

Diagnosis

Clinical

Aujeszky's disease should be suspected in pig herds with high mortality and CNS symptoms in young piglets, and lower mortality and respiratory signs in older animals. It should also be suspected in other species with intense pruritis and other typical CNS signs.

Differential diagnosis

In pigs, the differential diagnosis includes porcine polio-encephalomyelitis, classical swine fever, hemagglutinating encephalomyelitis infection, streptococcal meningoencephalitis, swine influenza, salt poisoning, hypoglycemia, poisoning by organic arsenic or mercury, and congenital tremor. Diseases that result in abortions may also need to be ruled out. In species other than pigs, rabies and scrapie must be considered.

Laboratory tests

Aujeszky's disease can be diagnosed by isolation of the pseudorabies virus, detection of viral DNA by polymerase chain reaction (PCR), or serology. Virus isolation is possible on a number of cell lines; porcine kidney (PK–15) cells are most often used. Latent virus can be difficult to isolate.

An alternative method is to identify viral DNA in secretions or organ samples with PCR. A fluorescent antibody test can detect virus antigens in the tonsils, pharyngeal mucosa, and brain.

Serologic tests include virus neutralization, enzyme–linked immunosorbent assay (ELISA), and latex agglutination tests. ELISAs can distinguish antibodies from a natural infection and antibodies that have been stimulated by gene–deleted vaccines. In species other than pigs, the animal often dies before mounting an antibody response.

Samples to collect

In live pigs, nasal swabs should be taken for virus isolation. The swabs should be placed in sterile saline with antibiotics or in virus transport medium. Pseudorabies virus may also be isolated from oropharyngeal fluid or biopsies of the tonsils.

At necropsy, the spleen, brain, lung, and tonsil are the preferred organs for virus isolation from pigs. Half of the brain (longitudinal section) and samples of the other organs should be collected aseptically. In latently infected pigs, virus isolation is most likely to be successful from the trigeminal ganglion. In other species, the section of the spinal cord that innervated the pruritic area should be collected. The pruritic area of the skin, together with the subcutaneous tissues, should also be submitted. Samples for virus isolation should be sent to the laboratory under cold conditions.

Samples submitted for histology should include brain, spinal cord, ganglia, tonsils, mesenteric lymph nodes, spleen, lung, kidney, and liver. Samples from the brain or the tonsils can be collected for fluorescent antibody tests. At least 10 ml of serum should also be collected for serology.

Recommended actions if Aujeszky's disease is suspected

Notification of authorities

Aujeszky's disease is a reportable disease in the United States. Specific guidelines for each state should be consulted. If Aujeszky's disease should be reported immediately to state or federal authorities upon diagnosis or suspicion of the disease:
Federal: Area Veterinarians in Charge (AVICs):
http://www.aphis.usda.gov/vs/area_offices.htm
State Veterinarians:
http://www.aphis.usda.gov/vs/sregs/official.html

Quarantine and disinfection

A voluntary eradication program for Aujeszky's disease is in progress in the United States; vaccination, quarantine of infected herds, depopulation, and disinfection are cornerstones of this plan. The pseudorabies virus is susceptible to orthophenylphenols and quaternary ammonium compounds. It is also inactivated by sunlight, drying, and high temperatures.

Public health

The symptoms of pseudorabies have not been seen in humans. Seroconversion does occur.

For more information

World Organization for Animal Health (OIE)
http://www.oie.int

OIE Manual of Standards
http://www.oie.int/eng/normes/mmanual/a_summry.htm
OIE International Animal Health Code
http://www.oie.int/eng/normes/mcode/A_summry.htm

References

"Aujeszky's Disease." In *Manual of Standards for Diagnostic Tests and Vaccines*. Paris: World Organization for Animal Health, 2000, pp. 245–257.

"Pseudorabies." In *The Merck Veterinary Manual*, 8th ed. Edited by S.E. Aiello and A. Mays. Whitehouse Station, NJ: Merck and Co., 1998, pp. 964–966.

"Pseudorabies (Aujeszky's Disease)." Pork News and Views 1996 July/August. Accessed 9 Oct 2001. http://www.gov.on.ca/OMAFRA/english/livestock/swine/news/julaug96.html.

"Accelerated Pseudorabies Eradication Program." July 2001 United States Department of Agriculture Animal and Plant Health Inspection Service. Accessed 9 Oct 2001. http://www.aphis.usda.gov/oa/apep/.

"Pseudorabies Eradication Program Report: Updated Report, May 2005." United States Department of Agriculture. Animal and Plant Health Inspection Service. Accessed 12 Jan 2006. http://www.aphis.usda.gov/vs/nahps/pseudorabies/update.html.

Avian Influenza, Highly Pathogenic

Fowl Plague

Importance

Highly pathogenic avian influenza (HPAI) is a serious and often fatal infection in domestic poultry. An epidemic can cause significant economic damage. A 1983–1984 outbreak in the northeastern United States resulted in federal control costs of nearly $65 million, the destruction of more than 17 million birds, and a 30% increase in retail egg prices. Eradication of highly pathogenic avian influenza from domestic poultry is possible, but there is always the possibility of reintroduction through migratory waterfowl, other wild birds, and pet birds.

Etiology

Avian influenza results from infection by type A influenza viruses (family Orthomyxoviridae). Numerous avian influenza viruses exist, but only viruses with certain virulence characteristics (pathogenicity in birds or cell cultures and/or specific genetic sequences) are designated highly pathogenic avian influenza. Two surface antigens, hemagglutinin (H) and neuraminidase (N), are used to classify the viruses into serotypes. Although there are 16 recognized hemagglutinin subtypes of avian influenza, only the H5 and H7 subtypes have been associated with the HPAI phenotype. Most of the H5 and H7 avian influenza viruses that are isolated are classified as low pathogenic, although some have the potential to mutate to the HPAI form of the virus. Avian influenza viruses are also involved in the production of new mammalian strains of influenza virus through genetic reassortment.

Species affected

Type A influenza viruses from all species are similar, but the viruses typically will have higher specificity for one species or related groups of animals. Therefore, human influenza viruses typically infect only humans. With birds, similar host specificity is observed, although some generalization according to families of birds can be made. For example, the gallinaceous birds, including chickens, turkeys, quail, and pheasant often have a severe fatal infection with HPAI viruses, but the same viruses may cause only minor disease when they infect ducks, geese and other waterfowl. In some outbreaks, a virus may affect only one species of birds present on a farm. Avian influenza viruses can also be isolated from apparently healthy migratory waterfowl, sea birds, shore birds, imported pet birds, and ratites. Birds other than domestic poultry often do not show clinical symptoms of HPAI.

Geographic distribution

Highly pathogenic avian influenza viruses can be found worldwide. Outbreaks have occurred in Australia, Cambodia, Chile, China, Croatia, England, Korea, Indonesia, Ireland, Italy, Malaysia, Mexico, Mongolia, the Netherlands, Pakistan, Romania, Russia, Scotland, Thailand, Turkey, Ukraine, the United States and Vietnam.

In early 2004, widespread outbreaks of HPAI (H5N1) occurred in poultry in Asia (Cambodia, China, Indonesia, Japan, Laos, South Korea, Thailand and Vietnam). By March 2004, the outbreak was reported to be under control. Since late June 2004, however, new outbreaks of a H5N1 (HPAI) virus have been reported in poultry in China, Indonesia, Romania, Thailand, Turkey, Ukraine and Vietnam and in wild migratory birds in China, Croatia, Mongolia and Russia. Human, feline and possibly swine infections and deaths have been associated with some of these outbreaks.

Transmission

Avian influenza viruses appear to spread to poultry from migratory waterfowl. The feces contain large amounts of virus, which can infect a new host. Once the virus has spread from the natural reservoir to chickens and turkeys, the virus can spread on the farm by both the aerosol route and the fecal–oral route because of the close proximity of the birds. The low pathogenic form of the virus, under some circumstances, can mutate to the highly pathogenic form of the virus. Vertical transmission is unlikely because infected embryos rarely survive and hatch.

Fomites and infected birds can transmit the disease between flocks. In one outbreak in Pennsylvania, the virus may have been spread by garbage flies. The spreading of manure onto agricultural fields has also been a likely source of disease spread.

Incubation period

The incubation period is 1 to 7 days.

Clinical signs

The clinical signs of highly pathogenic avian influenza include marked depression with ruffled feathers, excessive thirst, inappetence, and watery diarrhea that progresses from bright green to white. In some cases, sudden death may be seen with few clinical signs.

In mature chickens, the combs are often swollen and may be cyanotic at the tip or contain ecchymoses and necrotic foci. The wattles are often swollen and may be cyanot. Congestion, swelling, or hemorrhages can be seen on the conjunctivae, edema may occur around the eyes and on the neck, and the legs may have diffuse areas of hemorrhage. Coughing, sneezing, and nasal discharge may also be seen. Egg production stops; the last eggs laid often have no shells. Death is common, but severely affected hens occasionally recover.

In broilers, the clinical signs may include severe depression, inappetence, facial and neck edema, neurologic signs including torticollis and ataxia, and death.

Similar symptoms are seen in turkeys. Swollen sinuses are seen occasionally in turkeys.

Although ducks and geese develop viremia, clinical signs are usually minimal. In rare cases the viruses cause neurological signs like torticollis and depression. Some mortality, especially in geese, has been observed in both natural and experimental infections.

Post mortem lesions

During necropsy, excessive fluid may flow from the nares and oral cavity. Subcutaneous edema may be present on the head and neck, and petechial hemorrhages may be found on the inside of the keel. The conjunctivae can be severely congested and may contain petechiae. Very small petechiae are sometimes found on the abdominal fat, serosal surfaces, and peritoneum; epicardial hemorrhages are often prominent. The mucosa of the proventriculus, gizzard, and intestines may contain hemorrhages. The kidneys are often severely congested and occasionally plugged with white urate deposits. Either hemorrhagic tracheitis or a normal trachea with excessive mucus may be seen. Lungs are often edematous and congested or hemorrhagic. In laying hens, the ovary can be hemorrhagic or degenerated and contain necrotic foci, the peritoneal cavity may contain yolk, and there may be severe airsacculitis and peritonitis. In young birds and birds with peracute disease, the only significant lesions may be dehydration and severe congestion of the muscles.

The post–mortem lesions in domestic turkeys are similar to those in chickens but may not be as severe.

Morbidity and mortality

Morbidity and mortality often approach 100% in domestic poultry. Any survivors are usually in poor condition and do not begin laying again for several weeks.

A vaccine for the H5 serotype has recently been licensed by APHIS for limited use in case of an outbreak. No commercially available vaccine can be purchased in the U.S. at this time.

Diagnosis

Clinical

Highly pathogenic avian influenza should be suspected when severe depression, inappetence, and a drastic drop in egg production are followed by sudden deaths in the flock. Facial edema, swollen and cyanotic combs and wattles, and petechial hemorrhages on the internal organs support this diagnosis.

Differential diagnosis

The differential diagnosis includes exotic Newcastle disease (END), infectious laryngotracheitis, and acute bacterial diseases including fowl cholera and *Escherichia coli* infections.

Laboratory tests

Avian influenza is usually diagnosed by virus isolation in embryonated fowl eggs or by reverse–transcription polymerase chain reaction (RT–PCR) tests. Virus isolation can be confirmed by agar gel immunodiffusion (AGID) tests, enzyme–linked immunosorbent assays (ELISAs). The isolate is subtyped with antisera against the hemagglutinin and neuraminidase antigens. Highly pathogenic strains are identified by their lethality in susceptible chickens and genetic sequence.

Serology can also be helpful in diagnosis. AGID tests are commonly used for surveillance for any AI infection in poultry. ELISA tests are also available. However, not all species of birds make precipitating antibodies. Hemagglutination inhibition tests are also used, but are subtype specific and may miss some infections.

Samples to collect

Before collecting or sending any samples from animals with a suspected foreign animal disease, the proper authorities should be contacted. Samples should only be sent under secure conditions and to authorized laboratories to prevent the spread of the disease. Some isolates of the avian influenza virus may be zoonotic; samples should be collected and handled with all appropriate precautions.

For virus isolation from live birds, tracheal and cloacal swabs should be collected. If this is not feasible, samples of fresh feces may also yield virus. Oronasal and cloacal swabs or intestinal contents should be taken from dead birds. The trachea, spleen, lung, air sac, kidney, liver, heart, intestines, and brain may also be sampled. Samples should be taken from several birds, as many may not yield virus.

For transport to the laboratory, the swabs should be placed in virus transport media (brain heart infusion media with or without antibiotics). With large numbers of samples, oropharyngeal or cloacal swabs from up to five birds may be pooled in one tube of broth (do not mix oropharyngeal and cloacal swabs in the same tube). Alternatively, samples of tissues (approximately 0.5 cubic cm each) can be collected and placed into the virus transport medium. The samples should be sent to the laboratory on wet ice. If shipment will be delayed for more than 24 hours, the specimens should be quick–frozen and not allowed to thaw during shipment. Blood should also be taken from several birds for serology.

Recommended actions if highly pathogenic avian influenza is suspected

Notification of authorities

Highly pathogenic avian influenza must be reported promptly to state or federal authorities upon diagnosis or suspicion of the disease.

Federal: Area Veterinarians in Charge (AVICs):
http://www.aphis.usda.gov/vs/area_offices.htm
State Veterinarians:
http://www.aphis.usda.gov/vs/sregs/official.html

Quarantine and disinfection

To control an outbreak of highly pathogenic avian influenza, the premises must be thoroughly cleaned and disinfected. Insects and mice on the premises should be eliminated, then the flock depopulated and the carcasses destroyed by burying, composting, or rendering. Once the birds have been killed, the manure and feed should be removed down to a bare concrete floor. If the floor is earthen, one inch or more of soil should also be removed. The manure can be buried at least five feet deep. It may also be composted for 90 days or longer, depending on the environmental conditions. The compost should be tightly covered with black polyethylene sheets to prevent entry of birds, insects, and rodents. Feathers can be burned or composted; alternatively, they may be removed and the area wet down with disinfectant.

High–pressure spray equipment should be used to clean all equipment and building surfaces. Once all surfaces are clean and free of all organic material, the entire premises should be sprayed with an approved residual disinfectant. Many disinfectants are usually effective for AI.

Public health

Avian influenza viruses were once thought to be nonpathogenic for humans; however, in 1997, 18 people were infected and six people died from an H5 avian influenza virus in Hong Kong. Additional cases of human infection in Hong Kong and China have also been reported since the 1997 outbreak. Prior to this outbreak, only sporadic cases of human infection with avian influenza virus had been reported.

During the 2003 outbreak of H7N7 avian influenza in the Netherlands, 86 people were diagnosed with infection with the poultry virus. Most of the cases had only symptoms of conjunctivitis, although several people had influenza–like illness, and one veterinarian died from complications related to the H7N7 infection.

The 2004-2005 avian influenza (H5N1) outbreak in Asia impacted human health. Between December 2003 and November 29, 2005, 133 human cases and 68 deaths were confirmed in Thailand, Vietnam, Cambodia, Indonesia, and China. Most cases occurred as a result of people having direct or close contact with infected poultry or contaminated surfaces. Person-to-person transmission during this outbreak has been rare and has not continued beyond one person.

For More Information

World Organization for Animal Health (OIE)
http://www.oie.int
OIE Manual of Standards
http://www.oie.int/eng/normes/mmanual/a_summry.htm

OIE International Animal Health Code
http://www.oie.int/eng/normes/mcode/A_summry.htm
USAHA Foreign Animal Diseases Book
http://www.vet.uga.edu/vpp/gray_book/FAD/

References

Beard, C.W. Avian influenza. In *Foreign Animal Diseases*. Richmond, VA:United States Animal Health Association, 1998; 71–80.

Centers for Disease Control and Prevention. Key facts about avian influenza (Bird Flu) and avian influenza A (H5N1) virus. January 10, 2006. Accessed Jan. 12, 2006. http://www.cdc.gov/flu/avian/gen_info/facts.htm.

Influenza. In Aiello SE, Mays D, editors. The *Merck Veterinary Manual*. 8th ed. Whitehouse Station, NJ:Merck and Co., 1998; 1983.

World Health Organization for Animal Health (OIE). Highly pathogenic avian influenza. In *Manual of Standards for Diagnostic Tests and Vaccines*. Paris:World Organization for Animal Health, 2000; 212–220.

United States Department of Agriculture. Animal and Plant Health Inspection Service Web site. Highly pathogenic avian influenza. May 2001. Accessed Oct 24, 2001. http://www.aphis.usda.gov/oa/pubs/avianflu.html.

Bluetongue

Sore Muzzle, Pseudo Foot and Mouth Disease, Muzzle Disease

Importance

Bluetongue is an insect–borne viral disease of ruminants; among domestic animals, clinical disease is seen most often in sheep. This disease can result in significant morbidity; affected sheep may have erosions and ulcerations on the mucous membranes, dyspnea, or lameness from muscle necrosis and inflammation of the coronary band. Affected animals may slough their hooves and surviving animals can lose part or all of their wool. Some strains of the virus can result in mortality rates as high as 50%.

Etiology

Bluetongue results from infection by the bluetongue virus, an orbivirus in the family Reoviridae. Twenty–four serotypes have been identified worldwide; five have been isolated in the United States.

Species affected

Bluetongue virus infects ruminants including sheep, goats, cattle, buffalo, deer, antelope, bighorn sheep, and North American elk. Clinical disease is seen often in sheep, occasionally in goats, and rarely in cattle. In Africa, some large carnivores have antibodies to bluetongue, and, in the United States, a contaminated vaccine resulted in some abortions in dogs.

Geographic distribution

Bluetongue has been found in Africa, Europe, the Middle East, the South Pacific, North America, South America, and parts of Asia. In the United States, the distribution of the vector limits infections to the southern and western states.

Transmission

Bluetongue virus is transmitted by biting midges in the genus *Culicoides*. In the United States, *Culicoides varipennis* var *sonorensis* is the principal vector. Ticks or sheep keds can be mechanical vectors but are probably of minor importance in disease transmission. Bluetongue is not a contagious disease; however, virus can be spread mechanically on surgical equipment and needles. Bluetongue virus can be found in semen, but venereal spread does not appear to be a major route of infection.

Incubation period

In sheep, the incubation period is usually 5 to 10 days. Cattle can become viremic starting at 4 days post–infection, but rarely develop symptoms. Animals are usually infectious to the insect vector for several weeks.

Clinical signs

In sheep, the clinical signs may include fever, excessive salivation, depression, dyspnea, and panting. Initially, animals have a clear nasal discharge; later, the discharge becomes mucopurulent and dries to a crust around the nostrils. The muzzle, lips, and ears are hyperemic and the lips and tongue may be very swollen. The tongue is occasionally cyanotic and protrudes from the mouth. The head and ears may also be edematous. Erosions and ulcerations are often found in the mouth; these lesions may become extensive and the mucous membranes may become necrotic and slough. The coronary bands on the hooves are often hyperemic and the hooves painful; lameness is common and animals may slough their hooves if they are driven. Pregnant ewes may abort their fetuses, or give birth to "dummy" lambs. Additional clinical signs can include torticollis, vomiting, pneumonia, or conjunctivitis. The death rate varies with the strain of virus. Three or four weeks after recovery, some surviving sheep can lose some or all of their wool.

Infections in cattle are usually subclinical; often, the only signs of disease are changes in the leukocyte count and a fluctuation in rectal temperature. Rarely, cattle have mild hyperemia, vesicles, or ulcers in the mouth, hyperemia around the coronary band, hyperesthesia, or a vesicular and ulcerative dermatitis. The skin may have thick folds, particularly in the cervical region. The external nares may contain erosions and a crusty exudate. Temporary sterility may be seen in bulls. Infected cows may give birth to calves with hydranencephaly or cerebral cysts. Cattle that have clinically apparent disease may develop severe breaks in the hooves several weeks after infection; such breaks are usually followed by foot rot.

In pronghorn antelope and whitetail deer, the most common symptoms are hemorrhages and sudden death. Infections in goats are usually subclinical, similar to disease in cattle.

Post mortem lesions

In sheep, the face and ears are often edematous. A dry, crusty exudate may be seen on the nostrils. The coronary bands of the hooves are often hyperemic; petechial or ecchymotic hemorrhages may be present and extend down the horn. Petechiae, ulcers and erosions are common in the oral cavity, particularly on the tongue and dental pad, and the oral mucous membranes may be necrotic or cyanotic. The nasal mucosa and pharynx may be edematous or cyanotic and the trachea hyperemic and congested. Froth is sometimes seen in the trachea and fluid may be found in the thoracic cavity. Hyperemia and occasional erosions may be seen in the reticulum and omasum. Petechiae, ecchymoses, and necrotic foci may be found in the heart. In some cases, hyperemia, hemorrhages, and edema are found throughout the internal organs. Hemorrhage at the base of the pulmonary artery is particularly characteristic of this disease. The intermuscular fascial planes may be expanded by edema fluid, and the skeletal muscles may have focal hemorrhages or necrosis.

In deer, the most prominent lesions are widespread petechial to ecchymotic hemorrhages. More chronically infected deer may have ulcers and necrotic debris in the oral cavity and lesions on the hooves, including severe fissures or sloughing.

Morbidity and mortality

In sheep, the severity of disease varies with the breed of sheep, strain of virus, and environmental stress. Morbidity can be up to 100% and mortality is usually 0% to 50%. Similar morbidity and mortality rates are seen in bighorn sheep.

Most infections in cattle, goats, and North American elk are asymptomatic. In cattle, morbidity may be up to 5%, but death is rare. In some animals, lameness and poor condition can persist for some time.

Infections are usually severe in whitetail deer and pronghorn antelope. In these two species, morbidity rates are as high as 100% and mortality is usually 80% to 90%.

Vaccines are available, but are specific for each serotype. Vaccines can cause fetal malformations during the first 100 days of gestation in ewes and may be able to recombine with field strains to produce new strains of virus.

Diagnosis

Clinical

Bluetongue should be suspected when typical clinical signs are seen during seasons when insects are active. A recent history of wasting and foot rot in the herd supports the diagnosis.

Differential diagnosis

The differential diagnosis includes foot and mouth disease, vesicular stomatitis, peste de petits ruminants, plant photosensitization, malignant catarrhal fever, bovine virus diarrhea, infectious bovine rhinotracheitis, parainfluenza–3 infection, contagious ecthyma (contagious pustular dermatitis), sheep pox, foot rot, and *Oestrus ovis* infestation.

Laboratory tests

Bluetongue can be diagnosed by isolating the virus in cell cultures or embryonated chicken eggs. Appropriate cell cultures include mouse L, baby hamster kidney (BHK)–21, African green monkey kidney (Vero), and *Aedes albopictus* (AA) cells. Isolation in embryonated eggs is more sensitive than isolation in cell culture. Virus identity is confirmed by antigen–capture enzyme–linked immunosorbent assay (ELISA), immunofluorescence, immunoperoxidase, or virus neutralization tests.

Polymerase chain reaction (PCR) techniques are widely used to identify the virus in clinical samples. These techniques allow for rapid diagnosis and can identify the virus serogroup and serotype.

Bluetongue can also be diagnosed by animal inoculation studies in sheep, suckling mice, or hamsters. Virus isolation is particularly valuable when the virus titer is very low.

Serology is sometimes used for diagnosis. Antibodies appear 7 to 14 days after infection and are usually long–lasting. Available serologic tests include agar gel immunodiffusion (AGID), competitive ELISA, and virus neutralization. Complement fixation is also used in some countries. The AGID and ELISA tests can identify serogroup–specific antibodies.

Samples to collect

A human infection has been documented in one laboratory worker; reasonable precautions should be taken while working with this virus.

Blood samples (for virus isolation) and serum should be collected from several live animals. Spleen, bone marrow, or both are the tissues of choice at necropsy. Other authorities recommend spleen, heart, and mesenteric lymph nodes. Blood and serum should be collected from lambs with congenital disease; spleen, lung, and brain tissue should also be sent, if they are available. All samples should be transported cold but not frozen and sent to the laboratory as soon as possible.

Recommended actions if bluetongue is suspected
Notification of authorities

Bluetongue is a reportable disease in many states. State authorities should be consulted for more specific information.

Federal: Area Veterinarians in Charge (AVICs):

Quarantine and disinfection

Bluetongue is transmitted by insect vectors and is not contagious by casual contact. Disinfectants cannot prevent the virus from being transmitted between animals; however, where disinfection is warranted, sodium hypochlorite or 3% sodium hydroxide are effective. Insect control is important in limiting the spread of the disease; synthetic pyrethroids or organophosphates are effective against *Culicoides*. Moving animals into barns in the evening can also reduce the risk of infection.

Public health

Bluetongue is not a significant threat to human health. However, one human infection has been documented in a laboratory worker and reasonable precautions should be taken while working with this virus.

For more information

World Organization for Animal Health (OIE)
http://www.oie.int
OIE Manual of Standards
http://www.oie.int/eng/normes/mmanual/a_summry.htm
OIE International Animal Health Code
http://www.oie.int/eng/normes/mcode/A_summry.htm
USAHA Foreign Animal Diseases Book
http://www.vet.uga.edu/vpp/gray_book/FAD/
Animal Health Australia. The National Animal
Health Information System (NAHIS)
http://www.aahc.com.au/nahis/disease/dislist.asp

References

Abraham, G., J. Morrison, C. Mayberry, B. Cottam, and R. Gobby. "*Australian Veterinary Emergency Plan* (Ausvetplan 2000) Operational Procedures Manual. Decontamination." Agriculture and Resource Management Council of Australia and New Zealand 2000. 14 December 2001. http//www.aahc.com.au/ausvetplan/decfnl2.pdf.

Blackwell, J.H. "Cleaning and Disinfection." In *Foreign Animal Diseases*. Richmond, VA: United States Animal Health Association, 1998, pp. 445–448.

"Bluetongue." Animal Health Australia. The National Animal Health Information System (NAHIS). 11 December 2001. http//www.brs.gov.au/usr–bin/aphb/ahsq?dislist=alpha.

"Bluetongue." In *Manual of Standards for Diagnostic Tests and Vaccines*. Paris: World Organization for Animal Health, 2000, pp. 153–167.

"Bluetongue." In *The Merck Veterinary Manual*, 8th ed. Edited by S.E. Aiello and A. Mays. Whitehouse Station, NJ: Merck and Co., 1998, pp. 520–521.

"Guidelines for the management of a suspected outbreak of foreign disease at federally–inspected slaughter establishments." Canadian Food Inspection Agency 14 December 2001. http//www.inspection.gc.ca/english/anima/meavia/mmopmmhv/chap9/9.1–3e.shtml.

Stott, J.L. "Bluetongue and Epizootic Hemorrhagic Disease." In *Foreign Animal Diseases*. Richmond, VA: United States Animal Health Association, 1998, pp. 106–117.

Boophilus annulatus
Cattle Tick, Cattle Fever Tick, American Cattle Tick

Importance

Boophilus annulatus is a hard tick found most often on cattle. It can transmit babesiosis (*Babesia bigemina* and *Babesia bovis* infections) and anaplasmosis (infection by *Anaplasma marginale*). Heavy tick burdens on infested animals can decrease production and damage hides.

Species affected

The preferred hosts for this species are cattle.

Geographic distribution

B. annulatus is found in subtropical and tropical regions. This tick is endemic in the southern regions of the former U.S.S.R., Africa, the Middle East, the Near East, the Mediterranean, and Mexico. It has been eradicated from North America, but can be sometimes found in Texas or California, in a buffer quarantine zone along the Mexican border.

Life cycle

B. annulatus is a one–host tick; all stages are spent on one animal. The eggs hatch in the environment and the larvae crawl up grass or other plants to find a host. They may also be blown by the wind. In the summer, *B. annulatus* ticks can survive for as long as 3 to 4 months without feeding. In cooler temperatures, they may live without food for up to 6 months.

Newly attached ticks are usually found on the softer skin inside the thigh, flanks, and forelegs. They may also be seen on the abdomen and brisket.

Identification

Boophilus annulatus is a member of the family Ixodidae (hard ticks). Hard ticks have a dorsal shield (scutum) and their mouthparts (capitulum) protrude forward when they are seen from above. *Boophilus* ticks have a hexagonal basis capitulum. The spiracular plate is rounded or oval and the palps are very short, compressed, and ridged dorsally and laterally. Males have adanal shields and accessory shields. The anal groove is absent or indistinct in females, and faint in males. There are no festoons or ornamentation.

Recommended actions if *Boophilus annulatus* is suspected

Notification of authorities

Suspected or known *B. annulatus* infestations should be reported immediately to state or federal authorities.
Federal: Area Veterinarians in Charge (AVICs):
http://www.aphis.usda.gov/vs/area_offices.htm
State Veterinarians:
http://www.aphis.usda.gov/vs/sregs/official.html

Control measures

Farms and ranches with *B. annulatus* infestations are placed under quarantine for 6 to 9 months. A single acaricide treatment can destroy all of the ticks on an animal, but will not prevent reinfestation. Cattle that have had direct or presumed contact with *B. annulatus* must be dipped at regular intervals for at least a year.

Public health

B. annulatus can spread babesiosis to susceptible (usually splenectomized) humans.

For more information

World Organization for Animal Health (OIE)
http://www.oie.int
OIE International Animal Health Code
http://www.oie.int/eng/normes/mcode/A_summry.htm
USAHA Foreign Animal Diseases Book
http://www.vet.uga.edu/vpp/gray_book/FAD/

U.S. Department of Agriculture, Animal and Plant Health Inspection Service (USDA APHIS) http://www.aphis.usda.gov.

Identification of the Paralysis Tick *I. holocyclus* and Related Ticks http://members.ozemail.com.au/~norbertf/identification.htm

References

"*Boophilus* spp." In *The Merck Veterinary Manual*, 8th ed. Edited by S.E. Aiello and A. Mays. Whitehouse Station, NJ: Merck and Co., 1998, pp. 674–675.

"Controlling Cattle Fever Ticks." February 2001 United States Department of Agriculture, Animal and Plant Health Inspection Service. 29 November 2001. http//www.aphis.usda.gov/oa/pubs/fscfever.html.

Corwin, R.M. and J. Nahm. "*Boophilus* spp." 1997 University of Missouri College of Veterinary Medicine. 29 November 2001 http//www.parasitology.org/Arthropods/Arachnida/Boophilus.htm.

"Identification of the paralysis tick *I. holocyclus* and related ticks. February 2001 New South Wales Department of Agriculture. 29 November 2001. http//members.ozemail.com.au/~norbertf/identification.htm.

Boophilus microplus

Southern Cattle Tick, Cattle Tick

Importance

Boophilus microplus is a hard tick that can be found on many hosts including cattle, buffalo, horses, donkeys, goats, sheep, deer, pigs, and dogs. It can transmit babesiosis (*Babesia bigemina* and *Babesia bovis* infections) and anaplasmosis (infection by *Anaplasma marginale*). Heavy tick burdens on infested animals can decrease production and damage hides.

Species affected

B. microplus infests mainly cattle, deer, and buffalo, but can also be found on horses, goats, sheep, donkeys, dogs and pigs.

Geographic distribution

B. microplus can be found worldwide in subtropical and tropical regions. This tick is endemic in the Indian region, much of Asia, northeastern Australia, Madagascar, parts of Africa, the Caribbean, and many countries in South and Central America, including Mexico. It has been eradicated from North America, but can be sometimes found in Texas or California, in a buffer quarantine zone along the Mexican border.

Life cycle

B. microplus is a one–host tick; all stages are spent on one animal. The eggs hatch in the environment and the larvae crawl up grass or other plants to find a host. They may also be blown by the wind. In the summer, *B. microplus* can survive for as long as 3 to 4 months without feeding. In cooler temperatures, they may live without food for up to 6 months.

Newly attached ticks are usually found on the softer skin inside the thigh, flanks, and forelegs. They may also be seen on the abdomen and brisket.

Identification

Boophilus microplus is a member of the family Ixodidae (hard ticks). Hard ticks have a dorsal shield (scutum) and their mouthparts (capitulum) protrude forward when they are seen from above. *Boophilus* ticks have a hexagonal basis capitulum. The spiracular plate is rounded or oval and the palps are very short, compressed, and ridged dorsally and laterally. Males have adanal shields and accessory shields. The anal groove is absent or indistinct in females, and faint in males. There are no festoons or ornamentation.

B. microplus adults have a short, straight capitulum. The legs are pale cream and there is a wide space between first pair of legs and the snout. The body is oval to rectangular and the shield is oval and wider at the front. The snout is short and straight.

The nymphs of this species have an orange–brown scutum. The body is oval and wider at front. The body color is brown to blue–gray, with white at the front and sides.

B microplus larvae have a short, straight capitulum and a brown to cream body. Larvae have 6 legs instead of 8.

Recommended actions if *Boophilus microplus* is suspected

Notification of authorities

Suspected or known *B. microplus* infestations should be reported immediately to state or federal authorities.

Federal: Area Veterinarians in Charge (AVICs): http://www.aphis.usda.gov/vs/area_offices.htm

State Veterinarians: http://www.aphis.usda.gov/vs/sregs/official.html

Control measures

Farms and ranches with *B. microplus* infestations are placed under quarantine for 6 to 9 months. A single acaricide treatment can destroy all of the ticks on an animal, but will not prevent reinfestation. Cattle that have had direct or presumed contact with *B. microplus* must be dipped at regular intervals for at least a year.

Public health

B. microplus can spread babesiosis to susceptible (usually splenectomized) humans.

For more information

World Organization for Animal Health (OIE) http://www.oie.int

OIE International Animal Health Code http://www.oie.int/eng/normes/mcode/A_summry.htm

USAHA Foreign Animal Diseases Book http://www.vet.uga.edu/vpp/gray_book/FAD/

U.S. Department of Agriculture, Animal and Plant Health Inspection Service (USDA APHIS) http://www.aphis.usda.gov

Distinguishing Common Ticks on the East Coast of Australia http://members.ozemail.com.au/~norbertf/common.htm

Identification of the Paralysis Tick *I. holocyclus* and Related Ticks http://members.ozemail.com.au/~norbertf/identification.htm

Larval Stages of the Paralysis Tick *Ixodes holocyclus*, the Cattle Tick *Boophilus microplus* and the Bush Tick *Haemaphysalis longicornis* http://members.ozemail.com.au/~norbertf/larvae.htm

Nymphal Stages of the Paralysis Tick *Ixodes holocyclus*, the Cattle Tick *Boophilus microplus* and the Bush Tick *Haemaphysalis longicornis* http://members.ozemail.com.au/~norbertf/nymphs.htm

References

"*Boophilus* spp." In *The Merck Veterinary Manual*, 8th ed. Edited by S.E. Aiello and A. Mays. Whitehouse Station, NJ: Merck and Co., 1998, pp. 674–675.

"Controlling Cattle Fever Ticks." February 2001 United States Department of Agriculture, Animal and Plant Health Inspection Service. 29 November 2001. http//www.aphis.usda.gov/oa/pubs/fscfever.html.

Corwin, R.M. and J. Nahm. "*Boophilus* spp." 1997 University of Missouri, College of Veterinary Medicine. 29 November

2001. http//www.parasitology.org/Arthropods/Arachnida/
Boophilus.htm.

"Distinguishing Common Ticks on the East Coast of Australia."
February 2001. New South Wales Department of Agriculture. 29 November 2001. http//members.ozemail.com.
au/~norbertf/common.htm.

"Identification of the Paralysis Tick *I. holocyclu*s and Related
Ticks." February 2001 New South Wales Department of
Agriculture. 29 November 2001. http//members.ozemail.
com.au/~norbertf/identification.htm.

"Larval Stages of the Paralysis Tick *Ixodes holocyclus*, the Cattle
Tick *Boophilus microplus* and the Bush Tick *Haemaphysalis longicornis*."
February 2001 New South Wales Department of Agricul-
ture. 29 November 2001. http//members.ozemail.com.
au/~norbertf/larvae.htm>.

"Nymphal Stages of the Paralysis Tick *Ixodes holocyclus*, the Cattle
Tick *Boophilus microplus* and the Bush Tick *Haemaphysalis longicornis*." February 2001 New South Wales Department of
Agriculture. 29 November 2001. http//members.ozemail.
com.au/~norbertf/nymphs.htm>.

Botulism

*Bulbar Paralysis, Lamziekte, Limberneck, Loin
Disease, Shaker Foal Syndrome, Toxicoinfectious
Botulism, Western Duck Sickness*

Importance

Botulism, caused by a *Clostridium botulinum* neurotoxin, can
affect many species of mammals, birds, and fish. Among animals,
this disease is seen most often in waterfowl, poultry, mink, cattle,
sheep, horses, and some species of fish; an estimated 10 to 50
thousand wild waterfowl are killed annually by botulism. A form
of botulism also appears to be responsible for the shaker foal
syndrome in horses. In humans, *C. botulinum* can cause descending
flaccid paralysis, generally beginning with the cranial nerves and
– if left untreated – progressing through the body causing respiratory and limb paralysis. Death due to respiratory failure occurs in
approximately 5% of human cases. Botulinum toxins can be used
as a bioterrorist weapon spread by aerosol, or contamination of
food or drink, therefore all cases should be reported immediately
and thoroughly investigated. Naturally caused cases of botulism
are rare in domestic mammals in the United States; cases in wildfowl and poultry are more common.

Etiology

Clostridium botulinum is a spore–forming, anaerobic bacterium
which produces a potent neurotoxin. Botulism can result from
the ingestion of preformed toxin or the growth of *C. botulinum*
in anaerobic tissues. Seven types of botulism toxin are known,
designated by the letters A through G. Types A, B, E and F cause
illness in humans. Type C is the most common cause of botulism
in animals. Type D is sometimes seen in cattle and dogs, and type
B can occur in horses. Types A and E are found occasionally in
mink and birds. Type G rarely causes disease, although a few cases
have been seen in humans. All types of botulinum toxin produce
the same disease; however, the toxin type is important if antiserum
is used for treatment.

Species affected

Many species of mammals and birds, as well as some fish, can
be affected by botulism. Clinical disease is seen most often in wildfowl, poultry, mink, cattle, sheep, horses, and some species of fish.

Dogs, cats, and pigs are relatively resistant; botulism is seen occasionally in dogs and pigs but has not been reported from cats.

Geographic distribution

C. botulinum is found in the soil worldwide. In ruminants,
botulism mainly occurs in areas where phosphorus or protein
deficiencies are found. Botulism is seen regularly in cattle in South
Africa and sheep in Australia. This disease is rare in ruminants
in the United States, although a few cases have been reported in
Texas and Montana.

Transmission

Although *C. botulinum* and its spores are widely distributed in
soils, the intestinal tracts of fish and mammals, and the gills and
viscera of shellfish, the bacteria can only grow under anaerobic
conditions. Botulism occurs when animals ingest the preformed
toxins in food or *C. botulinum* spores germinate in anaerobic tissues
and produce toxins as they grow.

Preformed toxins can be found in a variety of sources, including decaying vegetable matter (grass, hay, grain, spoiled silage) and
carcasses. Carnivores usually ingest the toxins in contaminated
meat such as chopped raw meat or fish. Ruminants in phosphorus–deficient areas may chew bones and scraps of attached meat;
a gram of dried flesh can have enough botulinum toxin to kill a
cow. Ruminants may also be fed hay or silage contaminated by the
toxin–containing carcasses of birds or mammals. Horses usually
ingest the toxin in contaminated forage. Birds can ingest the toxins
in maggots that have fed on contaminated carcasses or in dead
invertebrates from water with decaying vegetation. Cannibalism
and contaminated feed may also result in cases in poultry.

The toxicoinfectious form of botulism occurs when an anaerobic wound is contaminated with *C. botulinum*. Sites predisposed to
C. botulinum infection can include gastrointestinal ulcers, abscesses
in the navel, liver, or lungs, and skin or muscle wounds. This form
of botulism appears to be responsible for shaker foal syndrome in
horses. Toxicoinfectious botulism is also seen in chickens, when
broilers are intensively reared on litter; the cause of this phenom-
enon is unknown.

Incubation period

The incubation period can be 2 hours to 2 weeks; in most
cases, the symptoms appear after 12 to 24 hours. Mink are often
found dead within 24 hours of ingesting the toxin.

Clinical signs

Botulism is characterized by progressive motor paralysis. Typical clinical signs may include muscle paralysis, difficulty chewing
and swallowing, visual disturbances, and generalized weakness.
Death usually results from paralysis of the respiratory or cardiac
muscles.

Ruminants

In cattle, the symptoms may include drooling, restlessness,
incoordination, urine retention, dysphagia, and sternal recumbency.
Laterally recumbent animals are usually very close to death. In
sheep, the symptoms may include drooling, a serous nasal discharge, stiffness, and incoordination. Abdominal respiration may
be observed and the tail may switch on the side. As the disease
progresses, the limbs may become paralyzed and death may occur.

Horses

The clinical signs in horses are similar to cattle. The symptoms
may include restlessness, knuckling, incoordination, paralysis of
the tongue, drooling, and sternal recumbency. The muscle paralysis
is progressive; it usually begins at the hindquarters and gradually
moves to the front limbs, head, and neck.

The shaker foal syndrome is usually seen in animals less than 4
weeks old. The most characteristic signs are a stilted gait, muscle
tremors, and the inability to stand for more than 4 to 5 minutes.
Other symptoms may include dysphagia, constipation, mydriasis,

and frequent urination. In the later stages, foals usually develop tachycardia and dyspnea. Death generally occurs 24 to 72 hours after the initial symptoms and results from respiratory paralysis. Some foals are found dead without other clinical signs.

Pigs

Pigs are relatively resistant to botulism. Reported symptoms include anorexia, refusal to drink, vomiting, pupillary dilation, and muscle paralysis.

Foxes and Mink

During outbreaks of botulism, many animals are typically found dead, while others have various degrees of paralysis and dyspnea. The clinical picture is similar in commercially raised foxes.

Birds

In poultry and wild birds, flaccid paralysis is usually seen in the legs, wings, neck, and eyelids. Wildfowl with paralyzed necks may drown. Broiler chickens with the toxicoinfectious form may also have diarrhea with excess urates.

Post mortem lesions

There are no distinct, diagnostic post mortem lesions. Respiratory paralysis may cause nonspecific signs in the lungs. In the shaker foal syndrome, the most consist lesions are excess pericardial fluid with strands of fibrin, pulmonary edema, and congestion.

Morbidity and mortality

Botulism is common in wild waterfowl; an estimated 10 to 50 thousand wild birds are killed annually. In some large outbreaks, a million or more birds may die. Ducks appear to be affected most often. Botulism also affects commercially raised poultry. In chickens, the mortality rate varies from a few birds to 40% of the flock. Some affected birds may recover without treatment.

Botulism seems to be relatively uncommon in most domestic mammals; however, in some parts of the world, epidemics with up to 65% morbidity are seen in cattle. The prognosis is poor in large animals that are recumbent. In cattle, death generally occurs within 6 to 72 hours after sternal recumbency. Most dogs with botulism recover within 2 weeks.

Diagnosis

Clinical

A presumptive diagnosis of botulism may be made with the clinical signs and history. If possible, the diagnosis should be confirmed with testing (see below).

Differential diagnosis

Other causes of motor paralysis should be ruled out in all species. In poultry, mild infections characterized by leg paralysis should be differentiated from Marek's disease, drug or chemical toxicity, and skeletal abnormalities. In waterfowl, the differential diagnosis includes fowl cholera and chemical toxicity, particularly lead poisoning.

Laboratory tests

Botulism can be difficult to diagnose, as the toxin is not always found in clinical samples or the feed. Diagnosis is often a matter of excluding other diseases. A definitive diagnosis can be made if botulinum toxin is identified in the feed, stomach or intestinal contents, vomitus or feces. The toxin is occasionally found in the blood in peracute cases. Botulinum toxin can be detected by a variety of techniques, including enzyme–linked immunosorbent assays (ELISAs), electrochemiluminescent (ECL) tests and mouse inoculation or feeding trials. The toxins can be typed with neutralization tests in mice.

In toxicoinfectious botulism, the organism can be cultured from tissues. *C. botulinum* is an anaerobic, Gram positive, spore–forming rod. On egg yolk medium, toxin–producing colonies usually display surface iridescence that extends beyond the colony.

Samples to collect

Serum, feces, gastric fluid, intestinal contents, and food suspected of contamination can be submitted for testing. Cultures may also be taken from infected wounds. Samples should be kept refrigerated.

Recommended actions if botulism is suspected

Notification of authorities

Local, state and federal authorities should be notified of any possible cases of botulism.

Federal: Area Veterinarians in Charge (AVICs):
http://www.aphis.usda.gov/vs/area_offices.htm
State Veterinarians:
http://www.aphis.usda.gov/vs/sregs/official.html

Quarantine and disinfection

Quarantine is not necessary. Botulism is not communicable by casual contact but, in some cases, tissues from dead animals can be toxic if ingested by other animals.

Botulinum toxins are large, easily denatured proteins. They can be inactivated by exposure to sunlight, chemical disinfection with 0.1% sodium hypochlorite or 0.1 N NaOH, or heating to 80°C for 30 minutes or 100°C for 10 minutes. Chlorine and other disinfectants can destroy the toxins in water. The vegetative cells of *Clostridium botulinum* are susceptible to many disinfectants, including 1% sodium hypochlorite and 70% ethanol. The spores are resistant to environmental conditions but can be destroyed by moist heat (120°C for at least 15 min).

Public health

In humans, botulism is classified into three forms: foodborne, wound, and infant or intestinal botulism. Foodborne botulism is caused by ingestion of neurotoxins when food is not properly handled to control bacterial growth. Inadequate heating during canning or food preparation is the most common cause. Wound botulism is caused by contamination with soil and insufficient cleansing of wounds allowing *C. botulinum* spores to germinate in an anaerobic environment and produce toxin. Injectable drug users have an increased risk of wound botulism. Intestinal botulism generally occurs in children less than a year of age. It is caused by the ingestion of *C. botulinum* spores which germinate in the intestinal tract and produce toxin. Although honey is the most well known source of botulism in infants, many foods can potentially contain spores from the soil. Adults with altered gastrointestinal microflora are also susceptible to this form of botulism.

Foodborne and wound botulism cause a symmetrical, descending, flaccid paralysis. The cranial nerves are generally affected first causing double vision, blurred vision, drooping eyelids, slurred speech, difficulty swallowing, and dry mouth. Constipation or diarrhea, and vomiting may also be seen initially. The signs progress to paralysis of respiratory muscles, arms, and legs. Wound botulism is very similar to foodborne infections; however, gastrointestinal signs are not usually present and patients may have a wound exudate or develop a fever. Infants with botulism show similar signs with lethargy, poor feeding, constipation, drooping eyelids, difficulty swallowing, loss of head control, progressive weakness or paralysis, and respiratory depression or arrest. The onset may be gradual or sudden.

Public education on proper handling of food, refrigeration and home canning techniques helps to prevent cases of foodborne botulism. Early identification and treatment of the disease are important in recovery. In the United States where treatment is readily available, the case fatality rate for this form is 5% to 10%. Death is usually caused by respiratory failure. Early treatment with botulinum antitoxin may help to prevent progression of paralysis. Recovery can take months to years. The case fatality rate for hospitalized cases of infant botulism is less than 1%. Some suggest botulism may be the cause for up to 5% of sudden infant death syndrome (SIDS) cases.

For more information

Centers for Disease Control and Prevention (CDC)
http://www.cdc.gov/ncidod/dbmd/diseaseinfo/
botulism_t.htm
Material Safety Data Sheets-Canadian Laboratory
Centre for Disease Control
http://www.phac-aspc.gc.ca/msds-ftss/index.html
USAMRIID's Medical Management of Biological
Casualties Handbook
http://www.vnh.org/BIOCASU/toc.html
U.S. FDA Foodborne Pathogenic Microorganisms and Natural
Toxins Handbook (Bad Bug Book)
http://vm.cfsan.fda.gov/~mow/intro.html

References

"Botulinum." In *Medical Management of Biological Casualties Handbook*, 4th ed. Edited by M. Kortepeter, G. Christopher, T. Cieslak, R. Culpepper, R. Darling J. Pavlin, J. Rowe, K. McKee, Jr., E. Eitzen, Jr. Department of Defense, 2001. 10 Dec 2002 http//www.vnh.org/BIOCASU/17.html.

"Botulism." Centers for Disease Control and Prevention (CDC), June 2002. 10 Dec 2002. http//www.cdc.gov/ncidod/dbmd/diseaseinfo/botulism_t.htm.

"Botulism." In *Control of Communicable Diseases Manual*, 17th ed. Edited by J. Chin. Washington, D.C.: American Public Health Association, 2000, pp. 70–75.

"Botulism." In *The Merck Veterinary Manual*, 8th ed. Edited by S.E. Aiello and A. Mays. Whitehouse Station, NJ: Merck and Co., 1998, pp. 442–444; 916; 1315; 1362; 1969–1970.

"*Clostridium botulinum.*" In *Foodborne Pathogenic Microorganisms and Natural Toxins Handbook*. U.S. Food & Drug Administration, Center for Food Safety & Applied Nutrition, Feb 2002. 12 Dec 2002. http//www.cfsan.fda.gov/~mow/chap2.html

Herenda, D., P.G. Chambers, A. Ettriqui, P. Seneviratna, and T.J.P. da Silva. "Botulism." In *Manual on Meat Inspection for Developing Countries*. FAO Animal Production and Health Paper 119. 1994 Publishing and Multimedia Service, Information Division, FAO, 12 Dec 2002. http//www.fao.org/docrep/003/t0756e/T0756E03.htm#ch3.3.2.

"Material Safety Data Sheet – *Clostridium botulinum.*" January 2001. Canadian Laboratory Centre for Disease Control. 10 Dec 2002 http//www.phac-aspc.gc.ca/msds-ftss/index.html.

Solomon H.M. and T. Lilly, Jr. "*Clostridium botulinum.*" In *Bacteriological Analytical Manual Online*, 8th ed. U.S. Food and Drug Administration, January 2001. 12 Dec 2002. http//vm.cfsan.fda.gov/~ebam/bam–17.html.

Wells C.L. and T.D. Wilkins. "*Clostridia*: sporeforming anaerobic bacilli." In *Medical Microbiology*. 4th ed. Edited by Samuel Baron. New York; Churchill Livingstone, 1996. 10 Dec 2002. http//www.gsbs.utmb.edu/microbook/ch018.htm.

Weber, J.T., C.L. Hatheway and M.E. St. Louis. "Botulism" In *Infectious Diseases*, 5th ed. Edited by P.D. Hoeprich, M.C. Jordan, and A.R. Ronald. Philadelphia: J. B. Lippincott Company, 1994, pp. 1185–1194.

Bovine Babesiosis
Tick Fever, Texas Fever, Piroplasmosis, Redwater

Importance

Bovine babesiosis is a tick–borne infection with significant morbidity and mortality. The economic losses from this disease can be considerable. In 1906, $130 million was lost to tick infestation and endemic bovine babesiosis in the southern United States. In today's economy, this would represent more than a billion dollars. Babesiosis and its vectors were eradicated in the United States by 1943; however, the disease is still widespread in other parts of the world and reintroduction is a significant threat.

Etiology

Babesiosis results from infection by protozoa in the genus *Babesia* (order Piroplasmida, phylum Apicomplexa). *Babesia bovis* and *B. bigemina* are the most important species in cattle. Infections with *B. divergens*, *B. major*, *B. ovate*, and *B. jakimovi* are also seen.

Species affected

Cattle *Babesia* are largely host specific. *B. bovis* is found in cattle, water buffalo, and African buffalo. Infection in the latter two species is uncommon and they are not likely to be reservoirs for the disease. *B. bigemina* is found in cattle and buffalo. *B. jakimovi* can infect cattle, the Tartarean roe deer, Asian elk, and reindeer. *B. divergens*, *B. major*, and *B. ovate* also infect cattle.

Geographic distribution

Bovine babesiosis can be found wherever the tick vectors exist, but is most common in the tropics. *B. bovis* and *B. bigemina* are particularly important in Asia, Africa, Central and South America, southern Europe, and Australia. These two species and their vectors were formerly endemic throughout much of the southern United States, but now are found only in a quarantine buffer zone along the Mexican border. *B. divergens* is an important parasite in the United Kingdom and northwestern Europe. *B. major* is also seen in the United Kingdom and northern Europe, and *B. ovate* is found in Japan. *B. jakimovi* causes Siberian piroplasmosis.

Transmission

Babesia parasites are spread through the bite of infected ticks. Ticks become infected when they feed on infected cattle and can pass the parasites to their larvae. Larval ticks transmit *B. bovis*, while adult and nymphal ticks transmit *B. bigemina*. *Boophilus microplus* is the major vector in tropical and subtropical regions. *Ixodes ricinus* transmits *B. divergens* in northwestern Europe. *Haemaphysalis*, *Rhipicephalus*, and other species of *Boophilus* may also transmit *Babesia*. Biting flies and fomites contaminated by infected blood can act as mechanical vectors. Cattle and infected ticks are thought to be the major reservoirs of infection. *B. bigemina* can be passed transovarially through several generations.

Incubation period

The symptoms of *B. bigemina* infections usually appear 2 to 3 weeks after tick infestation; *B. bovis* takes slightly longer. After direct inoculation of blood, the incubation period is 4 to 5 days for *B. bigemina* and 10 to 12 days for *B. bovis*. Large inocula can result in shorter incubation times.

Clinical signs

Young animals are fairly resistant to infection with *Babesia* and are often asymptomatic. In older animals, *B. bigemina* is considered to be less virulent than *B. bovis*; however, strains can vary considerably in pathogenicity. Relatively innocuous isolates of *B. bigemina* are common in Australia, but highly pathogenic strains are found in Africa. Typically, animals infected with *B. bigemina* develop anorexia and a high fever, with rectal temperatures up to 41.5°C (106.7°F). Animals may separate from the herd, stand with an arched back, and display a roughened coat, dyspnea, and tachycardia. At the start of an infection, the mucus membranes are usually red and injected. As the disease progresses, they become pale from anemia. The anemia often develops rapidly and is frequently accompanied by hemoglobinuria and hemoglobinemia. The anemic crisis usually passes within a week. Central nervous system signs are not common during *B. bigemina* infections.

B. bovis is generally more virulent than *B. bigemina*. Cattle infected with *B. bovis* usually develop a high fever, anorexia, depression, ataxia, and circulatory shock. Hemoglobinuria and hemoglobinemia are less common than in *B. bigemina* infections. Sequestration of infected erythrocytes in brain capillaries may result in incoordination, teeth grinding, and mania. Animals may be found on the ground with the involuntary movements of the legs. Death often follows CNS signs.

Infection with *B. divergens* or *B. jakimovi* results in clinical symptoms similar to *B. bigemina*. Central nervous system signs are rare in *B. divergens* infections. *B. major* is nonpathogenic under most conditions, and *B. ovate* is mildly pathogenic.

Post mortem lesions

In cattle that die soon after infection, post–mortem lesions are mainly related to intravascular hemolysis. The lungs are often congested and edematous. Serosanguineous fluid and petechial hemorrhages may be visible in the pericardial sac. Other internal lesions include an enlarged, icteric liver, a distended gallbladder containing dark green bile, and a markedly enlarged spleen with a dark, pulpy consistency. Icterus and submucosal hemorrhages may be seen on the abomasal and intestinal mucosa. The urinary bladder often contains reddish–brown urine. The blood may be thin and watery. Jaundice is often present in the connective tissues. The lymph nodes are edematous and may contain petechiae.

Cattle that have died after a longer illness are often icteric and emaciated. The blood is thin and watery, the intermuscular fascia edematous, and the kidneys pale and often edematous. The liver is yellowish–brown, and flakes of semisolid material may be found in the bile. Either hemorrhagic or normal urine may be present in the urinary bladder. The spleen is enlarged but usually firmer than in acute babesiosis. Subepicardial petechial hemorrhages may also be seen.

Morbidity and mortality

Mortality in *B. bigemina* infections is highly variable. Both treatment and previous exposure can affect the outcome. Up to half of all fully susceptible adults die without treatment, but most animals raised in endemic areas survive the infection. Once hemoglobinuria develops, the prognosis is guarded. Infections with *B. bovis* are generally more severe and CNS signs suggest a poor prognosis.

Infected cattle can be treated with a variety of drugs. Cattle can develop lifelong resistance to a species after infection. Some degree of protection may also develop against other *Babesia* species. Vaccines are available in some countries against selected strains.

Animals that survive an episode of babesiosis usually experience loss of condition and a slow recovery, with severe weight loss, a drop in milk production, and possibly abortion.

Diagnosis

Clinical

Babesiosis should be suspected in cattle with fever, anemia, jaundice, and hemoglobinuria in endemic areas, particularly if there are signs of erythrocyte hemolysis.

Differential diagnosis

The differential diagnosis for bovine babesiosis includes anaplasmosis, trypanosomiasis, theileriosis, bacillary hemoglobinuria, hemobartonellosis, leptospirosis, and eperythrozoonosis. Rabies, other encephalitides, and toxins must also be considered in cattle exhibiting nervous signs.

Laboratory tests

Babesiosis is diagnosed by identification of the parasites in blood or tissue smears, positive serologic tests, or transmission experiments.

Parasites are found most easily during acute infections. *Babesia* organisms can be detected under oil immersion (minimum x8 eyepiece and x60 objective lens) in erythrocytes in blood and tissue smears. *B. bovis* can be hard to find in blood samples; brain biopsies may be helpful in detecting this species.

In chronic infections, parasites are uncommon in blood samples and diagnosis is usually made by serology. Antibodies to *Babesia* are detected with an indirect fluorescent antibody (IFA) test or ELISA.

Carriers may be identified by transfusing blood into a test animal. In vitro culture can also be helpful. DNA probes and PCR have occasionally been used.

Samples to collect

Before collecting or sending any samples from animals with a suspected foreign animal disease, the proper authorities should be contacted. Samples should only be sent under secure conditions and to authorized laboratories to prevent the spread of the disease. *B. bovis* and *B. divergens* have been implicated in rare human infections; samples should be collected and handled with all appropriate precautions.

Both thin blood films and organ smears should be taken from dead animals. Organ smears should be taken from (in order of preference) cerebral cortex, kidney, liver, lung, and bone marrow. Slides should be air–dried, fixed in absolute methanol (5 minutes for organ smears, 1 minute for blood smears), and stained for 20 to 30 minutes with 10% Giemsa. Diagnosis is unreliable in animals that have been dead for more than 24 hours; however, parasites can sometimes be found for 24 hours or more in the blood from the lower leg.

Thick and thin blood films should be taken from live animals. Six blood smears should be made for each animal. If possible, blood should be taken from the capillaries in the ear or tail. *B. bovis* parasites are most readily detected in capillary blood, but *B. bigemina* and *B. divergens* are found throughout the vasculature. Blood films should be stained as soon as possible. Thin blood films should be stained as described above; thick blood films should be air–dried, heat–fixed for 5 minutes, and stained with 5% Giemsa for 20 to 30 minutes. If samples of capillary blood are not available, blood may be collected into an anticoagulant. EDTA can be used; however, heparin can affect staining and is not recommended.

Serum can be collected for IFA or ELISA detection of antibodies.

Recommended actions if bovine babesiosis is suspected

Notification of authorities

Bovine babesiosis must be reported immediately to state or federal authorities.

Federal: Area Veterinarians in Charge (AVICs):
  http://www.aphis.usda.gov/vs/area_offices.htm
State Veterinarians:
  http://www.aphis.usda.gov/vs/sregs/official.html

Quarantine and disinfection

Disinfectants and sanitation are not generally effective against the spread of this disease. However, preventing the transfer of blood from one animal to another is vital.

Public health

B. bovis and *B. divergens* have been implicated in rare human infections. Most cases developed in splenectomized or otherwise immunodeficient individuals. These infections were often fatal.

For more information

World Organization for Animal Health (OIE)
http://www.oie.int
OIE Manual of Standards
http://www.oie.int/eng/normes/mmanual/a_summry.htm
OIE International Animal Health Code
http://www.oie.int/eng/normes/mcode/A_summry.htm
USAHA Foreign Animal Diseases Book
http://www.vet.uga.edu/vpp/gray_book/FAD/
How to Make Organ Smears for Tick fever Diagnosis
http://www.dpi.qld.gov.au/tickfever/1619.html

References

"Bovine Babesiosis." In *Manual of Standards for Diagnostic Tests and Vaccines*. Paris: World Organization for Animal Health, 2000, pp. 412–422.

"Bovine Babesiosis." In *The Merck Veterinary Manual*, 8th ed. Edited by S.E. Aiello and A. Mays. Whitehouse Station, NJ: Merck and Co., 1998, pp. 23–25.

"How to Make Organ Smears for Tick Fever Diagnosis." 28 Aug. 2001 Queensland Government Department of Primary Industries. 29 Aug 2001. http//www.dpi.qld.gov.au/tickfever/1619.html

Kuttler, K.L. "Bovine Babesiosis." In *Foreign Animal Diseases*. Richmond, VA: United States Animal Health Association, 1998, pp. 81–105.

Bovine Ephemeral Fever

Bovine Epizootic Fever, Ephemeral Fever, 3-Day Sickness, 3-Day Stiffsickness, Dragon Boat Disease

Importance

Bovine ephemeral fever is an economically important disease in cattle. Its impact includes lost production – decreased milk production, abortion, temporary infertility in bulls, and prolonged recovery in some animals – as well as trade restrictions. Although mortality is usually low, cattle in good condition are usually affected more severely; mortality rates can be higher than 30% in very fat cattle.

Etiology

Bovine ephemeral fever is caused by the ephemeral fever virus (also known as bovine ephemeral fever virus). This arthropod–borne rhabdovirus is antigenically related to several nonpathogenic viruses, including Kimberley virus, Berrimah virus, and Adelaide River virus. It is also related to the Kotonkan and Puchong viruses, which cause diseases similar to ephemeral fever. Antibodies against related viruses are not protective against bovine ephemeral fever.

Species affected

Only cattle (*Bos taurus*, *Bos indicus*, and *Bos javanicus*) and water buffalo develop bovine ephemeral fever, but asymptomatic infections have been seen in hartebeest, waterbuck, wildebeest, and perhaps goats. Antibodies have also been found in Cape buffalo, as well as deer and antelope in Africa and deer in Australia.

Geographic distribution

Bovine ephemeral fever is endemic in a belt of temperate, subtropical, and tropical countries in Africa, Australia, and Asia. This disease occurs in all of Africa and in Asian countries south of a line that includes Israel, Iraq, Iran, Syria, India, Pakistan, Bangladesh, southern and central China, and southern Japan through Southeast Asia to Australia.

Transmission

The vector for bovine ephemeral fever is not proven, but the disease appears to be spread mainly by mosquitoes. Ephemeral fever virus has been isolated from *Culex* and *Anopheles* mosquitoes in Australia, and from *Culicoides* biting midges in Africa and Australia. The timing of outbreaks supports mosquitoes as a vector. The disease can also be spread by intravenous inoculation of small amounts of blood. Bovine ephemeral fever is not transmitted by close contact, bodily secretions, or aerosol droplets. The virus does not seem to be transmitted in semen and is rapidly inactivated in meat. Carriers are not known to occur.

Incubation period

In experimental infections, the incubation period is usually 2 to 4 days, with a few infections developing up to 9 days. The natural incubation period is probably similar.

Clinical signs

The clinical signs of bovine ephemeral fever are generally transient but severe. Infected cattle usually develop a biphasic or triphasic fever, with temperature peaks approximately 12 to 18 hours apart. During the first fever, milk production in lactating cows often drops dramatically, but other clinical signs are mild. During the second fever, the symptoms are more severe. Animals may have an increased heart rate, tachypnea, depression, anorexia, ruminal atony, serous or mucoid discharges from the nose and eyes, salivation, muscle twitching, waves of shivering, joint pain, stiffness, and shifting lameness. There may also be submandibular edema or patchy edema on the head. Many animals become recumbent for eight hours to days. Some may temporarily lose their reflexes and be unable to rise. These clinical signs can be exacerbated by severe environmental stress or forced exercise.

Most animals begin to improve a day or two after the first symptoms appear, and recover completely within another one to two days. Lactating cows and animals in good condition are usually affected more severely and may take up to a week to recover. Complications are uncommon but can include temporary or permanent paralysis, gait impairments, aspiration pneumonia, emphysema, and the subcutaneous accumulation of air along the back. Temporary infertility may develop in bulls, and abortions can occur in cows. In recovered animals, milk production is decreased by 10% to 15% for the rest of the lactation, but usually returns to normal after subsequent pregnancies. Death may occur during either the febrile or recovery stages.

Post mortem lesions

The most obvious lesion in bovine ephemeral fever is a small amount of fibrin–rich fluid in the pleural, peritoneal, and pericardial cavities. Variable amounts of fluid may also be found in the joint capsules. Serofibrinous polysynovitis, polyarthritis, polytendovaginitis, and cellulitis are common. Patchy edema may be apparent in the lungs and lymphadenitis is often seen. Petechial hemorrhages or edema may be found in the lymph nodes. Areas of focal necrosis in the major muscle groups are common.

Morbidity and mortality

In outbreaks of bovine ephemeral fever, the morbidity rate may be as high as 80%. The average mortality rate is 1% to 2%, but can be higher in animals in good condition. In some outbreaks in very fat cattle, the outcome may be fatal in more than 30%.

Although treatment is usually not necessary, anti–inflammatory drugs and calcium borogluconate injections are effective. Good immunity is seen after an infection, and vaccines of varying efficacy are available.

Diagnosis

Clinical

Bovine ephemeral fever should be suspected in cattle that develop severe but transient symptoms including a biphasic (or multiphasic) fever and temporary paralysis or recumbency. This disease may be difficult to diagnose when a single animal is affected.

Differential diagnosis

Bovine ephemeral fever in a single animal can be confused with early Rift Valley fever, heartwater, bluetongue, botulism, babesiosis, or blackleg. The salivation may also resemble foot and mouth disease, but no vesicles are found.

Laboratory tests

Most cases of bovine ephemeral fever are confirmed by serology. A rising titer should be demonstrated with either a virus neutralization test or enzyme–linked immunosorbent assay (ELISA). Cross–reactions are sometimes seen to related viruses such as Kimberley virus.

Virus isolation from the blood can be tried, but often fails. Suitable cultures include BHK–21, bovine kidney, hamster lung, Vero, and *Aedes albopictus* cell lines, or hamster lung tissue culture. The virus is usually identified by immunofluorescence.

Bovine ephemeral fever can also be confirmed by inoculating susceptible cattle with uncoagulated whole blood. Unweaned mice may also be used.

Samples to collect

Before collecting or sending any samples from animals with a suspected foreign animal disease, the proper authorities should be contacted. Samples should only be sent under secure conditions and to authorized laboratories to prevent the spread of the disease.

Blood samples should be collected during a fever spike and one to two weeks later. The samples should include at least 20 ml of clotted blood for serology and 5 ml of anticoagulated blood (an anticoagulant other than EDTA should be used). Two smears should be made from the unclotted blood and air–dried; the rest of the sample should be submitted for virus isolation. For faster confirmation, samples should be taken from animals in various stages of the disease.

Recommended actions if bovine ephemeral fever is suspected

Notification of authorities

Bovine ephemeral fever should be reported immediately to state or federal authorities.

Federal: Area Veterinarians in Charge (AVICs):
http://www.aphis.usda.gov/vs/area_offices.htm
State Veterinarians:
http://www.aphis.usda.gov/vs/sregs/official.html

Quarantine and disinfection

Sodium hypochlorite and other disinfectants effectively destroy ephemeral fever virus; however, disinfection is relatively unimportant in preventing the spread of this virus. The ephemeral fever virus is not spread by casual contact or in secretions and is rapidly inactivated in the muscles of carcasses after death. Contact with potential insect vectors must be avoided.

Public health

There is no evidence that humans can be infected by the ephemeral fever virus.

For more information

World Organization for Animal Health (OIE)
http://www.oie.int
OIE International Animal Health Code
http://www.oie.int/eng/normes/mcode/A_summry.htm

USAHA Foreign Animal Diseases Book
http://www.vet.uga.edu/vpp/gray_book/FAD/

References

"Ephemeral Fever." In *The Merck Veterinary Manual*, 8th ed. Edited by S.E. Aiello and A. Mays. Whitehouse Station, NJ: Merck and Co., 1998, pp. 528–529.

Nandi, S., and B.S. Negi. "Bovine Ephemeral Fever: a Review." *Comparative Immunology, Microbiology, and Infectious Diseases* 22 (1999): 81–91.

St. George, T.D. "Bovine Ephemeral Fever." In *Foreign Animal Diseases*. Richmond, VA: United States Animal Health Association, 1998, pp. 118–128.

Bovine Spongiform Encephalopathy

Mad Cow Disease

Importance

Bovine spongiform encephalopathy (BSE, "mad cow disease") is a transmissible spongiform encephalopathy (TSE) that affects cattle. TSEs are progressive and fatal neurodegenerative diseases. There are multiple TSEs which affect different species of animals including scrapie in sheep, transmissible mink encephalopathy (TME, mink scrapie), feline spongiform encephalopathy (FSE), chronic wasting disease (CWD) in deer and elk, and a spongiform encephalopathy of exotic ruminants. These diseases were once thought to be entirely species specific, but it now appears that some agents can cross species barriers. In the United Kingdom, factors leading to the BSE epidemic may have been responsible for concurrent outbreaks of FSE in cats and spongiform encephalopathy in exotic ruminants. BSE has also been linked to a variant of Creutzfeldt–Jakob disease (CJD) in humans.

Etiology

BSE is thought to be caused by prions, a proteinaceous infectious particle that is smaller than the smallest known virus. Prions have not been completely characterized and a minority opinion is that BSE may be caused by virinos or retroviruses. The BSE agent is extremely resistant to the treatments that ordinarily destroy bacteria, spores, viruses, and fungi and can survive in tissue post–mortem.

Species affected

BSE is seen in cattle and can be experimentally transmitted to cats, mink, mice, pigs, sheep, goats, marmosets and cynomolgus monkeys.

Geographic distribution

Since the diagnosis of the first cases of BSE in the United Kingdom in 1986, infected indigenous cattle have since found in Austria, Belgium, Canada, Czech Republic, Denmark, Finland, France, Germany, Greece, Ireland, Israel, Italy, Japan, Liechtenstein, Luxembourg, Netherlands, Poland, Portugal, Slovakia, Slovenia, Spain, Switzerland, and the United States. Cases have also been seen in imported cattle in the Falkland Islands and Oman. BSE has never been detected in Australia, New Zealand, Central America or South America.

Transmission

BSE seems to be transmitted orally. The BSE agent is found mainly in nervous tissues. In naturally infected cattle, it has been detected only in the brain, spinal cord, and retina. In experimentally infected calves, it is also seen in the distal ileum. This agent has never been found in muscle, blood, or milk, and natural infections do not seem to spread laterally between cattle. The offspring of BSE-infected cattle have an increased risk of developing BSE, but it is not known whether this is due to vertical transmission or another mode of transmission.

There are several hypotheses on the actual origins of the BSE agent. Some sources suggest that this agent has been present in cattle since the 1970s, and may have resulted from a genetic mutation in cattle. An alternative hypothesis is that it mutated from the agent that causes scrapie, and crossed species when sheep tissues were fed to cattle in MBM. A recently published report suggests that the BSE agent may have been a mutant of a human TSE agent. This agent is thought to have been present in raw mammalian materials imported from the Indian subcontinent and used to make MBM.

The first cases of BSE appeared in the U.K. in the 1980s. By the end of 1987, the Central Veterinary Laboratory of the State Veterinary Service concluded that the cause of the reported cases of BSE was the consumption of meat-and-bone meal (MBM), which was made from animal carcasses and incorporated into cattle feed. At first it was thought that cattle were becoming infected from scrapie-contaminated sheep tissues and that the MBM had become infectious because rendering methods that had previously inactivated the conventional scrapie agent were changed. However, the theory that BSE resulted from changes in rendering methods is probably not correct because rendering methods have never been capable of completely inactivating TSEs. The BSE agent was probably amplified when BSE-contaminated cattle carcasses and wastes were used to make MBM, which was then fed to cattle.

Incubation period

All TSEs have incubation periods of months or years. The incubation period of BSE is more than a year and often several years. The peak incidence of disease occurs in 4 to 5 year old cattle.

Clinical signs

Bovine spongiform encephalopathy is usually insidious in onset and tends to progress slowly. The clinical signs are neurologic and once the symptoms appear, the disease is relentlessly progressive and fatal. The clinical signs of BSE may include hyperesthesia, hindlimb ataxia, pelvic swaying, hypermetria, tremors, falling, and behavioral changes such as apprehension, nervousness, and occasionally frenzy. Intense pruritus is not usually seen. Nonspecific symptoms include loss of condition, weight loss, and decreased milk production. Decreased rumination, bradycardia, and altered heart rhythms have also been reported. The disease progresses to recumbency and coma, and death occurs weeks to months later. Rare cases may develop acutely and progress rapidly within days.

Post mortem lesions

The only gross lesions found are nonspecific; there may be emaciation or wasting of the carcass in some cases. The typical histopathologic lesions are confined to the central nervous system. Neuronal vacuolation and non–inflammatory spongiform changes in the gray matter are characteristic. Amyloid plaques are rarely seen in BSE cases. Lesions are usually but not always bilaterally symmetrical.

Morbidity and mortality

BSE is always fatal once the symptoms appear. In 1992, the annual incidence of BSE in United Kingdom cattle was 1%; however, the number of cases has been decreasing in recent years. The peak incidence in the UK occurred in January 1993 with 1,000 new cases every week.

Diagnosis

Clinical

BSE should be suspected in animals that develop a slowly progressive, fatal neurologic disease.

Differential diagnosis

The differential diagnosis of BSE includes nervous ketosis, hypomagnesemia, listeriosis, polioencephalomalacia, rabies, brain tumor, spinal cord trauma, and lead poisoning.

Laboratory tests

BSE is diagnosed by detecting PrP^{Sc} (a disease–specific isoform of the membrane protein PrP) in the central nervous system. Accumulations of PrP^{Sc} can be found in unfixed brain extracts by immunoblotting and in fixed brains by immunohistochemistry. The diagnosis can also be confirmed by finding characteristic fibrils of PrP^{Sc} (scrapie–associated fibrils) with electron microscopy in brain extracts. Some of these tests can be used on frozen or autolyzed brains. BSE can be detected by transmission studies in mice. However, an incubation period of several months often makes this technique impractical for diagnosis. New commercial tests to detect BSE (PrP^{Sc}) in cattle brain samples include a modified immunoblot, a chemiluminescent ELISA test, a sandwich immunoassay, and a two–site noncompetitive immunometric procedure. Serology is not useful for diagnosis, as antibodies are not made against the BSE agent.

Since the first BSE case was discovered in the U.S. in December 2003, at least five rapid diagnostic tests have been licensed for use. These rapid tests can detect the prion before the spongiform holes develop in the brain and before the animal becomes clinical. However, it is not known how much prion protein has to be present to be detected. The rapid tests have shown very good sensitivity and specificity. Three of the tests underwent the same laboratory verification process, and all were able to correctly identify 1,000 negative samples and 300 positive samples. However, there has been little information made available about false positives and false negatives when the tests have been used on large numbers of samples in a surveillance program. It should be understood that a test result is influenced not only by the test used, but also the collection of an appropriate sample and use of proper procedure.

Samples to collect

Before collecting or sending any samples from animals with a suspected foreign animal disease, the proper authorities should be contacted. Samples should only be sent under secure conditions and to authorized laboratories to prevent the spread of the disease. Samples should be collected and handled with all appropriate precautions.

For post–mortem examination, the whole brain, brain stem, or medulla should be removed as soon as possible after death for histopathology. For specific PrP detection, the caudal medulla at the obex should be removed and refrigerated soon after death.

Recommended action if BSE is suspected

Notification of authorities

BSE is a reportable exotic disease and authorities must be notified immediately of any suspicious cases.

Federal: Area Veterinarians in Charge (AVICs):
   http://www.aphis.usda.gov/vs/area_offices.htm
State Veterinarians:
   http://www.aphis.usda.gov/vs/sregs/official.html
For the latest information regarding BSE, please visit the USDA APHIS website at http://www.aphis.usda.gov/lpa/issues/bse/bse.html

Quarantine and disinfection

BSE does not appear to spread laterally, but once an animal is found positive the whole herd is quarantined and trace backs will occur. The prototype agent, scrapie, is highly resistant to disinfectants, heat, ultraviolet radiation, ionizing radiation, and formalin, especially if it is in tissues, dried organic material or at a very high titer. A single porous load autoclave cycle of 134–138°C for 18 minutes has been recommended for inactivation, however, this temperature range may not completely inactivate the prion protein. Infectious tissues should either be autoclaved under the same conditions or incinerated.

Sodium hypochlorite and sodium hydroxide are effective chemical disinfectants; sodium hypochlorite containing 2% available chlorine or 2–N sodium hydroxide should be applied for more than 1 hour at 20°C and overnight for equipment. These recommended decontamination measures will reduce titers but may be incompletely effective if dealing with high titer material, when the agent is protected within dried organic matter, or in tissue preserved in aldehyde fixatives. The prion protein may survive in tissues post–mortem after a wide range of rendering processes. Related hamster scrapie infectivity can survive interment in soil for 3 years and dry heat of 1 hour at temperatures as high as 360°C. (Information obtained from OIE website at http://www.oie.int/eng/maladies/fiches/a_B115.htm.)

Rendering at 133°C at 3 bar pressure for a minimum of 20 minutes is used in Great Britain in order to dispose of the infected carcasses. Many medical experts recommend the use of disposable instruments in neurosurgery if the risk of contacting highly infective CJD tissue is high. Equipment used for brain biopsies in the U.K. is quarantined until a diagnosis is confirmed because risk of CJD spread is too high to try and disinfect to reuse those instruments.

U.S. prevention and control prior to December 2003

The U.S. Department of Agriculture (USDA) has a number of stringent safeguards in place to prevent the spread of BSE in this country. In 1989, importation bans on live ruminants and restrictions on most ruminant products from countries where BSE had been diagnosed (including the U.K.) were initiated. These were expanded to include all European countries in December 1997. Additionally, active targeted surveillance measures for BSE have been implemented in the U.S. since 1990. Efforts focused on animals of highest risk. These include adult animals exhibiting any sign of neurological disease or distress, non–ambulatory ("downer") animals, rabies–negative cattle, as well as cattle that die on farms (added in 2002). In 2003, approximately 20,000 head of cattle were tested for BSE, which was 47 times more samples than recommended by OIE guidelines.

In August 1997, FDA initiated regulations, known as the "animal feed rule," to further enhance BSE prevention efforts. The rule prohibits the feeding of most mammalian material to ruminant animals, including cattle. The regulation exempts the following products: blood and blood byproducts, milk products, pure porcine and pure equine proteins, plate waste, tallow, gelatin and non–mammalian protein (Poultry, marine, vegetable). Additionally, it regulates the process and control system for producing feed for ruminants so it does not contain the prohibited mammalian tissue (i.e., brain, eyes, spinal cord, etc.). On December 7, 2000, the USDA prohibited importation of all rendered animal protein products, regardless of species, from any European country.

Prevention measures for the human food chain are also in place. Since 2002, FSIS has prohibited any spinal cord tissue from inclusion in products produced by advanced meat recovery (AMR) processing and labeled as "meat". Routine sampling of product was initiated by FSIS in March 2003 to ensure the regulation was followed. AMR is an industrial technology that removes muscle tissue from the bone of beef carcasses under high pressure without incorporating bone material when operated properly.

The U.S. BSE response plan

In 1990, the Animal and Plant Health Inspection Service (APHIS) of USDA developed an initial plan to respond to confir-

mation of BSE in the United States. The BSE Emergency Disease Guideline includes a step–by–step plan of action to address identification of suspect animals, laboratory confirmation, epidemiologic investigation, animal and herd disposition activities, as well as communication and notification plans. The guideline was updated, revised and approved by officials at all levels of APHIS, Food Safety Inspection Service (FSIS), and USDA in 1996.

APHIS and FSIS investigators also receive comprehensive training in the detection and diagnosis of BSE. Prior to slaughter, any animal with neurological conditions is inspected by FSIS and considered suspect for BSE. The carcass is condemned and not allowed for use in the human food chain. The brain tissue is forwarded to APHIS' National Veterinary Services Laboratory (NVSL) for histopathology, immunohistochemistry, and immunoblotting. If a presumptive diagnosis of BSE is suggested, the sample is then hand carried by a NVSL pathologist to the BSE world reference laboratory in the United Kingdom for confirmation. Within 24 hours upon confirmation of a case of BSE, the Office of International Epizooties (OIE) is notified. Notification protocols for all agencies involved in the response plan are then initiated by NVSL. The VS Area Veterinarian-in-Charge (AVIC), in cooperation with State animal health authorities, coordinates any field activities and the suspect animal's herd of origin is quarantined.

U.S. response to first case of BSE

On December 23, 2003, the USDA reported the first presumptive case of BSE in the U.S. It was discovered in a "downer" dairy cow in the state of Washington that had been sent to slaughter. In accordance with the U.S. BSE response plan, brain tissue was forwarded to the NVSL. Upon finding a presumptive positive result, tissue was hand delivered to the BSE world reference laboratory in Weybridge, England. Additionally, samples were forwarded to the National Animal Disease Center (NADC) and the Meat Animal Research Center for further diagnostics and DNA testing. On December 25, the UK world reference laboratory confirmed the diagnosis of BSE. Upon completion of DNA testing, the positive cow was identified as one imported from a dairy farm in Alberta, Canada.

Even though effective safeguard measures were already in place in the U.S., the Secretary of Agriculture, Ann Veneman, announced on December 30, 2003, additional safeguards being implemented due to an abundance of caution, to further strengthen protections against BSE in the U.S. These additional safeguards include the following:

1) All downer cattle presented for slaughter will be banned from the human food chain. Additionally any suspect cattle (i.e., adults with neurological conditions) will be held until BSE tests are confirmed negative;
2) Specified risk material (SRM) will also be prohibited from the human food chain. This material includes the skull, brain, trigeminal ganglia, eyes, vertebral column, spinal cord and dorsal root ganglia of cattle over 30 months of age. Additionally, the distal ileum and tonsils (which is already prohibited) from all cattle are prohibited;
3) Additional process controls were also determined for AMR systems. Prior regulations prohibited spinal cord tissue in product going into the human food chain, which is routinely verified by FSIS officials through testing of product. Regulations have now been expanded to prohibit dorsal root ganglia, skull, as well as any spinal cord tissue in processing;
4) The use of air–injection stunning of cattle at slaughter has also been prohibited immediately to reduce the potential of brain tissue being dislocated into the tissue of carcasses;
5) Additionally, a national animal identification plan (which was previously being developed) will begin immediate implementation.

The Secretary has also appointed an international panel of scientific experts to provide an objective review of the U.S. response actions to this case, as well as areas of potential improvement.

In June 2005, the USDA reported the first case of BSE in an animal born in the U.S. The infected cow was a 12-year old Brahma cross that had been born and raised in Texas. It was sold in a livestock sale in November 2004, and was dead on arrival at a packing plant. The carcass, which had been sent on to a pet food factory, was tested for BSE and incinerated rather than being used. Although the first test results from this animal, done in the U.S., were conflicting, a sample sent to a BSE reference laboratory in the UK was positive. APHIS, the Food and Drug Administration, Texas Animal Health Commission and Texas Feed and Fertilizer Control Service conducted a joint investigation to determine the source of the infection and test this animal's cohorts and recent offspring. All adult animals that had left this farm after 1990, and the two calves born to the infected cow within two years of its death were traced. Most of these animals had been slaughtered, died or were presumed to be dead, although a few animals were untraceable. One surviving animal was tested and found to be negative, and another was determined to be of no interest because of its age. As the BSE-infected cow had been born before the 1997 ban on meat-and-bone-meal, it appears to have been infected from that source.

Public health

Current thinking is that people who ingest BSE contaminated food products may develop variant Creutzfeldt-Jakob disease (vCJD). The incubation period for vCJD is unknown because it is a relatively new disease, but it is likely that it is many years or decades. Therefore, a person who develops vCJD likely would have consumed an infected product or products many years earlier.In contrast to classic CJD, vCJD in the UK predominantly affects young people with 28 years as the mean age at death. The mean duration of illness is 14.1 months for vCJD. The disease has atypical clinical features (as compared to CJD), with prominent psychiatric or sensory symptoms at the time of clinical presentation. Onset of neurological abnormalities with vCJD is delayed and includes ataxia within weeks or months. Dementia and myoclonus occur later in the illness. Affected persons generally become completely immobile and mute at the end stage of the disease. There is no known effective treatment for vCJD. There is experimental treatment taking place with quinicrine. Supportive treatment and symptomatic care are recommended.

From 1996 (when the first suspected cases of vCJD occurred) to November 2005, a total of 185 cases of vCJD have been reported worldwide; of these, 158 cases have occurred in the U.K. Other cases have been reported in other countries, including the U.S. Many of these cases were in individuals likely exposed to the BSE agent while residing in the U.K. There have been no confirmed cases of vCJD originating in the United States.

For more information

World Organization for Animal Health (OIE)
　　http://www.oie.int
OIE Manual of Standards
　　http://www.oie.int/eng/normes/mmanual/a_summry.htm
United States Department of Agriculture, Animal and Plant Health Inspection Service
　　http://www.aphis.usda.gov/lpa/issues/bse/bse.html
United States Food and Drug Administration
　　http://www.fda.gov/oc/opacom/hottopics/bse.html
Centers for Disease Control and Prevention
　　http://www.cdc.gov/ncidod/dvrd/bse/index.htm
Canadian Food Inspection Agency
　　http://www.inspection.gc.ca/english/anima/heasan/disemala/disemalae.htm

Animal Health Australia. The National Animal Health Information System
　　http://www. aahc.com.au/nahis/disease/dislist.asp

References

"Bovine spongiform encephalopathy." Animal Health Australia. The National Animal Health Information System (NAHIS). Accessed 7 November 2001. http://www.brs.gov.au/usr–bin/aphb/ahsq?dislist=alpha.

"Bovine spongiform encephalopathy." In *Manual of Standards for Diagnostic Tests and Vaccines*. Paris: Office International des Epizooties, 2000, pp.

"Bovine spongiform encephalopathy." In *The Merck Veterinary Manual*, 8th ed. Edited by S.E. Aiello and A. Mays. Whitehouse Station, NJ: Merck and Co., 1998, pp. 897–8.

Irani, D.N. "Bovine spongiform encephalopathy." Johns Hopkins Department of Neurology. Resource on Prion Diseases. Accessed 7 November 2001. http://www.jhu–prion.org/animal/ani–bse–hist.shtml.

"Transmissible spongiform encephalopathies." July 2000 United States Department of Agriculture Animal and Plant Health Inspection Service (APHIS). Accessed 7 November 2001 at http://www.aphis.usda.gov/oa/pubs/fstse.html.

Bovine spongiform encephalopathy (BSE) response plan summary. United States Department of Agriculture. Accessed 29 December 2003. http://cofcs66.aphis.usda.gov/lpa/issues/bse/bsesum.pdf.

"Federal agencies take special precautions to keep "mad cow disease" out of the United States". U.S. Department of Health and Human Services Fact Sheet. August 2001. Accessed 30 December 2003. http://www.cfsan.fda.gov/~lrd/hhsbse2.html.

"Evaluation of the potential for bovine spongiform encephaloptahy in the United States. United States Department of Agriculture and Harvard Center for Risk Analysis. Accessed November 26, 2001. http://www.aphis.usda.gov/lpa/issues/bse/risk_assessment/mainreporttext.pdf.

"Veneman annouces additional protection measures to guard against BSE." United States Department of Agriculture. News Release December 30, 2003. http://www.usda.gov/news/relaeses/2003/12/0449.html.

"Bovine spongiform encephalopathy (BSE). Overview." United States Department of Agriculture Animal Plant and Health Inspection Service (APHIS). Accessed 29 December 2003. http://www.aphis.usda.gov/lpa/issues/bse/bse–overview.html.

"Bovine spongiform encephalopathy (BSE). Surveillance." United States Department of Agriculture Animal Plant and Health Inspection Service (APHIS). Accessed at 29 December 2003. http://www.aphis.usda.gov/lpa/issues/bse/bse–surveillance.html.

"Report on Food and Drug Administartion Dallas District investigation of bovine spongiform encephalopathy event in Texas 2005." Department of Health and Human Services, U.S. Food and Drug Administartion. Accessed Aug 30, 2005. http://www.fda.gov/cvm/texasfeedrpt.htm.

"Press Release: Investigation results of Texas cow that tested positive for bovine spongiform encephalopathy (BSE)." U.S. Department of Agriculture. Release Number 0336.05. Accessed Aug. 30, 2005. http://www.usda.gov/wps/portal/!ut/p/_s.7_0_A/7_0_1OB/.cmd/ad/.ar/sa.retrievecontent/.c/6_2_1UH/.ce/7_2_5JM/.p/5_2_4TQ/.d/l/_th/J_@_(D/_s.7_0_A/7_0_1OB?PC_7_2_5JM_contentid=2005/08/0336.xml&PC_7_2_5JM_navtype=RT&PC_7_2_5JM_parentnav=LATEST_RELEASE&PC_7_2_5JM_navid=NEWS_RELEASE#7_2_5JM.

"The BSE inquiry: The report. A report to the Minister of Agriculture, Fisheries and Food, the Secretary of State for Health and the Secretaries of State for Scotland, Wales and

Northern Ireland." Lord Phillips, chair. London: Her Majesty's Stationery Office; 2000. Report no HC 887-1. Crown copyright. Accessed Jan 2006. http://www.bseinquiry.gov.uk/report/. Accessed Jan 2006.

"Bovine spongiform encephalopathy factsheet." United States Department of Agriculture Animal and Plant Health Inspection Service (APHIS). Accessed Jan 2006. http://www.aphis.usda.gov/lpa/pubs/fsheet_faq_notice/fs_ahbse.html.

Balter M. Intriguing clues to a scrapie-mad cow link. *Science.* 2001;292(5518):827-9.

Colchester AC, Colchester NT. The origin of bovine spongiform encephalopathy: the human prion disease hypothesis. *Lancet.* 2005 Sep 3-9;366(9488):856-61.

"Probable variant Creutzfeldt-Jakob disease in a U.K citizen who had temporaliy reside in Texas, 2001-2005." Centers for Disease Control and Prevention. Accessed Jan 2006. http://www.cdc.gov/ncidod/dvrd/vcjd/other/probablevcjd_texas2001_2005_111805.htm.

Belay ED, Sejvar JJ, Shieh WJ, Wiersma ST, Zou WQ, Gambetti P, Hunter S, Maddox RA, Crockett L, Zaki SR, Schonberger LB. Variant Creutzfeldt-Jakob disease death, United States. *Emerg Infect Dis* 2005; 11(9):1351-1354.

Bovine Tuberculosis

Importance

Bovine tuberculosis is a significant zoonosis that can spread to humans through aerosols and by ingestion of raw milk. In developed countries, eradication efforts have significantly reduced the prevalence of this disease, but reservoirs in wildlife make complete eradication difficult. Bovine tuberculosis is still common in less developed countries, and economic losses can occur in cattle and African buffalo from deaths, chronic disease, and trade restrictions. Infections may also be a serious threat to endangered species.

Etiology

Bovine tuberculosis results from infection by *Mycobacterium bovis*, a Gram positive, acid–fast bacterium.

Species affected

Cattle and buffalo are considered to be the maintenance hosts for *M. bovis*. Infections have also been described in numerous other domestic and wild animals including sheep, goats, horses, pigs, deer, antelope, dogs, cats, ferrets, camels, foxes, mink, badgers, rats, primates, llamas, kudus, elands, tapirs, elk, elephants, sitatungas, oryxes, addaxes, rhinoceroses, opossums, ground squirrels, otters, seals, hares, moles, raccoons, coyotes, lions, tigers, leopards, and lynx. Most of these species are considered to be spill–over hosts; however, some can act as wildlife reservoirs. Known reservoir hosts include brush–tailed opossums in New Zealand, badgers in the United Kingdom and Ireland, deer in the United States, bison in Canada, and greater kudu, common duiker, African buffalo, warthogs, and Kafue lechwe in Africa.

Geographic distribution

Tuberculosis has been found worldwide. Eradication programs are in progress or nearing completion in a number of countries in Europe, as well as the United States, Canada, Japan, and New Zealand. A few countries including Australia, Denmark, Sweden, Norway, and Finland are considered to be free of bovine tuberculosis.

Transmission

Tuberculosis can be transmitted either by the respiratory route or ingestion. In cattle, aerosol spread is more common. In pigs, ingestion is frequent. Cutaneous, genital, and congenital infections have been seen but are rare. Infectious bacteria can be shed in the respiratory secretions, feces, milk, and in some individuals in the urine, vaginal secretions, or semen. Not all infected animals transmit the disease. Asymptomatic and anergic carriers occur.

M. bovis can survive for several months in the environment, particularly in cold, dark, and moist conditions.

Incubation period

The clinical signs usually take months to develop. Infections can also remain dormant for years and reactivate during periods of stress or in old age.

Clinical signs

Bovine tuberculosis is usually a chronic debilitating disease, but can occasionally be acute and rapidly progressive. Early infections are often asymptomatic. In the late stages, common symptoms include progressive emaciation, a low–grade fluctuating fever, weakness, and inappetence. Animals with pulmonary involvement usually have a moist cough that is worse in the morning, during cold weather, or exercise, and may have dyspnea or tachypnea. In some animals, the retropharyngeal or other lymph nodes enlarge and may rupture and drain. Greatly enlarged lymph nodes can also obstruct blood vessels, airways, or the digestive tract. If the digestive tract is involved, intermittent diarrhea and constipation may be seen. Lesions are sometimes found on the female genitalia but are rare on the male genitalia. In cats, skin lesions similar to those of feline leprosy may be seen.

Post mortem lesions

Bovine tuberculosis is characterized by the formation of tuberculous granulomas (tubercles) where bacteria have localized. These granulomas are usually yellowish and caseous, caseo–calcareous, or calcified, and are often encapsulated. In some species such as deer, lesions resemble abscesses more than typical tubercles. Occasional tubercles may appear purulent. Granulomas are most often found in the mediastinal, retropharyngeal, and portal lymph nodes. They are also common in the lung, spleen, liver, and the surfaces of body cavities. In disseminated cases, multiple small granulomas may be found in numerous organs. Many infected cattle have only a few lesions at necropsy.

Morbidity and mortality

Bovine tuberculosis is often a sporadic disease, with many infections confined to one or two animals in a herd. In two studies of transmission from naturally infected reactor cattle, 0% to 40% of susceptible contacts became infected and 0% to 10% developed gross lesions. The severity of disease varies with the dose of infectious organisms and individual immunity. Infected animals may remain asymptomatic, become ill only after stress or in old age, or develop a fatal, chronically debilitating disease. In developed countries, most reactors are detected during routine testing and mortality from tuberculosis is rare.

Drug treatment can be effective but does not always eliminate the infection and is not available in all countries.

Diagnosis

Clinical

Tuberculosis can be difficult to diagnose based only on the clinical signs. In developed countries, few infections become symptomatic; most are diagnosed by routine testing or found at the slaughterhouse.

Differential diagnosis

The differential diagnosis includes contagious bovine pleuropneumonia, *Pasteurella* or *Corynebacterium pyogenes* pneumonia, aspiration pneumonia (often secondary to Chronic Wasting Disease in cervids), traumatic pericarditis, caseous lymphadenitis or melioidosis in small ruminants, and chronic aberrant liver fluke infestation.

Laboratory tests

In live cattle, tuberculosis is usually diagnosed in the field with the tuberculin skin test. Occasionally, the sputum and other body fluids may be collected for microbiological examination. Post–mortem, bovine tuberculosis can be diagnosed by histopathology, microscopic demonstration of acid–fast bacilli, isolation of mycobacteria on selective culture media, and identification by biochemical tests. Slides may be stained with the Ziehl/Neelsen stain, a fluorescent acid–fast stain, or immunoperoxidase techniques. DNA probe/polymerase chain reaction (PCR) methods have also been described. Very rarely, guinea–pig inoculation may be necessary before isolation and identification of the organism.

New diagnostic blood tests include the lymphocyte proliferation assay, the gamma–interferon assay, and enzyme–linked immunosorbent assays (ELISAs). The gamma interferon test is only useful in members of the Bovidae, but the lymphocyte proliferation test and ELISA may be used in other zoo animals and wildlife. These tests are not used routinely for diagnosis in cattle.

All procedures for bacterial culture should be done in a biological safety cabinet, as the bacteria may survive in heat fixed smears or become aerosolized during specimen preparation.

Samples to collect

Bovine tuberculosis is a zoonotic disease; samples should be collected and handled with all appropriate precautions.

The tuberculin (delayed hypersensitivity) test is the standard method of diagnosis in live cattle and the prescribed test for international trade. The comparative intradermal tuberculin test can be used to distinguish between infections with *M. bovis* and sensitization to other *Mycobacteria* species. Variations such as the thermal test and Stormont test have also been used. False negative reactions may occur in animals that have poor immunity or are anergic, old, or have recently calved. In some cases, blood samples may be taken for diagnostic blood tests. Samples for the gamma interferon test must be transported to the laboratory promptly, as this test must be started within eight hours of blood collection.

At necropsy, samples for culture should be taken from abnormal lymph nodes and affected organs such as the lungs, liver, and spleen. If an animal reacted on the tuberculin test but there are no gross lesions, samples should be taken from the retropharyngeal, bronchial, mandibular, supramammary, and mediastinal lymph nodes, some of the mesenteric lymph nodes, and the liver. These specimens should be shipped to the laboratory quickly. If shipping must be delayed, the samples can be refrigerated or frozen. If refrigeration or freezing is not feasible, 0.5% (w/v) boric acid may be added for periods of a week or less. Specimens should also be collected for histopathology. All samples must be wrapped securely and comply with all biosafety regulations to prevent human infections.

Recommended actions if bovine tuberculosis is suspected

Notification of authorities

Bovine tuberculosis is a reportable disease. State authorities should be consulted for specific regulations.

Federal: Area Veterinarians in Charge (AVICs):
http://www.aphis.usda.gov/vs/area_offices.htm
State Veterinarians:
http://www.aphis.usda.gov/vs/sregs/official.html

Quarantine and disinfection

Control measures usually include early diagnosis with the tuberculin test, segregation or slaughter of infected animals, and tracing and containment of animals that have been in contact with reactors.

M. bovis is relatively resistant to disinfectants and requires long contact times for inactivation. Effective disinfectants include 5% phenol, iodine solutions with a high concentration of available iodine, glutaraldehyde, and formaldehyde. In environments with low concentrations of organic material, 1% sodium hypochlorite with a long contact time is also effective. This organism is also susceptible to moist heat.

Public health

M. bovis can infect humans, primarily by ingestion of raw (unpasteurized) milk or dairy products but also through aerosols and breaks in the skin. Infections in humans may result in asymptomatic infections, pulmonary tuberculosis, or disseminated infections. The symptoms of pulmonary infection can include fever, cough, chest pain, cavitation, hemoptysis, and fibrosis. Untreated infections may be fatal. *M. bovis* is classified as a risk group 3 pathogen.

For more information

World Organization for Animal Health (OIE)
http://www.oie.int
OIE Manual of Standards
http://www.oie.int/eng/normes/mmanual/a_summry.htm
OIE International Animal Health Code
http://www.oie.int/eng/normes/mcode/A_summry.htm
Michigan Bovine Tuberculosis Eradication Project
http://www.bovinetb.com/
Manual for the Recognition of Exotic Diseases of Livestock. FAO/SPC Animal Health Information System
http://www.spc.int/rahs/
Material Safety Data Sheet–*Mycobacterium tuberculosis, Mycobacterium bovis*. Canadian Laboratory Centre for Disease Control
http://www.phac-aspc.gc.ca/msds-ftss/index.html

References

"Bovine Tuberculosis." Animal Health Australia. The National Animal Health Information System (NAHIS). 2 November 2001 http//www.aahc.com.au/nahis/disease/dislist.asp

"Bovine Tuberculosis." In *Manual of Standards for Diagnostic Tests and Vaccines*. Paris: World Organization for Animal Health, 2000, pp. 359–370.

"Bovine Tuberculosis." September 1995. USDA Animal and Plant Health Inspection Service. 5 November 2001. http://www.aphis.usda.gov/oa/pubs/fsbtb.html>.

Cousins D.V. "*Mycobacterium bovis* infection and control in domestic livestock." *Rev. Sci. Tech.* 20, no. 1 (2001): 71–85.

Garner G. and P. Saville. "Bovine Tuberculosis." In *Manual for the Recognition of Exotic Diseases of Livestock*. FAO/SPC Animal Health Information System. 5 November 2001 http//panis.spc.org.fj>.

"Material Safety Data Sheet –*Mycobacterium tuberculosis, Mycobacterium bovis*." March 2001. Canadian Laboratory Centre for Disease Control. 1 November 2001. http://www.hc–sc.gc.ca/pphb–dgspsp/msds–ftss/msds103e.html.

"Pathogenesis and Diagnosis of Infections with *M. bovis* in Cattle (Appendix C)." March 2000 The Independent Scientific Group on Cattle TB (ISG). 6 November 2001. http://www.defra.gov.uk/animalh/tb/isg/report/annexc.shtml.

"Press Release of 4 January 2000. Update on Wildlife Diseases." January 2000 Office International des Epizooties. 6 November 2001. http://www.oie.int/eng/press/A_000104.htm.

"Trends and Sources of Zoonotic Agents in Animals, Feeding Stuffs, Food and Man in the European Union and Norway in 1999." European Commission Health and Consumer Protection Directorate–General. 6 November 2001. http//europa.eu.int/comm/food/fs/sfp/mr/mr08_en.pdf.

"Tuberculosis." In *The Merck Veterinary Manual*, 8th ed. Edited by S.E. Aiello and A. Mays. Whitehouse Station, NJ: Merck and Co., 1998, pp. 489–493.

"World Bovine Tuberculosis Multiannual Animal Disease Status." Office International des Epizooties. 6 November 2001. http//www.oie.int/hs2/sit_mald_freq_pl.asp?c_cont=6&c_mald=35.

Brucellosis

*Malta Fever, Mediterranean Fever, Undulant Fever,
Enzootic Abortion, Contagious Abortion,
Bang's Disease*

Importance

Brucellosis is a zoonotic disease that can cause chronic painful illness in humans if not treated. It also can have great economic impact by limiting transport of infected animals and products. Brucella can be transmitted through unpasteurized milk and dairy products to the general public. Aerosol transmission makes this organism a possible candidate for bioterrorist attack.

Etiology

There are six known bacterial species in the genus *Brucella*: *Brucella abortus, B. melitensis, B. suis, B. ovis, B. canis,* and *b. neotomae.* Organisms in this genus are gram–negative coccobacilli or short rods. *B. abortus* usually causes brucellosis in cattle, bison and water buffalo. *B. melitensis* is the most important species in sheep and goats, and *B. suis* in pigs. *B. ovis* can cause infertility in rams. *B. neotomae* is found in American wood rats. *B. abortus, B. melitensis, B. suis* and, rarely, *B. canis*, are zoonotic.

Species affected

Most species of *Brucella* are primarily associated with certain hosts; however, infections can also occur in other species, particularly when they are kept in close contact. *Brucella melitensis* mainly infects sheep and goats, but has also been seen in cattle and dogs. *Brucella abortus* is found in cattle, bison, and water buffalo and occasionally in sheep, goats, and dogs. *B. suis* is transmitted most significantly by pigs, though some variants are found in other species including hares, rodents, reindeer, caribou, Arctic foxes, and wolves. *B. ovis* is seen in sheep, *B. canis* in dogs and *B. neotomae* in American wood rats. *Brucella* infection can also be seen in other wild species including bison, elk, deer, moose, camels, and water buffalo. Horses in contact with infected cows can develop fistulous withers or poll evil; the infecting organism is most often *Brucella abortus.*

Geographic distribution

Brucellosis is found worldwide, but is well controlled in most developed countries. It still presents a problem in Africa, the Middle East, Central Asia, Southeast Asia, South America, and some Mediterranean countries.

B. melitensis is particularly common in Latin America, central Asia, the Mediterranean, and around the Arabian Gulf. This species does not seem to occur in northern Europe, Southeast Asia, Australia, or New Zealand. *B. ovis* is seen in Australia, New Zealand, and many other sheep–raising regions, including the United States. *B. suis* can be found worldwide, but the infection rate is high only in parts of South America and Southeast Asia, and in feral pigs in Australia and the southeastern United States. *B. abortus* has been eradicated from Japan, Canada, northern Europe, Australia, and New Zealand. In humans, brucellosis is rare in Europe, Canada, and United States but occurs regularly in the Middle East, the Mediterranean, Mexico, and Central America.

Transmission

Among animals, *Brucella* is usually transmitted by contact with the placenta, fetus, fetal fluids, and vaginal discharges from infected animals. Animals are infectious after either an abortion or a full–term parturition. Bacteria can also be found in the blood, urine, milk, and semen; shedding in milk and semen can be prolonged or lifelong. Infection occurs by ingestion and through mucous membranes, broken skin, and possibly intact skin. The mammary gland can be infected by direct contact; in cattle, the udder can be colonized by *B. abortus, B. melitensis* or *B. suis* on the hands of farm workers. *B. suis, B. ovis* and *B. canis* can be spread venereally; vene-

real transmission of *B. abortus* can occur but is rare. Some *Brucella* species can be transmitted vertically.

Brucella can be spread on fomites. In conditions of high humidity, low temperatures, and no sunlight, these organisms can remain viable for several months in water, aborted fetuses, manure, wool, hay, equipment, and clothes. *Brucella* is destroyed by several hours of exposure to direct sunlight.

Incubation period

The period between infection and reproductive signs is variable. In cattle, abortions and stillbirths usually occur 2 weeks to 5 months after infection.

Clinical signs

Brucellosis in cattle

In cattle, *B. abortus* causes abortions, stillbirths, and weak calves; abortions usually occur during the second half of gestation. The placenta may be retained and lactation may be decreased. Generally after the first abortion, the cow goes on to have subsequent normal pregnancies, though she still can shed the organism in milk and uterine discharges. Testicular abscesses or orchitis are sometimes seen in bulls. Arthritis can develop after long–term infections. Systemic signs do not usually occur.

Brucellosis in sheep and goats

In sheep and goats, *B. melitensis* can cause abortion, retained placenta, orchitis, and epididymitis. Abortions usually occur late in gestation in sheep and during the fourth month of gestation in goats. In goats, mastitis and lameness may be seen. Arthritis is rare in sheep.

B. ovis affects sheep but not goats. This organism can cause epididymitis, orchitis, and impaired fertility in rams. Initially, only poor quality semen may be seen; later, lesions may be palpable in the epididymis and scrotum. The testes may atrophy permanently. Abortions, placentitis, and perinatal mortality can be seen but are uncommon. Systemic signs are rare.

Brucellosis in pigs

In pigs, the most common symptom is abortion, which can occur at any time during gestation, and weak or stillborn piglets. Vaginal discharge is often minimal and the abortions may be mistaken for infertility. Temporary or permanent orchitis can be seen in boars. Boars can also excrete *B. suis* asymptomatically in the semen and sterility may be the only sign of infection. Swollen joints and tendon sheaths or lameness can occur in both sexes. Less common signs include posterior paralysis, metritis, and abscesses in other parts of the body. Although some pigs recover, others remain permanently infected. Fertility can be permanently impaired.

Brucellosis in horses

In horses, *B. abortus* and occasionally *B. suis* can cause inflammation of the supraspinous or supra–atlantal bursa; this syndrome is known, respectively, as fistulous withers or poll evil. The bursal sac becomes distended by a clear, viscous, straw–colored exudate and develops a thickened wall. It can rupture, leading to secondary inflammation. In chronic cases, nearby ligaments and the dorsal vertebral spines may become necrotic. *Brucella*–associated abortions are rare in horses.

Brucellosis in dogs

B. canis causes abortions, stillbirths, and infertility in dogs. Most infections are seen in kennels. Abortions usually occur during the last trimester and are followed by a prolonged vaginal discharge. Infected dogs may have lymphadenitis, epididymitis, periorchitis, and prostatitis. Fever is not usually seen.

Post mortem lesions

At slaughter, signs of infection including bacteria, purulent lesions, and granulomas may be present in the reproductive tract, mammary tissues, or articular tissues, as well as spleen, liver, lymph nodes, kidneys, and lungs.

The ruminant fetus may be autolyzed, normal, or have evidence of bronchopneumonia. In cattle, acute or chronic placentitis is sometimes seen. The cotyledons may be red, yellow, normal, or necrotic. The intercotyledonary region is typically leathery, with a wet appearance and focal thickening. Placentitis, with edema and necrosis of the cotyledons and a thickened and leathery intercotyledonary region, can also be seen in sheep infected with *B. melitensis*. The placenta is usually normal in goats. Fetal and placental lesions are rare in pigs infected with *B. suis*, but the fetus may be autolyzed.

Morbidity and mortality

In previously unexposed and unvaccinated cattle, infections spread rapidly with many abortions. Endemic herds will show only sporadic signs and cows may abort their first pregnancies. In dogs, up to 75% fewer puppies may be weaned from affected kennels. Ruminants usually abort only during their first gestation, but abortions can occur repeatedly in affected dogs. In pigs, the abortion rate is 0% to 80%. Fertility can be permanently impaired after infections with some species of *Brucella*. Deaths are rare in adult animals.

Diagnosis

Clinical

All abortions in cattle should be treated as suspected brucellosis and should be investigated. Cattle herds with brucellosis typically have multiple late–term abortions. In dogs, brucellosis should be considered when abortions are seen during the last trimester or when male dogs develop epididymitis and testicular atrophy.

Differential diagnosis

Other diseases causing abortion in the various species should be considered. In cattle, the differentials may include trichomoniasis, vibriosis, leptospirosis, listeriosis, infectious bovine rhinotracheitis, and various mycoses. In female dogs, brucellosis can resemble infections with beta–hemolytic streptococci or *Escherichia coli*.

Laboratory tests

Stained slides of infected materials may be indicative of brucellosis, but definitive diagnosis is made by culture and identification of the organism.

Serology

In cattle, serological screening tests may be done using complement fixation, ELISA, or rose Bengal tests. Increases in antibody titers may be seen with acute cases, but are not useful in chronic or recurrent cases. The milk ring test can be used to screen bulk milk samples for brucellosis.

In sheep and goats, *B. melitensis* can be diagnosed with buffered *Brucella* antigen tests (BBAT, also known as the card and plate agglutination tests) or complement fixation. ELISAs are being developed. The bulk milk ring test is not used in small ruminants. *B. ovis* infections can be diagnosed by ELISA, complement fixation, hemagglutination inhibition, indirect agglutination, and gel diffusion tests.

The tube or slide agglutination and gel diffusion tests are generally used in dogs. Nonspecific agglutination sometimes occurs but can be eliminated by pretreatment with 2–mercaptoethanol.

Serology is less reliable in pigs. Conventional serologic tests can misdiagnose *B. suis* infections in individual pigs; these tests are considered to be more reliable for a herd diagnosis. The BBATs are used most often; complement fixation or other serum agglutination tests may also be available. ELISA techniques and fluorescence polarization assays have been developed and may be more effective than other serologic tests.

Other tests

Immunofluorescent techniques can detect *B. abortus* in the placenta and fetus or *B. ovis* in the semen. A brucellin allergic skin test is sometimes used to test pigs for *B. suis* or unvaccinated sheep and goats for *B. melitensis*. This assay is generally a herd test. Polymerase chain reaction (PCR) techniques have also been developed for some species.

Samples to collect

Brucellosis is highly infectious to humans; samples should be collected and handled with all appropriate precautions.

Stomach contents from aborted fetuses are especially useful in diagnosis, as are other fetal tissues, placenta, and abortion material. Other samples of use include lymph nodes, spleen, liver, milk, semen, infected lesions from post mortem examination, blood, and serum. Repeated sampling of the semen may be necessary in *B. ovis* infections, as this organism is shed intermittently. Blood can be cultured from dogs; this species can be bacteremic for as long as 18 months after infection.

Recommended actions if brucellosis is suspected

Notification of authorities

Brucellosis is a notifiable disease in the U.S. All cases should be reported to the local health authority, state or federal veterinarians.
Federal: Area Veterinarians in Charge (AVICs):
http://www.aphis.usda.gov/vs/area_offices.htm
State Veterinarians:
http://www.aphis.usda.gov/vs/sregs/official.html

Quarantine and disinfection

Quarantine and slaughter of infected animals in necessary to eradicate the disease. Any area exposed to infected animals and their discharges should be thoroughly cleaned and disinfected. The *Brucella* organism can survive for months in the environment, but is destroyed by heat and sun exposure.

Public health

Brucellosis is highly pathogenic to humans and is one of the most easily acquired laboratory infections. In humans, brucellosis can be caused by *B. abortus*, *B. melitensis*, *B. suis* and, rarely, *B. canis*. *B. abortus* and *B. melitensis* vaccines are also pathogenic for people. Exposure is generally occupational in laboratory workers, veterinarians, and others in contact with infected animals. Ingestion of unpasteurized dairy products is also a concern is some areas.

The disease in humans often shows influenza–like signs with intermittent fever, malaise, generalized aching, bacteremia, and granulomatous lesions in internal organs. The duration can vary from several days or months to a year or longer, sometimes with permanent consequences. Severe complications can occur involving the musculoskeletal, cardiovascular, genitourinary, and central nervous systems. In humans, the case–fatality rate in untreated cases is less than 2%, and death is usually caused by endocarditis.

For more information

World Organization for Animal Health (OIE)
http://www.oie.int
OIE Manual of Standards
http://www.oie.int/eng/normes/mmanual/a_summry.htm
Brucellosis in Sheep and Goats (*Brucella melitensis*) European Commission Health and Consumer Protection Directorate General
http://europa.eu.int/comm/food/fs/sc/scah/out59_en.pdf
Centers for Disease Control and Prevention (CDC).
Brucellosis information
http://www.cdc.gov/ncidod/dbmd/diseaseinfo/brucellosis_t.htm
Manual for the Recognition of Exotic Diseases of Livestock. A Reference Guide for Animal Health Staff. Food and Agricul-

ture Organization of the United Nations
http://www.spc.int/rahs/

Material Safety Data Sheets –Canadian Laboratory Centre for Disease Control
http://www.phac-aspc.gc.ca/msds-ftss/index.html

USAMRIID's Medical Management of Biological Casualties Handbook
http://www.vnh.org/BIOCASU/toc.html

References

Alton G.G. and J.R.L. Forsyth. "*Brucella*." In *Medical Microbiology*. 4th ed. Edited by Samuel Baron. New York; Churchill Livingstone, 1996. 15 Dec 2002. http//www.gsbs.utmb.edu/microbook/ch028.htm.

"Bacterial infections caused by Gram–negative bacilli. Enterobacteriaceae." In *The Merck Manual*, 17th ed. Edited by M.H. Beers and R. Berkow. Whitehouse Station, NJ: Merck and Co., 1999. 8 Nov 2002. http://www.merck.com/pubs/mmanual/section13/chapter157/157d.htm.

"Bovine brucellosis." In *Manual of Standards for Diagnostic Tests and Vaccines*. Paris: World Organization for Animal Health, 2000, pp. 328–345.

"Brucellosis (*Brucella melitensis, abortus, suis,* and *canis*). Centers for Disease Control and Prevention, June 2002. 16 Dec 2002. http//www.cdc.gov/ncidod/dbmd/diseaseinfo/brucellosis_t.htm.

"Brucellosis." In *Medical Management of Biological Casualties Handbook*, 4th ed. Edited by M. Kortepeter, G. Christopher, T. Cieslak, R. Culpepper, R. Darling J. Pavlin, J. Rowe, K. McKee, Jr., E. Eitzen, Jr. Department of Defense, 2001. 16 Dec 2002 http//www.vnh.org/BIOCASU/7.html.

"Brucellosis." In *The Merck Veterinary Manual*, 8th ed. Edited by S.E. Aiello and A. Mays. Whitehouse Station, NJ: Merck and Co., 1998, pp. 991; 993; 994; 996; 998–1002; 1043.

"Brucellosis in sheep and goats (*Brucella melitensis*)." July 2001. European Commission Health and Consumer Protection Directorate General. 17 Dec 2002. http//europa.eu.int/comm/food/fs/sc/scah/out59_en.pdf.

"Caprine and ovine brucellosis (excluding *B. ovis*)." In *Manual of Standards for Diagnostic Tests and Vaccines*. Paris: World Organization for Animal Health, 2000, pp. 467–489.

"Control of Communicable Diseases." Edited by J. Chin. American Public Health Association, 2000, pp. 75–78.

"Fistulous withers and poll evil." In *The Merck Veterinary Manual*, 8th ed. Edited by S.E. Aiello and A. Mays. Whitehouse Station, NJ: Merck and Co., 1998, p. 762.

Garner G., P. Saville and A. Fediaevsky. "Brucellosis (Canine)." In *Manual for the Recognition of Exotic Diseases of Livestock. A Reference Guide for Animal Health Staff*. Food and Agriculture Organization of the United Nations. Secretariat of the Pacific Community, Dec 2002. 17 April 2003. http//www.spc.int/rahs/Manual/Canine–Feline/BRUCELLOSIS(CANINE)E.HTM.

Garner G., P. Saville and A. Fediaevsky. "Brucellosis (Bovine)." In *Manual for the Recognition of Exotic Diseases of Livestock. A Reference Guide for Animal Health Staff*. Food and Agriculture Organization of the United Nations. Secretariat of the Pacific Community, Dec 2002. 17 April 2003. http//www.spc.int/rahs/Manual/BOVINE/BRUCELLOSISE.HTM.

Herenda, D., P.G. Chambers, A. Ettriqui, P. Seneviratna, and T.J.P. da Silva. "Brucellosis." In *Manual on Meat Inspection for Developing Countries*. FAO Animal Production and Health Paper 119. 1994 Publishing and Multimedia Service, Information Division, FAO, 17 Dec 2002. http//www.fao.org/docrep/003/t0756e/T0756E03.htm#ch3.3.7.

"Material Safety Data Sheet –*Brucella* spp." Canadian Laboratory Centre for Disease Control, January 2001. 16 Dec 2002. http//www.phac-aspc.gc.ca/msds-ftss/index.html.

Plommet M., Diaz R. and J–M. Verger. "Brucellosis." In *Zoonoses*. Edited by S.R. Palmer, E.J.L. Soulsby and D.I.H Simpson. New York: Oxford University Press, 1998, pp. 23–35.

"Porcine brucellosis." In *Manual of Standards for Diagnostic Tests and Vaccines*. Paris: World Organization for Animal Health, 2000, pp. 623–629.

Chlamydiosis (Avian)

Psittacosis, Ornithosis

Importance

Avian chlamydiosis is a bacterial infection that may cause severe disease in some birds and be carried asymptomatically by others. Chlamydiosis can result in serious economic losses in turkey or duck operations. It is also a significant human zoonosis. Many infections spread to humans from pet birds (particularly psittacine birds), turkeys, or ducks. Untreated cases may be fatal.

Etiology

In birds, chlamydiosis results from infection by *Chlamydophila psittaci* (order Chlamydiales, family Chlamydiaceae). This organism, previously known as *Chlamydia psittaci*, is a Gram negative, coccoid, obligate intracellular bacterium. There are at least six avian serotypes.

Species affected

Avian chlamydiosis occurs in most birds, but is particularly common in psittacine birds, pigeons, doves, and mynah birds. This disease is sometimes seen in ducks and turkeys but only rarely in chickens.

Geographic distribution

Avian chlamydiosis can be found worldwide. *C. psittaci* is particularly common in psittacine birds in tropical and subtropical regions. This disease is present in the United States. In a 1982 survey, *C. psittaci* was isolated from 20% to 50% of necropsied pet birds in California and Florida.

Transmission

C. psittaci is transmitted frequently by the inhalation of infectious dust and occasionally by ingestion. Fomites can also spread chlamydiosis, and biting insects, mites, and lice may be important in mechanical transmission. Birds can be asymptomatic carriers; carriers shed *C. psittaci* intermittently, particularly when stressed. One form of the organism, the elementary body, can survive in dried feces for months.

Incubation period

The incubation period in cage birds is usually 3 days to several weeks. However, in latent infections, active disease may be seen years after infection.

Clinical signs

In turkeys, ducks, and pigeons, the clinical signs can include depression, ruffled feathers, weakness, inappetence, weight loss, nasal discharge, respiratory distress, yellowish–green or green diarrhea, and unilateral or bilateral conjunctivitis. Egg production is decreased. Nervous signs may be seen, including transient ataxia in pigeons and trembling or gait abnormalities in ducks.

In pet birds, common symptoms include anorexia, weight loss, diarrhea, yellowish droppings, sinusitis, respiratory distress, nervous signs, and conjunctivitis. Asymptomatic infections and mild infections with diarrhea or mild respiratory signs may also be seen. Residual disturbances in feathering may be apparent in survivors.

Post mortem lesions

Post–mortem lesions in birds can include pneumonia, airsacculitis, hepatitis, myocarditis, epicarditis, nephritis, peritonitis, and splenitis. In turkeys, an enlarged and congested spleen may be the only lesion. Wasting, vascular congestion, fibrinous airsacculitis, fibrinous pericarditis, fibrinous pneumonia with congestion of the lungs, or fibrinous perihepatitis may also be seen in turkeys. In pigeons, common lesions include hepatomegaly, airsacculitis, enteritis, and conjunctivitis with swollen and encrusted eyelids. The spleen may rupture. In cage birds, the liver may be enlarged and yellow with focal necrosis. The spleen is often enlarged, with white foci. Airsacculitis, pericarditis, and congestion of the intestinal tract can also be seen in this species.

Morbidity and mortality

Morbidity and mortality vary with the host species and pathogenicity of the serotype. Young birds tend to be more susceptible than older birds. In turkeys, serovar D strains cause 50% to 80% morbidity and 10% to 30% mortality. In broiler turkeys, up to 80% of infections with this serovar may be fatal. Other serovars in turkeys usually result in 5% to 20% morbidity, with mortality under 50%. In ducks, morbidity may be up to 80% and mortality 0% to 40%. Concurrent infections or stress increase the severity of the disease.

Antibiotics are effective in treating the symptoms of chlamydiosis, but do not always eliminate infections in birds.

Diagnosis

Clinical

Chlamydiosis can be difficult to diagnose; however, it should be considered in a bird that is lethargic and has nonspecific signs of illness. A high index of suspicion should be maintained in recently purchased pet birds.

Differential diagnosis

In turkeys, the differential diagnosis includes influenza, aspergillosis, fowl cholera, and *Mycoplasma gallisepticum* infections. In cage birds, infections with herpesviruses, paramyxovirus, influenza, and the Enterobacteriaceae should be considered. Samples from all birds should be cultured for *Salmonella*, *Pasteurella*, *Mycoplasma*, and other bacteria and viruses.

Laboratory tests

Chlamydiosis is usually diagnosed by isolating *C. psittaci* from affected birds. *C. psittaci* can be isolated in embryonated eggs, laboratory animals, or cell cultures of buffalo green monkey (BGM), African green monkey (Vero), McCoy, or L cells. The organisms can be identified by direct immunofluorescence or other staining techniques. A single negative culture may be misleading, as carrier birds may shed *C. psittaci* only intermittently. Treatment with antibiotics during the 2 to 3 weeks before testing may also lead to false negatives.

Chlamydiosis can also be diagnosed by demonstrating *C. psittaci* in tissues, feces, or exudates by histochemical or immunohistochemical staining. Antigen capture enzyme–linked immunosorbent assays (ELISAs) are also used, but may lack sensitivity or cross–react with other Gram negative bacteria. Polymerase chain reaction (PCR) and polymerase chain reaction/ restriction fragment length polymorphism (PCR–RFLP) assays have been described.

Serology is occasionally helpful. At least a four–fold rise in titer should be seen in paired samples. Complement fixation is the standard test. Other assays include ELISA, latex agglutination (LA), elementary body agglutination (EBA), micro–immunofluorescence (MIFT), and agar gel immunodiffusion tests. The EBA test detects IgM only and can be used to diagnose current infections.

Samples to collect

Chlamydiosis is a zoonotic disease; samples should be collected and handled with all appropriate precautions.

In live birds, pharyngeal and nasal swabs should be taken. Feces, cloacal swabs, conjunctival scrapings, and peritoneal exudate may also be submitted. Post–mortem samples from acute cases should include whole blood and samples of ocular exudates, nasal exudates, and the fibrinous or inflammatory exudates around organs. Tissue samples should also be collected from the lung, kidney, spleen, liver, and pericardium. If diarrhea is present, the colon contents or feces should be cultured. Samples for bacterial isolation must be collected aseptically and placed in sucrose/phosphate/glutamate (SPG) medium for transport. Serum may also be collected for serology. To prevent human infections, samples should be wrapped securely and shipped in conformation with all biohazard regulations.

Recommended actions if chlamydiosis is suspected

Notification of authorities

Chlamydiosis is a reportable disease. State authorities should be consulted for more specific information.

Federal: Area Veterinarians in Charge (AVICs):
http://www.aphis.usda.gov/vs/area_offices.htm
State Veterinarians:
http://www.aphis.usda.gov/vs/sregs/official.html

Quarantine and disinfection

C. psittaci is a contagious disease; birds must be quarantined during treatment. While a bird is being treated, the premises should be cleaned and disinfected frequently to eliminate infectious dust. The circulation of feathers and dust should also be minimized. When handling infected birds or cleaning cages, handlers should wear protective clothing, gloves, a paper surgical cap, and a respirator with at least a N95 rating.

Dead birds should be immersed in disinfectant solutions to prevent infectious dust from spreading in the air. Carcasses must be wet with detergent and water or disinfectant during necropsy. Potentially infectious material, including carcasses, should be examined in a laminar flow hood or while wearing the proper protective equipment.

C. psittaci is susceptible to quaternary ammonium compounds, chlorophenols, iodophore disinfectants, formaldehyde, 80% isopropyl alcohol, or a 1:100 dilution of household bleach.

Public health

Human infections usually occur by inhalation and often develop after contact with pet birds or poultry. Human chlamydiosis varies from a mild, flu–like infection with a fever, shivering, headaches, anorexia, sore throat, and photophobia to a serious atypical pneumonia with a dry cough and dyspnea. More rarely, a severe systemic illness with endocarditis, myocarditis, and renal complications may develop. Encephalitis, meningitis, and myelitis have also been seen. Treated cases are rarely fatal.

For more information

World Organization for Animal Health (OIE)
http://www.oie.int
OIE Manual of Standards
http://www.oie.int/eng/normes/mmanual/a_summry.htm
OIE International Animal Health Code
http://www.oie.int/eng/normes/mcode/A_summry.htm
Material Safety Data Sheet – *Chlamydia psittaci* at Canadian Laboratory Centre for Disease Control
http://www.phac-aspc.gc.ca/msds-ftss/index.html

References

"Avian Chlamydiosis." In *Whiteman and Bickford's Avian Disease Manual*, 4th ed. Edited by B.R. Charlton et al. Kennett Square, Pa: American Association of Avian Pathologists, 1996, pp. 68–71.

"Avian Chlamydiosis." In *Manual of Standards for Diagnostic Tests and Vaccines*. Paris: World Organization for Animal Health, 2000, pp. 679–690.

"Chlamydiosis." In *The Merck Veterinary Manual*, 8th ed. Edited by S.E. Aiello and A. Mays. Whitehouse Station, NJ: Merck and Co., 1998, pp. 1300–1301.

"Chlamydiosis." In *Poultry Diseases*, 4th ed. Edited by F.T.W. Jordan and M. Pattison. London: W.B. Saunders, 1996, pp. 94–99.

Gerlach, H. "*Chlamydia.*" In *Clinical Avian Medicine and Surgery*. Edited by G.J. Harrison and L. Harrison. Philadelphia: W.B. Saunders, 1986, pp. 457–463.

Johnston W.B., M. Eidson, K.A. Smith, and M.G. Stobierski. "Compendium of chlamydiosis (psittacosis) control, 1999." Psittacosis Compendium Committee, National Association of State Public Health Veterinarians. *Journal of the American Veterinary Medical Association* 214, no. 5 (1999):640–646.

"Material Safety Data Sheet –*Chlamydia psittaci.*" January 2001. Canadian Laboratory Centre for Disease Control. 1 November 2001. http//www.phac-aspc.gc.ca/msds-ftss/index.html.

Vanrompay D., R. Ducatelle, and F. Haesebrouck. "Chlamydia psittaci infections: a review with emphasis on avian chlamydiosis." *Veterinary Microbiology* 45, no. 2–3 (1995):93–119.

Classical Swine Fever

Hog Cholera, Peste du Porc,
Colera Porcina, Virusschweinepest

Importance

Classical swine fever is a serious and highly contagious viral disease of pigs. Acute or chronic infections occur; both are usually fatal. In herds infected with less virulent isolates, the only symptom may be poor reproductive performance or a failure to thrive. A wide range of clinical signs and a similarity to other diseases can make classical swine fever challenging to diagnose.

Etiology

Classical swine fever results from infection by classical swine fever virus (CSFV), (genus *Pestivirus*, family Flaviviridae). This virus is also known as hog cholera virus. Only one serotype has been found. The CSF virus is very similar to the bovine viral diarrhea (BVD) virus that affects cattle.

Species affected

Classical swine fever affects domestic and wild pigs.

Geographic distribution

Classical swine fever is found in East and Southeast Asia, the Indian subcontinent, China, East and Central Africa, and most of South and Central America. This disease has been eradicated from the United States, Canada, New Zealand, and Australia. Most of Western Europe is free of classical swine fever; however, foci of infection remain in Germany and some countries of Eastern Europe.

Transmission

Classical swine fever is highly contagious. Virus transmission is mainly oral; CSFV is often spread by feeding uncooked contaminated garbage. Animals can also be infected through the mucus membranes, conjunctiva, and skin abrasions. Aerosol spread is sometimes seen in confined spaces; however, the virus does not travel long distances in the air. Infected carrier sows may give birth to persistently infected pigs. Mechanical spread by fomites and insects occurs.

Infected pigs are the only reservoir of virus. Blood, secretions and excretions, and tissues contain infectious virus. CSFV is moderately fragile in the environment, but can remain infectious for months in refrigerated meat and years in frozen meat. It can survive in contaminated pens and on fomites for as long as two weeks.

Incubation period

Variable incubation periods have been published, ranging from 2 to 14 days.

Clinical signs

The clinical signs of classical swine fever vary with the strain of virus and susceptibility of the pigs. More virulent strains cause acute disease; less virulent strains can result in a high percentage of chronic, mild, or asymptomatic infections.

In acute classical swine fever, common clinical signs include a high fever, dullness, weakness, drowsiness, huddling, anorexia, an unsteady gait, conjunctivitis, and constipation followed by diarrhea. Several days after the first symptoms appear, the abdomen, inner thighs, and ears may develop a purple discoloration. Convulsions may be seen in the terminal stages. Pigs with acute classical swine fever often die within one to two weeks.

The symptoms of chronic disease include intermittent fever, anorexia, periods of constipation or diarrhea, stunted growth, and alopecia. Immunosuppression may lead to concurrent infections. The symptoms of chronic infections can wax and wane for weeks to months and may affect only a few animals in the herd. Chronic infections are almost always fatal.

Reproductive symptoms may also be seen. Virulent strains can cause abortions or the death of piglets soon after birth. Less virulent strains of CSFV may result in stillbirths or mummification. Some piglets are born with a congenital tremor or congenital malformations of the visceral organs and central nervous system. Other piglets are asymptomatic but persistently infected. These animals are persistently viremic and become clinically ill after several months. They may have mild anorexia, depression, stunted growth, dermatitis, diarrhea, conjunctivitis, ataxia, or paresis, and may die. In some breeding herds infected by less virulent strains, poor reproductive performance is the only sign of disease.

Post mortem lesions

The lesions of classical swine fever are highly variable. In acute disease, the most common lesion is hemorrhage. The skin may be discolored purple and the lymph nodes may be swollen and hemorrhagic. Petechial or ecchymotic hemorrhages can often be seen on serosal and mucosal surfaces, particularly the kidney, urinary bladder, epicardium, larynx, trachea, intestines, subcutaneous tissues, and spleen. Straw–colored fluid may be found in the peritoneal and thoracic cavities and the pericardial sac. Necrotic foci are common in the tonsils. Splenic infarcts are occasionally seen. The lungs may be congested and hemorrhagic. In some acute cases, lesions may be absent or inconspicuous.

The lesions of chronic disease are less severe and may be complicated by secondary infections. In addition, necrotic foci or "button" ulcers may be found in the intestinal mucosa, epiglottis and larynx.

In congenitally infected piglets, common lesions include cerebellar hypoplasia, thymic atrophy, ascites, and deformities of the head and legs.

Morbidity and mortality

Both morbidity and mortality are high in acute infections. The mortality rate in acute cases can reach 90%. Chronic infections are also fatal in most cases.

Vaccines may be available in some areas. Vaccines can protect animals from clinical disease, but do not prevent infections. Good vaccination programs can eventually eliminate the infection in herds.

Diagnosis

Clinical

Classical swine fever should be suspected in pigs with signs of septicemia and a high fever, particularly if uncooked scraps have been fed, unusual biological products have been used, or new animals have been added to the herd. Differentiation from other diseases may be difficult without laboratory testing. In acute outbreaks, the likelihood of observing the characteristic necropsy lesions is better if 4 or 5 pigs are examined.

Differential diagnosis

The differential diagnosis includes African swine fever, porcine dermatitis and nephropathy syndrome, erysipelas, eperythrozoonosis, salmonellosis, actinobacillosis, Glasser's disease (*Haemophilus para suis* infection), thrombocytopenic purpura, warfarin poisoning, Aujeszky's disease, heavy metal poisoning, and salt poisoning. Pigs congenitally infected with bovine viral diarrhea (BVD) virus may look very similar to pigs with classical swine fever.

Laboratory tests

Classical swine fever can be diagnosed by detecting the virus or its antigens in whole blood or tissue samples. Virus antigens are detected by direct immunofluorescence or enzyme–linked immunosorbent assays (ELISAs). CSFV is differentiated from other pestiviruses by immunofluorescence testing with monoclonal antibodies. The virus can also be isolated in several cell lines including PK–15 cells; it is identified by direct immunofluorescence or peroxidase staining. Reverse transcriptase polymerase chain reaction (RT–PCR) tests are available.

Serology is used for diagnosis and surveillance. The most commonly used tests are virus neutralization tests, including the fluorescent antibody virus neutralization (FAVN) test, the neutralizing peroxidase–linked assay (NPLA), and ELISAs. Antibodies usually develop during the third week after infection, but cannot be reliably detected until 30 days after infection. They persist for life. Antibodies against ruminant pestiviruses may be found in breeding animals; only tests that use monoclonal antibodies can differentiate between these viruses and CSFV.

Samples to collect

Before collecting or sending any samples from animals with a suspected foreign animal disease, the proper authorities should be contacted. Samples should only be sent under secure conditions and to authorized laboratories to prevent the spread of the disease.

Samples should be taken from at least 4 pigs. In live pigs, whole blood is preferred but tonsil biopsies are sometimes useful. Serum samples should be taken from recovered animals or sows that have been in contact with suspected cases.

At necropsy, the tonsils should be submitted for virus isolation or antigen detection. Other organs to collect include the submandibular and mesenteric lymph nodes, spleen, kidneys, and the distal part of the ileum. Samples for antigen detection and virus isolation should be refrigerated but not frozen; they should be kept cold during shipment to the laboratory. A complete set of tissues, including the whole brain, should be submitted in 10% buffered formalin for histology.

Recommended actions if classical swine fever is suspected

Notification of authorities

Classical swine fever should be reported immediately upon diagnosis or suspicion of the disease.

Federal: Area Veterinarians in Charge (AVICs):
http://www.aphis.usda.gov/vs/area_offices.htm
State Veterinarians:
http://www.aphis.usda.gov/vs/sregs/official.html

Quarantine and disinfection

CSFV is moderately fragile in the environment. This virus is sensitive to drying and ultraviolet light and is rapidly inactivated by a pH less than 3. Sodium hypochlorite and phenolic compounds are effective disinfectants. CSFV can survive for long periods in meat, but is destroyed by cooking.

During outbreaks, confirmed cases and contact animals may be slaughtered and aquarantine imposed. Vaccination may be used as a tool to assist in controlling an outbreak and eradicating the disease. In countries free of classical swine fever, periodic serologic sampling is necessary to monitor for the potential reintroduction of disease.

Public health

Classical swine fever does not affect humans.

For more information

World Organization for Animal Health (OIE)
http://www.oie.int
OIE Manual of Standards
http://www.oie.int/eng/normes/mmanual/a_summry.htm
OIE International Animal Health Code
http://www.oie.int/eng/normes/mcode/A_summry.htm
USAHA Foreign Animal Diseases Book
http://www.vet.uga.edu/vpp/gray_book/FAD/
Animal Health Australia. The National Animal Health
Information System (NAHIS)
http://www.aahc.com.au/nahis/disease/dislist.asp

References

Blackwell, J.H. "Cleaning and Disinfection." In *Foreign Animal Diseases*. Richmond, VA: United States Animal Health Association, 1998, pp. 445–448.

"Classical Swine Fever (Hog Cholera)." In *Manual of Standards for Diagnostic Tests and Vaccines*. Paris: World Organization for Animal Health, 2000, pp. 199–211.

Dulac, G.C. "Hog Cholera." In *Foreign Animal Diseases*. Richmond, VA: United States Animal Health Association, 1998, pp. 273–282.

"Hog Cholera." In *The Merck Veterinary Manual*, 8th ed. Edited by S.E. Aiello and A. Mays. Whitehouse Station, NJ: Merck and Co., 1998, pp. 509–512.

"Hog Cholera." Animal Health Australia. The National Animal Health Information System (NAHIS). 24 Oct 2001. http//www.aahc.com.au/nahis/disease/dislist.asp.

Contagious Agalactia

Importance

Contagious agalactia can cause serious economic losses in sheep and goats from mastitis, polyarthritis, and keratoconjunctivitis. Mortality may be as high as 10% to 20% in some outbreaks. This disease is infectious; the causative organism can be shed in milk, other secretions, urine, and feces, and may be present in water, feed, and other fomites. Some outbreaks may affect most of the animals on a farm.

Etiology

Typically, contagious agalactia is caused by infection with *Mycoplasma agalactiae*. However, animals with very similar symptoms may be infected with *M. capricolum capricolum*, *M. putrefasciens*, *M. mycoides capri*, or the "large colony" type of *M. mycoides mycoides* instead. Such atypical infections appear to be much more common in goats than sheep. Some authorities consider infections with all of these agents to be contagious agalactia; others prefer to reserve the term for infections with *M. agalactiae*. Until this issue has been resolved, reports of contagious agalactia outbreaks should specify the species involved.

Species affected

Contagious agalactia affects sheep and goats. Goats appear to be particularly susceptible to the disease.

Geographic distribution

Contagious agalactia caused by *M. agalactiae* is important in the former Soviet Union, India, Pakistan, the Near East, and in the Mediterranean region of Europe, Asia, and North Africa. It has also been found in South America, South Africa, and Australia. Three isolations of *M. agalactiae* have been reported from the United States but these North American strains did not seem to cause significant disease.

Transmission

Animals infected with *M. agalactiae* shed the organisms in urine, feces, and secretions including milk. *M. agalactiae* can be shed during more than one lactation; between lactations, the organisms can survive in the supramammary lymph nodes. Asymptomatic or chronically infected carriers may be infectious for months.

Most cases of contagious agalactia develop at parturition or soon after. Most infections develop when an animal ingests contaminated milk, either directly or in feed or water. Animals may also ingest mycoplasmas in urine, feces, nasal, or ocular discharges, or inhale contaminated dust. *M. agalactiae* can enter the teat opening directly during milking. It can also spread on fomites. Although mycoplasmas are usually thought to be fragile and short–lived in the environment, some *M. agalactiae* have been reported to survive for long periods in the soil, dung, or secretions. Survival appears to be particularly likely if the temperature is low.

Incubation period

The incubation period in natural infections is highly variable, from 7 to 56 days.

Clinical signs

Infections with *M. agalactiae* may be asymptomatic, mild, acute, or chronic. Acute cases begin with a transient fever followed by malaise, poor appetite, and mastitis. The udder is hot and swollen; either one or both glands can be affected. Characteristically, the milk is greenish–yellow or grayish–blue; the consistency is watery at first, then lumpy. Lactation diminishes and may completely stop. Eventually, the udder atrophies and becomes flabby and fibrosed. Polyarthritis is common, and may be the major symptom in male goats. Lameness and swelling are particularly noticeable in the tarsal and carpal joints. The animal may become unable to stand or walk. Keratoconjunctivitis develops in approximately half of all infections. It is usually temporary, but occasionally results in blindness in one or both eyes. Abortions can occur in pregnant animals and kids may develop pneumonia. *M. agalactiae* may also cause granular vulvovaginitis in goats.

Post mortem lesions

Characteristically, female animals have catarrhal mastitis with primary inflammation of the interstitial tissues. Animals in later stages may have secondary acinar involvement. Fibrosis or parenchymatous atrophy may be seen. In both males and females with acute disease, congestion of the musculature, spleen, and liver may be found. Arthritis with periarticular edema is common, particularly in the carpal joints. The synovial membranes may be hyperemic, and the joint cavities may contain hemorrhagic or turbid fluid. Serous or mucopurulent conjunctivitis may be present, as well as keratitis or corneal ulceration.

Morbidity and mortality

Most cases of contagious agalactia develop during or soon after parturition. In serious disease outbreaks, the majority of suscep-

tible animals may become ill. Mortality is usually 20% or less, but may be higher if secondary bacterial pneumonia develops.

Antibiotics can result in symptomatic improvement, but may not be effective against joint infections and rarely eliminate the infection. Vaccines are available in some countries, but inactivated vaccines are generally not very effective. Live vaccines may prevent symptoms, but do not stop infections or shedding of virulent mycoplasmas. Vaccine organisms may be shed in the milk. In endemic areas, sanitary precautions can decrease the incidence of disease. Removal of newborns from the dam can also be effective.

Diagnosis

Clinical

Contagious agalactia should be suspected in animals with mastitis and decreased milk production, keratoconjunctivitis, and arthritis, particularly when these symptoms develop near the time of parturition.

Differential diagnosis

The differential diagnosis includes infections with *Pasteurella haemolytica*, *Streptococcus* species, *Staphylococcus* species, caprine arthritis encephalitis virus, or *Erysipelothrix rhusiopathiae*. *M. capricolum capricolum*, *M. putrefasciens*, *M. mycoides capri*, and the "large colony" type of *M. mycoides mycoides* should also be considered, particularly in goats.

Laboratory tests

Contagious agalactia is identified by isolation of the causative organism, followed by serologic confirmation of its identity. *M. agalactiae* can be grown on media containing heart–infusion broth, yeast extract, horse or pig serum, and ampicillin or cycloserine. Typical fried egg colonies are seen on solid media. Culture may take 2 to 3 weeks. Isolates are identified serologically with the disk growth inhibition test, film inhibition test, or indirect fluorescent antibody test.

Polymerase chain reaction (PCR) techniques and immunoblotting have also been used to identify *M. agalactiae*.

Serology can be useful during confirmed outbreaks. The most commonly used test is complement fixation. Other serologic tests include enzyme–linked immunosorbent assay (ELISA), "film and spots" inhibition, and indirect hemagglutination.

Samples to collect

Before collecting or sending any samples from animals with a suspected foreign animal disease, the proper authorities should be contacted. Samples should only be sent under secure conditions and to authorized laboratories to prevent the spread of the disease.

In live animals, the preferred samples for culture are milk, aspirated joint fluid, and nasal exudate. Mycoplasmas can also be isolated from blood samples during acute disease. In addition, they may be found in swabs from the eyes, urine, and feces. Serum should be collected for serology.

The optimal samples from dead animals are the udder and its associated lymph nodes, joint fluid, and samples from lung lesions. Some authorities also recommend blood, urine, liver, spleen, and other organs. Samples for culture should be collected aseptically and placed in transport medium (heart infusion broth, 20% serum, 10% yeast extract, and benzylpenicillin). They should be kept cool and quickly transported to the laboratory on wet ice. If samples must be held for more than a few days, they may be frozen.

Recommended actions if contagious agalactia is suspected

Notification of authorities

Contagious agalactia should be reported immediately to state or federal authorities.

Federal: Area Veterinarians in Charge (AVICs):
   http://www.aphis.usda.gov/vs/area_offices.htm
State Veterinarians:
   http://www.aphis.usda.gov/vs/sregs/official.html

Quarantine and disinfection

M. agalactiae is contagious to contact animals and can also be spread on fomites. The organism can be inactivated by sodium hypochlorite (30 ml of household bleach in 1 gallon of water), 2% sodium hydroxide (pH 12.4), 1% formalin, cresol, sodium carbonate (4% anhydrous or 10% crystalline with 1% detergent), and ionic and nonionic detergents.

Public health

There is no evidence that *M. agalactiae* is a threat to human health.

For more information

World Organization for Animal Health (OIE)
   http://www.oie.int
OIE Manual of Standards
   http://www.oie.int/eng/normes/mmanual/a_summry.htm
OIE International Animal Health Code
   http://www.oie.int/eng/normes/mcode/A_summry.htm
USAHA Foreign Animal Diseases Book
   http://www.vet.uga.edu/vpp/gray_book/FAD/

References

Maré, C. John. "Contagious Agalactia of Sheep and Goats." In *Foreign Animal Diseases*. Richmond, VA: United States Animal Health Association, 1998, pp. 147–153.

"Contagious Agalactia." In *Manual of Standards for Diagnostic Tests and Vaccines*. Paris: World Organization for Animal Health, 2000, pp. pp. 490–496.

"Contagious Agalactia." In *The Merck Veterinary Manual*, 8th ed. Edited by S.E. Aiello and A. Mays. Whitehouse Station, NJ: Merck and Co., 1998, pp. 1003–1004.

Contagious Bovine Pleuropneumonia

Importance

Contagious bovine pleuropneumonia (CBPP) causes lung and occasionally joint disease. Economic losses can be significant due to high infectivity and the presence of chronic subclinical carriers. The response to antibiotic treatment can be incomplete, creating chronic carriers; therefore slaughter is generally recommended for infected animals. Humans have not been found to be susceptible to contagious bovine pleuropneumonia.

Etiology

Mycoplasma mycoides mycoides small–colony type (SC type) is the causative agent of contagious bovine pleuropneumonia. *M. mycoides mycoides* large–colony type is not pathogenic in cattle, but in sheep and goats can cause septicemia, polyarthritis, mastitis, encephalitis, conjunctivitis, hepatitis, and occasionally pneumonia. Contagious caprine pleuropneumonia is caused by a different *Mycoplasma* agent (see the contagious caprine pleuropneumonia fact sheet).

Species affected

The genus *Bos* (including European breeds *Bos taurus*) and zebu (*Bos indicus*) cattle are the main hosts for contagious bovine pleuropneumonia. European breeds seem to be more susceptible than African breeds. Animals less than 3 years old are also more susceptible. Bison and yak have been infected in zoos, and infections have been reported in water buffalo (*Bubalus bubalis*). Wild bovids and camels are resistant.

Geographic distribution

Contagious bovine pleuropneumonia is endemic in Africa, the Middle East, and parts of Asia (especially India and China). Contagious bovine pleuropneumonia is not currently found in the Western hemisphere. The United States has been CBPP–free since 1893.

Transmission

Close contact is necessary for transmission, which occurs primarily through the inhalation of infected droplets from a coughing animal. The organism is also present in saliva, urine, fetal membranes, and uterine discharges. Transplacental infection has been known to occur. Introduction of a carrier animal to a susceptible herd is the most common cause of outbreaks.

Incubation period

The incubation period for contagious bovine pleuropneumonia can be long (20 to 123 days). After experimental direct tracheal infection, the clinical signs appear in 2 to 3 weeks.

Clinical signs

In adult animals, lethargy, anorexia and fever are the first signs of CBPP, followed by cough. The signs progress to include thoracic pain, dyspnea, an increased respiratory rate, and elbow abduction. Animals with chronic infections have less obvious signs of pneumonia, but may cough with exercise. These animals are often thin and may have a recurrent mild fever. Infected calves commonly have polyarthritis with or without pneumonia. Joints may be warm and swollen and extremely painful.

Post mortem lesions

The post mortem lesions of CBPP include thickening and consolidation of lung tissues with extensive fibrin accumulation on pleural surfaces and within interlobular septa. Lesions are frequently unilateral. Large amounts of straw–colored fluid may be present in the thoracic cavity and pericardial sac. A characteristic marbled appearance of the affected lungs is caused by the presence of both acute and chronic lesions in the interlobular septa. Fibrin is progressively replced by fibrous connective tissue over time. Encapsulated pulmonary sequestra (necrotic lung tissue) can be found even in recovered animals. The organism can survive for many months within these sequestra. In calves with polyarthritis, joints are filled with abundant fibrin.

Morbidity and mortality

Morbidity and mortality rates vary greatly. Morbidity increases with close confinement. Mortality can be affected by secondary factors such as nutrition and parasitism and can range from 10% to 70%.

Diagnosis

Clinical

Contagious bovine pleuropneumonia is difficult to diagnose based on clinical signs alone as there can be many causes of severe pneumonia in cattle. Animals with CBPP frequently present with unilateral pneumonia. In a herd with signs of pneumonia in adults and polyarthritis in calves, CBPP should be considered. Post mortem lesions may be more useful in the diagnosis.

Differential diagnosis

Differentials for acute infections include acute bovine pasteurellosis (mannheimiosis) and pleuropneumonia resulting from mixed infections. Bovine mannheimiosis generally spreads more rapidly through a herd and primarily affects young animals. Chronic infections should be differentiated from caseonecrotic bronchopneumonia associated with *Mycoplasma bovis* infection, hydatid cyst, actinobacillosis, tuberculosis, and bovine farcy.

Laboratory tests

Mycoplasma mycoides mycoides is isolated and identified by metabolic and growth inhibition tests, MF–dot test and polymerase chain reaction. Serological tests include complement fixation (used only for herds, not individual diagnosis), competitive ELISA (under validation by International Atomic Energy Agency and several reference laboratories) and hemagglutination. An agglutination test is available for use in active outbreaks at the herd level.

Samples to collect

Before collecting or sending any samples from animals with a suspected foreign animal disease, the proper authorities should be contacted. Samples should only be sent under secure conditions and to authorized laboratories to prevent the spread of the disease.

Samples include lung lesions, pleural fluids, lymph nodes, and lung tissue exudate. These should be not be frozen for isolation of the organism. Acute and convalescent serum samples can also be tested.

Recommended actions if contagious bovine pleuropneumonia is suspected

Notification of authorities

Contagious bovine pleuropneumonia should be reported immediately to state or federal authorities upon diagnosis or suspicion of the disease.

Federal: Area Veterinarians in Charge (AVICs):
http://www.aphis.usda.gov/vs/area_offices.htm
State Veterinarians:
http://www.aphis.usda.gov/vs/sregs/official.html

Quarantine and disinfection

Quarantine of exposed and infected animals is recommended along with testing and slaughter of infected animals. Antibiotic treatment is not effective due to the sequestration of the organism. *M. mycoides mycoides* (SC type) may survive in the environment for a few days, but does not survive in meat or meat products. It is inactivated by common disinfectants. The organism survives well with freezing.

Public health

Humans have not been found to be susceptible to *Mycoplasma mycoides mycoides*.

For more information

World Organization for Animal Health (OIE)
http://www.oie.int
OIE Manual of Standards
http://www.oie.int/eng/normes/mmanual/a_summry.htm
OIE International Animal Health Code
http://www.oie.int/eng/normes/mcode/A_summry.htm
USAHA Foreign Animal Diseases Book
http://www.vet.uga.edu/vpp/gray_book/FAD/

References

"Contagious Bovine Pleuropneumonia." In *Manual of Standards for Diagnostic Tests and Vaccines*. Paris: World Organization for Animal Health, 2000, pp.123–133.

"Contagious Bovine Pleuropneumonia." In *The Merck Veterinary Manual*, 8th ed. Edited by S.E. Aiello and A. Mays. Whitehouse Station, NJ: Merck and Co., 1998, pp. 1078–1079.

Brown, Corrie "Contagious Bovine Pleuropneumonia." In *Foreign Animal Diseases*. Richmond, VA: United States Animal Health Association, 1998, pp. 154–160.

"Contagious Bovine Pleuropneumonia." 30 Aug. 2000 Office International des Epizooties 16 Oct. 2001. http//www.oie.int/eng/maladies/fiches/a_A060.htm.

Contagious Caprine Pleuropneumonia

Importance

Contagious caprine pleuropneumonia (CCPP) is an extremely contagious disease of goats with acute signs of pneumonia and high mortality. Fibrinous pleuropneumonia is found at necropsy.

Etiology

Two organisms have been reported as the causative agents for contagious caprine pleuropneumonia. *Mycoplasma capricolum capripneumoniae*, commonly known as *mycoplasma* biotype F–38, is the most contagious and virulent of the two. *Mycoplasma mycoides capri* (type strain PG–3) also appears to cause the disease in goats, although much less commonly and with somewhat different signs.

Other mycoplasma organisms can cause pneumonia in goats, but are not considered to cause CCPP. *M. mycoides mycoides* large–colony type is pathogenic in sheep and goats and can cause septicemia, polyarthritis, mastitis, encephalitis, conjunctivitis, hepatitis, and occasionally pneumonia. *M. mycoides mycoides* small–colony type (SC type) is the causative agent of contagious bovine pleuropneumonia which produces similar signs in cattle to CCPP in goats. *M. capricolum capricolum*, closely related to *mycoplasma* F–38, causes mastitis, septicemia, and polyarthritis in goats and occasionally pneumonia. *M. mycoides mycoides* large–colony type and *M. capricolum capricolum* have been seen in North America.

Species affected

Goats are the only species known to be affected by *Mycoplasma* F–38. Sheep can be experimentally infected with *M. mycoides capri* and the organism can be transmitted from goats to sheep, however, sheep are not considered susceptible to natural disease.

Geographic distribution

Contagious caprine pleuropneumonia can be found in Africa, the Middle East, Eastern Europe, the former Soviet Union, and the Far East. Neither of the causative organisms has been found in North America.

Transmission

Transmission of CCPP is by direct contact through inhalation of infected respiratory droplets. *Mycoplasma* F–38 is much more contagious than *M. mycoides capri*. Carrier animals may shed more organisms after times of stress and sudden changes in climate.

Incubation period

The incubation period is often 6 to 10 days, though it is sometimes as long as 3 to 4 weeks.

Clinical signs

Signs of classical CCPP, caused by *Mycoplasma* F–38, are distinctly respiratory. They include very high fever (106°F/ 41°C), lethargy, anorexia, coughing, and labored respiration. Frothy nasal discharge and stringy saliva may also be seen. Acute cases generally die within 7 to 10 days. Chronic cases occur when animals have some resistance through previous exposure. These animals are more likely to survive and become carriers.

M. mycoides capri infection is often more generalized with septicemia. The reproductive, gastrointestinal, and respiratory systems are commonly affected.

Post mortem lesions

Post mortem lesions seen with *Mycoplasma* F–38 infections are limited to the lungs. They include fibrinous pneumonia with straw–colored fluid in the thorax, and pea–sized yellow colored nodules with surrounding congestion as the disease progresses. The lesions may involve one or both lungs and adhesions to the chest wall may occur with thickened pulmonary pleura. Unlike contagious bovine pleuropneumonia, there is no thickening of the interlobular tissue.

M. mycoides capri can cause encephalitis, meningitis, lymphadenitis, splenitis, genitourinary tract inflammation, and intestinal lesions. Lung lesions when present are more similar to contagious bovine pleuropneumonia; often, unilateral, fibrinous pneumonia with hepatization and dilated interlobular septa is seen.

Morbidity and mortality

Morbidity is often 100% and mortality may be 70% to 100%. Close confinement increases the spread of disease. Morbidity and mortality are higher with *Mycoplasma* F–38 infection than *M. mycoides capri*.

Diagnosis

Clinical

Severe respiratory disease in goats with high morbidity and mortality along with characteristic post mortem lesions are highly suspicious for contagious caprine pleuropneumonia.

Differential diagnosis

Differentials should include other causes of pneumonia such as pasteurellosis and peste des petits ruminants.

Laboratory tests

A definitive diagnosis of *Mycoplasma* F–38 infection is made by isolation and identification of the organism. Immunofluorescence, growth or metabolic inhibition tests, and polymerase–chain–reaction (PCR) can be used for identification. Serological tests for antibodies to *Mycoplasma* F–38 include complement fixation (CF), passive hemagglutination (PH), and enzyme–linked immunosorbent assay (ELISA). Serological tests are generally used on a herd basis and not for individual diagnosis. Whole blood or serum can be used in the field to detect antibodies to *Mycoplasma* F–38 using the latex agglutination test.

Samples to collect

Before collecting or sending any samples from animals with a suspected foreign animal disease, the proper authorities should be contacted. Samples should only be sent under secure conditions and to authorized laboratories to prevent the spread of the disease.

Samples for culture include lung lesions, swabs of major bronchi, and tracheobronchial or mediastinal lymph nodes. Samples should be collected aseptically and placed in a transport medium such as heart infusion broth, 20% serum, 10% yeast extract, and benzylpenicillin at 250 to 1000 IU/ml. Refrigeration and shipping on wet ice is necessary. Samples should be frozen if they will not reach the laboratory within a few days. Blood may also be collected for serological diagnosis.

Recommended actions if contagious caprine pleuropneumonia is suspected

Notification of authorities

State and federal veterinarians should be immediately informed of any suspected cases of contagious caprine pleuropneumonia.

Federal: Area Veterinarians in Charge (AVICs):
http://www.aphis.usda.gov/vs/area_offices.htm
State Veterinarians:
http://www.aphis.usda.gov/vs/sregs/official.html

Quarantine and disinfection

Testing, slaughter, and on–site quarantine are helpful in controlling the spread of contagious caprine pleuropneumonia. Vaccines are used in some countries.

Public health

Humans have not been found to be susceptible to infection with any of these mycoplasmas.

For more information

World Organization for Animal Health (OIE)
http://www.oie.int
OIE Manual of Standards
http://www.oie.int/eng/normes/mmanual/a_summry.htm
OIE International Animal Health Code
http://www.oie.int/eng/normes/mcode/A_summry.htm
USAHA Foreign Animal Diseases Book
http://www.vet.uga.edu/vpp/gray_book/FAD/

References

"Contagious Caprine Pleuropneumonia." In *Manual of Standards for Diagnostic Tests and Vaccines.* Paris: World Organization for Animal Health, 2000, pp. 503–514.

"Contagious Caprine Pleuropneumonia." In *The Merck Veterinary Manual,* 8th ed. Edited by S.E. Aiello and A. Mays. Whitehouse Station, NJ: Merck and Co., 1998, pp. 1109–1110.

Mare, C. John. "Contagious Caprine Pleuropneumonia." In *Foreign Animal Diseases.* Richmond, VA: United States Animal Health Association, 1998, pp. 161–169.

Contagious Equine Metritis

Importance

Contagious equine metritis (CEM) is a highly communicable venereal disease of horses. This disease can spread rapidly from a single carrier. Stallions are asymptomatic and may transmit the infection to the majority of mares they cover. Asymptomatic carrier mares can also infect stallions.

Infected mares develop an acute purulent metritis and fail to conceive, resulting in substantial economic losses. Additional economic costs include the cost of pre-breeding tests in endemic areas, as well as surveillance screening before importation into CEM-free countries. Immunity is weak, and animals may become infected repeatedly.

Etiology

Contagious equine metritis is caused by *Taylorella equigenitalis*, a fastidious microaerophilic gram-negative coccobacillus. Two types of strains exist, one sensitive and the other resistant to streptomycin. A small-colony variant may be particularly difficult to identify: its only distinguishing characteristic in culture is that the colonies are small and transparent.

In 1997 and 1998, an organism resembling *T. equigenitalis* was isolated during routine export testing from donkeys in California and Kentucky. The animals had no clinical signs. Following bacteriologic studies, this organism has been proposed as a new species, *Taylorella asinigenitalis*. *T. asinigenitalis* causes no apparent disease, but is contagious and induces an antibody response. This nonpathogenic organism can be distinguished from *T. equigenitalis* by a polymerase chain reaction (PCR) assay.

Species affected

Horses are the only species infected naturally by this organism. Thoroughbreds seem to be particularly susceptible. Donkeys have been infected under experimental conditions.

Geographic distribution

Taylorella equigenitalis has been reported mainly in the United Kingdom and Europe; however, this organism is difficult to grow in culture, and its geographic distribution is difficult to estimate accurately. Many countries have introduced strict import regulations to prevent its introduction. Contagious equine metritis has been eradicated from the United States.

Transmission

T. equigenitalis is transmitted mainly during mating, but may also be spread by artificial insemination or on mechanical vectors. The transmission rate is extremely high. Stallions are the most common source of the infection. In the stallion, the bacteria can persist for months or years on the surface of the penis (particularly the urethral fossa) and the smegma of the prepuce. Mares can also carry *T. equigenitalis* on the clitoris. Foals born to infected mares may become long-term asymptomatic carriers.

Incubation period

An inflammatory reaction begins 24 hours after colonization by the organism and reaches a peak after 10 days to 2 weeks. Clinically, the infection usually becomes apparent 10 to 14 days after breeding.

Clinical signs

Infected stallions display no clinical signs. Mares develop metritis and temporary infertility. The infection may be subclinical; the only symptom may be a return to estrus after a shortened estrus cycle. More severely affected mares develop a copious mucopurulent vaginal discharge 10 to 14 days after breeding. In an uncomplicated infection, the discharge is usually mucoid, purulent, and gray; mixed bacterial infections may result in a gray to yellow exudate. The discharge often disappears after a few days but the infection may persist for months. Most infected mares do not conceive. Those that do may abort or give birth to a foal that becomes a carrier at maturity. Chronically infected animals are asymptomatic.

Post mortem lesions

The most severe post-mortem lesions are usually found in the uterus. The endometrial folds may be swollen and edematous, and a mucopurulent exudate may be apparen. Edema, hyperemia, and a mucopurulent exudate may be seen on the cervix. Salpingitis and vaginitis also occur. Lesions are most apparent approximately 14 days after infection, then gradually decrease in severity over the next few weeks.

Morbidity and mortality

Fatal infections have not been seen. Morbidity is high; nearly every mare mated to an infected stallion will become infected. Most mares recover without incident but some can become carriers. Immunity after an infection is not complete, and mares can be infected repeatedly during a short period of time.

Infected animals can be treated with systemic antibiotics and disinfectant washing of the penis or clitoral area. Surgical excision of the clitoral sinuses can eliminate the organism in carrier mares.

Diagnosis

Clinical

Contagious equine metritis should be a consideration in mares that develop an abundant mucopurulent vaginal discharge 10 to 14 days after breeding. The disease may also be suspected in mares that return prematurely to estrus, particularly when several mares have the same symptoms after being mated to the same stallion.

Differential diagnosis

Pseudomonas aeruginosa and some capsule types of *Klebsiella pneumoniae* can cause outbreaks of endometritis. In general, most bacterial infections are not as contagious and produce a scantier discharge than contagious equine metritis.

Laboratory tests

Microscopic examination of Gram-stained smears of the uterine discharge may reveal numerous gram-negative coccobacilli (present individually or arranged end-to-end) and large numbers of inflammatory cells.

Definitive diagnosis is by isolation of the causative organism from swabs of the genital tract. Bacterial isolation should be performed by a laboratory experienced in isolating *T. equigenitalis*.

Stallions may also be bred to test mares and the test mares cultured for the causative organism. A recently developed PCR technique may be more sensitive than culture.

Serologic tests cannot reliably detect infections with *T. equigenitalis*. These assays should not be used instead of culture, but may be helpful as adjunct tests. Several antibody tests are available. Complement fixation can detect *T. equigenitalis* in mares from 15 to 45 days after infection, but becomes unreliable thereafter. Other tests include the rapid plate agglutination (RPA), antiglobulin, enzyme-linked immunosorbent assay (ELISA), passive hemagglutination (PHA), and agar-gel diffusion tests. Serologic tests are not useful in stallions, since stallions do not produce detectable antibodies to *T. equigenitalis*.

Samples to collect

Before collecting or sending any samples from animals with a suspected foreign animal disease, the proper authorities should be contacted. Samples should only be sent under secure conditions and to authorized laboratories to prevent the spread of the disease.

T. equigenitalis can be isolated from vaginal discharges. In suspect mares, swabs should be taken from the clitoral fossa, sinuses, and endometrium (if possible, during estrus). In stallions, swabs should be taken from the urethra, urethral fossa, penile sheath, and pre-ejaculatory fluid. No antibiotics should be used for at least seven days before the sample is taken.

Swabs should be placed in a transport medium with activated charcoal (for example, Amies medium) to absorb bacterial products that may inhibit the growth of *T. equigenitalis* . Samples should be kept cool and transported to the laboratory within 24 to 48 hours.

Recommended actions if contagious equine metritis is suspected

Notification of authorities

Contagious equine metritis must be reported to state or federal authorities immediately upon diagnosis or suspicion of the disease.

Federal: Area Veterinarians in Charge (AVICs):
http://www.aphis.usda.gov/vs/area_offices.htm
State Veterinarians:
http://www.aphis.usda.gov/vs/sregs/official.html

Quarantine and disinfection

Taylorella equigenitalis is susceptible to most common disinfectants, including chlorhexidine, ionic and nonionic detergents, and sodium hypochlorite (30 ml of household bleach in 1 gal of water).

Public health

There is no evidence of human infection with this organism.

For more information

World Organization for Animal Health (OIE)
http://www.oie.int
OIE Manual of Standards
http://www.oie.int/eng/normes/mmanual/a_summry.htm
OIE International Animal Health Code
http://www.oie.int/eng/normes/mcode/A_summry.htm
USAHA Foreign Animal Diseases Book
http://www.vet.uga.edu/vpp/gray_book/FAD/

References

"Contagious Equine Metritis." In *Manual of Standards for Diagnostic Tests and Vaccines*. Paris: World Organization for Animal Health, 2000, pp. 522-527.

"Contagious Equine Metritis." In *The Merck Veterinary Manual*, 8th ed. Edited by S.E. Aiello and A. Mays. Whitehouse Station, NJ: Merck and Co., 1998, pp. 1019-1020.

"Disease Information." 1 September 2000 Vol. 13, no. 34. Office International des Epizooties 28 Aug. 2001. http//www.oie.int/eng/info/hebdo/AIS_29.HTM#Sec0.

Swerczek, T.W. "Contagious Equine Metritis." In *Foreign Animal Diseases*. Richmond, VA: United States Animal Health Association, 1998, pp. 170-181.

Dourine

Covering Disease, Morbo Coitale Maligno, Slapsiekte, el Dourin, Mal de Coit, Beschalseuche, Sluchnaya Bolyezn

Importance

Dourine is a serious, often chronic, venereal disease of horses in Asia, Africa, South America, and southeastern Europe. This infection can result in neurologic signs and emaciation, and the mortality rates are high. No vaccine is available, and treatment with drugs may result in inapparent carriers.

Etiology

Dourine is caused by infection with the protozoal parasite *Trypanosoma equiperdum* (subgenus *Trypanozoon*, Salivarian section). This parasite can periodically replace its major surface glycoprotein antigen and evade immune responses. Strains vary in their pathogenicity.

Species affected

Dourine mainly affects horses, donkeys, and mules. The disease is generally more severe in improved breeds of horses, and milder in native ponies, donkeys, and mules. Various laboratory animals, including rats, can also be infected. Zebras have tested positive by serology, but there is no conclusive evidence of infection. Horses and donkeys appear to be the only natural reservoir for *T. equiperdum*. Male donkeys can be asymptomatic carriers.

Geographic distribution

Dourine was once widespread, but has been eradicated from a number of countries. Currently, the disease is endemic in most of Asia, northern and southern Africa, South America, and southeastern Europe.

Transmission

Unlike other trypanosomal infections, dourine is transmitted almost exclusively during breeding. Transmission from stallions to mares is more common, but mares can also transmit the disease to stallions. *T. equiperdum* can be found in the vaginal secretions of infected mares and the seminal fluid, mucous exudate of the penis, and sheath of stallions. Periodically, the parasites disappear from the genital tract and the animal becomes noninfectious for weeks to months. Noninfectious periods are more common late in the disease.

Rarely, infected mares pass the infection to their foals, either before birth or through the milk. These infected foals can spread the organism when they mature. Other means of transmission may also be possible, but there is no evidence that arthropod vectors play any role in transmission.

Incubation period

The incubation period is a few weeks to several years.

Clinical signs

Dourine is characterized mainly by swelling of the genitalia, cutaneous plaques, and nervous signs. The symptoms vary with the virulence of the strain, the nutritional status of the horse, and stress factors. The clinical signs wax and wane, and may be precipitated by stress. Stages of exacerbation, tolerance, and relapse can occur several times before the animal either recovers or dies.

In mares, the first symptom is usually a mucopurulent vaginal discharge. The vulva becomes edematous; this swelling may extend along the perineum to the ventral abdomen and mammary gland.

Vulvitis, vaginitis with polyuria, and signs of discomfort may be seen. The genital region, perineum, and udder may become depigmented. Abortion can occur with more virulent strains.

In stallions, the first symptoms are edema of the prepuce and glans penis. Paraphimosis may occur. The swelling may spread to the scrotum, perineum, ventral abdomen and thorax. Vesicles or ulcers may be seen on the genitalia; when they heal, these ulcers can leave permanent white scars (leukodermic patches). Edematous patches called "silver dollar plaques" (up to 5-8 cm diameter and 1 cm thick) may appear on the skin, particularly over the ribs. These cutaneous plaques usually last for 3 to 7 days and are pathognomonic for the disease. They do not occur with all strains.

Nervous signs can develop soon after the genital edema or weeks to months later. Restlessness and weight shifting from one leg to another is often followed by progressive weakness, incoordination, and eventually paralysis. Other clinical signs may include anemia, conjunctivitis, keratitis, intermittent fever, and emaciation. Dourine also results in a progressive loss of condition, predisposing animals to other diseases.

Post mortem lesions

Anemia, cachexia, and genital edema are often seen postmortem. The edema, which may be indurated, can extend to the ventral abdomen. Gelatinous exudates can often be seen under the skin. In stallions, the scrotum, sheath, and testicular tunica may be thickened and infiltrated. The testes may be embedded in sclerotic tissue and may not be recognizable. In mares, a gelatinous infiltrate may thicken the vulva, vaginal mucosa, uterus, bladder, and mammary glands. The lymph nodes (particularly in the abdominal cavity) may be enlarged, soft, and possibly hemorrhagic. The perineural connective tissue can be infiltrated with edematous fluid and the spinal cord may be surrounded by a serous infiltrate. A soft, pulpy, or discolored spinal cord may be noted, particularly in the lumbar or sacral regions.

Morbidity and mortality

The likelihood of infection with *T. equiperdum* depends on whether the infected host is in an infectious or noninfectious stage. The severity and duration of this disease vary with the virulence of the strain, the nutritional status of the host, and stress factors. The prevalent southern African strain results in a chronic, mild disease that may last for up to 10 years. In South America, Asia, and Europe, dourine tends to be more acute. In South America, the disease often lasts only one to two months.

Estimates of the mortality rate range from 50% to nearly 100%. Apparent recoveries have been questioned by some, in view of the long course of the disease and the waxing and waning symptoms. In endemic areas, drug treatment may be possible; however, treatment may result in inapparent disease carriers. No vaccine is available.

Diagnosis

Clinical

Symptoms suggestive of dourine include genital edema and neurologic signs. "Silver dollar plaques," if present, are pathognomonic. This disease can be hard to diagnose, as the clinical signs may be difficult to identify. Diagnosis is particularly difficult in the early stages or during latent infections.

Differential diagnosis

The differential diagnosis includes coital exanthema, surra, anthrax, equine infectious anemia, equine viral arteritis, and purulent endometritis such as contagious equine metritis.

Laboratory tests

Dourine is usually diagnosed by serology combined with clinical signs. The complement fixation test is the prescribed test for international trade, but uninfected animals (particularly donkeys and mules) often have inconsistent or nonspecific reactions. Indirect fluorescent antibody tests may help to resolve these cases. Other serologic tests include the enzyme linked immunosorbent assay (ELISA), radioimmunoassay, counter immunoelectrophoresis, and agar gel immunodiffusion (AGID). A recently developed test can distinguish equine piroplasmosis, dourine, and glanders by immunoblotting.

Definitive diagnosis is by identification of the parasite; however, the organisms are extremely difficult to find. A small number of trypanosomes may be found in the lymph, edematous fluids of the external genitalia, vaginal mucus, and fluid content of plaques. Organisms may sometimes be found in the urethral or vaginal mucus collected in vaginal or preputial washings or scrapings. On rare occasions, the trypanosomes can be found in thick blood films; however, the parasites are often undetectable in the blood. The success rate can be improved by centrifuging a blood sample and examining the re-centrifuged plasma.

Samples to collect

Before collecting or sending any samples from animals with a suspected foreign animal disease, the proper authorities should be contacted. Samples should only be sent under secure conditions and to authorized laboratories to prevent the spread of the disease.

Serum, whole blood in EDTA, and blood smears should be submitted. If silver dollar plaques are present, the skin over a plaque should be washed, shaved, and dried, and the fluid should be aspirated with a syringe to look for trypanosomes.

Recommended actions
if dourine is suspected

Notification of authorities

Dourine must be reported to state or federal authorities immediately upon diagnosis or suspicion of the disease.
Federal: Area Veterinarians in Charge (AVICs):
http://www.aphis.usda.gov/vs/area_offices.htm
State Veterinarians:
http://www.aphis.usda.gov/vs/sregs/official.html

Quarantine and disinfection

T. equiperdum cannot survive outside a living organism, and dies quickly with its host.

Public health

There is no evidence that *T. equiperdum* can infect humans.

For more information

World Organization for Animal Health (OIE)
http://www.oie.int
OIE Manual of Standards
http://www.oie.int/eng/normes/mmanual/a_summry.htm
OIE International Animal Health Code
http://www.oie.int/eng/normes/mcode/A_summry.htm
USAHA Foreign Animal Diseases Book
http://www.vet.uga.edu/vpp/gray_book/FAD/

References

"Dourine." In *Manual of Standards for Diagnostic Tests and Vaccines*. Paris: World Organization for Animal Health, 2000, pp. 528-534.

"Dourine." In *The Merck Veterinary Manual*, 8th ed. Edited by S.E. Aiello and A. Mays. Whitehouse Station, NJ: Merck and Co., 1998, pp. 35-36.

Gilbert, R.O. "Dourine." In *Foreign Animal Diseases*. Richmond, VA: United States Animal Health Association, 1998, pp. 182-188.

"Emergency Situations. Guidelines for the management of a suspected outbreak of foreign disease at federally-inspected slaughter establishments." Canadian Food Inspection Agency. 11 Sept. 2001. http//www.inspection.gc.ca/english/anima/meavia/mmopmmhv/chap9/9.1-3e.shtml.

Enterovirus Encephalomyelitis

Teschen Disease, Talfan Disease, Poliomyelitis Suum, Benign Enzootic Paresis

Importance

Enterovirus encephalomyelitis is a neurologic disease of pigs caused by at least nine serotypes of porcine enterovirus. Most of these viruses are widely distributed and cause mild disease in young pigs; however, the most virulent form, called Teschen disease, is highly contagious and severe and can affect pigs of all ages. Although many of the porcine enteroviruses can be found in the United States, Teschen disease does not occur in the U.S.

Etiology

Enterovirus encephalomyelitis can be caused by a number of porcine enteroviruses (genus *Enterovirus*, family Picornaviridae). The most virulent form, Teschen disease, results from infection by strains of porcine enterovirus serotype 1 (PEV–1). Less severe forms, including Talfan disease (benign enzootic paresis) and poliomyelitis suum, can be caused by strains of PEV–1, 2–6, 8, 12 or 13.

Species affected

Enterovirus encephalomyelitis is seen only in pigs.

Geographic distribution

The highly virulent strain of PEV–1 responsible for Teschen disease has been found in Central and Eastern Europe, Uganda, and Madagascar. Serious outbreaks were seen in Europe in the 1940s and 1950s, but no outbreaks of Teschen disease have been reported worldwide for a number of years.

The milder forms of disease are found worldwide. Most if not all herds of swine are endemically infected with several serotypes of porcine enterovirus. Clinical disease is infrequent in the United States.

Transmission

Porcine enteroviruses can be found in the intestines and oral secretions. Transmission is by the fecal–oral route. The viruses can be spread by direct or indirect contact and on fomites, including contaminated swill. Convalescent animals can shed small amounts of virus in the feces for up to 7 weeks. Porcine enteroviruses are highly resistant to inactivation; they can be found in the environment for more than 5 months and can survive in liquid manure for prolonged periods.

Incubation period

The incubation period for natural enterovirus encephalomyelitis infections is approximately 14 days. The neurologic signs of Teschen disease appear 5 to 7 days after experimental inoculation of piglets with the virulent 'Zabreh' strain.

Clinical signs

The clinical signs of Teschen disease typically include fever, anorexia, depression, incoordination, and ataxia, followed by painful hypersensitivity, paralysis, and death within 3 to 4 days. Muscle tremors, rigidity, nystagmus, seizures, changes in or loss of the voice, stiffness, opisthotonos, and clonic spasms of the legs may be seen. Affected pigs may grind their teeth, smack their lips, and squeal as if they are in pain. In the final stages of the disease, progressive paralysis develops, beginning in the hindquarters and ascending toward the head. During this stage, pigs may be hypothermic. Death is usually the result of the paralysis of the respiratory muscles. Animals that are mildly affected sometimes recover.

Enterovirus encephalitis caused by other strains of PEV is similar but milder.

Post mortem lesions

There are no characteristic gross lesions. In some cases, the cerebrospinal meninges and nasal mucosa may be congested.

Morbidity and mortality

Morbidity and mortality rates are high in Teschen disease: 70% to 90% of the pigs may die within a few days. The symptoms are usually most severe in animals less than 3 months old; however, any age can be affected. Talfan disease and other mild forms are less severe, with variable morbidity and mortality rates. These milder forms are usually seen in nursery– or finishing–age pigs.

There is no treatment for enterovirus encephalitis. Commercial vaccines may be available in Europe but are not marketed in the United States.

Diagnosis

Clinical

Teschen disease may be suspected in herds with encephalitis accompanied by high morbidity and mortality rates. Enterovirus encephalomyelitis cannot be differentiated from other forms of viral encephalomyelitis based on the clinical signs or gross pathology.

Differential diagnosis

The differential diagnosis includes Aujeszky's disease (pseudorabies), classical swine fever, Japanese encephalitis, hemagglutinating encephalomyelitis, bacterial meningoencephalitis, hypoglycemia, and poisoning from salt (water deprivation), lead, insecticides, or other toxins. Rabies, highly virulent strains of the porcine reproductive and respiratory syndrome (PRRS) virus, and edema disease (*Escherichia coli* enterotoxemia), may also be considered.

Laboratory tests

Enterovirus encephalomyelitis is diagnosed by histological examination of the brain and spinal cord, virus isolation from the central nervous system (CNS), or serology in convalescent pigs.

The cerebrum, cerebellum, diencephalon, medulla oblongata, and cervical and lumbar spinal cord are used for histological diagnosis. The typical microscopic lesions are inflammatory lesions with perivascular lymphocyte infiltration in the gray matter of the brain and spinal cord, particularly the ventral horns of the spinal cord, diencephalon, and cerebellum. In the later stages, the neurons degenerate and are replaced by glial connective tissue.

Porcine enteroviruses can be isolated from the brain or spinal cord in cell culture; cytopathic effects are seen in porcine kidney or testis cell cultures. As porcine enteroviruses are ubiquitous, virus isolation from tissues other than the central nervous system is not diagnostic. The viruses are identified and serotyped with virus neutralization tests, indirect immunofluorescence, and other serologic tests. Animal inoculation studies can be used to determine the pathogenicity of the isolate. A reverse–transcription polymerase chain reaction test (RT–PCR) has been developed but is not yet widely available.

Enterovirus encephalomyelitis can also be diagnosed by a four–fold rise in the PEV–1 titer. As PEV–1 infections can be widespread, a single titer is not diagnostic. Serologic tests include virus neutralization tests and enzyme–linked immunosorbent assay (ELISA).

Samples to collect

Before collecting or sending any samples from animals with a suspected foreign animal disease, the proper authorities should be contacted. Samples should only be sent under secure conditions and to authorized laboratories to prevent the spread of the disease.

The brain and spinal cord should be collected for virus isolation and histology. Both fresh tissues and samples preserved in equal parts isotonic saline and glycerol should be collected. Samples for virus isolation should be taken from pigs that have died very recently or were killed for necropsy. Paired serum samples may also be helpful.

Recommended actions if enterovirus encephalomyelitis is suspected

Notification of authorities

Teschen disease is reportable. Milder forms of enteroviral encephalitis are present in the United States; state or federal authorities should be consulted for more specific information on reporting porcine enteroviral diseases.

Federal: Area Veterinarians in Charge (AVICs):
http://www.aphis.usda.gov/vs/area_offices.htm
State Veterinarians:
http://www.aphis.usda.gov/vs/sregs/official.html

Quarantine and disinfection

Quarantine requirements and disinfection procedures may vary with the form of the disease. Porcine enteroviruses are resistant to heat, lipid solvents, and some disinfectants but can be inactivated by sodium hypochlorite or 70% ethanol. They can survive in pH 2 to 9. Viruses in manure can be inactivated by aeration, ionizing radiation, or anaerobic digestion.

Public health

The porcine enteroviruses responsible for enterovirus encephalomyelitis do not appear to be zoonotic.

For more information

World Organization for Animal Health (OIE)
http://www.oie.int
OIE Manual of Standards
http://www.oie.int/eng/normes/mmanual/a_summry.htm
OIE International Animal Health Code
http://www.oie.int/eng/normes/mcode/A_summry.htm
Manual for the Recognition of Exotic Diseases of Livestock
http://panis.spc.int/
Teschen disease. U.K. Department of Environment, Food and Rural Affairs (DEFRA)
http://www.defra.gov.uk/animalh/diseases/notifiable/disease/teschen.htm
Animal Health Australia. The National Animal Health Information System (NAHIS)
http://www.aahc.com.au/nahis/disease/dislist.asp
The Merck Veterinary Manual
http://www.merckvetmanual.com/mvm/index.jsp

References

Alvarez R. "Case study: Enteroviral polioencephalomyelitis in finishing–age pigs." In *Animal Disease Diagnostic Lab Newsletter*, Fall 2001. 6 March 2003. http://www.addl.purdue.edu/newsletters/2001/fall/ep.htm.

"Enterovirus encephalomyelitis." In *Manual for the Recognition of Exotic Diseases of Livestock: A Reference Guide for Animal Health Staff*. Food and Agriculture Organization of the United Nations, 1998. 3 March 2003. http//panis.spc.int/.

"Enterovirus encephalomyelitis." In *Manual of Standards for Diagnostic Tests and Vaccines*. Paris: Office International des Epizooties, 2000. 3 March 2003. http//www.oie.int/eng/normes/mmanual/A_00084.htm.

"Porcine enteroviral encephalomyelitis." In *The Merck Veterinary Manual*, 8th ed. Edited by S.E. Aiello and A. Mays. Whitehouse Station, NJ: Merck and Co., 1998, p. 925.

"Teschen disease." U.K. Department of Environment, Food and Rural Affairs (DEFRA), December, 2002. 6 March 2003. http//www.defra.gov.uk/animalh/diseases/notifiable/disease/teschen.htm.

Epizootic Hematopoietic Necrosis

Importance

Epizootic hematopoietic necrosis is a systemic disease that is highly fatal in redfin perch. Infections, with occasional deaths, also occur in rainbow trout. The causative virus remains infective for prolonged periods in water and dried films and is extremely resistant to disinfection. Closely related viruses cause epizootic hematopoietic necrosis in European catfish and sheatfish.

Etiology

Epizootic hematopoietic necrosis results from infection by epizootic hematopoietic necrosis virus (EHNV) or the closely related viruses European sheatfish virus (ESV) and European catfish virus (ECV). All three viruses are members of the genus *Ranavirus* and family Iridoviridae.

Species affected

EHNV infects redfin perch and rainbow trout. Experimental infections with this virus have been reported in Macquarie perch, mosquito fish, silver perch, mountain galaxias, Murray cod, and Atlantic salmon; natural infections have not been seen in any of these species. ESV and ECV are found in sheatfish and catfish.

Geographic distribution

EHNV is found only in Australia. ECV and ESV are endemic in Europe.

Transmission

The natural route of transmission is not known; however, infections can occur after bath inoculation and spread through the water is likely. Oral transmission probably occurs; fish develop gastrointestinal lesions after natural infections but not intraperitoneal inoculation. Infection through the gills or skin has not been ruled out. Carriers appear to exist for all three viruses.

EHNV is highly resistant to drying. This virus can remain infective for more than 97 days in the water and for at least 113 days in dried fish tissues. It can also survive for more than 300 days in cell cultures at 4°C, and for 2 years in fish tissues stored at −20°C. Given its resistance to drying and inactivation, transmission by fomites is likely.

Incubation period

The incubation period for EHNV infections is 3 to 10 days in water temperatures of 19–32°C, and up to 32 days in water temperatures of 8–10°C.

Clinical signs

The clinical signs in rainbow trout may include darkening of the body surface, inappetence, abdominal distension, and ataxia. Other symptoms reported in natural outbreaks are skin ulcers, flared opercula, and reddening at the base of the fins. In perch, sudden death is the most common sign. Depression, darkening of the body surface, erratic swimming, and erythema around the nostrils and brain region have also been seen. Hemorrhages may occur in the gills and at the base of the fins.

Post mortem lesions

Lesions in rainbow trout may include abdominal distension, serosanguineous ascitic fluid, and swelling of the spleen or kidney. Petechial hemorrhages have been seen on the viscera in a few fish. The gross lesions may be minimal in this species. In redfin perch, there may be swelling of the kidney or liver, hemorrhages at the base of the fins, and focal hemorrhages in the gills. The spleen is often swollen, but is occasionally pale and shrunken. Petechiae may be found on the viscera. Skin erosions, scleral hemorrhages, and exophthalmia have also been seen. Pale foci are sometimes found in the liver in redfin perch, but are rare in rainbow trout.

Morbidity and mortality

The temperature of the water affects the likelihood of infection. In rainbow trout, natural infections are seen in water temperatures between 11-17°C and experimental infections occur between 8-21°C. Disease is not seen in redfin perch when the water temperature is below 12°C. Poor water quality and external parasites have been associated with infections in rainbow trout.

Redfin perch are highly susceptible to infection with EHNV. During an initial epidemic, high mortality is seen in both adult and juvenile fish but, in endemic areas, most infections occur in juveniles. Infections in this species are usually fatal.

Rainbow trout are relatively resistant to EHNV infection; although the case fatality rate may be high, the mortality rate appears to be 3% to 4% or less. Infections occur in all sizes of rainbow trout, but death is more common in smaller fish (up to 125 mm fork–length).

High morbidity and mortality may be seen in ECV and ESV infections.

Diagnosis

Clinical

Epizootic hematopoietic necrosis should be suspected in redfin perch when an epidemic is characterized by sudden high mortality and necrosis of the renal hematopoietic tissue, spleen, liver, and pancreas. During outbreaks in rainbow trout, fewer fish may be affected.

Laboratory tests

Epizootic hematopoietic necrosis can be diagnosed by isolating EHNV, ECV, or ESV in cell cultures; appropriate cell lines include CHSE–214 (Chinook salmon embryo) or BF–2 (bluegill fry) cells. The identity of the virus is confirmed by immunofluorescence or an enzyme–linked immunosorbent assay (ELISA); antigen–capture ELISA is the method of choice. Electron microscopy may also be helpful in identification.

Virus antigens or nucleic acids can also be identified directly in tissues by immunofluorescence, ELISA, immunoblotting (Western blotting), or PCR. EHNV, ESV and ECV can be also be distinguished from other iridoviruses by sodium dodecyl sulphate–polyacrylamide gel electrophoresis (SDS–PAGE).

Serology may become effective in screening fish populations, but has not yet been validated for routine diagnosis. ELISAs for EHNV antibodies are being tested in rainbow trout.

Samples to collect

Before collecting or sending any samples from animals with a suspected foreign animal disease, the proper authorities should be contacted. Samples should only be sent under secure conditions and to authorized laboratories to prevent the spread of the disease.

If the fish are symptomatic, the samples to collect depend on the size of the fish. Small fish (less than or equal to 4 cm) should be sent whole. The viscera including the kidney should be collected from fish 4 to 6 cm long. The kidney, spleen, and liver should be sent from larger fish. Samples from asymptomatic animals should include the kidney, liver, spleen, and heart, as well as the ovarian fluid and milt at spawning. Samples should be taken from 10 diseased fish and combined to form pools with approximately 1.5 g of material (no more than 5 fish per pool).

The pools of organs or ovarian fluids should be placed in sterile vials. The samples may also be sent in cell culture medium or Hanks' basal salt solution with antibiotics. They should be kept cold (4°C) but not frozen. If the shipping time is expected to be longer than 12 hours, serum or albumen (5–10%) may be added to stabilize the virus. Ideally, virus isolation should be done within 24 hours after fish sampling.

Recommended actions if epizootic hematopoietic necrosis is suspected

Notification of authorities

Epizootic hematopoietic necrosis should be reported to state or federal authorities immediately upon diagnosis or suspicion of the disease.

Federal: Area Veterinarians in Charge (AVICs):
http://www.aphis.usda.gov/vs/area_offices.htm
State Veterinarians:
http://www.aphis.usda.gov/vs/sregs/official.html

Quarantine and disinfection

Quarantine is necessary for the control of outbreaks; epizootic hematopoietic necrosis is a contagious disease and asymptomatic carriers occur.

EHNV is highly resistant to drying and disinfection. In dried surface films, this virus can be destroyed by 70% ethanol for two hours but it is resistant to sodium hypochlorite. In liquid suspensions, EHNV can be destroyed by sodium hypochlorite, heating to 60°C for 15 minutes, or pH of 4.0 or 12.0. Farm equipment should be scrubbed to remove dried films, then disinfected with sodium hypochlorite. Lime may be effective in earthen ponds.

Public health

There is no indication that this disease is a threat to human health.

For more information

World Organization for Animal Health (OIE)
http://www.oie.int
OIE Diagnostic Manual for Aquatic Animal Diseases
http://www.oie.int/eng/normes/fmanual/A_summry.htm
OIE International Aquatic Animal Health Code (2001)
http://www.oie.int/eng/normes/fcode/a_summry.htm

References

"Epizootic Hematopoietic Necrosis." In *Diagnostic Manual for Aquatic Animal Diseases*. Paris: World Organization for Animal Health, 2000. http//www.oie.int/eng/normes/fmanual/A_00012.htm.

"Fish Health Management: Viral Diseases." In The *Merck Veterinary Manual*, 8th ed. Edited by S.E. Aiello and A. Mays. Whitehouse Station, NJ: Merck and Co., 1998, pp. 1291–1293.

"General Information." In *Diagnostic Manual for Aquatic Animal Diseases*. Paris: World Organization for Animal Health, 2000. http//www.oie.int/eng/normes/fmanual/A_00010.htm.

Langdon, J.S. "Experimental transmission and pathogenicity of epizootic haematopoietic necrosis virus (EHNV) in redfin perch, *Perca fluviatilis* (L.), and other teleosts." *J. Fish Dis.*, 12(1989):295–310.

Reddacliff, L.A. and R.J. Whittington. "Pathology of epizootic haematopoietic necrosis virus (EHNV) infection in rainbow trout (*Oncorhynchus mykiss* (Walbaum)) and redfin perch (*Perca fluviatilis* (L.))." *J. Comp. Pathol.* 115, no. 2 (1996):103–115.

Whittington R.J., A. Philby, G.L. Reddacliff and A.R. MacGown. "Epidemiology of epizootic haematopoietic necrosis virus (EHNV) infection in farmed rainbow trout, *Oncorhynchus mykiss* (Walbaum): findings based on virus isolation, antigen capture ELISA and serology." *J. Fish Dis.*17 (1994):205–218.

Whittington R.J. and G.L. Reddacliff G.L. "Influence of environmental temperature on experimental infection of redfin perch (*Perca fluviatilis*) and rainbow trout (*Oncorhynchus mykiss*) with epizootic haematopoietic necrosis virus, an Australian iridovirus." *Aust. Vet. J.* 72 (1995):421–424.

Epizootic Lymphangitis

Pseudoglanders, Pseudofarcy, Equine Blastomycosis, Equine Histoplasmosis, Equine Cryptococcosis, Histoplasmosis farciminosi, African Farcy

Importance

Epizootic lymphangitis is an economically important disease in some areas of the world, particularly where large numbers of horses, donkeys, or mules are assembled. This disease was a serious concern during the early twentieth century when large numbers of horses were stabled together. The causative organism, *Histoplasma capsulatum* var. *farciminosum*, does not currently exist in the United States.

Etiology

Epizootic lymphangitis results from infection by a dimorphic fungus, *Histoplasma capsulatum* var. *farciminosum*. This organism has also been known as *Histoplasma farciminosum*, *Cryptococcus farciminosis*, *Zymonema farciminosa*, and *Saccharomyces farciminosus*. *H. capsulatum* var. *farciminosum* exists as a yeast in tissues and a mycelium in the environment.

Species affected

Epizootic lymphangitis mainly affects horses, donkeys, and mules. Infections have also been reported in camels, cattle, and laboratory animals such as mice and rabbits.

Geographic distribution

Currently, epizootic lymphangitis is endemic in the Middle East, India, the Far East, and parts of Africa. In Africa, infections are most common in the north, but have also been seen in other parts of the continent. Sporadic cases have also been reported from other parts of the world.

Transmission

H. capsulatum var. *farciminosum* infects animals through open wounds. The skin form results from wound contamination by organisms in the soil. Biting flies in the genera *Musca* and *Stomoxys* are thought to spread the conjunctival form. Flies may also spread the skin form by feeding on infected open wounds. The pulmonary form, which is rare, probably develops when an animal inhales the organism.

In its saprophytic soil phase, *H. capsulatum* var. *farciminosum* is relatively resistant to environmental conditions. It can survive for many months in a warm, moist environment and may be spread on fomites such as grooming or harness equipment.

Incubation period

The incubation period is usually several weeks, but can be variable.

Clinical signs

The most common form of epizootic lymphangitis affects the skin and lymphatics, particularly on the extremities, chest wall, face, and neck. The first symptom is a painless, freely moveable, intradermal nodule, approximately 2 cm in diameter. This nodule enlarges and eventually bursts. In some cases, the lesions may be small and inconspicuous, and heal spontaneously. More often, the skin ulcers grow, with cycles of granulation, partial healing, and renewed eruptions. The surrounding skin becomes hard, variably painful, and swollen. The infection also spreads along the lymphatics, causing cord–like thickening of the lymphatic vessel and further skin involvement. These cycles of eruption and granulation gradually resolve, leaving only a scar. The process usually takes about 3 months. Epizootic lymphangitis sometimes spreads to the underlying joints and results in severe arthritis. Occasionally, conjunctivitis, keratoconjunctivitis, a serous or purulent nasal discharge, or pneumonia may also be seen. The lymph nodes may be enlarged, but fever is uncommon.

Post mortem lesions

On post–mortem examination, areas of skin and subcutaneous tissue are thickened, fibrous, and firm. Purulent foci may be noted on the cut surfaces. The lymphatic vessels are usually distended and contain purulent material. The regional lymph nodes are soft, swollen, and reddened and can contain purulent foci. Arthritis, periarthritis, or periostitis may be seen. On the nasal mucosa, multiple small gray–white nodules or ulcers with raised borders and granulating bases may be apparent. The lungs, spleen, liver, testes, and other internal organs can contain nodules and abscesses.

Morbidity and mortality

Morbidity is high when large numbers of animals are gathered together, but otherwise low. Death is uncommon.

Animals have been treated with sodium iodide, potassium iodide, and surgical excision combined with antifungal drugs, but the clinical signs may recur. Natural immunity is good, and both killed and live attenuated vaccines have been tried in some endemic areas.

Diagnosis

Clinical

Epizootic lymphangitis should be suspected in Equidae with skin nodules or ulcers and cycles of granulation, partial healing, and renewed eruptions. The symptoms are highly suggestive, but must be differentiated by laboratory tests from diseases such as glanders.

Differential diagnosis

Epizootic lymphangitis can resemble glanders, strangles, ulcerative lymphangitis, sporotrichosis, and histoplasmosis.

Laboratory tests

Epizootic lymphangitis is diagnosed by detecting *H. capsulatum* var. *farciminosum* in tissue sections or smears of lesions. Established lesions usually contain large numbers of yeasts. On a Gram–stained slide, the organism is a Gram–positive, approximately 2–5 μm diameter, pleomorphic, ovoid to globose structure. Organisms can also be detected in haematoxylin and eosin–stained tissue samples.

H. capsulatum var. *farciminosum* can be cultured from lesions approximately half of the time. Mycobiotic agar is the recommended medium; other media that may be used include Sabaraud's dextrose agar enriched with 2.5% glycerol, brain–heart infusion agar with 10% horse blood, and pleuropneumonia–like organism (PPLO) nutrient agar with 2% dextrose and 2.5% glycerol. Mycelial colonies develop in approximately 2 to 8 weeks at 26°C. The colonies are dry, granular, wrinkled, and yellow to dark brown. Aerial forms are rare. On microscopic examination, the hyphae are hyaline, septate, branched, pleomorphic, and Gram stain variable.

Antibodies have been detected by indirect and direct fluorescent antibody tests, enzyme–linked immunosorbent assay (ELISA), passive hemagglutination, and skin hypersensitivity tests. Inoculation of samples into immunosuppressed mice can also be used for diagnosis.

Samples to collect

Before collecting or sending any samples from animals with a suspected foreign animal disease, the proper authorities should be contacted. Samples should only be sent under secure conditions and to authorized laboratories to prevent the spread of the disease. Rare cases of human infections have been reported. Although the organism has not been unequivocally identified, precautions should be taken to prevent possible infection.

Samples should be collected from the suppurative and nodular lesions and placed in a liquid nutrient medium. They should be kept refrigerated and sent to the laboratory on wet ice as soon as possible. Air–dried smears from swabs of lesions should be prepared on glass slides for direct examination. Samples of lesions that include both viable and nonviable tissue should be placed in 10% buffered formalin. A sterile serum sample should also be submitted.

Recommended actions if epizootic lymphangitis is suspected

Notification of authorities

Epizootic lymphangitis must be reported to state or federal authorities immediately upon diagnosis or suspicion of the disease.

Federal: Area Veterinarians in Charge (AVICs):
http://www.aphis.usda.gov/vs/area_offices.htm
State Veterinarians:
http://www.aphis.usda.gov/vs/sregs/official.html

Quarantine and disinfection

Strict hygienic precautions are necessary to prevent the spread of this disease. In endemic areas, care should be taken to prevent spread the organism on grooming equipment or harnesses, and bedding should be burned. *H. capsulatum* can be inactivated by moist heat of 121°C for at least 15 minutes. It is also destroyed by 1% sodium hypochlorite, glutaraldehyde, formaldehyde, and phenolics. Its susceptibility to 70% ethanol is questionable.

In non–endemic areas, affected animals must be destroyed.

Public health

Rare cases of human infections have been reported. Although the organism has not been unequivocally identified, precautions should be taken to prevent possible infection.

For more information

World Organization for Animal Health (OIE)
http://www.oie.int
OIE Manual of Standards
http://www.oie.int/eng/normes/mmanual/a_summry.htm
OIE International Animal Health Code
http://www.oie.int/eng/normes/mcode/A_summry.htm
USAHA Foreign Animal Diseases Book
http://www.vet.uga.edu/vpp/gray_book/FAD/

References

"Epizootic Lymphangitis." In *Manual of Standards for Diagnostic Tests and Vaccines.* Paris: World Organization for Animal Health, 2000, pp. 601–606.

"Epizootic Lymphangitis." In *The Merck Veterinary Manual*, 8th ed. Edited by S.E. Aiello and A. Mays. Whitehouse Station, NJ: Merck and Co., 1998, pp. 466.

Gilbert, R.O. "Epizootic Lymphangitis." In *Foreign Animal Diseases.* Richmond, VA: United States Animal Health Association, 1998, pp. 201–206.

"Material Safety Data Sheet –*Histoplasma capsulatum.*" March 2001. Canadian Laboratory Centre for Disease Control. 10 Sept. 2001. http://www.phac-aspc.gc.ca/msds-ftss/index.html.

Equine Encephalomyelitis: Eastern, Western & Venezuelan

Eastern Equine Encephalomyelitis:EEE; Western Equine Encephalomyelitis: WEE; Venezuelan Equine Encephalomyelitis: VEE, VE, Peste Loca, Venezuelan Encephalitis, Venezuelan Equine Fever, Viral Encephalomyelitis

Importance

Eastern, Western, and Venezuelan equine encephalomyelitis are zoonotic diseases, caused by mosquito–transmitted viruses, that affect horses. The clinical signs may be mild to severe and include fever, encephalitis, and sometimes death.

Etiology

Eastern, Western, and Venezuelan equine encephalomyelitis viruses belong to the genus *Alphavirus* of the family Togaviridae. They are single–stranded RNA arboviruses.

The Venezuelan equine encephalomyelitis (VEE) complex is divided into epizootic and enzootic groups of viruses. The epizootic subtypes are responsible for most epidemics. They are highly pathogenic for horses and also cause illness in humans. Enzootic (sylvatic) subtypes are generally found in limited geographic areas, where they occur in natural cycles between rodents and mosquitoes. The enzootic subtypes can cause human disease. They are usually nonpathogenic for horses; however, in 1993 an enzootic variant was responsible for an outbreak of VEE among horses in Mexico.

Species affected

All of these encephalitis viruses can infect rodents, birds (poultry, game birds, and ratites as well as many species of wild birds), humans, and equines. Eastern equine encephalomyelitis (EEE) virus will also infect bats, reptiles, and amphibians, while Venezuelan equine encephalomyelitis (VEE) virus can additionally infect bats and marsupials.

Geographic distribution

All three viruses are limited to the Americas, with each virus infecting a different region. EEE is found in the eastern and north central United States and bordering areas in Canada, as well as a few areas of Central and South America and the Caribbean. WEE occurs in western and central USA, Canada, and parts of South America. VEE is endemic in northern South America, Trinidad, and Central America; epizootics occur in northern and western South America. In 1970–1971 an epizootic spread through Central America and into the USA. VEE is considered to be exotic in the U.S. and Canada, although low virulence strains of VEE virus are endemic in southern Florida.

Transmission

Eastern, Western, and Venezuelan equine encephalomyelitis viruses are transmitted in the saliva of mosquitoes that have been previously infected by biting viremic animals. Disease transmission is seasonal and dependent upon environmental conditions such as warm temperatures and standing water, which promote mosquito reproduction and development. EEE and WEE viruses primarily cycle between birds and mosquitoes, whereas VEE virus has a rodent–mosquito cycle. Human and equine hosts are dead–end hosts for EEE and WEE; however, horses are the major amplifying host for the epizootic subtypes of the VEE virus during epidemics.

During outbreaks of disease in game birds, EEE and WEE are introduced by mosquitoes, but transmission within the population may be primarily due to feather picking and cannibalism.

Incubation period

For EEE and WEE the incubation period is 5 to 15 days. VEE generally has an incubation of 2 to 6 days, but can occasionally become apparent after a single day.

Clinical signs

All three viruses cause similar clinical signs, which may range from very mild vague signs of fever, anorexia, and depression to encephalitic signs and sometimes death. Horses may become less responsive to stimuli or hyperexcitable, have unusual behavior, become blind or ataxic, or walk in small circles then progressively lose motor control. Affected animals may become prostrate, with violent, uncontrolled limb, head, mouth, and eye movements prior to death.

Post mortem lesions

Gross post–mortem lesions for the encephalitis viruses are non–specific. Mild to severe hemorrhages or necrosis of the brain and meninges may sometimes be noted.

The microscopic lesions are much more characteristic and suggest a severe inflammatory response in the grey matter. Neuronal degeneration with infiltration by polymorphonuclear leukocytes, diffuse and focal gliosis, and perivascular cuffing with lymphocytes and neutrophils are seen. Neuronophagia and liquefaction of the neuropil may also be present. The central nervous system (CNS) lesions are more severe in cases with a longer duration and progression of neurological signs. WEE causes focal brain lesions with lymphocytic infiltrates, while EEE lesions are generally more severe, found throughout the grey matter, and contain more neutrophils. With VEE, the CNS lesions tend to be more severe in the cerebral cortex and diminish towards the cauda equina.

Morbidity and mortality

In endemic areas, natural immunity decreases morbidity and mortality for all three viruses. EEE is often fatal in horses, while WEE may cause a subclinical or mild disease with less than 30% mortality. In susceptible populations, VEE can have a morbidity rate of 50% to 100% with a 50% to 90% mortality rate in horses. In endemic populations, morbidity may be only 10% to 40%.

Diagnosis

Clinical

Viral encephalomyelitis may be suspected in horses with acute neurological signs during times of mosquito activity, especially if multiple animals are showing signs. Other diseases may exhibit similar signs and the diagnosis must be confirmed with laboratory tests.

Differential diagnosis

The differential list for these encephalomyelitis viruses can be long due to non–specific clinical signs, but may include West Nile virus and other arboviral encephalomyelitides, African horse sickness, rabies, toxins, botulism, hepatoencephalopathy, and trauma. If neurological signs are absent, equine infectious anemia, colic, shock, and many other possibilities arise.

Laboratory tests

A definitive diagnosis is made by virus isolation and identification, or serology with paired serum samples. EEE virus can usually be isolated from the brain and sometimes other tissues of dead horses; however, WEE virus is rarely isolated. VEE virus can be isolated from blood or serum taken during the febrile phase. It is more difficult to isolate from the blood or brain samples of encephalitic animals.

The virus is grown in cell culture or laboratory animals. Identification can be made using complement fixation (CF), hemagglutination inhibition, plaque reduction neutralization (PRN), or immunofluorescence tests. Serologic tests include PRN, IgM capture enzyme–linked immunosorbent assay, hemagglutination inhibition, and CF tests. Serological diagnosis should take into account previous exposure or subclinical disease and current herd epidemiology and clinical signs.

Samples to collect

Before collecting or sending any samples from animals with suspected Venezuelan equine encephalomyelitis, the proper authorities should be contacted. Samples should only be sent under secure conditions and to authorized laboratories to prevent the spread of the disease. Eastern, Western, and Venezuelan encephalomyelitis are zoonotic diseases; samples should be collected and handled with all appropriate precautions.

Samples include heparinized blood and serum, with paired samples taken during acute and convalescent stages if possible. Viremia is highest during the febrile period and virus may be isolated from blood samples taken during this time. At necropsy, half the brain and a piece of pancreas should be kept unfixed, and a complete set of tissues should be fixed in 10% formalin.

Recommended actions if viral encephalomyelitis is suspected

Notification of authorities

Local health authorities and/or state veterinarians should be notified of any possible cases of Eastern, Western, or Venezuelan equine encephalomyelitis.

Federal: Area Veterinarians in Charge (AVICs):
http://www.aphis.usda.gov/vs/area_offices.htm
State Veterinarians:
http://www.aphis.usda.gov/vs/sregs/official.html

Quarantine and disinfection

These viruses are obligate intracellular parasites and do not survive in the environment. Transmission is dependent upon mosquito vectors, therefore mosquito control and the use of repellants and screens is most effective in reducing the incidence of disease in horses and humans.

Public health

Humans may have flu–like signs of a sudden fever, vomiting, stiff neck, frontal headache, dizziness, and lethargy. Some people may become disorientated and confused, and rapidly progress to stupor, coma, and death. In humans, EEE can cause severe disease with a mortality rate of approximately 65%. Survivors may have permanent neurological effects. WEE usually causes mild disease in humans, but may affect children more severely with a fatality rate of 3% to 14%. For VEE, as with WEE, most deaths occur in the very young and elderly.

Laboratory workers have a higher risk of infection with these arboviruses, especially through aerosol exposure. These people should be vaccinated and work only in certified biosafety cabinets in a biocontainment facility. Care should be taken when performing post–mortem examinations on animals suspected of having Eastern, Western, or Venezuelan equine encephalomyelitis. Residents and workers in agricultural communities and areas of new development can also be at higher risk for infection.

For more information

World Organization for Animal Health (OIE)
http://www.oie.int
OIE Manual of Standards
http://www.oie.int/eng/normes/mmanual/a_summry.htm
OIE International Animal Health Code
http://www.oie.int/eng/normes/mcode/A_summry.htm
USAHA Foreign Animal Diseases Book
http://www.vet.uga.edu/vpp/gray_book/FAD/
Centers for Disease Control and Prevention (CDC)
http://www.cdc.gov/ncidod/dvbid/arbor/arbdet.htm
Material Safety Data Sheets –Canadian Laboratory Centre for Disease Control
http://www.phac-aspc.gc.ca/msds-ftss/index.html
USAMRIID's Medical Management of Biological Casualties Handbook
http://www.vnh.org/BIOCASU/toc.html

References

"Equine Encephalomyelitis (Eastern and Western)." In *Manual of Standards for Diagnostic Tests and Vaccines*. Paris: World Organization for Animal Health, 2000, pp. 535–541.

"Venezuelan Equine Encephalomyelitis." In *Manual of Standards for Diagnostic Tests and Vaccines*. Paris: World Organization for Animal Health, 2000, pp. 595–600.

Leake, Colin J. "Mosquito–Borne Arboviruses." In *Zoonoses*, edited by S.R. Palmer, Lord Soulsby and D.I.H Simpson: Oxford University Press, New York, 1998, pp. 401–413.

"Arthropod–Borne Viral Diseases." In *Control of Communicable Diseases Manual*, 17th ed., edited by James Chin. Washington, D.C.: American Public Health Association, 2000, pp. 28–47.

Walton, T.E. "Venezuelan Equine Encephalomyelitis." In *Foreign Animal Diseases*. Richmond, VA: United States Animal Health Association, 1998, pp 406–414.

Equine Infectious Anemia

Swamp Fever, Mountain Fever, Slow Fever, Equine Malarial Fever, Coggins Disease

Importance

Equine infectious anemia (EIA) is a retroviral infection of horses that results in acute symptoms in some animals, and chronic fevers, anemia, edema, and cachexia in others. All infected horses, including those that are asymptomatic, become carriers and are infectious for life. Infected animals must either be destroyed or remain permanently isolated from other horses to prevent transmission.

Etiology

Equine infectious anemia is caused by equine infectious anemia virus (EIAV), a lentivirus (family Retroviridae) related to the human immunodeficiency virus. EIAV becomes incorporated into leukocyte DNA in both symptomatic and asymptomatic animals. This virus displays significant antigenic drift.

Species affected

Equine infectious anemia virus affects members of the Equidae.

Geographic distribution

Equine infectious anemia has been found worldwide. This virus exists in the United States.

Transmission

Equine infectious anemia is transmitted mechanically on the mouthparts of biting flies in the genus *Stomoxys* (horse flies and deer flies). Transmission is more common in the summer and in humid, swampy regions. EIA can also be spread on contaminated needles or surgical instruments, and passed from a mare to her foal in utero.

In infected horses, EIAV persists in the white blood cells for life. Horses with inapparent infections are less likely to transmit the disease than horses with chronic symptoms; after visiting an asymptomatic carrier, only one out of every 6 million flies is likely to become a vector.

Incubation period

The incubation period is usually one to three weeks, but may be as long as three months.

Clinical signs

The clinical signs of acute EIA are often nonspecific. In some acute cases, the only symptom noted is a fever which, in mild cases, can last less than 24 hours. Other clinical signs can include weakness, severe anemia, jaundice, tachypnea, petechiae on the mucus membranes, and blood–stained feces. Occasionally, death occurs during the acute infection. After the initial bout, most horses become asymptomatic carriers. Some develop recurring symptoms that vary from mild illness and failure to thrive to fever, depression, petechial hemorrhages on the mucus membranes, weight loss, anemia, dependent edema, and sometimes death. Inapparent infections may become symptomatic during concurrent illnesses, severe stress, or hard work.

Post mortem lesions

In acutely infected animals, the spleen and its associated lymph nodes are enlarged. In chronic infections, there may be emaciation, splenomegaly, pale mucous membranes, and enlarged abdominal lymph nodes. Edema is common, particularly in the limbs and along the ventral abdominal wall. Intravascular clotting and emboli are frequently seen in advanced cases. Some animals may have proliferative glomerulonephritis. Reticuloendothelial cell proliferation in multiple organs is common.

Morbidity and mortality

Morbidity varies with the geographic region. Morbidity is difficult to predict, as virus transmission depends on the number of flies, their habits, the number of times a fly bites the same or other horses, the density of the horse population, the amount of virus in the blood of the infected horse, and the quantity of blood transferred. Infection rates as high as 70% have been seen on farms where the disease has been endemic for many years. The mortality rate can be as high as 80% during the acute stage of experimental infections, if the dose of virus is high. However, deaths are uncommon in most natural infections.

No vaccine or treatment is available.

Diagnosis

Clinical

Equine infectious anemia should be suspected in individual horses with weight loss and intermittent fever. It should also be considered when several horses experience fever, anemia, edema, progressive weakness, or weight loss, particularly when new animals have been introduced into the herd or a member of the herd has died.

Differential diagnosis

The differential diagnosis includes other febrile illnesses, including anthrax, influenza, and equine encephalitis.

Laboratory tests

Equine infectious anemia is confirmed by serology. The agar gel immunodiffusion (Coggins) test is the "gold standard" used for confirmation of the disease. Enzyme–linked immunosorbent (ELISA) assays are also available. Positive results on ELISA are confirmed with the Coggins test, as false positives are sometimes seen. Antibodies may not be detected early in the disease.

Negative serologic tests are necessary for interstate movement of horses. State regulations vary, but many states require periodic tests, a single mandatory test, or tests before participation in organized activities.

Virus isolation is not usually required for a diagnosis, but it is occasionally done. The virus can be isolated by inoculating blood from a suspected carrier onto leukocyte cultures. Virus identity is confirmed by ELISA or immunofluorescence tests.

If the status of a horse cannot be determined by other methods, blood may be inoculated into a susceptible horse. Antibody status and clinical signs in the test animal should be monitored for at least 45 days.

Samples to collect

Serum should be collected for serology. Occasionally, unclotted blood may be collected for virus isolation or inoculation into a test animal.

Recommended actions if equine infectious anemia is suspected

Notification of authorities

Equine infectious anemia is a reportable disease in many states. Each state should be checked for specific regulations.

Federal: Area Veterinarians in Charge (AVICs):
http://www.aphis.usda.gov/vs/area_offices.htm
State Veterinarians:
http://www.aphis.usda.gov/vs/sregs/official.html

Quarantine and disinfection

Infected horses must be permanently isolated from other horses or euthanized. A reactor is usually marked with a brand, freezemarking, or a lip tattoo, and cannot be transported between states (except to its home farm, a slaughterhouse, or a diagnostic or research facility, under quarantine conditions). Foals born to infected mares should be isolated from other horses until maternal antibody disappears and the foal is determined to be free of infection.

Enveloped viruses such as EIAV can be destroyed by most common disinfectants.

Public health

There is no evidence that equine infectious anemia is a threat to humans.

For more information

World Organization for Animal Health (OIE)
http://www.oie.int
OIE Manual of Standards
http://www.oie.int/eng/normes/mmanual/a_summry.htm
OIE International Animal Health Code
http://www.oie.int/eng/normes/mcode/A_summry.htm
Animal Health Australia. The National Animal Health Information System (NAHIS)
http://www.aahc.com.au/nahis/disease/dislist.asp
Equine Infectious Anemia. American Association for Horsemanship Safety.
http://tarlton.law.utexas.edu/dawson/eia/eia.htm

References

"Code of Federal Regulations Title 9, Chapter I, Subchapter C. Interstate Transportation of Animals (including poultry) and Animal Products. Part 75 – Communicable Diseases In Horses, Asses, Ponies, Mules, and Zebras. Equine Infectious Anemia (Swamp Fever)." 26 Sept 2001. http//tarlton.law. utexas.edu/dawson/eia/us_eia.htm.

"Equine Infectious Anemia." American Association for Horsemanship Safety. 26 Sept 2001. http://tarlton.law.utexas. edu/dawson/eia/eia.htm.

"Equine Infectious Anemia." In *Manual of Standards for Diagnostic Tests and Vaccines*. Paris: World Organization for Animal Health, 2000, pp. 542–545.

"Equine Infectious Anemia." In *The Merck Veterinary Manual*, 8th ed. Edited by S.E. Aiello and A. Mays. Whitehouse Station, NJ: Merck and Co., 1998, pp. 499–500.

"Equine Infectious Anemia." In *Veterinary Virology*. Edited by F.A. Murphy, E.P.J. Gibbs, M.C. Horzinek, and M.J. Studdert. San Diego, CA: Academic Press, 1999, pp. 386–387.

"Equine Infectious Anemia." Oct. 1996. USDA APHIS VS CEAH, National Animal Health Monitoring System. 26 Sept 2001. http//www.aphis.usda.gov:80/oa/pubs/fseia.html>

Equine Piroplasmosis

Equine Babesiosis

Importance

Equine piroplasmosis is a tick–borne protozoal infection of horses. Piroplasmosis may be difficult to diagnose, as it can cause variable and nonspecific clinical signs. The symptoms of this disease range from acute fever, inappetence, and malaise, to anemia and jaundice, sudden death, or chronic weight loss and poor exercise tolerance. The disease may be fatal in up to 20% of previously unexposed animals. The tick vectors exist in the United States, and epidemics of piroplasmosis were seen in Florida in the 1960s.

Etiology

Equine piroplasmosis results from infection by the protozoa *Babesia caballi* or *B. equi* (phylum Apicomplexa). The two organisms may infect an animal concurrently.

Species affected

Equine piroplasmosis affects horses, mules, donkeys and zebras. Zebras are an important reservoir for infection in Africa.

Geographic distribution

Equine piroplasmosis is not endemic in Australia, Canada, England, Ireland, Japan and the United States. Epidemics were reported in Florida in 1961 and 1965, but after a 10–year eradication campaign, the United States appears to be free of this disease. *Babesia equi* infections have also been reported from Australia, but this parasite does not seem to have become endemic there.

Transmission

Babesia caballi and *Babesia equi* are transmitted by adult and nymphal ticks. *B. caballi* is spread by ticks in the genera *Dermacentor*, *Hyalomma*, and *Rhipicephalus*. *Dermacentor nitens*, *D. albipictus*, and *D. variabilis* can transmit this protozoan in the laboratory. Transovarial transmission occurs.

B. equi also appears to be spread by ticks in the genera *Dermacentor*, *Hyalomma*, and *Rhipicephalus*. The vectors for this disease in the Western Hemisphere have not been identified. *B. equi* does not appear to be passed transovarially.

Equine piroplasmosis can also be spread by contaminated needles and syringes. Intrauterine infection of the foal is fairly common, particularly with *B. equi*. After recovery, horses may become carriers for long periods of time.

Incubation period

The incubation period for *B. equi* infections is 12 to 19 days, and infections are more severe. For *B. caballi* infections, it is 10 to 30 days.

Clinical signs

The clinical signs of piroplasmosis are variable and often nonspecific. In rare peracute cases, animals may be found dead or dying. More often, piroplasmosis presents as an acute infection, with a fever, inappetence, malaise, labored breathing, congestion of the mucus membranes, and small, dry feces. Anemia, jaundice, hemoglobinuria, sweating, petechial hemorrhages on the conjunctiva, a swollen abdomen, and posterior weakness or swaying may be also seen. Subacute cases may have a fever (sometimes intermittent), inappetence, malaise, weight loss, signs of mild colic, and mild edema of the distal limbs. The mucus membranes can be pink, pale pink, or yellow, and may have petechiae or ecchymoses. In chronic cases, common symptoms include mild inappetence, poor exercise tolerance, weight loss, transient fevers, and an enlarged spleen (palpable on rectal examination). Foals infected in utero are usually weak at birth, and rapidly develop anemia and severe jaundice.

Post mortem lesions

In acute cases, the animal is usually emaciated, jaundiced, and anemic. The liver is typically enlarged and dark orange–brown. The spleen is enlarged, and the kidneys are pale and flabby. Petechial hemorrhages may be seen in the kidneys and subepicardial and subendocardial hemorrhages in the heart. There may also be edema in the lungs and signs of pneumonia.

Morbidity and mortality

The mortality rate can be up to 20% in previously unexposed animals. In endemic regions, equine piroplasmosis can be treated

with drugs; *B. equi* is usually less responsive to therapy than *B. caballi*. There is no vaccine.

Diagnosis

Clinical

Equine piroplasmosis should be suspected in horses with anemia, jaundice, and fever; however, the clinical signs are often variable and nonspecific.

Differential diagnosis

The differential diagnosis for piroplasmosis includes surra, equine infectious anemia, dourine, African horse sickness, purpura hemorrhagica, and various plant and chemical toxicities.

Laboratory tests

Equine piroplasmosis can be diagnosed by identification of the organisms in Giemsa stained blood or organ smears. *B. caballi* merozoites are joined at their posterior ends, while *B. equi* merozoites are often connected in a tetrad or "Maltese cross." Organisms can often be found in acute infections, but may be very difficult to find in carrier animals. In carriers, thick blood films can sometimes be helpful.

Because *Babesia* organisms can be difficult to detect in carriers, serology is often the diagnostic method of choice. Serologic tests include complement fixation, indirect fluorescent antibody (IFA), and enzyme–linked immunosorbent (ELISA) assays. The IFA test can distinguish between *B. equi* and *B. caballi*.

Other methods of diagnosis include DNA probes, in vitro culture, and the inoculation of a susceptible (preferably splenectomized) animal with blood from a suspected carrier. In addition, pathogen–free vector ticks can be fed on a suspect animal, and *Babesia* identified either in the tick or after the tick has transmitted the infection to a susceptible animal.

Samples to collect

Before collecting or sending any samples from animals with a suspected foreign animal disease, the proper authorities should be contacted. Samples should only be sent under secure conditions and to authorized laboratories to prevent the spread of the disease. Babesia equi has been implicated in human infections; samples should be collected and handled with all appropriate precautions.

Several thick and thin blood smears or an unclotted blood sample should be taken to detect *Babesia* organisms. If possible, blood samples should be collected during a rise in body temperature. Slides should be air–dried and fixed in methanol. Approximately 20 ml serum should also be taken for serology. For transmission tests to a susceptible horse, 500 ml uncoagulated blood (with antibiotics added) should be collected. Samples should be transported on wet ice or with frozen gel packs.

Recommended actions if equine piroplasmosis is suspected

Notification of authorities

Equine piroplasmosis should be reported immediately to state or federal authorities.

Federal: Area Veterinarians in Charge (AVICs):
http://www.aphis.usda.gov/vs/area_offices.htm
State Veterinarians:
http://www.aphis.usda.gov/vs/sregs/official.html

Quarantine and disinfection

Disinfectants and sanitation are not generally effective against the spread of tick–borne infections. However, preventing the transfer of blood from one animal to another is vital.

Public health

B. equi has been implicated in human infections.

For more information

World Organization for Animal Health (OIE)
http://www.oie.int

OIE Manual of Standards
http://www.oie.int/eng/normes/mmanual/a_summry.htm

OIE International Animal Health Code
http://www.oie.int/eng/normes/mcode/A_summry.htm

USAHA Foreign Animal Diseases Book
http://www.vet.uga.edu/vpp/gray_book/FAD/

Animal Health Australia. The National Animal Health
Information System (NAHIS)
http://www.aahc.com.au/nahis/disease/dislist.asp

References

Bruning, E. "Equine piroplasmosis. An update on diagnosis, treatment, and prevention." *British Veterinary Journal* 152 (1996):139–151.

"Babesiosis." In *The Merck Veterinary Manual*, 8th ed. Edited by S.E. Aiello and A. Mays. Whitehouse Station, NJ: Merck and Co., 1998, pp. 23–25.

"Equine Piroplasmosis." Animal Health Australia. 1996 The National Animal Health Information System (NAHIS). 3 Oct 2001. http//www.brs.gov.au/usr–bin/aphb/ahsq?dislist=alpha.

"Equine Piroplasmosis." In *Manual of Standards for Diagnostic Tests and Vaccines*. Paris: World Organization for Animal Health, 2000, pp. 558–564.

"Equine Piroplasmosis and the 1996 Atlanta Olympic Games." December 1995 United States Department of Agriculture Animal and Plant Health Inspection Service. 17 Oct 2001. http//www.aphis.usda.gov/oa/pubs/fsepiro.html.

Kuttler, K.L. "Babesiosis." In *Foreign Animal Diseases*. Richmond, VA: United States Animal Health Association, 1998, pp. 81–101.

Equine Viral Arteritis

Equine Typhoid, Epizootic Cellulites-Pinkeye, Epizootic Lymphangitis Pinkeye, Rotlaufseuche

Importance

Equine viral arteritis is an infectious disease of horses characterized by fever, depression, edema, conjunctivitis, nasal discharges, and abortions. Mortality is rare except in old, young, and debilitated horses, but economic losses can be significant. The economic impact includes decreased demand for carrier stallions as breeders, deaths in young foals, and abortions in 10% to 50% of susceptible mares.

Etiology

Equine viral arteritis is caused by equine arteritis virus, a RNA virus in the genus *Arterivirus* (family Arteriviridae). Isolates vary in the symptoms they produce.

Species affected

Equine arteritis virus is restricted to the Equidae. Antibodies to this virus have been found in horses, ponies, and zebras, and outbreaks have occurred in horses and ponies. The prevalence of the virus can vary significantly among horse breeds; Standardbreds are particularly susceptible.

Geographic distribution

Antibodies to equine viral arteritis have been found in most countries where testing has been done. Disease outbreaks are infrequent, but have been reported in the United States, Canada, Switzerland, Austria, the United Kingdom, and Poland.

Transmission

Equine arteritis virus can be transmitted by both the respiratory and the venereal route. Acutely affected horses excrete the virus in aerosols; aerosol transmission predominates when horses are gathered at racetracks, sales, shows, and other events. Venereal transmission from carrier stallions is particularly significant on breeding farms. Stallions appear to be the only carriers for the virus; carrier states have not been seen in mares, geldings, or sexually immature colts. Equine arteritis virus can also be carried on fomites. Mares infected late in pregnancy may give birth to foals infected in utero.

Incubation period

The incubation period for equine viral arteritis varies from 2 to 13 days. The average (mean) incubation period is 7 days.

Clinical signs

The symptoms of equine viral arteritis are generally more severe in old and young animals, and in horses in poor condition. The clinical signs of this disease can include fever, depression, anorexia, leukopenia, limb edema (particularly in the hindlimbs), and edema of the prepuce and scrotum. Other, less consistent, symptoms are lacrimation, conjunctivitis, photophobia, periorbital or supraorbital edema, nasal discharge, rhinitis, and edema of the ventral body wall. Some horses develop urticaria; the hives are most often localized to the head or neck, but are sometimes generalized. A stiff gait, ataxia, icterus, dyspnea, or diarrhea may also be seen. Abortions can occur; the rate may vary from less than 10% to greater than 50%. Abortions are not necessarily preceded by clinical disease.

Post mortem lesions

Edema, congestion, and hemorrhages are common in the subcutaneous tissues of the limbs and abdomen. Fluid accumulations may be seen in the peritoneal cavity, pleura, and pericardium. Edema and hemorrhages are often found in the thoracic and abdominal lymph nodes, as well as the small and large intestines (particularly the colon and cecum). In foals, pulmonary edema, interstitial pneumonia, emphysema, splenic infarcts, and enteritis have been seen. Aborted fetuses are usually partially autolyzed; the only visible abnormalities may be excessive fluid in the body cavities and interlobular interstitial pneumonia. Vascular lesions are not usually apparent in aborted fetuses.

Morbidity and mortality

In a 1998 survey of horses in the United States, 23.9% of unvaccinated Standardbreds, 4.5% of Thoroughbreds, 0.6% of Quarter horses, and 3.6% of Warmblood horses had antibodies to EVA. Approximately 30% of seropositive stallions are carriers. Mortality is rare, but can occasionally occur. Deaths are most likely in young foals that develop fulminating pneumonia or pneumoenteritis.

A modified live virus vaccine is commercially available. Only symptomatic treatment is available for infected horses.

Diagnosis

Clinical

Equine viral arteritis should be suspected in outbreaks of disease that include fever, depression, edema, conjunctivitis, nasal discharges, and abortions. The symptoms of this disease may be difficult to differentiate from other equine respiratory and non–respiratory illnesses.

Differential diagnosis

The differential diagnosis includes equine influenza, equine herpesvirus 1 and 4 infections, equine infectious anemia, African horse sickness, Getah virus infection, and purpura hemorrhagica and other streptococcal infections. Abortions caused by equine viral arteritis must be distinguished from abortions caused by equine herpesvirus 1 and 4 infections.

Laboratory tests

Equine viral arteritis can be diagnosed by virus isolation or serology. Equine arteritis virus may be found in nasal secretions, blood, semen, placenta, and a number of tissues and fluids post–mortem. Carrier stallions can often be identified by virus isolation from semen. Several cell lines are appropriate for virus isolation; early passage RK–13 cells are the system of choice.

Serologic tests include virus neutralization, complement fixation, agar gel immunodiffusion, indirect fluorescent antibody, and enzyme–linked immunosorbent (ELISA) assays. Virus neutralization tests are prescribed for international trade.

Polymerase chain reaction (PCR) techniques can also detect viral DNA in tissue samples and blood.

Samples to collect

In live animals, paired serum samples should be collected for serology. Nasopharyngeal and conjunctival swabs, and unclotted blood (with an anticoagulant other than heparin) should be collected for virus isolation or PCR. The samples for virus isolation should be taken as early as possible during the acute phase of the illness. Semen samples should be collected from suspect carrier stallions; these samples should contain the sperm–rich fraction of the ejaculate.

Post–mortem samples for virus isolation or PCR should include the placenta, body cavity fluids, lung, liver, spleen, and the lymph nodes associated with the respiratory and gastrointestinal system. Samples of these tissues should also be submitted for histopathology.

Recommended actions if equine viral arteritis is suspected

Notification of authorities

Equine viral arteritis is a reportable disease in many states. Each state should be checked for specific regulations.

Federal: Area Veterinarians in Charge (AVICs):
  http://www.aphis.usda.gov/vs/area_offices.htm
State Veterinarians:
  http://www.aphis.usda.gov/vs/sregs/official.html

Quarantine and disinfection

Equine viral arteritis is a contagious disease; quarantine of in–contact animals and disinfection are critical in preventing its spread. Enveloped viruses such as equine arteritis can be destroyed by most common disinfectants.

Public health

There is no indication that equine arteritis virus can infect humans.

For more information

World Organization for Animal Health (OIE)
  http://www.oie.int
OIE Manual of Standards
  http://www.oie.int/eng/normes/mmanual/a_summry.htm
OIE International Animal Health Code
  http://www.oie.int/eng/normes/mcode/A_summry.htm
U.S. Department of Agriculture, Animal and Plant Health Inspection Service. Equine Viral Arteritis (EVA) and the U.S. Horse Industry #N315.0400.
  http://www.aphis.usda.gov:80/vs/ceah/cahm/Equine/eq98eva.htm

References

"Equine Viral Arteritis." Animal Health Australia. 1996. The National Animal Health Information System (NAHIS). 3 Oct 2001. http//www.aahc.com.au/nahis/disease/dislist.asp.

"Equine Viral Arteritis." In *Manual of Standards for Diagnostic Tests and Vaccines*. Paris: World Organization for Animal Health, 2000, pp. 582–594.

"Equine Viral Arteritis." In *The Merck Veterinary Manual*, 8th ed. Edited by S.E. Aiello and A. Mays. Whitehouse Station, NJ: Merck and Co., 1998, pp. 500–502.

"Equine Viral Arteritis (EVA) and the U.S. Horse Industry #N315.0400." April 2000. USDA APHIS. 26 Sept. 2001. http://www.aphis.usda.gov:80/vs/ceah/cahm/Equine/eq98eva.htm.

Foot and Mouth Disease
Fiebre Aftosa

Importance

Foot and mouth disease (FMD) is highly contagious and can rapidly spread through a region if control and eradication practices are not put into place as soon as the disease is identified. Weight loss, poor growth, permanent hoof damage, and chronic mastitis are just some of the sequelae of infection. As a result, international trade embargoes could cause significant economic losses.

Etiology

The foot and mouth disease virus (FMDV) is in the family Picornaviridae, genus *Aphthovirus*. There are 7 immunologically distinct serotypes and over 60 subtypes. New subtypes occasionally develop spontaneously. The FMDV is inactivated at a pH below 6.5 or above 11. The virus can survive in milk and milk products when regular pasteurization temperatures are used. However, it is inactivated when ultra high-temperature pasteurization procedures are used. Virus stability increases at lower temperatures. It can survive in frozen bone marrow or lymph nodes. In organic material such as serum, the virus can survive drying. It can remain active for days to weeks in materials rich in organic matter under moist and cool temperatures. It is inactivated on dry surfaces and by UV radiation (sunlight).

Species affected

FMDV primarily affects cloven-hoofed domestic and wild animals, including cattle, pigs, sheep, goats, and water buffalo. Other susceptible species include hedgehogs, armadillos, nutrias, elephants, capybaras, rats, and mice.

Geographic distribution

Foot and mouth disease was found worldwide after World War II. The last U.S. outbreak was in 1929. Endemic areas are Asia, Africa, the Middle East, and parts of South America. Epidemics have occurred in recent years in Taiwan, South Korea, Japan, Mongolia, Uruguay, Russia, China, Britain, France, and The Netherlands. North and Central America, Australia, and New Zealand have been free for many years.

Transmission

Transmission primarily occurs by respiratory aerosols and direct or indirect contact with infected animals. Aerosol transmission requires proper temperature and humidity. Aerosol spread has occurred from bulk milk trucks. After inhalation of virus-rich aerosols, FMDV can survive for 24 hours in the human respiratory tract. Feeding of infected animal products such as meat, milk, bones, glands and cheese can also spread the disease. Contact with contaminated objects such as boots, hands or clothing can be a source of infection. Another source of infection is artificial insemination and contaminated biologicals and hormone preparations.

Sheep and goats are considered maintenance hosts. They can have very mild signs; therefore, diagnosis may be delayed allowing time for aerosol and contact spread and environmental contamination. In pigs, FMDV spreads rapidly since pigs exhale FMDV-laden aerosols that are thousands of times more concentrated than those of other species. Pigs are thus considered amplifying hosts. Cattle are considered 'indicators' of this disease because they generally are the first species to show signs of infection disease. Their lesions are more severe and progress more rapidly compared to other species.

Ruminants can carry the virus for long periods in their pharyngeal tissue. Recovered or vaccinated cattle exposed to diseased animals can be healthy carriers for 6 to 24 months. Sheep can be carriers for 4 to 6 months. Pigs are not carriers of FMDV. Some strains of the virus can affect one species more than others.

Incubation period

Animals in contact with clinically affected animals will generally develop signs of disease in 3 to 5 days. The virus can enter through damaged oral epithelium or the tonsils in pigs fed contaminated garbage. In this case signs can be seen in 1 to 3 days. Experimental exposure can elicit signs in 12 to 48 hours. Peak time of shedding of the virus and transmission usually occurs when vesicles rupture.

Clinical signs

Foot and mouth disease is characterized by fever and vesicles (blisters), which progress to erosions in the mouth, nares, muzzle, feet, or teats. Typical clinical signs include depression, anorexia, excessive salivation, serous nasal discharge, decreased milk production, lameness, and reluctance to move. Abortion may occur in pregnant animals due to high fever (FMD virus does not cross the placenta). Death in young animals is due to severe myocardial necrosis. In cattle, oral lesions are common with vesicles on the tongue, dental pad, gums, soft palate, nostrils, or muzzle. Hoof lesions are in the area of the coronary band and interdigital space. In pigs the hoof lesions are usually severe with vesicles on the coronary band, heel, and interdigital space. Vesicles can also be seen on the snout. Oral lesions are not as common as in cattle and are usually less severe. Drooling in pigs is rare. Sheep and goats show very mild, if any, signs of fever, oral lesions, and lameness. Animals generally recover in about 2 weeks with very low mortality in adult animals. Secondary infections may lead to a longer recovery time.

Post mortem lesions

The characteristic lesions of foot and mouth disease are single or multiple vesicles/bullae from 2 mm to 10 cm in diameter. Early lesions range from a small pale area to a fluid filled vesicle, sometimes coalescing with adjacent lesions to form bullae. The vesicles rupture, leaving red eroded areas, which may then be covered with a gray fibrinous coating. This coating becomes yellow, brown, or green and is replaced by new epithelium with a line of demarcation that gradually fades. Occasionally the fluid may escape through the epidermis instead of forming a vesicle. These "dry" lesions appear necrotic instead of vesicular. "Dry" lesions are more common in the pig oral cavity. Lesions at the coronary band progress similarly: the skin and hoof separate and, as healing occurs, a line showing evidence of coronitis appears on the hoof. Pigs may actually slough their claws in severe cases. "Tiger heart" lesions may also be seen; these lesions are characterized by a gray or yellow streaking in the myocardium caused by zones of degeneration and necrosis. Vesicular lesions may also be seen on the ruminal pillars.

Morbidity and mortality

Morbidity can be 100% in a susceptible population. Mortality is generally less than 1%. In younger animals or with more virulent strains mortality can be up to 40% increase.

Diagnosis

Clinical

Clinical signs of concurrent salivation and lameness with vesicles and/or erosions should make foot and mouth disease a differential consideration. Fever is often the first sign, so these animals should be carefully examined for early oral or digital lesions. The mouth of any lame animal, and the feet of animals with oral lesions or drooling, should also be checked. Teats of lactating females should be examined. Tranquilization may be necessary for a thorough examination as vesicles may be difficult to see. Laboratory testing is an absolute requirement to confirm FMDV infection as all vesicular diseases have almost identical clinical signs.

Differential diagnosis

The clinical signs of foot and mouth disease can be similar to vesicular stomatitis, swine vesicular disease, vesicular exanthema of swine, foot rot, traumatic stomatitis induced by poor quality feed, and chemical and thermal burns. In cattle, oral lesions seen later in the progression of FMD (erosions, ulcers) can resemble rinderpest, infectious bovine rhinotracheitis (IBR), bovine viral diarrhea (BVD), malignant catarrhal fever (MCF), and epizootic hemorrhagic disease. In sheep, these later lesions can resemble bluetongue, contagious ecthyma, and lip and leg ulceration.

Laboratory tests

FMDV can be identified using enzyme-linked immunosorbent assay (ELISA), complement fixation, and virus isolation. Virus isolation is done by inoculation of primary bovine thyroid cells and primary pig, calf and lamb kidney cells, inoculation of BHK-21 and IB-RS-2 cell lines, or inoculation of mice. ELISA and virus neutralization tests can be used to detect antibodies in serum. Virus isolation and identification must be performed on the initial case. Subsequently, antigen or nucleic acid detection can be used to diagnose additional cases in an outbreak.

Samples to collect

Before collecting or sending any samples from vesicular disease suspects, the proper authorities should be contacted. Samples should only be sent under secure conditions and to authorized laboratories to prevent spread of the disease. Since vesicular diseases can not be distinguished clinically, and some are zoonotic, samples should be collected and handled with all appropriate precautions.

Samples include vesicular fluid, the epithelium covering vesicles, esophageal-pharyngeal fluid, unclotted whole blood collected from febrile animals and fecal and serum samples from infected and non-infected animals.

Recommended actions if foot-and-mouth disease is suspected

Notification of authorities

A quick response is vitally important in containing an outbreak of foot and mouth disease. State and federal veterinarians should be immediately informed of any suspected vesicular disease.
Federal: Area Veterinarians in Charge (AVICs):
http://www.aphis.usda.gov/vs/area_offices.htm
State Veterinarians:
http://www.aphis.usda.gov/vs/sregs/official.html

Quarantine and disinfection

Suspected animals should be quarantined immediately and the premises should be disinfected. Sodium hydroxide (2%), sodium carbonate (4%), and citric acid (0.2%) are effective disinfectants. Less ideal disinfectants include iodophores, quaternary ammonium compounds, hypochlorite, and phenols, because they rapidly lose the ability to disinfect in the presence of organic matter. There are newer disinfectants that are better than and not as corrosive as some of these listed, included a chlorinated compound, Virkon-S®.

Vaccination

FMD vaccines, whether used prophylactically or for control of an outbreak, must closely match the type and subtype of the prevalent FMDV strain. With 7 serotypes, and more than 60 subtypes of FMDV, this task is one of the biggest challenges in FMD vaccination. Currently, there is no universal vaccine against FMD. The U.S., Canada, and Mexico maintain the North American FMD Vaccine Bank which contains vaccine strains for the most prevalent circulating serotypes in the world. The decision to use vaccination in control and eradication efforts is complex and depends upon scientific, economic, political, and societal factors specific to the outbreak situation. The final decision to use vaccination as an aid in controlling an outbreak of FMD in the U.S., Canada, or Mexico would be made by the Chief Veterinary Officer in each country.

Public health

FMDV infections in humans are rare, with just over 40 cases diagnosed since 1921. Vesicular lesions can be seen, but the signs are generally mild. Foot and mouth disease is not considered to be a public health problem.

For more information

World Organization for Animal Health (OIE)
> http://www.oie.int

OIE Manual of Standards
> http://www.oie.int/eng/normes/mmanual/a_summry.htm

OIE International Animal Health Code
> http://www.oie.int/eng/normes/mcode/A_summry.htm

USAHA Foreign Animal Diseases Book
> http://www.vet.uga.edu/vpp/gray_book/FAD/

CFSPH FAD Image Database
> http://www.cfsph.iastate.edu/DiseaseInfo/ImageDB/imagesFMD.htm

References

House, J. and C.A. Mebus. "Foot-and-mouth disease." In *Foreign Animal Diseases*. Richmond, VA: United States Animal Health Association, 1998, pp. 213-224.

"Foot and mouth disease." In *Manual of Standards for Diagnostic Tests and Vaccines*. Paris: World Organization for Animal Health, 2000, pp. 77-92.

Foot and Mouth Disease. Disease Lists and Cards. Office International des Epizooties. http//www.oie.int.

Fowl Typhoid

Importance

Fowl typhoid is an economically important disease of poultry and other birds, with high mortality in young birds. Hens may become chronic carriers and pass the disease to their embryos by egg transmission. Fowl typhoid has been eradicated from commercially raised poultry in the United States and many other developed countries, but may persist in backyard flocks.

Etiology

Fowl typhoid results from infection by *Salmonella gallinarum*, a Gram negative bacterial rod in the family Enterobacteriaceae (serogroup D).

Species affected

Chickens are the natural hosts for *S. gallinarum*; however, the disease can also affect turkeys, ducks, quail, guinea fowl, pheasants, pigeons, and grouse. Outbreaks have also been described in parrots, sparrows, ostriches, peafowl, and ring–necked doves, and cases have been seen in canaries and budgerigars.

Geographic distribution

Fowl typhoid is common in Mexico, Central and South America, Africa, and the Indian subcontinent. In the United States, Canada, Japan, Australia, and most countries in Western Europe, fowl typhoid has been eradicated from commercial poultry.

Although the disease may still be present in backyard flocks, no outbreak has been reported in the United States since 1980.

Transmission

Salmonella gallinarum is transmitted by both the respiratory and oral routes. Birds may become carriers and pass the organism to their offspring by egg transmission. Fomites, including contaminated feed, water, and litter, can also spread fowl typhoid, and wild birds, mammals, and insects may be important in mechanical transmission. *S. gallinarum* can survive in a favorable environment for several years.

Incubation period

The incubation period is usually 4 to 6 days.

Clinical signs

In chicks and poults, the clinical signs of fowl typhoid can include depression, loss of appetite, somnolence, droopy wings, huddling, dehydration, thirst, ruffled feathers, and weakness. Yellow or green diarrhea with pasting of the vent feathers is common, and there may be blindness or swelling of the joints. Birds that survive may be underweight and poorly feathered, and may not mature into productive adults.

In growing and adult birds, the disease can be inapparent. In symptomatic infections, the clinical signs may include a decreased appetite, depression, dehydration, weight loss, ruffled feathers, pale and shrunken combs, diarrhea, or a droopy appearance. There may also be a decrease in egg production or fertility.

Post mortem lesions

In young birds, the post–mortem lesions can include enteritis, dehydration, and anemia. The liver may be swollen, friable, and bile–stained and may contain white necrotic foci. The spleen is often enlarged and mottled, and the kidneys may be enlarged. Petechial hemorrhages can sometimes be found in the fat and musculature surrounding the internal organs, and the peritoneum, pericardium, and capsule of the liver may contain a fibrinous exudate. In some birds, there are white nodules in the epicardium, myocardium, pancreas, lung, gizzard, and sometimes the cecum; some of these nodules may resemble tumors. The joints may be swollen and contain a viscous creamy fluid. In turkeys, a characteristic sign is the appearance of small, white plaques visible through the wall of the intestine. In guinea fowl, the lesions often involve the respiratory tract.

In adult birds, the gross lesions may be minimal. In some animals, there may be a mottled pancreas, excess pericardial fluid, fibrinous pericarditis, or caseous granulomas in the lungs and air sacs. The testes sometimes contain white foci or nodules. Chronic carrier hens may have nodular or regressing ovarian follicles, or a few misshapen ova among normal ovules. In hens, caseous material is often found in the oviduct, and peritonitis, perihepatitis, or ascites may be seen.

Morbidity and mortality

Morbidity and mortality vary with the species, age, and breed of the birds, nutrition and management, and concurrent infections. Ducks, geese, and pigeons are relatively resistant to fowl typhoid. Among chickens, the White Leghorn breed appears to be more resistant than Rhode Island Reds or New Hampshires. The mortality rate can range from less than 1% to 100%; morbidity is usually somewhat higher. Mortality is usually highest in chicks and poults, particularly in 2 to 3–week old birds.

A vaccine is available. Antibiotics can reduce mortality, but do not eliminate the infection from the flock.

Diagnosis

Clinical

A tentative diagnosis can be made based on the clinical signs, flock history, mortality, and post–mortem lesions, but laboratory confirmation is essential.

Differential diagnosis

Fowl typhoid must be differentiated from infection with other species of *Salmonella*, *Mycoplasma synoviae*, *Staphylococcus aureus*, *Pasteurella multocida*, *Erysipelothrix rhusiopathiae*, and fungi including *Aspergillus*. The white nodules in chicks can be confused with Marek's disease. In adult carriers, local *S. gallinarum* infections may resemble infections by staphylococci, streptococci, coliform bacteria, other salmonellae, and *P. multocida*.

Laboratory tests

Fowl typhoid can diagnosed by the isolation of *S. gallinarum* from affected birds. This organism will grow on most standard nonselective aerobic media, as well as on MacConkey, brilliant green, desoxycholate citrate, and brilliant green sulphapyridine agars. *S. gallinarum* is a non–motile facultative anaerobe and grows best at 37°C. Colonies on nutrient agar are small (1–2 mm), circular, glistening, smooth, translucent, slightly raised, and entire after a 24 to 48 hour incubation. Treatment with antibiotics during the 2 to 3 weeks before testing may lead to false negatives. Further identification of the organism is by standard biochemical and serologic tests. Polymerase chain reaction (PCR) tests have also been used to detect *S. gallinarum*.

Fowl typhoid can also be diagnosed by serology. Agglutinating antibodies appear 3 to 10 or more days after infection. The rapid whole blood agglutination test can be used to immediately identify reactors in the field, but is not reliable in turkeys. Other serologic tests include the rapid serum agglutination test, tube agglutination, microagglutination, microantiglobulin, immunodiffusion, hemagglutination, and enzyme–linked immunosorbent (ELISA) assays. Cross–reactions with other species of *Salmonella*, particularly *S. enteritidis*, may occur. Testing for reactors should be repeated at 3 to 5 week intervals, as a single test may not detect all carrier birds.

Samples to collect

Before collecting or sending any samples from animals with a suspected foreign animal disease, the proper authorities should be contacted. Samples should only be sent under secure conditions and to authorized laboratories to prevent the spread of the disease.

Swabs or tissue samples should be collected for bacterial isolation. Samples can be taken from live birds, fresh carcasses, or freshly frozen carcasses. In live birds, swabs should be taken of the cloaca and conjunctivae. At necropsy, swabs may be used to sample the carcass or tissue samples can be collected aseptically from the spleen, liver, gall bladder, kidneys, heart, lungs, digestive tract, ova, testes, or affected joints. *S. gallinarum* can also be isolated from the contents of the intestine and cloaca. In carriers, *S. gallinarum* is most often recovered from the liver and feces. In asymptomatic birds, large amounts of homogenized tissues may be needed; the tissues can be pooled from different birds. Serum should also be collected for serology.

S. gallinarum can also be isolated from contaminated material in the birds' housing, transport boxes, or hatchers. Samples should include moist and dry litter, swabs from open drinkers, and aliquots of fluff, dust, and broken eggshells. Feed may also be collected for bacterial isolation; the total amount should be 25 to 100 grams. Eggs, embryos, and eggshell surfaces should be tested.

Recommended actions if fowl typhoid suspected

Notification of authorities

Fowl typhoid must be reported to state or federal authorities immediately upon diagnosis or suspicion of the disease.
> Federal: Area Veterinarians in Charge (AVICs):
> http://www.aphis.usda.gov/vs/area_offices.htm
> State Veterinarians:
> http://www.aphis.usda.gov/vs/sregs/official.html

Quarantine and disinfection

S. gallinarum can be inactivated by direct exposure to sunlight, heat treatment, phenol, formalin, dichloride of mercury, or potassium permanganate. Compounds that contain phenol are the most effective disinfectants under field conditions, but quaternary ammonium compounds and iodophores are also effective.

Public health

S. gallinarum is highly host adapted and is not considered to be a serious public health concern. In one survey, only 8 out of more than 450,000 isolations of *Salmonella* from humans were *S. gallinarum*. Whether these 8 isolates caused any symptoms in their hosts is unknown.

For more information

World Organization for Animal Health (OIE)
> http://www.oie.int
OIE Manual of Standards
> http://www.oie.int/eng/normes/mmanual/a_summry.htm
OIE International Animal Health Code
> http://www.oie.int/eng/normes/mcode/A_summry.htm
Mississippi State University Cooperative Extension Service
> http://www.msstate.edu/dept/poultry/disbact.htm

References

"Bacterial Diseases. Fowl Typhoid." 1997 Mississippi State University Cooperative Extension Service. 11 Oct. 2001. http://www.msstate.edu/dept/poultry/disbact.htm.

"Fowl Typhoid and Pullorum Disease." In *Manual of Standards for Diagnostic Tests and Vaccines*. Paris: World Organization for Animal Health, 2000, pp. 691–699.

"Fowl Typhoid." In *The Merck Veterinary Manual*, 8th ed. Edited by S.E. Aiello and A. Mays. Whitehouse Station, NJ: Merck and Co., 1998, pp. 1947–1948.

Shivaprasad, H.L. "Pullorum Disease and Fowl Typhoid." In *Diseases of Poultry*, 10th ed. Edited by B.W. Calnek. Ames, IA: Iowa State University Press, 1997, pp. 82–96.

Shivaprasad, H.L. "Fowl typhoid and pullorum disease." *Rev. Sci. Tech. Off. Int. Epiz.* 19, no. 2 (2000):405–424.

Glanders

Droes, Farcy, Malleus

Importance

Glanders is a highly contagious, potentially fatal zoonotic disease of horses, donkeys, and mules. The agent of this disease is a potential bioterrorist weapon.

Etiology

Glanders is caused by the bacteria *Burkholderia mallei,* previously known as *Pseudomonas, Pfeifferella, Loefflerella, Malleomyces, Actinobacillus, Corynebacterium, Mycobacterium,* and *Bacillus mallei*. It is closely related to *Burkholderia pseudomallei,* the cause of melioidosis.

Species affected

Horses, donkeys and mules are the primary species affected by *B. mallei*. Carnivores, especially cats and wild species, can be infected by eating contaminated meat. Laboratory rodents such as hamsters and guinea pigs are susceptible. Pigs, sheep, and cattle are resistant, but goats and camels can be infected. Humans are also susceptible to infection.

Geographic distribution

Previously worldwide in distribution, glanders has been eradicated from many countries by testing, slaughter, and import restrictions. It is still found in some Eastern European, African, Middle Eastern, and Asian countries, as well as Mexico and South America. Cross-reactions with *B. pseudomallei* make the distribution difficult to determine accurately.

Transmission

Transmission primarily occurs by the ingestion of nasal secretions from infected animals. Sharing water and feed troughs and nuzzling can spread the organism. Inhalation and cutaneous (through open wounds) transmission rarely occurs in animals.

Incubation period

In natural infections, the incubation period can be weeks to months. Experimental infection leads to fever after 3 days and other signs within a week.

Clinical signs

The clinical signs can be nasal, cutaneous, or pulmonary, which can all be seen in the same animal. Nasal signs include a highly infective yellow-green discharge with nodules and ulcers on the nasal mucosa. The ulcers may be severe, sometimes rupturing the septum. Ulcers heal leaving a stellate scar. The regional lymph nodes are often enlarged and may rupture. In the cutaneous form (Farcy), these nodules and ulcers are seen on the skin and exude a yellow discharge. The cutaneous lymphatic vessels may fill with the purulent exudate forming firm "Farcy pipes." Signs of the pulmonary form can range from inapparent or mild dyspnea to severe coughing. Infectious nodules are formed in the lungs leading to fever, weakness, and sometimes death. Nodules can also be found in the liver, spleen, or testes. Diarrhea and polyuria are sometimes seen. Chronic infections with slow progression of signs occur most often and can persist for years. Acute infections are seen more often in donkeys and mules than in horses and generally lead to death within a week.

Post mortem lesions

Nodular lesions can be found in the skin, nasal passages, lungs, or other internal organs. The nodules are generally 1 cm in diameter, gray or white in color with a surrounding area of hyperemia and edema. The nodules may be caseous or calcified. Ulcers may be present in the skin or nasal passages and stellate scarring can be seen as these ulcers heal. Lymphadenitis may be seen in associated lymph nodes or vessels.

Morbidity and mortality

Morbidity can be high when horses, mules and donkeys are in close contact. In China, 30% of horses were infected when large numbers of animals were gathered together in World War II. Acute infections are usually fatal within 1 to 2 weeks. Animals with the chronic form can sometimes survive for years.

Diagnosis

Clinical

Especially in endemic areas, typical nodules, ulcers and scars along with fever, weakness or respiratory difficulties may indicate glanders. Due to many inapparent and latent cases, testing is necessary to identify all infected animals.

Differential diagnosis

Differentials for glanders in Equidae include strangles, epizootic lymphangitis, ulcerative lymphangitis, melioidosis, and other causes of pneumonia, purulent sinusitis, and guttural pouch empyema. The skin lesions can be similar to dermatophilosis or dermatomycoses (i.e. sporotrichosis).

Laboratory tests

Smears from fresh exudates may reveal Gram-negative nonsporulating, nonencapsulated rods. Culture and identification can be used to confirm the diagnosis. Serological tests available include complement fixation and ELISA. These are quite sensitive and specific, except for their cross-reactivity with *B. pseudomallei*. False positives will occur in areas where melioidosis is endemic.

The mallein test can be used to identify infected animals. Mallein, a protein component of the organism, is injected into the dermis of the lower eyelid or administered in eyedrops. The protein elicits an allergic reaction in infected animals within 12 to 72 hours; the test is usually read at 48 hours. Mallein testing, especially repeated tests, may lead to seroconversion, causing uninfected animals to have a positive complement fixation test.

Samples to collect

Glanders is a zoonotic disease; samples should be collected and handled with all appropriate precautions. Samples should be well packaged, kept cool and labeled "Glanders suspect."

Samples should include serum, air-dried smears of exudate and sections of lesions, and including some in 10% buffered formalin.

Recommended actions if glanders is suspected

Notification of authorities

State and federal veterinarians should be notified of any suspected case of glanders.

Federal: Area Veterinarians in Charge (AVICs):
http://www.aphis.usda.gov/vs/area_offices.htm
State Veterinarians:
http://www.aphis.usda.gov/vs/sregs/official.html

Quarantine and disinfection

Burkholderia mallei is killed by direct sunlight, desiccation, and common disinfectants. The organism may live for several months in warm, moist conditions. To control the spread of disease, all contaminated bedding and food should be burned or buried, and all contact areas and objects including harnesses should be disinfected. Animals that test positive may be slaughtered. Susceptible animals should be removed for several months.

Public health

Glanders is an occupational concern for veterinarians, farriers, and other animal workers, as well as laboratory personnel. Infection with *B. mallei* is very painful and can be fatal. Humans can develop a chronic or acute form with nodules and abscessation similar to animals. Nodules may be seen on the face, legs, arms, and nasal mucosa, progressing to pyemia, metastatic pneumonia, and sometimes death. Without antibiotic treatment, disease in humans is usually fatal; untreated acute disease in humans has a 95% mortality rate within 3 weeks. With antibiotic treatment, the prognosis is much improved

For more information

World Organization for Animal Health (OIE)
http://www.oie.int
OIE Manual of Standards
http://www.oie.int/eng/normes/mmanual/a_summry.htm
OIE International Animal Health Code
http://www.oie.int/eng/normes/mcode/A_summry.htm
USAHA Foreign Animal Diseases Book
http://www.vet.uga.edu/vpp/gray_book/FAD/

Centers for Disease Control and Prevention (CDC)
    http://www.cdc.gov/ncidod/dbmd/diseaseinfo/glanders_
    t.htm
"Glanders and Melioidosis" in *e*Medicine
    http://www.emedicine.com/emerg/topic884.htm
Manual for the Recognition of Exotic Diseases of Livestock
    http://www.spc.int/rahs/

References

Gilbert, R.O. "Glanders" In *Foreign Animal Diseases*. Richmond,
    VA: United States Animal Health Association, 1998, pp. 245-
    252.
Blue, Sky R. In *Zoonoses*. Edited by S.R. Palmer, E.J.L. Soulsby and
    D.I.H Simpson. New York: Oxford University Press, 1998,
    pp. 105-108.
"Glanders." In *Manual of Standards for Diagnostic Tests and Vaccines*. Par-
    is: World Organization for Animal Health, 2000, pp. 576-581.

Heartwater

*Cowdriosis, Malkopsiekte, Pericardite Exsudative
Infectieuse, Hidrocarditis Infecciosa, Idropericardite
Dei Ruminanti*

Importance

Heartwater is one of the most important diseases of livestock
in Africa. This tick–borne illness is characterized by fever, rapid
respiration and anorexia, followed by neurologic symptoms. Infection is often fatal. Experimentally it has been demonstrated that
white–tailed deer are susceptible to infection, and also act as hosts
for the tick that transmits the disease; thus, heartwater has the
potential to become endemic in the United States.

Etiology

Heartwater results from infection by *Ehrlichia* (formerly *Cowdria) ruminantium*, a rickettsia (tribe Ehrlichia, family Rickettsiaceae).
This organism is pleomorphic, measuring from 400 to more
than 1,000 nm diameter. It is usually coccoid but occasionally
ring–formed. *E. ruminantium* is usually seen in clumps of several to
several thousand organisms in the cytoplasm of infected capillary
endothelial cells.

Strains of *E. ruminantium* vary in their pathogenicity. At least
one strain seems to be nonpathogenic for cattle; however, all
strains appear to be pathogenic for sheep and goats.

Species affected

Cattle, sheep, goats, and wild buffalo are severely affected by
heartwater, although in some indigenous African breeds of sheep
and goats, the symptoms are mild. Blesbok, wildebeest, guinea fowl,
leopard tortoises, and scrub hare are carriers. *E. ruminantium* can
also infect eland, springbok, antelope, white–tailed deer, ferrets, the
striped mouse, the albino mouse, and the multimammate mouse.

Geographic distribution

Heartwater is endemic in most of Africa south of the Sahara
desert, as well as in Madagascar, and in a few islands in the Caribbean. The disease has also been reported in Tunisia and the former
country of Yugoslavia.

Transmission

Heartwater can be transmitted by at least twelve species of
Amblyomma ticks. Ticks become infected as larvae or nymphs, and
can transmit the disease as nymphs or adults. Transovarial passage
does not occur.

A. variegatum (the tropical bont tick) is the major vector in
Africa and some parts of the Caribbean. Other vectors include
the bont tick *A. hebraeum* (in southern Africa), *A. lepidum* (in East
Africa and the Sudan), *A. astrion*, and *A. pomposum. A. sparsum, A.
gemma, A. cohaerans, A. marmoreum* and *A. tholloni* (the elephant tick)
are capable of transmitting experimental infections. Two North
American species, *A. maculatum* (the Gulf Coast tick) and *A. cajen-
nense*, can also transmit *E. ruminantium* in the laboratory, but neither
has been implicated in natural infections.

The Caribbean Amblyomma Program, established in 1995,
focuses on a regional approach to eradicating the tropical bont tick
on the 16 Caribbean islands where it is currently established. This
will help to prevent the introduction of heartwater into the U.S.

E. ruminantium is very fragile and does not survive outside a
host for more than a few hours at room temperature. However,
cows may transmit the infection to their calves in colostrum.

Incubation period

The incubation period in natural infections is usually 2 weeks,
but can be as long as a month. The incubation period after intravenous inoculation is 7 to 10 days in sheep and goats, and 10 to 16
days in cattle.

Clinical signs

Peracute disease is usually seen in Africa in non–native breeds
of sheep, cattle, and goats. Heavily pregnant cows are particularly
susceptible to this form. The clinical signs may include a fever,
severe respiratory distress, hyperesthesia, lacrimation, terminal
convulsions, and sudden death. Some breeds of cattle, including
Jerseys and Guernseys, may develop severe diarrhea as well. The
peracute form of heartwater is relatively rare.

The most common form of heartwater is acute disease. This
syndrome is seen in both non–native and indigenous cattle, sheep,
and goats. The symptoms begin with a sudden fever (up to 42°C),
anorexia, listlessness, and rapid respiration. Occasionally, animals
also have diarrhea. These symptoms are followed by nervous signs,
particularly chewing movements, protrusion of the tongue, twitching of the eyelids, and circling, often with a high–stepping gait.
Affected animals sometimes stand with their heads lowered and
legs apart. Some animals may become aggressive or anxious. As the
disease progresses, the neurologic signs become more severe, and
the animal goes into convulsions. In the terminal stages, galloping
movements, opisthotonos, hyperesthesia, nystagmus and frothing
at the mouth are common. Animals with the acute form of heartwater usually die within a week after the onset of the disease.

On rare occasions, heartwater appears as a subacute disease. In
this form, the clinical signs include a prolonged fever, coughing,
and mild incoordination. The animal either recovers or dies within
1 to 2 weeks.

Mild or subclinical infections are seen in calves less than 3 weeks
old, partially immune cattle or sheep, antelope, and some indigenous
breeds of sheep and cattle. The only symptom is a transient fever.
This form of the disease is known as "heartwater fever."

Post mortem lesions

The characteristic post–mortem lesion of heartwater is
hydropericardium, with straw–colored to reddish pericardial
fluid. Hydropericardium is more consistently found in sheep and
goats than in cattle. Other common lesions include pulmonary
and mediastinal edema, hydrothorax, and ascites. Subendocardial
petechial hemorrhages are frequent; submucosal and subserosal
hemorrhages may also be noted in other organs, especially the
abomasum. Animals may also have splenomegaly (more severe in
sheep and goats than in cattle), and edema and hemorrhages in
lymph nodes. Congestion, edema, and hemorrhages are sometimes
found in the brain.

Morbidity and mortality

Symptomatic infections in untreated non–native sheep, goats, and cattle are often fatal. In cattle, a mortality rate of 60% is common and, in Merino sheep, the death rate may be 80%. Angora goats are also extremely susceptible to this disease. Native animals are often more resistant to the infection; mortality in Persian or Afrikander sheep is only 6%.

Treatment with antibiotics is very effective, particularly when treatment is started soon after the symptoms appear. Immunization with virulent strains, followed by treatment with antibiotics, is often practiced in endemic areas and confers good immunity.

Diagnosis

Clinical

Heartwater should be suspected in animals with the typical clinical signs including fever, respiratory distress, characteristic nervous symptoms, and sudden death. The presence of *Amblyomma* ticks and typical post–mortem lesions support the diagnosis of heartwater.

Differential diagnosis

The peracute form of heartwater can be confused with anthrax. The acute form may resemble rabies, tetanus, bacterial meningitis or encephalitis, babesiosis, cerebral trypanosomiasis, or theileriosis. It must also be differentiated from poisoning with strychnine, lead, ionophores and other myocardial toxins, organophosphates, arsenic, chlorinated hydrocarbons, or some poisonous plants (*Cestrum laevigatum*, *Pavetta* species, and *Pachystigma* species). Accumulations of fluid similar to heartwater are also sometimes seen in heavy helminth infestations.

Laboratory tests

E. ruminantium is often diagnosed by microscopic examination of brain smears. The best samples are well–vascularized portions of the brain such as the cerebrum, cerebellum, or hippocampus. Brain smears are air dried, fixed with methanol, and stained with Giemsa. *E. ruminantium* will be seen as purplish–blue organisms among the capillary endothelial cells. The organisms can be found for two days in brains stored at room temperature and up to 34 days in refrigerated brains. The rickettsias can also be found in smears made from the intima of large blood vessels and during histopathologic examination of brain, renal glomeruli, and lymph nodes.

Heartwater can also be diagnosed in tissue samples with DNA probes. This method is effective in clinical cases, but is not sensitive enough to identify most carriers. Polymerase chain reaction (PCR) tests can detect clinical infections and some carriers.

Serologic tests include the indirect fluorescent antibody (IFA) test, enzyme–linked immunosorbent assays (ELISA), and immunoblotting (Western blotting). Cross–reactions with other *Ehrlichia* species occur in most of these tests, but the ELISAs that use recombinant antigens are more specific and reliable. Occasionally, the causative organism is isolated from the blood by cultivation on ruminant endothelial cells. Inoculation of fresh blood into a susceptible sheep or goat can also be used.

Samples to collect

Before collecting or sending any samples from animals with a suspected foreign animal disease, the proper authorities should be contacted. Samples should only be sent under secure conditions and to authorized laboratories to prevent the spread of the disease.

Samples from live animals should include 50 ml of heparinized blood and 10 ml serum. In addition, 10 ml of blood should be collected into heparin anticoagulant, then 10% DMSO should be added. Samples should be kept refrigerated and shipped with ice packs. From dead animals, a set of tissues in 10% buffered

formalin should be submitted, together with smears of the cerebral cortex or half of an unpreserved brain. Brain tissue can also be collected at necropsy by driving a large nail through the unopened skull, and aspirating a sample with a syringe. Another technique is to cut off the head and collect tissue through the foramen magnum with a curette.

Recommended actions if heartwater is suspected

Notification of authorities

Heartwater must be reported to state or federal authorities immediately upon diagnosis or suspicion of the disease.
Federal: Area Veterinarians in Charge (AVICs):
  http://www.aphis.usda.gov/vs/area_offices.htm
State Veterinarians:
  http://www.aphis.usda.gov/vs/sregs/official.html

Quarantine and disinfection

E. ruminantium cannot survive outside a living host for more than a few hours at room temperature. Control of this disease relies mainly on control of the tick vector with acaricides, and prevention of tick infection from infected animals. Transfer of blood between animals must also be avoided.

Public health

There is no indication that humans can be infected by *E. ruminantium*.

For more information

World Organization for Animal Health (OIE)
    http://www.oie.int
OIE Manual of Standards
    http://www.oie.int/eng/normes/mmanual/a_summry.htm
OIE International Animal Health Code
    http://www.oie.int/eng/normes/mcode/A_summry.htm
USAHA Foreign Animal Diseases Book
    http://www.vet.uga.edu/vpp/gray_book/FAD
The Caribbean Amblyomma Programme (CAP)
    http://forest.bio.ic.ac.uk/stvm/caribamb.htm

References

"Heartwater." In *Manual of Standards for Diagnostic Tests and Vaccines*. Paris: World Organization for Animal Health, 2000, pp. 304–312.

"Heartwater." In *The Merck Veterinary Manual*, 8th ed. Edited by S.E. Aiello and A. Mays. Whitehouse Station, NJ: Merck and Co., 1998, pp. 531–532.

Mare, C.J. "Heartwater." In *Foreign Animal Diseases*. Richmond, VA: United States Animal Health Association, 1998, pp. 253–264.

U.S. Department of Agriculture, Animal and Plant Health Inspection Service. December 4, 2003. http://www.aphis.usda.gov/mrpbs/manuals_guides/fy2001_reference_book/tropicalbonttick.pdf

Hemorrhagic Septicemia

Importance

Hemorrhagic septicemia is a highly fatal disease of cattle and water buffalo. In susceptible animals, the symptoms progress rapidly from dullness and fever to death within hours. Recovery is rare. In the United States, this disease appears to be endemic in one herd of bison but has not been seen in cattle.

Etiology

Hemorrhagic septicemia results from infection by 2 serotypes of *Pasteurella multocida*. Using agar gel immunodiffusion, these serotypes are known as B:2 or E:2. By agglutination, they are 6:B or 6:E. In newer classification schemes, the *Pasteurella multocida* strains that cause hemorrhagic septicemia (as well as most other *Pasteurella* infections) are *P. multocida multocida*.

Species affected

Epidemics of hemorrhagic septicemia mainly occur in cattle and buffalo; water buffalo are thought to be particularly susceptible. Infections occur infrequently in pigs, sheep, and goats. Cases have also been seen in bison, camels, elephants, horses, donkeys, deer, and yaks. Cattle, water buffalo, and bison appear to be the reservoirs of infection.

Geographic distribution

Hemorrhagic septicemia is an important disease in Asia, Africa, some countries in southern Europe, and the Middle East. The highest incidence is in Southeast Asia. The B:2 serotype has been seen in southern Europe, the Middle East, Southeast Asia, Egypt, and the Sudan. The E:2 serotype has been reported in Egypt, the Sudan, the Republic of South Africa, and several other African countries. Hemorrhagic septicemia also seems to be endemic in one herd of bison in the United States. Three confirmed outbreaks have been reported in these bison; however, there is no evidence that the disease spread to neighboring cattle. Neither serotype of *P. multocida* is known to occur in Australia, New Zealand, South America, or Central America.

Transmission

P. multocida is transmitted by direct contact with infected animals and on fomites. Cattle and buffalo become infected when they ingest or inhale the causative organism, which probably originates in the nasopharynx of infected animals. In endemic areas, up to 5% of cattle and water buffalo may normally be carriers. The carrier rate can increase to more than 20% for a few weeks after an outbreak.

The worst epidemics occur during the rainy season, in animals in poor physical condition. Stresses such as a poor food supply are thought to increase susceptibility to infection, and close herding and wet conditions seem to contribute to the spread of the disease. *P. multocida* can survive for hours and possibly days in damp soil or water. Viable organisms are not found in the soil or pastures after 2 to 3 weeks. Biting arthropods do not seem to be significant vectors.

Incubation period

In experimental infections with lethal doses, cattle or buffalo develop clinical signs within a few hours and die within 18 to 30 hours. In natural infections, the incubation period is usually 1 to 3 days but some animals can carry the organism for varying periods without symptoms.

Clinical signs

Most cases in cattle and buffalo are acute or peracute. A fever, dullness, and reluctance to move are the first symptoms. Salivation and a serous nasal discharge develop, and edematous swellings become apparent in the pharyngeal region. These swellings spread to the ventral cervical region and brisket. The mucous membranes are congested. Respiratory distress occurs, and the animal usually collapses and dies 6 to 24 hours after the first symptoms were seen. Either sudden death or a protracted course up to 5 days are also possible. Animals with clinical signs, particularly buffalo, rarely recover. Chronic cases do not seem to occur.

Post mortem lesions

At necropsy, widespread hemorrhages, edema, and hyperemia are seen. Swelling of the head, neck, and brisket occurs in nearly all cases. This edema consists of a coagulated serofibrinous mass with straw–colored or bloodstained fluid. Similar swellings can also be found in the musculature. Subserosal petechial hemorrhages may occur throughout the body, and the thoracic and abdominal cavities often contain blood–tinged fluid. Scattered petechiae may be visible in the tissues and lymph nodes, particularly the pharyngeal

and cervical nodes. These nodes are often swollen and hemorrhagic. Pneumonia or gastroenteritis occasionally occurs, but usually is not extensive. Atypical cases, with no throat swelling and extensive pneumonia, are sometimes seen.

Morbidity and mortality

Morbidity depends on immunity and environmental conditions, including both weather and husbandry. In endemic regions, 10% to 50% of cattle and buffalo become immune after exposure. Morbidity is higher when animals are herded closely, in poor condition, or exposed to wet conditions. Mortality is nearly 100% unless the animal is treated very early in the disease; few animals survive once they develop clinical signs.

Antibiotic treatment is effective if it is started very early, during the pyrexic stage. Various vaccines can provide protection for 6 to 12 months.

Diagnosis

Clinical

Hemorrhagic septicemia should be suspected in animals with a rapid course of infection, fever and edematous swellings in the throat, cervical, and parotid regions. A high herd incidence and high mortality in affected animals is also suggestive of this disease. In sporadic cases, hemorrhagic septicemia may be difficult to diagnose.

Differential diagnosis

The differential diagnosis includes other causes of sudden death such as lightning strikes, snakebite, blackleg, rinderpest, and anthrax. Acute salmonellosis and pneumonic pasteurellosis should also be considered.

Laboratory tests

Hemorrhagic septicemia is usually diagnosed by culturing the organism from affected animals. Success usually depends on collecting a fresh sample that is free from contaminating bacteria and post–mortem invaders. In Gram–stained blood or tissue smears, the organisms are Gram–negative, short, ovoid, coccoid forms with bipolar staining. Some pleomorphism can be expected. *P. multocida* can be grown on blood agar or casein/sucrose/yeast (CSY) agar. Fresh *P. multocida* colonies are smooth, grayish, translucent, glistening, and approximately 1 mm diameter after incubation on blood agar for 24 hours at 37°C. Larger colonies are seen on CSY agar, and smaller colonies may develop from old cultures. Biochemical tests are used for identification; the strains that cause hemorrhagic septicemia produce hyaluronidase. Immunologic tests to identify the E:2 and B:2 serotypes include a rapid slide agglutination test or indirect hemagglutination test for capsular typing, an agglutination test for somatic typing, agar gel immunodiffusion, and counter immunoelectrophoresis.

If in vitro culture is not successful, samples may be inoculated into a mouse and blood from the mouse used to identify the organism. Polymerase chain reaction techniques can also be used for detection and presumptive identification of the organism from clinical samples and pure or mixed bacterial cultures.

Serologic tests are not normally used for diagnosis; however, high titers (1:160 or higher by indirect hemagglutination) in surviving in–contact animals are suggestive of the disease.

Samples to collect

Before collecting or sending any samples from animals with a suspected foreign animal disease, the proper authorities should be contacted. Samples should only be sent under secure conditions and to authorized laboratories to prevent the spread of the disease.

There are no confirmed reports of human infections with *P. multocida* serotypes B:2 and E:2; however, other serotypes do cause human infections and precautions should be taken to avoid exposure.

P. multocida is not always found in blood samples before the terminal stage of the disease, and is not consistently present in nasal secretions. In freshly dead animals, a heparinized blood sample or swab should be collected from the heart within a few hours of death. A long bone freed of tissue should be taken from animals that have been dead for a long time. Other samples that have been used include liver, lung, kidney, spleen, ribs, and the tips of the ears. If a necropsy is not feasible, blood samples can be taken from the jugular vein by aspiration or incision. Blood samples should be placed in a standard transport medium and transported on ice.

Recommended actions if hemorrhagic septicemia is suspected

Notification of authorities

Hemorrhagic septicemia must be reported to state or federal authorities immediately upon diagnosis or suspicion of the disease.
Federal: Area Veterinarians in Charge (AVICs):
http://www.aphis.usda.gov/vs/area_offices.htm
State Veterinarians:
http://www.aphis.usda.gov/vs/sregs/official.html

Quarantine and disinfection

Hemorrhagic septicemia is contagious to contact animals and can be spread on fomites. The organisms can also survive for less than 2 to 3 weeks in damp soil and water. *P. multocida* is susceptible to mild heat (55°C) and most hospital disinfectants.

Public health

There are no confirmed reports of human infections with *P. multocida* serotypes B:2 and E:2; however, other serotypes do cause human infections and precautions should be taken to avoid exposure.

For more information

World Organization for Animal Health (OIE)
http://www.oie.int
OIE Manual of Standards
http://www.oie.int/eng/normes/mmanual/a_summry.htm
OIE International Animal Health Code
http://www.oie.int/eng/normes/mcode/A_summry.htm
USAHA Foreign Animal Diseases Book
http://www.vet.uga.edu/vpp/gray_book/FAD/

References

Carter, R.G.R. "Hemorrhagic Septicemia." In *Foreign Animal Diseases*. Richmond, VA: United States Animal Health Association, 1998, pp. 265–272.

Collins, F.M. "Pasteurella, Yersinia, and Francisella." In *Medical Microbiology*, 4th ed. Edited by S. Baron. April 2000. 7 Sept. 2001. http//www.gsbs.utmb.edu/microbook/.

"Hemorrhagic Septicemia." In *Manual of Standards for Diagnostic Tests and Vaccines*. Paris: World Organization for Animal Health, 2000, pp. 446–456.

"Hemorrhagic Septicemia." In *The Merck Veterinary Manual*, 8th ed. Edited by S.E. Aiello and A. Mays. Whitehouse Station, NJ: Merck and Co., 1998, pp. 532–534.

Hendra

*Equine Morbillivirus Pneumonia,
Acute Equine Respiratory Syndrome*

Importance

Hendra is an emerging infectious disease that has been found, to date, only in Australia. The disease appears to be spread from fruit bats (flying foxes) and can cause a highly fatal pneumonia in horses and cats. Hendra can also spread to humans and has been fatal in 2 of 3 cases diagnosed.

Etiology

Hendra is caused by the Hendra virus; a previously unknown virus placed in a new genus Henipavirus in the family Paramyxoviridae. Antibodies to the Hendra virus cross–react with the Nipah virus.

Species affected

Natural infections have been documented in horses and humans, and experimental infections in cats, horses, and guinea pigs. Fruit bats can be asymptomatic carriers. Dogs, mice, rats, rabbits, and chickens do not develop symptoms after inoculation and seroconversion has been seen only in rabbits.

Geographic distribution

Hendra has only been documented in Australia. Two outbreaks occurred from 1994 to 1995 and a single horse died of the disease in 1999 and in 2004. In surveys, no seropositive animals were found among 4000 Australian horses and 500 cats; however, antibodies to the virus were detected in fruit bats in Australia and Papua New Guinea.

Transmission

The Hendra virus does not appear to be highly contagious, and close contact seems to be necessary for it to spread. In infected horses, the virus has been isolated from the urine and oral cavity but not from nasal or rectal swabs. Experimentally infected cats shed the virus in urine, but not in nasal or oral secretions or feces. Aerosol transmission appears to be inefficient, but horses can become infected by ingesting the virus in contaminated feed. Human–to–human spread has not been seen.

In fruit bats, Hendra virus has been isolated from fetal tissues and blood. Vertical transmission has been documented in this species. Infected bat urine or an aborted bat fetus may have spread the virus to horses.

Incubation period

In natural infections, the incubation period in horses has been 8 to 16 days.

Clinical signs

In horses, the clinical signs include a fever, anorexia, depression, sweating, ataxia, and uneasiness. The respiration is rapid, shallow, and labored, and the mucus membranes may be congested. Jaundiced mucus membranes, mild neurologic signs, or subcutaneous edema may be seen. In natural but not experimental infections, animals often develop a copious frothy nasal discharge terminally. The clinical course is acute; deaths usually occur from one to three days after the onset of symptoms.

In cats, fever and increased respiratory rates are followed by severe illness and death within 24 hours.

Post mortem lesions

In horses, post–mortem lesions are found mainly in the lower respiratory tract. Marked subpleural edema, dilation of the pulmonary lymphatics, and congestion and ventral consolidation of the lungs are typical. Petechial hemorrhages have been seen on the pleural surfaces and patchy hemorrhages in the lung parenchyma. In natural infections, the airway often contains white or blood–tinged foam, and edema fluid oozes from cut tissues. Excess pleural and pericardial fluid, congested lymph nodes, and visceral edema may be seen. Scattered petechiae and ecchymoses may be found in the stomach, intestines, and perirenal tissues. Yellowing of the subcutaneous tissue is common.

In cats, typical lesions include severe pulmonary edema, hydrothorax, and edematous bronchial lymph nodes.

Morbidity and mortality

In the first Hendra outbreak, 13 of 20 symptomatic horses died. Nine horses at the same site did not become ill. In the second episode, 2 horses died of the disease. In the third episode, 1 of 2 horses sharing a paddock became ill and died of hendra; the other horse remained seronegative.

Vaccines and treatments for this disease have not been developed.

Diagnosis

Clinical

In endemic areas, Hendra should be suspected in horses that develop an acute respiratory disease with fever and high mortality.

Differential diagnosis

The differential diagnosis includes poisonings, circulatory catastrophes, shipping or transit fever, African horse sickness, Hantaan, equine influenza, equine herpesvirus 1 infection, anthrax, and botulism. Infections with *Yersinia*, *Pasteurella*, or *Legionella* species and *Streptobacillus moniliformis* should also be considered.

Laboratory tests

Hendra can be diagnosed by virus isolation, detection of nucleic acids or antigens, or demonstration of antibody. The virus can be isolated in a number of cell types, including Vero, BHK–21, MDCK, RK13, LLC–MK2, and MRC5 cell cultures. A marked cytopathic effect, with syncytia, is seen. Hendra virus can also be cultured in embryonated chicken eggs. Virus identity can be confirmed by molecular or serologic testing or electron microscopy.

Viral antigens can be detected by indirect immunoperoxidase or immunofluorescence assays on formalin–fixed tissues. A reverse–transcription polymerase chain reaction (RT–PCR) test has also been described. Antibodies can be detected by indirect immunofluorescence, immunoblotting, serum neutralization, and enzyme–linked immunosorbent (ELISA) assays.

Samples to collect

Before collecting or sending any samples from animals with a suspected foreign animal disease, the proper authorities should be contacted. Samples should only be sent under secure conditions and to authorized laboratories to prevent the spread of the disease. Appropriate precautions should be taken to prevent human infections during the collection and transport of specimens. Hendra has been classified as a Hazard Group 4 pathogen.

In live animals, virus isolation may not be reliable for diagnosis but can be attempted from the blood, bodily fluids, or tissues. Whenever possible, acute and convalescent sera should be collected for serology. Virus isolation is more likely to be successful in animals that have died from Hendra; at necropsy, samples of the lung, liver, spleen, and kidney should be collected aseptically. If neurologic signs were seen, samples should also be taken from the brain. A range of tissues, including lung and kidney, should be collected for histology. Samples for virus isolation should be transported to the laboratory as soon as possible and kept cold on wet ice or gel packs.

Recommended actions if Hendra is suspected

Notification of authorities

Hendra must be reported to state or federal authorities immediately upon diagnosis or suspicion of the disease.

Federal: Area Veterinarians in Charge (AVICs):
http://www.aphis.usda.gov/vs/area_offices.htm

State Veterinarians:
http://www.aphis.usda.gov/vs/sregs/official.html

Quarantine and disinfection

Hendra virus does not appear to be highly contagious. In Australia, outbreaks have been controlled by the destruction of seropositive horses and quarantines on horse movement in the area. This virus has been classified as a Hazard Group 4 pathogen;

infected animals and blood and tissue samples must be handled with appropriate biosecurity precautions.

Paramyxoviridae are enveloped viruses and can be readily inactivated by lipid solvents, non–ionic detergents, formaldehyde, oxidizing agents, and heat.

Public health

In two of the three outbreaks in horses, infections were also seen in humans. Three people were infected by the virus; all three had close contact with clinically ill horses or necropsied animals. The infections are thought to have occurred through contact with bodily fluids or aerosols. Two people developed a serious influenza–like disease, with fever, myalgia, and respiratory symptoms. One of the two died; the other recovered over the next six weeks. In the third case, a mild meningoencephalitic illness was followed by a long asymptomatic period then a fatal encephalitis.

There has been no evidence of seroconversion in people who are often in close contact with fruit bats.

For more information

World Organization for Animal Health (OIE)
http://www.oie.int

OIE International Animal Health Code
http://www.oie.int/eng/normes/mcode/A_summry.htm

Centers for Disease Control and Prevention (CDC)
http://www.cdc.gov/ncidod/diseases/index_eh.htm#h

Animal Health Australia. The National Animal Health Information System (NAHIS)
http://www.aahc.com.au/nahis/disease/dislist.asp

References

Barclay A.J. and D.J. Paton. "Hendra (equine morbillivirus)." *Vet. J.* 160, no. 3 (2000): 169–76.

"CDC Answers Your Questions About Hendra Virus." April 1999 Centers for Disease Control and Prevention. 2 November 2001. http//www.cdc.gov/ncidod/diseases/hendraq&a.htm.

"Hendra virus." Animal Health Australia. The National Animal Health Information System (NAHIS). 2 November 2001 http//www. aahc.com.au/nahis/disease/dislist.asp

Hooper P.T. and M.M. Williamson. "Hendra and Nipah virus infections." *Vet. Clin. North Am. Equine. Pract.* 16, no. 3 (2000): 597–603.

Hippobosca longipennis

Dog Fly, Louse Fly, Blind-fly

Importance

Hippobosca longipennis, the dog fly, is a blood–sucking parasite found mainly on carnivores. Its bites can be painful and irritating to some species. Heavy parasite burdens have been seen on dogs. Extensive blood loss or adverse effects from irritation are possible but have not been adequately documented. *H. longipennis* is an intermediate host for *Depetalonema dracunculoides*, a filarial parasite of dogs and hyenas. It is also a transport host for *Cheyetiella yasguri*, a mange mite of dogs. *H. longipennis* may be a vector of *Rickettsia conorii*, *Leishmania* species, or *Dermatophilus congolensis*; some authorities believe these last three relationships to be unlikely.

Species affected

Carnivores are the preferred host, as well as the only effective breeding host. *H. longipennis* has been found on cheetahs, lions, leopards, servals, African wild cats (*Felis silvestris libyca*), African civets, spotted hyenas, brown hyenas, dholes (*Canis adjustus*), Golden (Asiatic) jackals, black–backed jackals, African wild dogs (*Lycaeon pictus*), red foxes, bat–eared foxes, badgers, and domestic dogs. This parasite appears to be particularly common on cheetahs; 180 specimens were found on a single captive animal. Cheetahs do not appear to be bothered by the parasite. Although it has not yet been found on domestic cats, they can probably be infested as well. In Africa and the Middle East, *H. longipennis* is common on wild carnivores as well as domestic and feral dogs, but in Europe and the rest of Asia, it is seen mainly on dogs. There have also been occasional reports of infestations on antelopes, livestock, humans, and a bird; some of these parasites may have been incorrectly identified.

Geographic distribution

H. longipennis is most often found in open, dry, warm deserts and savannas; its distribution seems to be limited by low temperatures and high humidity. This fly appears to have originated in Africa, where it is widespread in all but the more humid west and central regions. It can also be found in suitable habitats in much of the European and Asian Palearctic Region south of about 45° north latitude. *H. longipennis* is occasionally reported from countries on the fringes of this range (e.g., Ireland, Germany, Poland, Taiwan, and Japan) but does not seem to have become permanently established there.

H. longipennis has probably entered the Americas many times without becoming established. The most serious incursion was in 1970, when infested cheetahs were imported from East Africa to the San Diego Zoo in California. The fly was not identified until 1972 and not fully eradicated until 1975. In the interim, other infested cheetahs were discovered in zoos in Georgia, Oregon, and Texas. They were also treated successfully. In 1983, *H. longipennis* flies were found in North Carolina on a shipment of bat–eared foxes from Africa. Outbreaks also occurred in Ireland in 1982 and Japan around 1990, both times on cheetahs imported from Namibia.

Life cycle

Female *H. longipennis* bear full–grown, mature larvae, one at a time. Shortly after larviposition, the larva pupariates. Populations may be able to survive adverse environmental conditions as diapausing puparia. The adult flies usually emerge in the morning, from 19 to 142 days after pupariation, depending on the climate and time of the year. The winged adults seek out suitable hosts and feed several times a day. On dogs, they prefer the ventral neck and front axillary regions. After approximately seven days, the flies mate on the host. The larvae develop internally for 3 to 8 days then the female deposits the larva on the soil, in cracks or crevices, under plants, or on debris. After larviposition, she returns to the host to feed and begin another larval maturation cycle. Individual females may live for 4 or 5 months, but about half that is more typical. Each female usually bears 10 to 15 offspring over a lifetime.

Identification

H. longipennis is a member of the family Hippoboscidae and order Diptera (suborder Cyclorrhapha). This fly is related to sheep keds. Hippoboscid flies have a sleek, dorsoventrally flattened head and body, powerful piercing–sucking mouthparts, and robust legs tipped with large, strong tarsal claws. The veins on their wings are crowded into the leading half of the wing.

Recommended actions if *Hippobosca longipennis* is suspected

Notification of authorities

H. longipennis infestations should be reported immediately to state or federal authorities. For identification, specimens should be sent to the USDA, APHIS, National Veterinary Services Laboratories in Ames, Iowa.

Federal: Area Veterinarians in Charge (AVICs):
http://www.aphis.usda.gov/vs/area_offices.htm
State Veterinarians:
http://www.aphis.usda.gov/vs/sregs/official.html

Control measures

In zoos, *H. longipennis* has been successfully eradicated from cheetahs and bat eared foxes by repeated insecticidal treatments. A carbaryl–sulfur dust formulation applied to the animals and their surroundings seems to be most effective. In some cases, full eradication has taken several years.

Public health

Humans are occasionally bitten; the bites have been described as either painless or as painful as a wasp or bee sting.

For more information

World Organization for Animal Health (OIE)
http://www.oie.int
OIE International Animal Health Code
http://www.oie.int/eng/normes/mcode/A_summry.htm
USAHA Foreign Animal Diseases Book
http://www.vet.uga.edu/vpp/gray_book/FAD/

References

"Adult flies (Diptera)." In *Veterinary Entomology: Arthropod Ectoparasites of Veterinary Importance.* Edited by R. Wall and D. Shearer. London: Chapman & Hall, 1997, pp. 117–120.

Bequaert, J. C. "The Hippoboscidae or louse–flies (Diptera) of mammals and birds. Part I. Structure, physiology and natural history." *Entomol. Amer.* (N. S.) 32 (1952):1–209; 33 (1953): 211–442.

Bequaert. J. C. "The Hippoboscidae or louse–flies (Diptera) of mammals and birds. Part II. Taxonomy, evolution and revision of American genera and species." *Entomol. Amer.* (N. S.) 34 (1954):1–232; 35 (1955):233–416; 36 (1956):417–611.

Hafez, M. and M. Hilali. "Biology of *Hippobosca longipennis* (Fabricius, 1805) in Egypt (Diptera: Hippoboscidae)." *Vet. Parasitol.* 4 (1978):275–288.

Keh, B., and R. M. Hawthorne. "The introduction and eradication of an exotic ectoparasitic fly, *Hippobosca longipennis* (Diptera: Hippoboscidae), in California." *J. Zoo–Anim. Med.* 8, no. 4 (1977):19–24.

Takaie, H, H, Hiramatsu, K. Tasaka, S. Shichiri, and F. Hashizaki. "*Hippobosca longipennis Fabricius* (Diptera: Hippoboscidae) from imported cheetahs." *J. Jap. Assoc Zool. Gardens Aquar.* 33, no.1 (1991):1–4.

Wilson, D.D. and R.A. Bram. "Foreign pests and vectors of arthropod–borne diseases." In *Foreign Animal Diseases.* Richmond, VA: United States Animal Health Association, 1998, pp. 225–239.

Infectious Hematopoietic Necrosis

Oregon Sockeye Salmon Disease, Columbia River Sockeye Disease, Sacramento River Chinook Disease

Importance

Infectious hematopoietic necrosis (IHN) can have a major economic impact on farms that rear salmon or freshwater rainbow trout. Outbreaks among wild salmon may also result in high mortality.

Etiology

Infectious hematopoietic necrosis is caused by infectious hematopoietic necrosis virus (IHNV), a member of the family Rhabdoviridae. Virus strains vary in their pathogenicity.

Species affected

Infectious hematopoietic necrosis affects rainbow trout, steelhead trout, Atlantic salmon, and Pacific salmon including chinook, sockeye, chum, yamame, amago, and coho. Pike fry can be experimentally infected.

Geographic distribution

Infectious hematopoietic necrosis is endemic along the Pacific Coast of North America, from the Sacramento River in California to Kodiak Island in Alaska. It has also been found in Minnesota, West Virginia, South Dakota, Idaho, and Colorado and has spread to continental Europe and Japan.

Transmission

Both diseased fish and asymptomatic carriers can transmit IHNV. Virus is shed in the feces, urine, sexual fluids, and external mucus. Particularly large amounts of virus are shed by juvenile fish. Transmission is mainly from fish to fish, primarily by direct contact but also through the water. The virus can also be spread in contaminated feed. Most infections are thought to occur through the gills or the digestive tract. Cases of "egg–associated" transmission have been reported and invertebrate vectors may exist.

Incubation period

The incubation period is 5 to 45 days.

Clinical signs

The clinical signs may include abdominal distension, exophthalmia, darkening of the skin, anemia, and fading of the gills. Long, semi–transparent fecal casts often trail from the anus. Hemorrhages are common at the base of the pectoral fins, the mouth, the skin posterior to the skull above the lateral line, the muscles near the anus, and the yolk sac in sac fry. In sac fry, the yolk sac often swells with fluid. Diseased fish move slowly, float with the current, and occasionally act as if they were suffering from cramps. In later stages, the fish tend to float on the surface, turn over, and occasionally swim frantically. Surviving fish often have scoliosis.

Post mortem lesions

The abdomen, stomach, and intestines often contain white to yellowish fluid. The kidney, liver, and heart are usually very pale. Necrosis is common in the kidney and spleen, and focal necrosis may be noted in the liver. Petechiae are common in the pyloric caeca, the spleen, the peritoneum, the intestines, and the membranes surrounding the heart and brain. Hemorrhages may be seen in the kidney, the peritoneum, and the swim bladder.

Morbidity and mortality

The water temperature influences infection; clinical disease is seen between 8°C and 15°C. Disease outbreaks almost always occur between the spring and early summer.

Mortality is high in fry and juvenile fish, but low in yearlings. The mortality rates in young Chinook salmon may be up to 60% and, in young Sockeye salmon, up to 90%. Resistance to infection increases in older fish, and disease is rare. Fish that survive infectious hematopoietic necrosis usually have good immunity, but some may become asymptomatic carriers. Asymptomatic infections may become clinical after handling or other stress.

Vaccination for this disease is still experimental.

Diagnosis

Clinical

Infectious hematopoietic necrosis should be suspected in rainbow trout or salmon with typical clinical symptoms and necropsy lesions. In some cases, the major symptom is a significant rise in mortality in young fish. Most outbreaks will be seen in the spring and early summer.

Laboratory tests

Infectious hematopoietic necrosis can be diagnosed by virus isolation in cell cultures; appropriate cell lines include EPC (*Epithelioma papulosum cyprini*) and BF–2 (bluegill fry) cells. Virus identity is confirmed by virus neutralization, immunofluorescence, enzyme–linked immunosorbent assay (ELISA), DNA probes, or polymerase chain reaction (PCR) tests.

Virus antigens or nucleic acids can also be identified directly in the tissues by immunofluorescence, ELISA, or PCR.

Serology may eventually become useful for screening fish populations, but has not yet been validated for routine diagnosis.

Samples to collect

If the fish are symptomatic, the samples to take depend on the size of the fish. Small fish (less than or equal to 4 cm) should be sent whole. The viscera including the kidney should be collected from fish that are 4 to 6 cm long. The kidney, spleen, and encephalon should be sent from larger fish. If the fish are asymptomatic, the samples should include the kidney, spleen, and encephalon, and the ovarian fluid at spawning. Samples should be taken from 10 diseased fish and combined to form pools with approximately 1.5 g of material (no more than 5 fish per pool).

The pools of organs or ovarian fluids should be placed in sterile vials. The samples may also be sent in cell culture medium or Hanks' balanced salt solution with antibiotics. They should be kept cold (4°C) but not frozen. If the shipping time is expected to be longer than 12 hours, serum or albumen (5–10%) may be added to stabilize the virus. Ideally, virus isolation should be done within 24 hours after fish sampling.

Recommended actions if infectious hematopoietic necrosis is suspected

Notification of authorities

Infectious hematopoietic necrosis should be reported to state or federal authorities immediately upon diagnosis or suspicion of the disease.

Federal: Area Veterinarians in Charge (AVICs):
http://www.aphis.usda.gov/vs/area_offices.htm
State Veterinarians:
http://www.aphis.usda.gov/vs/sregs/official.html

Quarantine and disinfection

Quarantine is necessary during outbreaks: infectious hematopoietic necrosis is a contagious disease and asymptomatic carriers occur. IHNV can be inactivated by temperatures of 60°C for 15 minutes. It is resistant to ethanol but sensitive to iodophor solutions.

Sterilizing the feed for at least 30 minutes at 60°C can reduce the risk of infection. Egg transmission can be decreased by disinfecting the surfaces of the eggs with an iodophor solution and incubating them in virus–free water. Outbreaks may be limited by raising the water temperature.

Public health

There is no indication that this disease is a threat to humans.

For more information

World Organization for Animal Health (OIE)
http://www.oie.int
OIE Diagnostic Manual for Aquatic Animal Diseases
http://www.oie.int/eng/normes/fmanual/A_summry.htm
International Aquatic Animal Health Code (2001)
http://www.oie.int/eng/normes/fcode/a_summry.htm

References

"Fish Health Management: Viral Diseases." In *The Merck Veterinary Manual*, 8th ed. Edited by S.E. Aiello and A. Mays. Whitehouse Station, NJ: Merck and Co., 1998, pp. 1291–1293.

"General Information." In *Diagnostic Manual for Aquatic Animal Diseases*. Paris: World Organization for Animal Health, 2000. http//www.oie.int/eng/normes/fmanual/A_00010.htm.

"Infectious Hematopoietic Necrosis." In *Diagnostic Manual for Aquatic Animal Diseases*. Paris: World Organization for Animal Health, 2000. http//www.oie.int/eng/normes/fmanual/A_00013.htm.

"Infectious Hematopoietic Necrosis (IHN)." In *Fish Diseases,* 5th ed. Edited by W. Schäperclaus, H. Kulow, and K. Schreckenbach. Rotterdam: A.A. Balkema, 1992, pp. 345–349.

"Infectious Hematopoietic Necrosis (IHN)." In *Infectious Diseases of Fish*. Edited by Shuzo Egusa. New Delhi, India: Amerind Pub. Co., 1992, pp. 20–35.

Influenza

Avian Influenza, Swine Influenza, Hog Flu, Pig Flu, Equine Influenza, Canine Influenza, Flu, Grippe

Importance

Influenza viruses are widespread in birds, swine, horses and humans. An equine influenza virus recently became established in dogs, resulting in the emergence of a new disease, canine influenza. In mammals, uncomplicated influenza has a high morbidity rate but most infections are self-limiting and nonfatal. However, in poultry, a form called highly pathogenic avian influenza (HPAI) is a serious disease with mortality and mortality rates up to 90% - 100%. HPAI, an exotic disease in the U.S., can devastate the poultry industry.

Rarely, avian and swine influenza viruses can infect humans. Most of these infections seem to be limited to conjunctivitis or mild respiratory disease but severe, fatal cases also occur. Severe disease has been reported most often with the highly pathogenic avian influenza viruses. Zoonotic influenza almost always seems to result from direct contact with infected animals or fomites, and the virus is not easily transmitted to other people. However, it would be possible for an animal influenza virus or a hybrid human/ animal influenza virus to become adapted to humans. Such an event would probably result in a human influenza pandemic.

Etiology

Viruses in the family Orthomyxoviridae cause influenza. There are three genera of influenza viruses: influenzavirus A, influenzavirus B and influenzavirus C. These viruses are also called type A, type B and type C.

Influenza A viruses

Influenza A viruses include the avian, swine, equine, and canine influenza viruses, as well as the human influenza A viruses. Influenza A viruses are classified into subtypes based on two surface antigens, hemagglutinin (H) and neuraminidase (N). There are 16 hemagglutinin antigens (H1 to H16) and 9 neuraminidase antigens (N1 to N9). These two proteins are involved in cell attachment and release from cells, and help determine the species specificity of a virus. They are also major targets for the immune response.

Subtypes of influenza A viruses are classified into strains. Strains of influenza viruses are described by their type, host, place of first isolation, strain number (if any), year of isolation, and antigenic subtype. For example, the prototype strain of the H7N7 subtype of equine influenza virus, first isolated in Czechoslovakia in 1956, is A/eq/Prague/56 (H7N7). For human strains, the host is typically omitted.

Antigenic shift and drift in influenza A viruses

Influenza A viruses change frequently. Strains gradually evolve as they accumulate point mutations during virus replication; this process is sometimes called 'antigenic drift.' A more abrupt change can occur during genetic reassortment. Reassortment is possible whenever two different influenza viruses infect a cell simultaneously; when the new viruses (the 'progeny') are assembled, they may contain some genes from one parent virus and some genes from the other. Reassortment between two different strains results in the periodic emergence of novel strains. Reassortment between subtypes can result in the emergence of a new subtype. Reassortment can also occur between the avian, swine, equine and human influenza A viruses. This type of reassortment can result in a 'hybrid' virus with, for example, both avian and human influenza virus proteins.

A sudden change in the subtypes found in host species is called an 'antigenic shift.' Antigenic shifts can result from three mechanisms: 1) genetic reassortment, 2) the direct transfer of a whole virus from one host species into another, or 3) the re-emergence of a virus that was found previously in a species but is no longer in circulation. Antigenic drift and antigenic shifts result in the periodic emergence of novel influenza viruses. By evading the immune response, these viruses can cause influenza epidemics and pandemics.

Avian influenza viruses

Avian influenza is caused by the avian influenza viruses. Avian influenza viruses are classified as either highly pathogenic avian influenza (HPAI) or low pathogenic avian influenza (LPAI) viruses, based on the genetic features of the virus and the severity of disease in poultry. To date, only subtypes that contained H5 or H7 have been highly pathogenic; subtypes that contained other hemagglutinins have been found only in the LPAI form. H5 and H7 LPAI viruses also exist, and can evolve into highly pathogenic strains.

Waterfowl, which seem to be the natural reservoirs for the type A influenza viruses, carry all of the known H and N antigens and, thus, all of the subtypes. In North America, H3, H4 and H6 viruses are found most often in wild ducks, but H5, H7 and H9 viruses are also found at low levels. Subtypes that have been found in ratites include H3N2, H4N2, H4N6, H5N2, H5N9, H7N1, H7N3, H9N2, H10N4 and H10N7. All were of low virulence for chickens. Isolates from cage birds usually contain H3 or H4.

In contrast to birds, only a few subtypes circulate in each species of mammal.

Human influenza viruses

Human influenza viruses are mainly found in humans, but they can also infect ferrets and sometimes swine. H1N1, H1N2 and H3N2 viruses are currently in general circulation. The H1N2 viruses appeared most recently. These viruses were first seen in human populations in 2001, probably as a result of genetic reassortment between the H3N2 and H1N1 viruses. H2N2 viruses circulated in the human population between 1957 and 1968.

Human influenza viruses change frequently as the result of antigenic drift, and occasionally as the result of antigenic shift. Epidemics occur every few years, as a result of small changes in the influenza viruses. Human pandemics, resulting from antigenic shifts, were most recently reported in 1918, 1957 and 1968.

Swine influenza viruses

Swine influenza is caused by the swine influenza viruses. There is less antigenic drift in these viruses than in the human viruses. The most common subtypes currently found in pigs are H1N1, H1N2 and H3N2. However, the situation is fairly complex, as two or more viruses of each subtype are circulating in swine populations.

One H1N1 virus circulating in the U.S. is the 'classical' H1N1 swine influenza virus. This virus, the first influenza virus known to have infected pigs, was originally found in swine populations in 1918. An 'avian-like' H1N1 virus circulates in both Europe and the U.S. This virus seems to be an avian influenza virus that was transmitted whole to pigs. It has, in some locations, replaced the classical H1N1 virus. In addition, a different 'avian-like' H1N1 virus is co-circulating with the classical H1N1 virus in pigs in Asia.

H3N2 viruses are found in pigs in the U.S. Midwest. These viruses are triple reassortants. They contain hemagglutinin and neuraminidase proteins from a human influenza virus, and internal proteins from the classical H1N1 swine influenza virus, an avian influenza virus, and a human influenza virus. H3N2 viruses are also found in Europe and Asia, but these viruses seem to be the result of reassortment between a human H3N2 virus, circulating there in pigs since the 1970s, and the H1N1 'avian-like' virus. The European H3N2 viruses contain human N3 and N2 proteins, and internal proteins from the avian virus.

The H1N2 virus in the U.S. is a reassortant of the classical H1N1 swine influenza virus and the triple reassortant H3N2 virus circulating in the U.S. The H1N2 virus in Europe is a reassortant of a human H1N1 virus and the European H3N2 virus.

Equine influenza viruses

Equine influenza is caused by the equine influenza viruses. There is less antigenic drift in equine viruses than human viruses. The two subtypes known to cause disease in horses are H7N7 (equine virus 1) and H3N8 (equine virus 2). The H7N7 virus is currently extinct or present at only very low levels in some parts of the world.

In 1989, a novel strain of equine influenza [A/eq/Jilin/89 (H3N8)] caused a serious epidemic, with high morbidity and mortality rates, in Chinese horses. This virus appears to be an avian influenza virus that was transmitted whole to horses. A related virus caused influenza in a few hundred horses the following year but there were no deaths. The H3N8 avian-like virus continued to circulate in horses in China for at least five years without further fatalities.

Canine influenza viruses

An H3N8 canine influenza virus has been reported in the U.S. This virus appears to be an equine influenza virus that recently jumped species, and bears a close resemblance to an isolate seen in horses in Wisconsin in 2004.

Influenza viruses in other species

H7N7 and H4N5 viruses, closely related to avian viruses, have been isolated from seals. In 1984, a H10N4 virus was isolated from mink during an epidemic in Sweden. This virus is also thought to have come from birds. A H5N1 avian influenza virus was recently isolated from sick domestic and zoo cats in Asia.

Influenza B and C viruses

Influenza B and C viruses mainly cause disease in humans, but are occasionally isolated from animals. Influenza B viruses are not categorized into subtypes, but are classified into strains. Influenza B viruses undergo antigenic drift but not antigenic shift. Antigenic drift is slower in these viruses than in influenza A viruses. Influenza C viruses are also classified only into strains and not into subtypes. Each strain is antigenically stable, and accumulates few changes over time. However, recent evidence suggests that reassortment occurs frequently between different strains of influenza C viruses.

Species affected

Avian influenza viruses

Avian influenza viruses mainly infect birds, but can also cause disease in horses, swine, mink, cats, marine mammals and humans. Poultry can develop serious or mild disease, depending on the subtype and strain of virus. In cage birds, most infections have been recorded in passerine birds. Psittacine birds are rarely affected.

Waterfowl appear to be the natural reservoirs for the influenza A viruses. Most, but not all, infections in wild birds are asymptomatic.

Swine influenza viruses

Swine influenza viruses mainly affect pigs but can also cause disease in turkeys and humans.

Equine influenza viruses

Equine influenza viruses mainly affect horses, donkeys and other Equidae. Antibodies to the equine H3N8 viruses have been

reported in humans. Recently, a H3N8 equine influenza virus appears to have jumped into dogs.

Canine influenza viruses

Canine influenza viruses have been reported only in dogs. To date, there have been no infections reported in other species, including humans.

Human influenza viruses

Human influenza viruses mainly cause disease in humans and ferrets. They can also infect pigs and have been reported in dogs, cattle and birds. Experimental infections have been reported in horses.

Influenza B and C viruses

Although influenza B and C viruses mainly infect humans, they are occasionally found in animals. Influenza B viruses can cause disease in ferrets and seals. They have also been isolated from pigs and a horse. Serologic evidence of infection has been found in pigs, dogs and horses.

Influenza C viruses have been isolated from humans and swine. These viruses can cause disease in experimentally infected dogs. Serologic evidence of infection has been found in pigs, dogs and horses.

Geographic distribution

Human and avian influenza viruses are found worldwide. Avian HPAI viruses have been eradicated from domestic poultry in most developed nations, but are found worldwide in waterfowl. Outbreaks of highly pathogenic avian influenza can occur in most countries, due to the transmission of avian influenza viruses from these reservoirs into domestic poultry. In 2004-2006, outbreaks of an avian influenza H5N1 (HPAI) virus occurred in poultry in Southeast Asia and spread into Europe. Human, feline and possibly porcine infections and deaths were associated with these outbreaks.

Swine influenza is common in North and South America, Europe and Asia and has been reported from Africa.

Equine influenza is found in most countries; only Australia, New Zealand and Iceland are known to be free from this disease. The H3N8 subtype is widespread in horse populations. The H7N7 subtype may be either extinct or present at only very low levels in some parts of the world, including North America and Europe. It can still be found at low levels in Central Asia.

The canine influenza virus has, to date, been found only in the U.S. Infections have been seen in the general canine population in Florida and, more recently, in New York and other states. In 2004 and 2005, infections were also reported in racing greyhounds in a number of states including Florida, Texas, Arkansas, Alabama, Arizona, West Virginia, Kansas, Iowa, Colorado, Rhode Island and Massachusetts.

Transmission

In mammals, the influenza viruses are transmitted in aerosols created by coughing and sneezing, and by contact with nasal discharges, either directly or on fomites. Close contact and closed environments favor transmission. In ferrets, *in utero* transmission can occur with high viremia after experimental infection.

In birds, avian influenza viruses are shed in the feces as well as in saliva and nasal secretions; fecal-oral transmission is the most common means of spread. Waterfowl can carry the avian influenza viruses asymptomatically and transmit them to poultry. These viruses have also been isolated from the water in ponds where ducks swim. In addition, avian influenza viruses have been found in the yolk and albumen of eggs from infected hens. Although these eggs are unlikely to hatch, broken shells could transmit the virus to other chicks in the incubator. Fomites can be important in transmission and flies may act as mechanical vectors.

Recently, avian influenza H5N1 was reported in domestic and zoo cats during an outbreak in Asia. The cats were all thought to have been infected by eating raw infected poultry. Experimental infections were established in cats by intratracheal inoculation with H5N1 viruses and by feeding them H5N1-infected chicks.

Transmission between species

Ordinarily, swine influenza viruses circulate only among pigs, equine influenza viruses among the Equidae, avian influenza viruses among birds, and human influenza viruses among humans. Occasionally, these viruses cross species barriers. Generally, the virus is not well adapted to the new host species and it does not undergo sustained transmission.

Rarely, transmission between species results in an epidemic in the new host. Generally, this requires a novel hemagglutinin and/or neuraminidase protein to evade the immune response, together with viral proteins that are well adapted to the new host's cells. Occasionally, a virus is transferred whole to the new host and can spread. This has occurred a few times when avian viruses infected mink, horses, seals and pigs. However, dissemination is more likely if the novel virus reassorts with a virus that that is already adapted to the host species. Reassortment can occur in the new host's own cells. It could also occur in an intermediate host, particularly a pig. Pigs have receptors that can bind swine, human, and avian influenza viruses. For this reason, they have been called 'mixing vessels' for the formation of new viruses. Reassortment is more likely if different species are kept in close proximity.

Incubation period

The incubation period is generally short in all species. The clinical signs usually appear within 1 to 3 days in horses, pigs or seals; incubation periods up to 7 days have been reported in horses. In poultry, the incubation period can be a few hours to a week. The incubation period for canine influenza is approximately 2 to 5 days.

Clinical signs

Avian influenza

The highly pathogenic avian influenza (HPAI) viruses cause severe disease in poultry. These viruses can cause serious infections in some species of birds on a farm while leaving others unaffected. The clinical signs are variable. The typical symptoms are those of a respiratory disease with sinusitis, lacrimation, edema of the head, cyanosis of the head, comb and wattle, and green to white diarrhea. Hemorrhagic lesions may be found on the comb and wattles of turkeys. Other signs may include anorexia, coughing, sneezing, blood-tinged oral and nasal discharges, ecchymoses on the shanks and feet, neurologic disease, decreased egg production, loss of egg pigmentation and deformed or shell-less eggs. Sudden death may occur with few other signs. Most of the flock usually dies. In ducks, the most common symptoms are sinusitis, diarrhea and increased mortality.

The low pathogenic (LPAI) viruses usually cause subclinical or mild illness. The symptoms may include decreased egg production or increased mortality rates. More severe disease, mimicking highly pathogenic avian influenza, can be seen if the birds are concurrently infected with other viruses or there are other exacerbating factors.

Avian influenza is often subclinical in wild birds, but some strains can cause illness and death.

Turkeys infected with swine influenza viruses may develop respiratory disease, have decreased egg production, or produce abnormal eggs.

Swine influenza

Swine influenza is an acute upper respiratory disease characterized by fever, lethargy, anorexia, weight loss and labored breathing. Coughing may be seen in the later stages of the disease. Sneezing, nasal discharge and conjunctivitis are less common symptoms. Abortions may also occur. Some virus strains can circulate in pigs with few or no clinical signs. Complications may include secondary bacterial or viral infections. Severe, potentially fatal bronchopneumonia is occasionally seen.

Equine influenza

Equine influenza usually spreads rapidly in a group of animals. In naïve horses, the first sign is usually a fever, followed by a deep, dry cough. Other symptoms may include a serous to mucopurulent nasal discharge, myalgia, inappetence and enlarged submandibular lymph nodes. There may be edema of the legs and scrotum, and spasmodic impaction colic has been reported. Animals with partial immunity can have milder, atypical infections with little or no coughing or fever. Healthy adult horses usually recover within 1 to 2 weeks, but the cough may persist longer. Secondary bacterial infections prolong recovery. Death in adult horses usually results from bacterial pneumonia, pleuritis or purpura hemorrhagica. Sequelae may include chronic pharyngitis, chronic bronchiolitis and emphysema. Interstitial myocarditis can occur during or after the infection. Young foals without maternal antibodies can develop a rapidly fatal viral pneumonia.

Horses experimentally infected with human influenza virus (H3N2 'Hong Kong') developed a mild febrile illness. The virus could be isolated for up to 5 days.

Influenza in dogs

Canine influenza is an emerging disease in dogs. The most common presentation resembles kennel cough. In this milder form, an initial fever is followed by a persistent cough and, sometimes, a purulent nasal discharge. The cough can last for up to 3 weeks regardless of treatment. The nasal discharge appears to resolve with antibiotics, suggesting that secondary bacterial infections may be important in this disease. More severely affected dogs exhibit a high fever (104-106°F) with an increased respiratory rate and other symptoms of pneumonia. Some dogs have been found dead peracutely with evidence of hemorrhages in the respiratory tract. Asymptomatic seroconversion has also been seen.

The clinical signs in dogs experimentally infected with influenza C virus included nasal discharge and conjunctivitis, which persisted for 10 days.

Influenza in ferrets

Ferrets are susceptible to the human influenza viruses. The symptoms may include fever, anorexia, depression, listlessness, sneezing, purulent nasal discharge and coughing. The infection is not usually fatal in adult animals, which generally recover in 5 days to 2 weeks. More severe or fatal disease can be seen in neonates.

Influenza in mink

In 1984, a H10N4 avian influenza virus caused an epidemic on 33 mink farms in Sweden. The symptoms included anorexia, sneezing, coughing, nasal and ocular discharges, and numerous deaths.

H5N1 influenza in cats

Influenza A was recently reported in cats. During an epidemic of H5N1 avian influenza in Asian poultry, there were anecdotal reports of fatal influenza in domestic cats, a white tiger and a clouded leopard. H5N1 avian influenza virus was isolated from these animals, which were all thought to have been infected by eating raw, infected poultry. Clinical signs in cats experimentally infected with the H5N1 virus included fever, lethargy, conjunctivitis, protrusion of the third eyelid and dyspnea. One cat died on the sixth day after inoculation; the remaining animals were euthanized and necropsied the following day.

Influenza in marine mammals

Influenza A viruses have been associated with outbreaks of pneumonia in seals and disease in a pilot whale. The viruses appeared to be of avian origin. The clinical signs in the seals included weakness, incoordination, dyspnea and swelling of the neck. A white or bloody nasal discharge was seen in some animals. In the single known case in a whale, the symptoms included extreme emaciation, difficulty maneuvering and sloughing skin.

Post mortem lesions

Avian influenza

The lesions in poultry are highly variable and can resemble other avian diseases. There may be subcutaneous edema of the head and neck, fluid in the nares and oral cavity, and severe congestion of the conjunctivae. Hemorrhagic tracheitis can be seen in some birds; in others, the tracheal lesions may be limited to excess mucoid exudate. Petechiae may be found throughout the abdominal fat, serosal surfaces and peritoneum. Hemorrhages may also be seen on the mucosa of the proventriculus, beneath the lining of the gizzard, and in the intestinal mucosa. The kidneys can be severely congested and are sometimes plugged with urate deposits. The ovaries may be hemorrhagic or degenerated, with areas of necrosis. The peritoneal cavity often contains yolk from ruptured ova. Severe airsacculitis and peritonitis may be seen in some birds. In birds that die peracutely and in young birds, the only lesions may be severe congestion of the musculature and dehydration.

Swine influenza

In uncomplicated infections, the gross lesions are mainly those of a viral pneumonia. Affected parts of the lungs are depressed and consolidated, dark red to purple red, and sharply demarcated. The lesions may be found throughout the lungs but are usually more extensive in the ventral regions. Other parts of the lungs may be pale and emphysematous. The airways are often dilated and filled with mucopurulent or blood-tinged, fibrinous exudate. The bronchial and mediastinal lymph nodes are typically enlarged. Severe pulmonary edema, or serous or serofibrinous pleuritis may also be seen. Some strains of swine influenza viruses produce more marked lesions than others. Generalized lymphadenopathy, hepatic congestion and pulmonary consolidation were reported in one outbreak of severe disease in swine.

Equine influenza

Interstitial pneumonia, pleuropneumonia, bronchitis, perivasculitis and interstitial myocarditis have been reported in fatal cases in horses.

Canine influenza

In fatal cases, hemorrhages may be found in the lungs, mediastinum and pleural cavity. On histologic examination, there may be tracheitis, bronchitis, bronchiolitis and suppurative bronchopneumonia.

Influenza in cats

The lesions reported in experimentally infected cats were multiple to coalescing foci of pulmonary consolidation. The lesions were similar whether the cats were infected intratracheally or by the ingestion of infected chicks.

Influenza in marine mammals

In seals, pneumonia with necrotizing bronchitis, bronchiolitis and hemorrhagic alveolitis have been reported. In a single case in a whale, the lungs were hemorrhagic and a hilar lymph node was greatly enlarged.

Morbidity and mortality

The severity of an influenza virus infection varies with the dose and strain of virus and the host's immunity. In mammals, uncomplicated infections are usually associated with high morbidity rates, low mortality rates and rapid recovery. Secondary bacterial infections can exacerbate the symptoms, prolong recovery and result in complications such as pneumonia.

Avian influenza

Avian influenza outbreaks occur in most countries including the U.S. Low pathogenic forms are seen most often, but outbreaks with the highly pathogenic H5 and H7 viruses are also reported periodically. In poultry, HPAI viruses are associated with very high morbidity and mortality rates, up to 90% - 100%. Any surviving birds are usually in poor condition. LPAI viruses usually result in mild or asymptomatic infections, but may also mimic HPAI viruses. Symptomatic infections and outbreaks have been reported in wild birds, but are unusual.

Swine influenza

Influenza is a major cause of acute respiratory disease in finishing pigs. Approximately 25% - 33% of 6-7 month old finishing pigs and 45% of breeding pigs have antibodies to the classical swine H1N1 virus in the U.S. High seroprevalence rates have also been reported in other countries.

Swine influenza viruses are usually introduced into a herd in an infected animal, and can survive in carrier animals for up to 3 months. In a newly infected herd, up to 100% of the animals may become ill but most animals recover within 5 to 7 days if there are no secondary bacterial infections or other complications. In uncomplicated cases, the case fatality rate varies from less than 1% to 3%. Once the virus has been introduced, it usually persists in the herd. Annual outbreaks are often seen. They occur mainly during the colder months. Many of the infections in endemically infected herds are subclinical; typical signs of influenza may occur in only 25% to 30% of the pigs. Maternal antibodies decrease the severity of disease in young pigs. Some viruses can infect the herd with few or no clinical signs.

Influenza epidemics can occur if a virus infects a population without immunity to the virus, or if the infection is exacerbated by factors such as poor husbandry, stress, secondary infections or cold weather. In the epidemic form, the virus spreads rapidly in pigs of all ages. In a 1918 epizootic, millions of pigs developed influenza, and thousands of the infections were fatal. Recently, a novel H3N2 entered pigs in the Midwest and has caused serious illness and reproductive losses in sows.

Pigs can also be infected with the human influenza A, B and C viruses. In the U.K., a study found antibodies to both swine and human influenza viruses in 14% of all pigs. Approximately 10% of the pigs were seropositive for influenza C viruses, but only sporadic infections with the human influenza B viruses were found. In Japan, a similar study found antibodies to the type C viruses in 19% of pigs.

Equine influenza

In horses, influenza outbreaks are not as seasonal as they are in pigs or humans. Instead, most outbreaks are associated with sales, races and other events where horses congregate. Widespread epidemics can be seen, with morbidity rates up to 60% - 90%, in naïve populations. In 1987, an equine influenza epidemic in India affected more than 27,000 animals and killed several hundred. In populations that have been previously exposed, cases are seen mainly in young and newly introduced animals.

Unless there are complications, healthy adult horses usually recover within 1-2 weeks, although coughing can persist. The H3N8 viruses usually cause more severe disease than the H7N7 viruses. Deaths are rare in adult horses, and are usually the result of secondary bacterial infections. Higher mortality rates have been reported in foals, animals in poor condition and donkeys. A rapidly fatal viral pneumonia may be seen in young foals with no maternal antibodies. In horses, tracheal clearance rates can be depressed for up to a month after infection.

Avian influenza viruses have rarely been reported in horses. In 1989, a novel strain of equine influenza [A/ eq/Jilin/89 (H3N8)] caused a serious epidemic in Chinese horses. The morbidity rate was 80% and the mortality rate was 20%. The virus appeared to be an avian influenza virus. A related virus caused influenza in a few hundred horses the following year but there were no deaths. The avian-like virus continued to circulate in horses for at least 5 years without further fatalities.

Canine influenza

Canine influenza was first reported in racing greyhounds and, at first, appeared to be confined to this breed. In 2004 and 2005, outbreaks of respiratory disease occurred in greyhounds at kennels and racetracks in 12 states including Florida, Texas, Arkansas, Alabama, Arizona, West Virginia, Kansas, Iowa, Colorado, Rhode Island and Massachusetts. The canine influenza virus was shown to be involved in some outbreaks and is presumed to have been responsible for the remainder. More recently, this disease has been seen in a variety of breeds at veterinary clinics and animal shelters in Florida and New York. All dogs regardless of breed or age are now considered to be susceptible. The canine population is not expected to have any naturally- acquired or vaccine-induced immunity to this new virus. In kennels, the infection rate may reach 100% and symptoms may be seen in 75% of the dogs infected. Most dogs are expected to develop the less severe form of the disease, and recover; however, a more severe form with pneumonia also occurs in a minority. In dogs with severe disease, the overall mortality rate is thought to be 1% - 5%.

Influenza in other mammals

In 1984, an outbreak with an avian H10N4 virus was reported on Swedish mink farms. The outbreak affected 33 farms and killed 3,000 mink. The morbidity rate was nearly 100%.

Fatal infections with an avian H5N1 virus were recently reported in three domestic cats, a white tiger and a clouded leopard. Experimental infections were also reported in 8 cats. The morbidity and mortality rates are unknown.

In seals, the case fatality rate was estimated to be 20% in one outbreak with a H7N7 virus, and 4% in an outbreak with a H4N5 virus. Explosive epidemics in seals are thought to be exacerbated by high population densities and unseasonably warm temperatures.

Diagnosis

Clinical

In horses, a rapidly spreading respiratory disease with a sudden onset of high fever, coughing, depression and weakness is suggestive of equine influenza. The clinical findings and course of the disease are also suggestive in swine influenza. In poultry, highly pathogenic avian influenza should be suspected in outbreaks with high morbidity and mortality rates. Low pathogenic avian influenza can be subclinical or mimic other diseases, and can be more difficult to diagnose.

Differential diagnosis

The differential diagnosis varies with the species and generally includes other respiratory diseases. In horses, these diseases include equine viral rhinopneumonitis and equine viral arteritis, among others. Swine influenza should be distinguished from diseases such as pasteurellosis, porcine reproductive and respiratory syndrome (PRRS), pseudorabies, chlamydial infections and *Haemophilus* infections. In poultry, highly pathogenic avian influenza may resemble acute fowl cholera or exotic Newcastle disease. In milder avian cases, a variety of respiratory diseases should be considered.

Laboratory tests

Avian influenza

Avian influenza is usually diagnosed by virus isolation in embryonated eggs. The virus is subtyped with immunodiffusion tests, or hemagglutination and neuraminidase inhibition tests. Virus inoculation into susceptible birds, together with genetic tests, is used to differentiate LPAI from HPAI viruses. Viral antigens can be detected with ELISAs, including a rapid test (Directigen® Flu A kit, Becton Dickinson Microbiology Systems). Reverse transcription polymerase chain reaction (RT-PCR) tests may be used to identify nucleic acids. Serological tests, including agar gel immunodiffusion, hemagglutination inhibition and ELISAs, may be used as supplemental tests.

Swine influenza

Swine influenza can be diagnosed by virus isolation, detection of viral antigens or nucleic acids, and serology. Mammalian influenza viruses can be isolated in embryonated chicken eggs or cell cultures. Isolated viruses are subtyped with hemagglutination inhibition and neuraminidase inhibition tests. Immunofluorescent techniques can detect antigens in fresh lung tissue, nasal epithelial cells or bronchoalveolar lavage. Other antigen tests include immunohistochemistry on fixed tissue samples, and ELISAs including the Directigen® Flu A test. RT-PCR assays are also available.

Serology on paired samples can diagnose swine influenza retrospectively. The hemagglutination inhibition test, which is subtype specific, is most often used. It may not detect new viruses. ELISA tests are also used. Rarely used serological tests in swine include agar gel immunodiffusion, the indirect fluorescent antibody test and virus neutralization.

Equine influenza

As in swine, equine influenza is confirmed by virus isolation, the detection of viral antigens or nucleic acids, or retrospectively by serology. The most commonly used serologic tests in horses are the hemagglutination inhibition test and a single-radial hemolysis (SRH) test. An ELISA that can distinguish natural from vaccine-induced antibodies is in development.

Canine influenza

At this time, canine influenza is mainly diagnosed by serology. Virus isolation may be useful in some cases. The virus can be isolated from the lung tissue samples taken post-mortem, but virus isolation has not been successful using pharyngeal swabs in live dogs.

Samples to collect

Before collecting or sending any samples from animals with a suspected foreign animal disease, the proper authorities should be contacted. Samples should only be sent under secure conditions and to authorized laboratories to prevent the spread of the disease.

Avian influenza

The avian influenza virus can be isolated from tracheal, oronasal or cloacal swabs in live birds, and pooled or individual organ samples (trachea, lungs, air sacs, intestine, spleen, kidney, brain, liver and heart) from dead birds. Feces can be substituted in small birds if cloacal samples are not practical. Serum can be collected for serology.

Swine influenza

The swine influenza viruses can be recovered from lung tissues at necropsy, or nasal or pharyngeal swabs from acutely ill pigs. Virus recovery is best from an animal with a fever, 24 to 48 hours after the onset of disease. Immunofluorescent techniques can detect antigens in fresh lung tissue, nasal epithelial cells or bronchoalveolar lavage. Immunohistochemistry on fixed tissue samples may also be available. Paired acute and convalescent serum samples should be taken to diagnose swine influenza retrospectively.

Equine influenza

In horses, peak virus shedding is thought to occur during the first 24 to 48 hours of fever, and samples for virus isolation should be taken then. As in swine, a serological diagnosis requires paired acute and convalescent samples.

Canine influenza

Paired serum samples should be submitted, if possible, for serology. Since canine influenza is an emerging disease, most dogs are not expected to have pre-existing titers to the canine influenza virus; however, single titers are still considered to be less useful. The virus can be isolated from the lung tissue samples taken post-mortem, but virus isolation has not been successful using pharyngeal swabs in live dogs. Pharyngeal swabs or tracheal wash samples taken from febrile dogs very early in the course of the disease might be more successful.

Recommended actions if influenza is suspected
Notification of authorities
Highly pathogenic avian influenza should be reported immediately to state or federal authorities upon diagnosis or suspicion of the disease.

Equine influenza, swine influenza, canine influenza and low-pathogenic avian influenza are endemic in the U.S.; however, canine influenza is an emerging disease and low pathogenic avian influenza in poultry flocks may result in regulatory action. State authorities should be consulted for specific information on reporting requirements for these four diseases.

Federal Area Veterinarians in Charge (AVIC):
  http://www.aphis.usda.gov/vs/area_offices.htm
State Veterinarians:
  http://www.aphis.usda.gov/vs/sregs/official.html

Quarantine and disinfection
Influenza viruses are contagious by aerosols or direct contact with nasal secretions. In general, the influenza viruses are relatively labile, but can persist for several hours in dried mucus. Avian influenza viruses (H7N2, LPAI) can persist for up to 2 weeks in feces and on cages. They can also survive for up to 32 days at 15–20°C, and at least 20 days at 28–30°C, but are inactivated more quickly when mixed with chicken manure. HPAI viruses can survive indefinitely when frozen.

During an outbreak of influenza among mammals, quarantine or isolation of infected animals helps prevent virus dissemination. Rest decreases virus shedding in horses. In poultry, outbreaks of highly pathogenic avian influenza are managed by quarantine, depopulation, cleaning and disinfection, and surveillance around the affected flocks. Influenza viruses can be transmitted on fomites, and strict hygiene is necessary to prevent virus transmission by this route. Infected facilities should be cleaned and disinfected after the outbreak. The influenza viruses are susceptible to a variety of disinfectants including 1% sodium hypochlorite, 70% ethanol, glutaraldehyde, formaldehyde and lipid solvents. They can also be inactivated by heat of 56°C for a minimum of 30 min, radiation or pH 2.

Inactivated influenza vaccines are available for pigs, horses and, in some countries, birds. The vaccines do not always prevent infection, but the disease is usually milder if it occurs. In the U.S., avian influenza vaccines are used most often in turkeys and are intended only to prevent infection by LPAI viruses. HPAI vaccines are not used routinely in the U.S. or most other countries. A "DIVA" (differentiating infected from vaccinated animals) strategy has been successfully used to control a low pathogenicity avian influenza outbreak in Italy. This strategy depends on using an inactivated vaccine containing the homologous H type and a heterologous N type. Vaccinated birds that subsequently become infected can be detected by testing for antibodies to the N type of the field strain.

Influenza vaccines are changed periodically to reflect the current subtypes and strains in a geographic area. In general, swine and equine viruses display less antigenic drift than human viruses and these vaccines are changed less often. Avian vaccines are usually autogenous or from viruses of the same subtype or hemagglutinin type.

Public health
Nearly all cases of influenza in people are caused by the human influenza viruses. However, zoonotic infections with the swine and avian influenza viruses have also been reported.
Avian influenza virus infections in humans
Transmission of the avian influenza viruses to people is rare, and has been reported only with the H5, H7 and H9 viruses. Most infections have been the result of direct contact with infected poultry or fomites, but during a 2003 outbreak in the Netherlands, three human infections occurred in family members of infected poultry workers. The virus subtype was H7N7. No case of sustained person-to-person transmission with the avian viruses has been reported in recent epidemics. However, there is evidence that the severe human pandemic in 1918 was caused by an avian influenza virus (H1N1) that became adapted to humans.

Healthy children and adults, as well as those with chronic medical conditions, have been affected by the avian influenza viruses. While some infections have been limited to conjunctivitis and/or typical influenza symptoms, others were serious or fatal. Viral pneumonia, acute respiratory distress syndrome, severe bronchointerstitial pneumonia, multiple organ dysfunction and other severe or fatal complications have been reported. In one fatal case, the initial symptoms were limited to a persistent high fever and headache, and respiratory disease was not seen until later. The HPAI viruses appear to cause more severe disease than the LPAI viruses.

The following human infections were reported between 1997 and 2005:

- In 1997, 18 human infections were reported in association with a H5N1 avian influenza virus outbreak in poultry in Hong Kong. The symptoms included fever, sore throat and cough and, in some cases, severe respiratory distress and viral pneumonia. Eighteen people were hospitalized and 6 died.
- In 1999, avian influenza (H9N2) was confirmed in 2 children in Hong Kong. The illnesses were mild and both children recovered. No other cases were found. Six unrelated H9N2 infections were also reported from mainland China in 1998-99; all 6 people recovered.
- In 2002, antibodies to an avian H7N2 virus were found in 1 person after an outbreak in poultry in Virginia.
- In 2003, 2 avian influenza H5N1 infections were reported in a Hong Kong family that had traveled to China. One of the 2 people died. Another family member died of a respiratory illness while in China, but no testing was done.
- In 2003, a H9N2 avian influenza virus infection was confirmed in a child in Hong Kong. The child was hospitalized but recovered.
- Cases of conjunctivitis have been reported after contact with H7N7 avian viruses in infected seals.
- In 2003, a H7N2 infection with respiratory signs was reported in a patient in New York. The person, who had serious underlying medical conditions, was hospitalized but recovered.
- In 2003, 347 total and 89 confirmed human infections were associated with an outbreak of avian H7N7 influenza virus in poultry in the Netherlands. Most cases occurred in poultry workers, but 3 family members also became ill. In 78 of the confirmed cases, conjunctivitis was the only sign of infection. Two people had influenza symptoms such as fever, coughing and muscle aches. Five had both conjunctivitis and influenza-like illnesses. (Four cases were classified as "other.") A single death occurred in an otherwise healthy veterinarian who developed acute respiratory distress syndrome and other complications. His initial symptoms included a persistent high fever and headache but no signs of respiratory disease. The virus isolated from the fatal case had accumulated a significant number of mutations, while viruses from most of the other individuals had not.
- In 2004, 2 cases of conjunctivitis and flu-like symptoms were confirmed in poultry workers in Canada. Both people recovered after treatment with an antiviral drug. Ten other infections were suspected but not confirmed; these cases included both conjunctivitis and upper respiratory symptoms. All of the infections were associated with a H7N3 virus outbreak in poultry.
- In 2004 and 2005, human illness and deaths were associated with widespread outbreaks of avian influenza (H5N1) among poultry in Asia. By October 2005, 118 confirmed human

cases and 61 human deaths from avian influenza had been reported to the World Health Organization (WHO).

The control of epidemics in poultry decreases the risk of exposure for humans. People working with infected birds should follow good hygiene practices and wear protective clothing, including boots, coveralls, gloves, face masks and headgear. In addition, the WHO recommends prophylaxis with antiviral drugs in people who cull birds infected with H5N1 HPAI viruses. To prevent reassortment between human and avian influenza viruses, people in contact with infected birds should be vaccinated against human influenza. They are also discouraged from having contact with sick birds while suffering flu symptoms.

Swine influenza virus infections in humans

Infections with swine influenza viruses have been reported sporadically in humans in the U.S., Europe and New Zealand. Recent serologic evidence suggests that swine influenza infections may occur regularly in people who have contact with pigs; however, relatively few infections have been documented. Person-to-person transmission with this virus appears to be limited and uncommon. One college student transmitted the virus to his roommate, who remained asymptomatic. Limited person-to-person transmission was also reported in 1976, when approximately 500 military recruits in Fort Dix, New Jersey were infected with a swine influenza virus. Although this virus spread to a limited extent on the base, which contained approximately 12,000 people, it did not spread to the surrounding community.

It is not known whether the symptoms of a zoonotic swine influenza virus infection differ significantly from human influenza. Most humans infected with the swine influenza viruses have had mild disease or been asymptomatic, but three deaths were reported: one in a young boy who was immunosuppressed, one in a military recruit and one in a pregnant woman who developed pneumonia. Swine influenza virus infections in humans may be underreported if they resemble human influenza.

Reported cases of influenza caused by swine influenza viruses include the following:

- A self-limiting illness with flu symptoms was reported in a college student. There was evidence that his roommate had been infected but remained asymptomatic.
- An infection with flu symptoms including diarrhea was reported in a young boy, who recovered. There was no evidence of spread to his family.
- Swine influenza virus was isolated from an immunocompromised child with pneumonia who died. Serologic evidence of possible infection was found in five contacts, but the infection did not spread further.
- A localized outbreak was reported at Fort Dix, New Jersey. A swine influenza virus was isolated from five recruits with respiratory disease, including one who died of pneumonia. Approximately 500 people were seropositive.

Equine influenza virus infections in humans

Antibodies to the equine H3N8 viruses have been reported in humans, but there are no reported cases of natural human disease. Volunteers inoculated with an equine virus became ill, and virus could be isolated for up to 10 days.

For more information

Animal Health Australia. The National Animal Health Information System (NAHIS)
http://www.aahc.com.au/nahis/disease/dislist.asp
Centers for Disease Control and Prevention (CDC)
http://www.cdc.gov/flu/
Material Safety Data Sheets – Canadian Laboratory Center for Disease Control
http://www.phac-aspc.gc.ca/msds-ftss/index.html
Medical Microbiology
http://www.gsbs.utmb.edu/microbook

OIE Manual of Diagnostic Tests and Vaccines for Terrestrial Animals
http://www.oie.int/eng/normes/mmanual/a_summry.htm
Prevention and Control of Influenza. Recommendations of the Advisory Committee on Immunization Practices
http://www.cdc.gov/mmwr/preview/mmwrhtml/rr5306a1.htm
The Merck Manual
http://www.merck.com/pubs/mmanual/
The Merck Veterinary Manual
http://www.merckvetmanual.com/mvm/index.jsp
USAHA Foreign Animal Diseases Book
http://www.vet.uga.edu/vpp/gray_book/FAD/
World Organization for Animal Health (OIE)
http://www.oie.int/

References

Abbott, A. Human fatality adds fresh impetus to fight against bird flu. *Nature* 2003;423:5.

Acha, P.N., Szyfres, B. (Pan American Health Organization [PAHO]). *Zoonoses and communicable diseases common to man and animals*. Volume 2. Chlamydiosis, rickettsioses and viroses. 3rd ed. Washington DC: PAHO; 2003. Scientific and Technical Publication No. 580. Influenza; p. 155-172.

Aiello, S.E., Mays, A., editors. *The Merck Veterinary Manual*. 8th ed. Whitehouse Station, NJ: Merck and Co; 1998. Equine influenza; p. 1084-1085.

Aiello, S.E., Mays, A., editors. *The Merck Veterinary Manual*. 8th ed. Whitehouse Station, NJ: Merck and Co; 1998. Ferrets: Influenza; p. 1332.

Aiello, S.E., Mays, A., editors. *The Merck Veterinary Manual*. 8th ed. Whitehouse Station, NJ: Merck and Co; 1998. Influenza (Fowl plague); p. 1983.

Aiello, S.E., Mays, A., editors. *The Merck Veterinary Manual*. 8th ed. Whitehouse Station, NJ: Merck and Co; 1998. Marine mammals: Influenza virus; p. 1359-1360.

Aiello, S.E., Mays, A., editors. *The Merck Veterinary Manual*. 8th ed. Whitehouse Station, NJ: Merck and Co; 1998. Swine influenza; p. 1106-1107.

Alexander, D.Y. A review of avian influenza [monograph online]. Available at: http://www.esvv.unizh.ch/gent_abstracts/Alexander.html. Accessed 30 Aug 2004.

American Veterinary Medical Association. Canine influenza virus emerges in Florida [online]. J Am Vet Med Assoc News Express. Sept. 22, 2005. Available at: http://www.avma.org/onlnews/javma/oct05/ x051015b.asp. Accessed 27 Sept 2005.

Beard, C.W. Avian influenza. In: *Foreign Animal Diseases*. Richmond, VA: United States Animal Health Association; 1998. p. 71-80.

Brown, I.H. (OIE/FAO/EU International Reference Laboratory for Avian Influenza). Influenza virus infections of pigs. Part 1: swine, avian & human influenza viruses [monograph online]. Available at: http://www.pighealth.com/influenza. htm. Accessed 23 Aug 2004.

Brown, I.H., Harris, P.A., Alexander, D.J. Serological studies of influenza viruses in pigs in Great Britain 1991-2 [abstract]. *Epidemiol Infect* 1995;114:511-520.

Canadian Laboratory Centre for Disease Control. Material Safety Data Sheet – Influenza virus [online]. Office of Laboratory Security; 2001 Sept. Available at: http://www.hc-sc.gc. ca/pphb-dgspsp/msds-ftss/index.html#menu. Accessed 24 Aug June 2004.

Capua, I., Marangon, S. Vaccination policy applied to the control of avian influenza in Italy. In Brown, F., Roth J.A. editors. *Vaccines for OIE List A and Emerging Animal Diseases*. Dev Biol. Basel, Karger 2003;114:213-219.

Carey, S. UF researchers: equine influenza virus likely cause of Jacksonville greyhound deaths [online]. News Releases, University of Florida College of Veterinary Medicine. Available at: http://www.vetmed.ufl.edu/pr/nw_story/greyhds.htm. Accessed 27 Sept 2005.

Centers for Disease Control and Prevention [CDC]. Avian flu [online]. CDC. Available at: http://www.cdc.gov/flu/avian/index.htm. Accessed 24 Aug 2004

Centers for Disease Control and Prevention [CDC]. Influenza. Information for health care professionals [online]. CDC; 2004. Available at: http://www.cdc.gov/fl u/professionals/background.htm. Accessed 24 Aug 2004.

Centers for Disease Control and Prevention [CDC]. Update on avian influenza A (H5N1) [online]. CDC; 2004 Aug. Available at: http://www.cdc.gov/fl u/avian/ professional/han081304.htm. Accessed 24 Aug 2004.

Chen, H., Deng, G., Li, Z., Tian, G., Li, Y., Jiao, P., Zhang, L., Liu, Z., Webster, R.G., Yu, K. The evolution of H5N1 influenza viruses in ducks in southern China. *Proc Natl Acad Sci USA* 2004;101:10452-10457.

Cornell University College of Veterinary Medicine. Canine influenza virus detected [online]. Animal Health Diagnostic Center announcements. Sept 21, 2005. Available at http://www.diaglab.vet.cornell.edu/news.asp. Accessed 27 Sept 2005.

Cornell University College of Veterinary Medicine. Samples for detecting the presence of canine influenza virus [online]. Animal Health Diagnostic Center announcements. Sept 21, 2005. Available at: http://www.diaglab.vet.cornell.edu/news.asp. Accessed 27 Sept 2005.

Couch, R.B. Orthomyxoviruses [monograph online]. In Baron S, editor. *Medical Microbiology*. 4th ed. New York: Churchill Livingstone; 1996. Available at: http://www.gsbs.utmb.edu/microbook/. Accessed 23 Aug 2004.

Crawford, P.C., Dubovi, E.J., Castleman, W.L., Stephenson, I., Gibbs, E.P.J., Chen, L., Smith, C., Hill, R.C., Ferro, P., Pompey, J., Bright, R.A., Medina, M-J., Johnson, C.M., Olsen, C.W., Cox, N.J., Klimov, A.I., Katz, J.M., Donis, R.O. Transmission of equine influenza virus to dogs. *Science* 2005 Sep 26; [Epub ahead of print]. Available at: http://www.sciencemag.org/cgi/rapidpdf/ 1117950v1. Accessed 27 Sept 2005.

Dacso, C.C., Couch, R.B., Six, H.R., Young. J.F., Quarles, J.M., Kasel, J.A. Sporadic occurrence of zoonotic swine influenza virus infections. *J Clin Microbiol*.1984;20:833-5.

Daly, J.M., Mumford, J.A. Influenza infections [online]. In: Lekeux, P., editor. *Equine respiratory diseases*. Ithaca NY: International Veterinary Information Service [IVIS]; 2001. Available at: http://www.ivis.org/special_books/Lekeux/toc.asp. Accessed 10 May 2004.

Enserink, M., Kaiser, J. Avian flu finds new mammal hosts. *Science* 2004;305:1385.

Enserink, M. Flu virus jumps from Horses to Dogs [monograph online]. *Science Now*. 26 September 2005. Available at: http://sciencenow.sciencemag.org/ cgi/content/full/2005/926/2. Accessed 27 Sept 2005.

Fenner, F., Bachmann, P.A., Gibbs, E.P.J., Murphy, F.A., Studdert, M.J., White, D.O. *Veterinary virology*. San Diego, CA: Academic Press Inc.; 1987.Orthomyxoviridae; p. 473-484.

Fouchier, R.A.M., Schneeberger, P.M., Rozendaal, F.W., Broekman, J.M., Kemink, S.A.G., Munster, V., Kuiken, T., Rimmelzwaan, G.F., Schutten, M., van Doornum, G.J.J., Koch, G., Bosman, A., Koopmans, M., Osterhaus, A.D.M.E. Avian influenza A virus (H7N7) associated with human conjunctivitis and a fatal case of acute respiratory distress syndrome. *Proc Natl Acad Sci USA*. 2004;101:1356–1361.

Greenbaum, E., Morag, A., Zakay-Rones, Z. Isolation of influenza C virus during an outbreak of influenza A and B viruses. *J Clin Microbiol* 1998;36:1441-1442.

Hanson, B.A., Stallknecht, D.E., Swayne, D.E., Lewis, L.A., Senne, D.A. Avian influenza viruses in Minnesota ducks during 1998–2000. *Avian Dis* 2003;47(3 Suppl):867-71.

Harper, S.A., Fukuda, K., Uyeki, T.M., Cox, N.J., Bridges, C.B. Prevention and control of influenza. Recommendations of the Advisory Committee on Immunization Practices (ACIP) *Morb Mortal Wkly Rep*. 2004;53(RR-6):1-40. Available at: http://www.cdc. gov/mmwr/preview/mmwrhtml/rr5306a1.htm. Accessed 25 Aug 2004.

Heinen, P. Swine influenza: a zoonosis. Vet Sci Tomorrow [serial online]. 2003 Sept 15. Available at: http://www.vetsite.org/publish/articles/000041/print.html. Accessed 26 Aug 2004.

Hinshaw, V.S., Bean, W.J., Webster, R.G., Rehg, J.E., Fiorelli, P., Early, G., Geraci, J.R., St Aubin, D.J. Are seals frequently infected with avian influenza viruses? *J Virol*. 1984;51(3):863-865.

International Committee on Taxonomy of Viruses [ICTV]. Universal Virus Database, version 3. 00.046. Orthomyxoviridae [online]. ICTV; 2003. Available at: http://www.ncbi.nlm.nih.gov/ICTVdb/ICTVdB. Accessed 25 Aug 2004.

Jakeman, K.J., Tisdale, M, Russell, S., Leone, A., Sweet C. Efficacy of 2'-deoxy-2'-fluororibosides against influenza A and B viruses in ferrets. *Antimicrob Agents Chemother*. 1994;38:1864-1867.

Janke, B.H. Relative Prevalence of Reassortants and Subtypes. Twelfth Annual Swine Disease Conference for Swine Practitioners. College of Veterinary Medicine, Iowa State University, Ames, Iowa. Nov. 11-12, 2004.

Karasin, A.I., Schutten, M.M., Cooper, L.A., Smith, C.B., Subbarao, K., Anderson, G.A., Carman, S., Olsen, C.W. Genetic characterization of H3N2 influenza viruses isolated from pigs in North America, 1977-1999: evidence for wholly human and reassortant virus genotypes. *Virus Res.* 2000;68:71-85.

Kimura, H., Abiko, C, Peng, G., Muraki,Y., Sugawara, K., Hongo, S., Kitame, F., Mizuta, K., Numazaki, Y., Suzuki, H., Nakamura, K. Interspecies transmission of influenza C virus between humans and pigs. *Virus Res.* 1997;48:71-79.

Kuiken, T., Rimmelzwaan, G., van Riel, D., van Amerongen, G., Baars, M., Fouchier, R., Osterhaus, A. Avian H5N1 influenza in cats. *Science* [serial online]. 2004; 10.1126/science.1102287. Available at: http://www.sciencemag.org/cgi/rapidpdf/1102287v1.pdf. Accessed 3 Sept 2004.

Lamb, S., McElroy, T. Bronson alerts public to newly emerging canine flu. Florida Department of Agriculture and Consumer Services, Department Press Release. Sept. 20, 2005. Available at: http://doacs.state.fl .us/ press/2005/09202005.html. Accessed 27 Sept 2005.

Lu, H., Castro, A.E., Pennick, K., Liu, J., Yang, Q., Dunn, P., Weinstock, D., Henzler, D. Survival of avian influenza virus H7N2 in SPF chickens and their environments. *Avian Dis* 2003;47(3 Suppl):1015-1021.

Manuguerra, J.C., Hannoun, C., Simon, F., Villar, E,, Cabezas, J.A. Natural infection of dogs by influenza C virus: a serological survey in Spain [abstract]. *New Microbiol* 1993;16:367-371.

Matsuzaki, Y., Mizuta, K., Sugawara, K., Tsuchiya, E., Muraki, Y., Hongo, S., Suzuki, H., Nishimura, H.. Frequent reassortment among influenza C viruses. *J. Virol* 2003;77: 871–881.

Matsuzaki, Y., Sugawara, K., Mizuta, K., Tsuchiya, E., Muraki, Y., Hongo,S., Suzuki, H., Nakamura, K.. Antigenic and genetic characterization of influenza C viruses which caused two outbreaks in Yamagata City, Japan, in 1996 and 1998. *J Clin Microbiol* 2002;40:422-429.

Michigan Department of Agriculture, Animal Industry Division. Ferret health advisory sheet. 2 p. Available at: http://www.michigan.gov/documents/MDA_FerretHealthAdvisorySheet_31881_7.pdf. Accessed 20 Aug 2004.

Myers, K.P., Olsen, C,W,, Setterquist, S.F., Capuano, A.W., Donham, K.J., Thacker, E.L., Merchant, J.A., Gray, G.C. Are swine workers in the United States at increased risk of infection with zoonotic influenza virus? *Clin Inf Dis* 2006:42:14-21.

National Institute of Allergy and Infectious Diseases [NIAID], National Institutes of Health [NIH]. Flu drugs [online]. NIAID, NIH; 2003 Feb. Available at: http://www.niaid.nih. gov/factsheets/fludrugs.htm. Accessed 30 Aug 2004.

Office International des Epizooties [OIE]. *Manual of Diagnostic Tests and Vaccines for Terrestrial Animals.* OIE; 2004. Highly pathogenic avian influenza. Available at: http://www.oie.int/eng/normes/ mmanual/A_summry.htm. Accessed 23 Aug 2004.

Office International des Epizooties [OIE]. *Manual of Diagnostic Tests and Vaccines for Terrestrial Animals.* OIE; 2004. Swine influenza. Available at: http://www.oie.int/eng/normes/ mmanual/A_summry.htm. Accessed 23 Aug 2004.

Olsen, C.W., Brammer, L., Easterday, B.C., Arden, N., Belay, E., Baker, I., Cox, N.J. Serologic evidence of H1 swine influenza virus infection in swine farm residents and employees. *Emerg Infect Dis* 2002;8:814-9.

Panigrahy, B., Senne, D.A., Pedersen, J.C. Avian influenza virus subtypes inside and outside the live bird markets, 1993-2000: a spatial and temporal relationship. *Avian Dis* 2002;46:298-307.

Patriarca, P.A., Kendal, A.P., Zakowski, P.C., Cox, N.J., Trautman, M.S., Cherry, J.D., Auerbach, D.M., McCusker, J., Belliveau, R.R., Kappus, K.D. Lack of significant person- to-person spread of swine influenza-like virus following fatal infection in an immunocompromised child. *Am J Epidemiol* 1984;119:152-158.

Promed Mail. Influenza, canine-USA (multistate). October 2, 2005. Archive Number 20051002.2883. Available at http://www. promedmail.org. Accessed 3 Oct 2005.

Randolph, R.W. Medical and surgical care of the pet ferret: Influenza. In: Kirk RW, editor. *Current Veterinary Therapy X.* Philadelphia: WB Saunders; 1989. p. 775.

Reid, A.H., Taubenberger, J.K. The origin of the 1918 pandemic influenza virus: a continuing enigma. *J Gen Virol* 2003;84:2285-2292.

Sweet, C., Smith, H.. Pathogenicity of influenza virus. *Microbiol Rev.* 1980:44; 303-330.

Taubenberger, J.K., Reid, A.H., Lourens, R.M., Wang, R., Jin, G., Fanning, T.G. Characterization of the 1918 influenza virus polymerase genes. *Nature* 2005 Oct 6;437(7060):889-893.

U.S. Department of Agriculture, Animal and Plant Health Inspection Service, Veterinary Services [USDA APHIS, VS]. Highly pathogenic avian influenza. A threat to U.S. poultry [online]. USDA APHIS, VS; 2002 Feb. Available at: http://www.aphis. usda.gov/oa/pubs/avianflu.html. Accessed 30 Aug 2004.

World Health Organization [WHO]. Avian influenza fact sheet; 2004 Jan. Available at: http://www.who. int/csr/don/2004_ 01_15/en/. Accessed 30 Aug 2004.

World Health Organization. Cumulative number of confirmed human cases of avian influenza A/(H5N1) reported to WHO. Available at: http://www.who.int/csr/disease/avi- an_influenza/country/cases_table_2005_10_20_/en/index. html. Accessed 20-October- 2005.

Yamaoka, M., Hotta, H., Itoh, M., Homma, M. Prevalence of antibody to influenza C virus among pigs in Hyogo Prefecture, Japan. *J Gen Virol* 1991;72:711-4.

Ixodes ricinus

European Castor Bean Tick, Castor Bean Tick, Sheep Tick

Importance

Ixodes ricinus is a hard tick that infests livestock, deer, dogs, and a wide variety of other species including humans. This tick has long mouthparts that can make its bites painful and annoying; the bites can also become secondarily infected by bacteria. Feeding by large numbers of ticks may result in anemia. *I. ricinus* can also transmit numerous diseases including babesiosis (*Babesia divergens* and *Babesia bovis* infections), louping ill, tick–borne encephalitis, rickettsial tick borne fever of sheep, Lyme disease, Crimean–Congo hemorrhagic fever, and Bukhovinian hemorrhagic fever. It can also spread *Anaplasma marginale*, *Coxiella burnetii*, and *Ehrlichia phagocytophila*.

Species affected

Adult *I. ricinus* feed on large mammals such as cattle, sheep, and deer. The larvae of this species feed on small reptiles, mammals, and birds and the nymphs parasitize small and medium–sized vertebrates. In endemic areas, dogs and cats can be infested.

Geographic distribution

I. ricinus can be found in cool, relatively humid, shrubby or wooded pastures, gardens, floodplains, and forests. This tick is endemic in most of Europe, parts of Asia, and North Africa.

Life cycle

I. ricinus is a 3–host tick. The larvae feed on small reptiles, mammals, and birds and the nymphs parasitize small and medium–sized vertebrates. The adult ticks feed only on large mammals, including cattle, sheep, and deer. *I. ricinus* ticks are often found around the mouth, ears, and eyelids of sheep, dogs, and cats, and around the udder and axillary region of cattle.

The life cycle of *I. ricinus* usually takes 2 to 4 years to complete. This tick can only survive in areas with high humidity and is not usually active in the summer. Ticks that do not feed in the spring do not usually survive the summer.

Identification

I. ricinus is a member of the family Ixodidae (hard ticks). Hard ticks have a dorsal shield (scutum) and their mouthparts (capitulum) protrude forward when they are seen from above. *Ixodes* ticks have long mouthparts but no eyes. They are inornate and have no festoons. The anal groove is distinct and surrounds the anus anteriorly. *Ixodes* are sexually dimorphic: the stigmatic (spiracular) plates are oval in males, but circular in females. The ventral surface of the male has seven non–projecting, armor like plates.

Adult *I. ricinus* are red–brown; however, the female ticks are light gray when engorged. Before feeding, the males are approximately 2.5–3 mm long and the females 3–4 mm long. When they are engorged, the females can be as long as 1 centimeter. In this species, a spur is found on the posterior internal angle of the coxa of the first pair of legs; this spur overlaps the coxa of the second pair of legs. The tarsi are moderately long and tapering.

Recommended actions if *Ixodes ricinus* is suspected
Notification of authorities

Known or suspected *I. ricinus* infestations should be reported immediately to state or federal authorities.

Federal: Area Veterinarians in Charge (AVICs):
http://www.aphis.usda.gov/vs/area_offices.htm
State Veterinarians:
http://www.aphis.usda.gov/vs/sregs/official.html

Control measures

Acaricides can eliminate these ticks from the animal, but do not prevent reinfestation. Three–host ticks spend at least 90% of their life cycle in the environment rather than on the host animal; ticks must be controlled in the environment to prevent their spread.

Public health

All stages of *I. ricinus* will feed on humans, and their bite can be painful. This tick can also transmit several diseases that affect humans, including Crimean–Congo hemorrhagic fever and Lyme disease.

For more information

World Organization for Animal Health (OIE)
http://www.oie.int

OIE International Animal Health Code
http://www.oie.int/eng/normes/mcode/A_summry.htm

USAHA Foreign Animal Diseases Book
http://www.vet.uga.edu/vpp/gray_book/FAD/

Identification of the Paralysis Tick *I. holocyclus* and Related Ticks
http://members.ozemail.com.au/~norbertf/identification.htm

Hard Ticks (photographs) from the University of Edinburgh
http://www.nhc.ed.ac.uk/collections/ticks/hard.htm#Amblyomma

References

"Disease Information." 2001 Merial. 3 December 2001. http//nz.merial.com/farmers/sheep/disease/haema.html.

"Identification of the Paralysis Tick *I. holocyclus* and Related Ticks." February 2001 New South Wales Department of Agriculture. 29 November 2001. http//members.ozemail.com.au/~norbertf/identification.htm.

"*Ixodes.*" In *Veterinary Entomology: Arthropod Ectoparasites of Veterinary Importance*. Edited by R. Wall and D. Shearer. London: Chapman & Hall, 1997, pp. 117–120.

"*Ixodes* spp." In *The Merck Veterinary Manual*, 8th ed. Edited by S.E. Aiello and A. Mays. Whitehouse Station, NJ: Merck and Co., 1998, pp. 679–680.

Wilson, D.D. and R.A. Bram. "Foreign Pests and Vectors of Arthropod–Borne Diseases." In *Foreign Animal Diseases*. Richmond, VA: United States Animal Health Association, 1998, pp. 225–239.

Japanese Encephalitis

Japanese B Encephalitis,
Arbovirus B, Mosquito-borne Encephalitis Virus

Importance

Japanese encephalitis is a mosquito–borne viral infection of horses, pigs, and humans. In countries where it is endemic, the virus causes reproductive failure (stillbirth, mummification, embryonic death, and infertility) in pigs and encephalitis in horses. Japanese encephalitis is a significant zoonosis: in humans, it can result in a serious and potentially fatal encephalitis. In 1924, an epidemic in Japan was responsible for 4,000 deaths. The likelihood that this disease could become endemic in the United States, if introduced, is unknown.

Etiology

Japanese encephalitis is caused by infection with a mosquito–borne *flavivirus*, the Japanese encephalitis virus (family Flaviviridae, genus *Flavivirus*). Two subtypes of the virus exist, Nakayama and JaGar–01. The Japanese encephalitis virus is related to the St. Louis encephalitis virus, Murray Valley virus, and West Nile virus.

Species affected

The Japanese encephalitis virus can infect horses, pigs, humans, cattle, bats, reptiles, and various species of birds. Under experimental conditions, *Culex tritaeniorhynchus* can transmit the virus between horses; under natural conditions, humans and horses appear to be dead–end hosts. Cattle are often infected in endemic regions, but do not become ill or develop viremia. Swine develop clinical signs and also amplify the virus.

Geographic distribution

Japanese encephalitis virus infections can be found throughout the temperate and tropical regions of Asia. The first human cases were found in Japan in the late 1800s. Vaccination and the use of agricultural pesticides have made Japanese encephalitis rare in Japan; however, a growing number of cases have been seen in horses and humans in China, India, Nepal, the Philippines, Sri Lanka, and northern Thailand. Human infections are occasionally found in Indonesia and northern Australia.

Transmission

The Japanese encephalitis virus can be transmitted by mosquitoes in the genera *Culex* and *Aedes*. The most important vectors are *Culex tritaeniorhynchus*, *C. annulus*, *C. fuscocephala*, *C. gelidus*, and mosquitoes in the *C. vishnui* complex. Birds may help to spread the infection to mammals; in Japan, herons and egrets help to maintain the virus cycle in nature. Swine can amplify the virus.

In temperate regions of Asia, a yearly cycle of infection is seen: mosquitoes appear in late spring, horses and swine become infected in late summer, and human cases peak during August and September. How the virus survives during the winter is unknown. It may be maintained in mosquitoes, either by transovarial passage or during hibernation. Bats might also be able to carry the virus for long periods of time.

Incubation period

The incubation period in horses is 8 to 10 days. The incubation period in pregnant swine is uncertain; however, exposure early in gestation seems to increase the chance that the litter will be affected.

Clinical signs

In horses, most infections are subclinical. Horses with clinical signs resemble animals with Western equine encephalomyelitis or Eastern equine encephalomyelitis, but the mortality rate is relatively low. The symptoms may include a fever, impaired locomotion, stupor, and teeth grinding. Blindness, coma, and death are possible. In some cases, the only symptoms may be a fever and short period of lethargy.

The most common symptom of Japanese encephalitis in pigs is the birth of stillborn or mummified fetuses, usually at term. Piglets born alive often have tremors and convulsions and die soon after birth.

Post mortem lesions

Only nonspecific post–mortem lesions are seen in horses, similar to the signs in animals that die from Eastern or Western equine encephalomyelitis.

The fetuses from infected sow are often stillborn or mummified. Hydrocephalus, cerebellar hypoplasia, and spinal hypomyelinogenesis may be seen.

Morbidity and mortality

Inapparent infections are common in horses; mortality in this species is approximately 5% or less. The mortality rate is high in piglets born to infected sows, but close to zero in adult pigs.

Vaccines are available for swine in Japan and Taiwan and are expected to provide good immunity.

Diagnosis

Clinical

Japanese encephalitis should be suspected in horses with fever and the symptoms of a central nervous system (CNS) disease. The principal sign in pigs is the birth of a litter with a large number of stillborn or weak piglets. In temperate regions, the disease is most common in the late summer and early autumn.

Differential diagnosis

In horses, the different diagnosis includes toxic encephalopathies and viral encephalitides such as rabies, West Nile, Eastern, Western, and Venezuelan equine encephalitis, and Murray Valley encephalitis.

In pigs, other causes of reproductive failure or encephalitis in newborns such as PRRS virus, porcine parvovirus, pseudorabies virus should be ruled out. Nipah resembles Japanese encephalitis in humans but, unlike Japanese encephalitis, this disease also affects adult pigs.

Laboratory tests

Japanese encephalitis can be diagnosed by virus isolation. The virus is isolated from blood, spinal cord samples, or portions of the corpus striatum, cortex, or thalamus of the brain. Samples are inoculated into 2 to 4 day old mice and the virus is identified by hemagglutination inhibition. Japanese encephalitis virus may also be identified by infection of cell cultures (chicken embryo or hamster kidney cells, or the mosquito cell line C3/36). Virus isolation from sick or dead horses is often unsuccessful.

Serology may also aid in diagnosis. A significant rise in titer should be seen with paired samples from the acute and convalescent stages. Serologic tests include the plaque reduction virus neutralization test, hemagglutination inhibition, and complement fixation. In horses, specific IgM and IgG antibodies can also be detected in the cerebrospinal fluid with enzyme immunoassays and are good evidence of infection.

Samples to collect

Before collecting or sending any samples from animals with a suspected foreign animal disease, the proper authorities should be contacted. Samples should only be sent under secure conditions and to authorized laboratories to prevent the spread of the disease. Biocontainment conditions are required for all potentially infectious material from a Japanese encephalitis case. Human encephalitis has been seen after infection through a scratch.

Brains should be submitted from animals with encephalitis; half should be fixed in 10% formalin and the other half unfixed. Paired serum samples should be taken at least 14 days apart for serology. In horses, cerebrospinal fluid should be submitted for virus–specific IgM and IgG. All samples must be kept cool. Samples to be saved for later virus isolation should be frozen to –80°C.

Recommended actions if Japanese encephalitis is suspected

Notification of authorities

Japanese encephalitis must be reported to state or federal authorities immediately upon diagnosis or suspicion of the disease.

Federal: Area Veterinarians in Charge (AVICs):
http://www.aphis.usda.gov/vs/area_offices.htm
State Veterinarians:
http://www.aphis.usda.gov/vs/sregs/official.html

Quarantine and disinfection

Biosafety level 3 practices are recommended for investigators working with this virus. Japanese encephalitis virus is inactivated by 70% ethanol, 2% glutaraldehyde, 3–8 % formaldehyde, 1% sodium hypochlorite, iodine, phenol iodophors, and organic solvents/detergents. It is also sensitive to heat, ultraviolet light, and gamma irradiation.

Public health

In humans, Japanese encephalitis virus infections range from a febrile headache syndrome to an acute and possibly fatal encephalitis. The infection is usually more severe in infants and the elderly. Mortality is 5% to 40%. Parkinsonism, convulsive disorders, paralysis, neuropsychiatric sequelae, or mental retardation are seen after 45% to 70% of severe cases.

For more information

World Organization for Animal Health (OIE)
http://www.oie.int
OIE Manual of Standards
http://www.oie.int/eng/normes/mmanual/a_summry.htm
OIE International Animal Health Code
http://www.oie.int/eng/normes/mcode/A_summry.htm
USAHA Foreign Animal Diseases Book
http://www.vet.uga.edu/vpp/gray_book/FAD/
Material Safety Data Sheet for Japanese Encephalitis Virus.
Canadian Laboratory Centre for Disease Control
http://www.phac-aspc.gc.ca/msds-ftss/index.html

References

"Japanese Encephalitis." In *Manual of Standards for Diagnostic Tests and Vaccines*. Paris: World Organization for Animal Health, 2000, pp. 607–614.

"Material Safety Data Sheet–Japanese Encephalitis." March 2001. Canadian Laboratory Centre for Disease Control. 29 Aug 2001. http//www.phac-aspc.gc.ca/msds-ftss/index.html.

Shope, R.E. "Japanese Encephalitis." In *Foreign Animal Diseases*. Richmond, VA: United States Animal Health Association, 1998, pp. 283–291.

Uppal, PK. "Emergence of Nipah virus in Malaysia." *Ann. N. Y. Acad. Sci.*, 916 (2000):354–357

Leishmaniasis

Cutaneous leishmaniasis:
Chiclero ulcer, Buba, Espundia, Pain-bois, Uta, Oriental sore, Aleppo boil, Baghdad sore, Delhi sore, Other local names

Visceral leishmaniasis:
Kala-azar, Black fever, Dum-dum fever, Sikari disease, Burdwan fever, Shahib's disease, Febrile tropical splenomegaly, Infantile splenic fever

Importance

Leishmaniasis is zoonotic disease caused by the protozoans of the genus *Leishmania*. These parasites are most commonly transmitted by insect-vectors, sandflies, and can affect humans and some animal species. As reservoir hosts, dogs and a variety of wild animals can be an indirect source of infection for humans.

Leishmaniasis is typically classified by the clinical presentation and can involve a variety of cutaneous or visceral manifestations. Factors determining the form of disease include the leishmanial species involved, the sandfly species involved, the geographic location [Old World (Eastern Hemisphere) or New World (the Americas)], and the immune response of the host.

Among domestic animals, the disease occurs most often in dogs, but cats and horses can also be affected. Human leishmaniasis may manifest in either a cutaneous or visceral form. Unlike human disease, infected dogs usually have both visceral and cutaneous involvement. Rarely, ocular manifestations may occur. In dogs, diagnosis and treatment can be difficult, as leishmaniasis can mimic other diseases and relapses are common after treatment.

Etiology

Leishmaniasis results from infection by species and subspecies of *Leishmania*, a protozoan parasite of the family Trypanosomatidae (order Kinetoplastida). *Leishmania* are diphasic protozoa; cycling between the vertebrate host and sandfly vector in either the promastigote or amastigote form. Both stages are capable of replication.

There are over 30 species of *Leishmania;* at least 20 species and subspecies are pathogenic for mammals, including humans. The different species are morphologically indistinguishable, but can be differentiated by biochemical methods.

Some of the *Leishmania* species are grouped into "complexes" based on molecular, biochemical and immunological similarities. This evaluation has found *L. infantum* and *L. chagasi* to be genetically identical and are now regarded as the same species.

In humans, Old World cutaneous leishmaniasis is predominantly caused by *Leishmania tropica* complex. Causative agents for New World cutaneous leishmaniasis include the *L. mexicana* complex and the *L. braziliensis* complex. Visceral leishmaniasis is usually caused by *L. chagasi/L. infantum*, in the Americas (New World) and *L. donovani* or *L. chagasi/L. infantum* in the Eastern Hemisphere (Old World). Dogs are most commonly infected with *L. infantum*.

Species affected

Leishmaniasis usually affects canids (including dogs, foxes, and jackals), humans, some rodents, marsupials, sloths, anteaters, and hyraxes. Cats, horses and other Equidae, and non-human primates are occasionally infected.

Infected mammals, including humans, can serve as a reservoir host. Disease varies with the reservoir host, species of *Leishmania* involved and the geographic region. The reservoirs may include dogs and wild canids, wild rodents, marsupials (opossum), sloths, anteaters and humans.

Geographic distribution

Infections in animals are often, but not always, seen in similar geographic regions to human leishmaniasis. Most affected countries are in the tropic and subtropics. Leishmaniasis are spread in large parts of Central and South America, Africa, Asia and the Mediterranean. More than 90% of the world's visceral leishmaniasis cases are in India, Bangladesh, Nepal, Sudan and Brazil. More than 90% of the cutaneous leishmaniasis cases have been reported from Brazil and Peru (New World) and from some Middle Eastern countries (Old World).

Disease from *Leishmania* species are sometimes classified by the location they are found; Old World leishmaniasis most commonly occur in countries of the Eastern Hemisphere, while New World leishmaniasis primarily occur in the Americas. This is principally due to the presence of the specific sandfly vector and reservoirs needed for the propagation of the parasite. Old World leishmaniasis is transmitted by *Phlebotomus* sandflies, while New World leishmaniasis is spread by sandflies from the genus *Lutzomyia*.

Endemic canine, but not human, leishmaniasis has been reported from parts of the United States. In 2000, leishmaniasis was diagnosed in and found to be established in a northeastern U.S. foxhound kennel; cases have been reported in a variety of other states, including Oklahoma, Ohio, Texas, Michigan, New York and Alabama.

Transmission

Leishmaniasis parasites are usually transmitted indirectly between hosts by Phlebotomidae sandflies of the genera *Phlebotomus* and *Lutzomyia*. The sandflies, which are biological vectors, have a flight range of a few kilometers and are usually most active at dawn and dusk. The disease is seasonal, and cases fluctuate with changes in the vector populations. Female sandflies are bloodsuckers and while feeding on an infected reservoir host, will suck up free *Leishmania* amastigotes or parasitized host cells. The parasite then transforms, in the midgut of the sandfly, to a promastigote, which multiplies rapidly (binary fission). When the sandfly feeds again, the promastigotes are injected into the new host.

Horizontal transmission can occur between dogs, presumably by bites, but appears to be rare.

Incubation period

The incubation period in dogs can vary from 3 months to several years. Incubation periods up to 7 years have been reported.

Clinical signs

Dogs

The symptoms of leishmaniasis in dogs are variable and can mimic other infections. Chronic systemic disease usually develops however, asymptomatic infections also occur. In dogs, both visceral and cutaneous manifestations may be found simultaneously; unlike humans, separate cutaneous and visceral syndromes are not seen. Any dog with cutaneous lesions should be presumed to have visceral involvement, since the parasites are usually disseminated throughout the body before the skin lesions develop.

The most common visceral signs seen are anorexia, weight loss, decreased exercise tolerance and muscle atrophy. Clinical signs may also include intermittent fever, anemia, local or generalized lymphadenopathy, and splenomegaly. Less commonly diarrhea, vomiting, melena, renal or liver failure, epistaxis, polyuria-polydipsia, sneezing, lameness (due to polyarthritis or myositis), ascites, and chronic colitis may occur.

Almost 90% of dogs with overt leishmaniasis will have cutaneous involvement. Signs most commonly seen include: non-pruritic exfoliative dermatitis, especially around the eyes, on the face, ears, or feet. These areas may also be alopecic with silvery white scales. Additional signs that may be noted include marked wasting of the temporal muscles, abnormally long and brittle nails, nasal or digital hyperkeratosis, or interdigital ulcers. In more advanced cases, cutaneous lesions can develop into pruritic nodules, ulcers, or scabs.

Ocular lesions are less commonly seen. The lesions are non-specific and may occur independently from systemic signs or can be seen after treatment. The most common ocular signs are blepharitis, conjunctivitis, keratitis, and anterior uveitis. Some animals may have mucocutaneous ulcers, nodules or pustular eruptions at the eyelid margins, keratoconjunctivitis, uveitis, or panopthalmitis.

Equidae

Horses, donkeys, and other Equids may develop nodules and occasionally scabs or ulcers, on or around the earflap.

Cats

Cats are rarely infected. In most infected cats, the lesions are limited to crusted cutaneous ulcers, usually found on the lips, nose, eyelids, or pinnae. Visceral lesions and signs are rare.

Rodents and other wild animals

Infections are often inapparent in rodents and other wild animal hosts; however, the *L. mexicana* complex may produce swellings, with hair loss or ulcers, at the base of the tail, ears or toes. The *L. braziliensis* complex can produce systemic infections in wild hosts, usually without skin lesions.

Post mortem lesions

The gross lesions are highly variable and may be minimal. Lesions may include cachexia, generalized lymphadenopathy, hepatosplenomegaly, areas of alopecia with desquamation on the head and trunk, and cutaneous ulcers or nodules. Ulcers and petechiae are occasionally seen on the mucous membranes. Small, light colored nodular foci (granulomas) may be found in a variety of organs, including the kidney, liver, and pancreas.

Morbidity and mortality

In dogs, infections vary from asymptomatic to symptomatic and may be fatal. More than 50% of all infected dogs are asymptomatic. These dogs may 1) progress towards overt disease, 2) remain asymptomatic for prolonged periods or life, or 3) heal spontaneously.

Diagnosis

Clinical

Recognition of leishmaniasis can be difficult. The clinical signs are variable and can mimic other diseases. Most dogs have a history of travel to an endemic area in the past 6 to 7 years.

Differential diagnosis

The differential diagnosis varies with the specific symptoms, and may include pemphigus foliaceous, demodicosis, zinc-responsive dermatosis, systemic lupus erythematosus, vasculitis, cutaneous lymphoma, necrolytic migratory erythema (hepatocutaneous), and sebaceotis adenitis.

Laboratory tests

In dogs, leishmaniasis is usually diagnosed by direct observation of the parasites, using Giemsa or proprietary quick stains, in smears, bone marrow aspirates, tissue biopsies, or skin scrapings from lesions. The *Leishmaniasis* amastigotes are round to oval parasites, with a round basophilic nucleus and a small rod-like kinetoplast. They are found in macrophages or freed from ruptured cells. Immunohistochemistry and polymerase chain reaction (PCR) techniques are also used.

Leishmania species can also be isolated by inoculation into hamsters or cultured in a variety of media including Novy-Mac-Neil-Nicole (NMN) medium, brain–heart infusion (BHI) medium, Evan's modified Tobie's medium (EMTM), or Schneider's *Drosophila* medium. Diagnosing leishmaniasis by culture requires 5 to 30 days, while animal inoculation can take weeks or months. The species, subspecies, and/or strain is identified by specialized techniques including isoenzyme analysis, immunofluorescence, immunoradiometric assays, immunohistochemistry, kinetoplast DNA restriction endonuclease analysis, or PCR.

Serology, including the indirect fluorescent antibody test, direct agglutination, enzyme-linked immunosorbent assay (ELISA), counterimmunoelectrophoresis, or immunoblotting may also be useful. Antibodies are not always found in animals that only have localized skin lesions. The delayed hypersensitivity test, which is used in humans, is not useful for dogs.

Samples to collect

In dogs, the parasites may be found in smears from lymph nodes or spleen, bone marrow aspirates, tissue biopsies, or skin scrapings from lesions. If isolation is attempted from the lymph nodes, multiple aspirates taken from different enlarged lymph nodes can increase the chance of a diagnosis. Organisms may also be found in ocular lesions, particularly in granulomas. Serum should be taken for serology.

Recommended actions if leishmaniasis is suspected

Notification of authorities

Leishmaniasis has been seen in some but not all states of the U.S. State authorities should be consulted for specific information on reporting requirements.

Quarantine and disinfection

Leishmaniasis is usually transmitted by the bite of sandflies. Insect repellents and insecticides can help prevent bites by sandflies. In endemic regions, susceptible animals should be kept indoors from an hour before sunset to an hour after dawn during the vector season. Horizontal transmission can occur between dogs but appears to be rare.

Leishmania species can be inactivated by 1% sodium hypochlorite, 2% glutaraldehyde, or formaldehyde. They are also susceptible to heat (50-60°C).

Vaccines are not available.

Public health

Leishmaniasis in humans manifests as either the cutaneous or visceral form, depending on the *Leishmania* species involved. Some texts also distinguish a mucocutaneous form. The incubation period can vary from 2 to 6 months, or in some cases be a long as years.

The parasite is most commonly spread by sandfly vectors, however, person-to-person transmission has been reported and may occur through vertical transmission, venereal transmission, or blood transfusion.

Cutaneous Leishmaniasis

Cutaneous leishmaniasis is most commonly caused by species of the *L. tropica* complex, *L. mexicana* complex and the *L. brazilensis* complex. The cutaneous form can affect the skin, mucous membranes, or both tissues. Initial lesions are pruritic, erythematous lesions, which develop into papules then into painless ulcers. Lesions may be single or multiple and vary in distribution from localized to diffuse. Some forms may spread via the lymphatics to other parts of the body and produce secondary lesions on the skin or mucosa. Lesions typically heal spontaneously within weeks or months, but can persist up to a year or longer. Some forms leave permanent scars. Atypical signs, with frequent relapses, are seen in AIDS patients.

In the mucocutaneous form caused by *L. braziliensis braziliensis* (espunda), the initial lesion is a papule, which develops into a painless ulcer. The ulcer seldom heals spontaneously; instead, it metastasizes to various mucocutaneous regions, including the nasal septum, mouth, nasopharynx, and sometimes the genitalia. This form rarely heals spontaneously, and mucocutaneous lesions in the nasopharynx can be fatal.

Visceral Leishmaniasis

Visceral leishmaniasis is usually caused by *L. chagasi/L. infantum*, and *L. donovani*. The visceral form may be acute or insidious in onset with a chronic course. The chronic form is typically seen in long-time residents of endemic regions. In some cases, a primary granuloma appears before the systemic signs. The typical clinical signs include a prolonged undulant fever, splenomegaly, hepatomegaly, and abdominal distension. Additional signs may include a cough, diarrhea, lymphadenopathy, secondary infections, anemia, edema, emaciation, darkening of the skin, and petechiae or hemorrhages on the mucous membranes. Visceral infections caused by *L. donovani* may be asymptomatic or mild.

Skin lesions can occur concurrently with the systemic signs or after treatment of Old World leishmaniasis; they are rarely seen in New World (the Americas) cases. Visceral leishmaniasis has a high mortality rate if left untreated. Some patients may recover spontaneously, however the percentage is unknown.

Treatment

In immunocompetent individuals, visceral or cutaneous leishmaniasis can usually be treated effectively with antimonial drugs. However, the visceral form is often resistant to treatment. In some countries, people may be vaccinated with a virulent strain of *L. major* (part of the *L. tropica* complex) in an inconspicuous area of the body, to prevent the development of cutaneous leishmaniasis scars on the face.

For more information

Centers for Disease Control and Prevention (CDC)
http://www.cdc.gov/ncidod/dpd/parasites/leishmania/default.htm
International Veterinary Information Service (IVIS).
http://www.ivis.org
Leishmania.co.uk
http://www.leishmania.co.uk

Material Safety Data Sheets - Canadian Laboratory Centre for Disease Control
http://www.phac-aspc.gc.ca/msds-ftss/index.html

Medical Microbiology
http://www.gsbs.utmb.edu/microbook

Ocular manifestations of canine leishmaniasis. In: *Proceedings from the 27th World Small Animal Veterinary Association [WSAVA] World Congress*, 2002; Grenada
http://www.vin.com/proceedings/Proceedings.plx?CID=WSAVA2002

Office International des Epizooties (OIE). Manual of Standards for Diagnostic Tests and Vaccines
http://www.oie.int/eng/normes/mmanual/a_summry.htm

The Merck Manual
http://www.merck.com/pubs/mmanual/

The Merck Veterinary Manual
http://www.merckvetmanual.com/mvm/index.jsp

References

Acha, P.N., Szyfres, B. (Pan American Health Organization [PAHO]). *Zoonoses and Communicable Diseases Common to Man and Animals.* Volume 3. Parasitoses. 3rd ed. Washington DC: PAHO; 2003. Scientific and Technical Publication No. 580. Cutaneous leishmaniasis; p. 38-49; 86-95.

Aiello, S.E., Mays, A. Editors. *The Merck Veterinary Manual.* 8th ed. Whitehouse Station, NJ: Merck and Co.; 1998. Visceral leishmaniasis; p 566-567.

Anonymous. Diagnosing leishmaniasis [online]. Leishmania.co.uk; 2004 Jan. Available at: http://www.leishmania.co.uk/info/diagnosis.html. Accessed 19 May 2004.

Canadian Laboratory Centre for Disease Control. Material Safety Data Sheet - *Leishmania* spp [online]. Office of Laboratory Security. 2001 March. Available at: http://www.hc-sc.gc.ca/pphb-dgspsp/msds-ftss/index.html#menu. Accessed 8 May 2004. http://www.phac-aspc.gc.ca/msds-ftss/msds94e.html on 24 Jan 2006.

Centers for Disease Control [CDC]. Leishmaniasis. CDC; Available at: http://www.dpd.cdc.gov/dpdx/HTML/Leishmaniasis.htm. Accessed 3 June 2004.

Ferrer, L. The pathology of canine leishmaniasis [online]. In: *Canine leishmaniasis: moving towards a solution. Proceedings of the Second International Canine Leishmaniasis Forum*; 2002 February 6-9; Sevilla, Spain. Boxmeer, The Netherlands: Intervet International; 2002. Available at: http://www.diagnosticoveterinario.com/proceedings/2nd%20Proc%20IntCanLforum%202002.pdf. Accessed 19 May 2004.

Glaser, T.A., Baatz, J.E., Kreishman, G.P., Mukkada, A.J. pH homeostasis in *Leishmania donovani* amastigotes and promastigotes. *Proc Natl Acad Sci USA* 1988;85(20):7602-7606.

Gradoni, L. The diagnosis of canine leishmaniasis [online]. In: *Canine leishmaniasis: moving towards a solution. Proceedings of the Second International Canine Leishmaniasis Forum*; 2002 February 6-9; Sevilla, Spain. Boxmeer, The Netherlands: Intervet International; 2002. Available at: http://www.diagnosticoveterinario.com/proceedings/2nd%20Proc%20IntCanLforum%202002.pdf. Accessed 19 May 2004.

Krauss, H., Weber, A, Appel, M., Enders, B., Isenberg, H.D., Schiefer, H.G., Slenczka, W., von Graevenitz, A., Zahner, H. *Zoonoses: Infectious Diseases Transmissible from Animals to Humans.* 3rd edition. Washington DC: ASM Press;2003.pp. 282-293.

Muller, G.H., Kirk, R.W., Scott, D.W. *Small Animal Dermatology.* 4th ed. Philadelphia: WB Saunders; 1989. Leishmaniasis; p 293-294.

Office International des Epizooties [OIE]. *Manual of Diagnostic Tests and Vaccines for Terrestrial Animals.* 5th ed. Paris: OIE; 2004. Leishmaniosis. Forthcoming.

Roze, M. Ocular manifestations of canine leishmaniasis. Diagnosis and treatment [online]. In: *Proceedings from the 27th World Small Animal Veterinary Association [WSAVA] World Congress*; 2002 Oct 3-6; Granada, Spain. Available at: http://www.vin.com/proceedings/Proceedings.plx?CID=WSAVA2002. Accessed 19 May 2004.

Schantz, P., Steurer, F., Jackson, J., Rooney, J., Akey, B., Duprey, Z., Breitschwerdt, E., Rowton, E., Gramiccia, M. Emergence of visceral leishmaniasis in dogs in North America [online]. In: *Leishmaniasis Seminar WorldLeish 2*; 2001 May 20-24; Crete, Greece. Available at: htttp://www.leish.intervet.it/pdf/creta.pdf. Accessed 19 May 2004.

Slappendel, R.J., Ferrer, L. Leishmaniasis. In: *Infectious Diseases of the Dog and Cat.* 2nd ed. Green CE, editor; Philadelphia: Saunders; 1998.

Strauss-Ayali, D., Baneth, G. Canine visceral leishmaniasis. In: *Recent Advances in Canine Infectious Diseases* [monograph online]. Carmichael L, editor. Ithaca NY: International Veterinary Information Service [IVIS]; 2001 Available at: http://www.ivis.org/advances/Infect_Dis_Carmichael/toc.asp. Accessed 10 May 2004.

Trees, A.J., Howman, P.J., Bates, P., Noyes, H.A., Pratlong, F., Blakely, J., Niles, J., Guy, M.W. Autochthonous canine leishmaniosis in the United Kingdom [online]. In: *Leishmaniasis Seminar WorldLeish 2*; 2001 May 20-24; Crete, Greece. Available at: htttp://www.leish.intervet.it/pdf/creta.pdf. Accessed 19 May 2004.

Louping Ill

Ovine Encephalomyelitis, Infectious Encephalomyelitis of Sheep, Trembling-Ill

Importance

Louping ill is a viral infection that can affect a variety of species, but is most significant in sheep. This tick–borne infection can be asymptomatic or mild, or may result in serious neurologic symptoms and death. Losses can be significant in young adult animals with declining passive immunity, as well as in mature sheep moved into endemic areas. There is no treatment.

Etiology

Louping ill results from infection by a single–stranded, neurotropic, RNA virus (family Flaviviridae, genus *Flavivirus*). The strains of louping ill virus do not vary significantly in their pathogenicity.

Species affected

Louping ill is most prevalent in sheep, which seem to be the principal maintenance host. Louping ill can also affect cattle, goats, horses, pigs, dogs, deer, red grouse, and ptarmigan. This virus infects a number of small mammals including shrews, wood mice, voles, and hares. Humans seem to be an accidental host.

Geographic distribution

Louping ill can be found throughout the upland areas of Scotland, Northern Ireland, Cornwall, and Wales. It has also been found in Norway. A closely related disease of sheep is reported from Bulgaria, Turkey, and the Basque region in Spain. None of the known vectors of louping ill virus are found in the United States.

Transmission

Louping ill virus can be transmitted by several species of ticks, including *Rhipicephalus appendiculatus, Ixodes persulcatus, Haemaphysalis anatolicum*, and *I. ricinus. I. ricinus* is thought to be the natural vector of this disease. Peak disease incidence follows seasonal tick activity; louping ill is most common between April and June, and in September.

Louping ill virus is also shed in the milk of sheep and goats. Virus transmission can be demonstrated in kids that nurse from infected goats, but not in lambs that suckle infected sheep. Louping ill virus can also be transmitted to various host species after exposure to infective aerosols and by parenteral routes. Spread on fomites has been documented.

Incubation period

The incubation period for louping ill is 6 to 18 days.

Clinical signs

In sheep, the early clinical signs of louping ill are fever, depression, anorexia, and sometimes constipation. This initial phase may be mild or inapparent. A second fever spike occurs about 5 days after the symptoms first appear; at this time, the virus either enters the central nervous system (CNS) or the animal recovers without further signs. The early symptoms of CNS involvement include muscle tremors, incoordination, ataxia, hyperesthesia, profuse salivation, protrusion of the tongue, champing of the jaws and the development of a characteristic hopping "louping gait." As the disease progresses, additional symptoms appear; they may include head pressing, paraplegia, convulsions, opisthotonos, and coma. Death is common. Surviving animals may have residual CNS deficits. Concurrent infections with *Cytoecetes plagocytoplila* or *Toxoplasma gondii* can significantly increase the pathogenicity of louping ill virus, probably by suppressing the immune system.

Lambs born to non–immune ewes may develop a peracute form of the disease. These animals may die within 2 days after the first symptoms appear.

Louping ill in cattle, horses, and pigs is similar to the disease in sheep. The symptoms in cattle typically include a staggering gait, head pressing, hyperexcitability, recumbency, and convulsions, followed by death. The clinical signs in piglets may include ataxia, muscle spasms, aimless movement, head pressing, and convulsions. Louping ill is rare in horses, and most cases seem to be subclinical.

Post mortem lesions

The only gross lesion on post–mortem is congestion of the meningeal vessels. Secondary pneumonia may be seen. On histology, severe meningoencephalomyelitis is apparent, with gliosis, perivascular infiltration, and neuronal degeneration.

Morbidity and mortality

Morbidity and mortality vary with immune status and other factors. Morbidity is usually low in mature sheep in endemic areas. Mortality ranges from 5% to 10% in adult sheep that have been previously exposed to the virus, to 60% in newly introduced animals. In endemic areas, most deaths occur in animals less than 2 years old. Lambs born in these areas are usually immune for the first year of life. At the end of the year, passive immunity declines and morbidity and mortality increase. Concurrent infections with tick–borne fever or toxoplasmosis, or environmental stress can significantly increase the development of encephalitis and mortality.

A vaccine is available. Treatment is not effective in sheep with CNS signs, but cattle may respond to supportive and symptomatic care.

Diagnosis

Clinical

Louping ill should be suspected in sheep with fever and signs of cerebellar and cerebral disease, particularly when the flock has recently been introduced to tick–infested pastures.

Differential diagnosis

The differential diagnosis in sheep includes scrapie, pregnancy toxemia, maedi–visna, tetanus, rabies, hydatid disease, listeriosis, hypocalcemia, tick pyremia, hypocuprosis, heavy metal toxicity, and poisoning by a variety of plant toxins. In cattle, the differential diagnosis includes listeriosis, malignant catarrhal fever, bovine spongiform encephalopathy, rabies, pseudorabies, hypomagnesemia, hypocalcemia, acute lead poisoning, and toxic plants.

Laboratory tests

Louping ill can be diagnosed by virus isolation, detection of virus antigens, or serology. Virus isolation from the blood can be successful during the acute phase of the disease, but is usually unsuccessful after the neurologic signs appear. Virus may also be isolated from necropsy samples of the brain and spinal cord. Louping ill virus can be isolated in embryonated eggs, primary pig kidney or chicken embryo cell cultures, or suckling mice. The virus is identified by serum neutralization.

Virus antigens can be detected by immunostaining of formalin–fixed brain or by a reverse transcriptase polymerase chain reaction (RT–PCR) assay.

Serologic tests include hemagglutination–inhibition, serum neutralization, and an enzyme–linked immunosorbent assay (ELISA). A complement fixation test is available, but rarely used; complement–fixing antibodies are transient and develop only late in the course of the disease.

Samples to collect

Before collecting or sending any samples from animals with a suspected foreign animal disease, the proper authorities should be contacted. Samples should only be sent under secure conditions and to authorized laboratories to prevent the spread of the disease. Louping ill is a zoonotic disease; samples should be collected and handled with all appropriate precautions.

For virus isolation, approximately 20 ml of uncoagulated blood should be collected during the acute stage of the disease, before the neurologic signs appear. Virus isolation is optimal during the first 3 to 4 days after the onset of the fever. Louping ill virus can often be isolated from the brain and spinal cord of sheep at necropsy; this is not as successful in cattle. For virus isolation from the nervous system, sterile unfixed samples of the brain and spinal cord should be placed in 50% glycerol and normal saline or frozen on dry ice. Samples for virus isolation should be transported to the laboratory as soon as possible.

Paired serum samples should be collected for serology. Half of the brain and pieces of the spinal cord should also be submitted for histology, in 10% formalin.

Recommended actions if louping ill is suspected

Notification of authorities

A diagnosis or suspicion of louping ill should be reported immediately to state or federal authorities.

Federal: Area Veterinarians in Charge (AVICs):
http://www.aphis.usda.gov/vs/area_offices.htm
State Veterinarians:
http://www.aphis.usda.gov/vs/sregs/official.html

Quarantine and disinfection

Prevention of infection of tick vectors is critical. Louping ill virus can also be spread in milk or contaminated tissues, and by fomites. Enveloped viruses such as louping ill virus are generally susceptible to most common disinfectants.

Public health

Humans can be infected by the louping ill virus after aerosol exposure, contamination of skin wounds, or tick bites. Transmission by ingesting milk from infected sheep or goats may be possible. Humans with louping ill can develop an illness that resembles influenza or polio, a biphasic encephalitis, or a hemorrhagic fever.

For more information

World Organization for Animal Health (OIE)
http://www.oie.int

OIE International Animal Health Code
http://www.oie.int/eng/normes/mcode/A_summry.htm

USAHA Foreign Animal Diseases Book
http://www.vet.uga.edu/vpp/gray_book/FAD/

Animal Health Australia. The National Animal Health
Information System (NAHIS)
http://www. aahc.com.au/nahis/disease/dislist.asp

References

"Louping Ill." Animal Health Australia. 1996 The National Animal Health Information System (NAHIS). 3 Oct 2001. http//www. aahc.com.au/nahis/disease/dislist.asp.

"Louping Ill." In *The Merck Veterinary Manual*, 8th ed. Edited by S.E. Aiello and A. Mays. Whitehouse Station, NJ: Merck and Co., 1998, pp. 945–946.

Timoney, P.J. "Louping ill." In *Foreign Animal Diseases*. Richmond, VA: United States Animal Health Association, 1998, pp. 292–302.

Lumpy Skin Disease

Pseudo-urticaria, Neethling Virus Disease,
Exanthema Nodularis Bovis, Knopvelsiekte

Importance

Lumpy skin disease is a pox viral disease of cattle that can cause mild to severe signs including fever, nodules in the skin, mucous membranes and internal organs, skin edema, lymphadenitis, and sometimes death. Economic concerns are decreased milk production, abortion, infertility, weight loss, poor growth, and damaged hides.

Etiology

Lumpy skin disease (LSD) is caused by a virus in the family Poxviridae, genus *Capripoxvirus*. It is closely related antigenically to sheep and goat pox virus. These viruses cannot be differentiated using routine serological testing.

Species affected

Lumpy skin disease is primarily a disease of cattle (*Bos taurus*, zebus, and domestic buffaloes), but the LSD virus can also infect oryx (*Oryx beisa*), giraffe (*Giraffe camelopardalis*), and impala (*Aepyceros melampus*), as well as sheep and goats experimentally.

Geographic distribution

Lumpy skin disease is generally confined to Africa. An outbreak occurred in Israel in 1989; the disease was eradicated by slaughter and vaccination.

Transmission

Transmission of the LSD virus is primarily by biting insects, particularly mosquitoes (e.g. *Culex mirificens* and *Aedes natrionus*) and flies (e.g. *Stomoxys calcitrans* and *Biomyia fasciata*). Epidemics occur in the rainy seasons. Direct contact is also a minor source of infections. Virus can be present in cutaneous lesions, saliva, nasal discharge, milk, semen, muscles, spleen, and lymph nodes. The virus can survive in desiccated crusts for up to 35 days. There is no carrier state.

Incubation period

The incubation period varies from 2 to 5 weeks.

Clinical signs

The clinical signs can range from inapparent to severe. Host susceptibility, dose, and route of virus inoculation affect the severity of disease. *Bos taurus* are more susceptible than *Bos indicus* and young calves often have more severe disease. The first sign is usually fever, which may be transitory or last up to 2 to 4 weeks.

Skin nodules of 1–5 cm diameter generally occur within 2 days of the initial fever. These nodules may become painful and develop a characteristic inverted conical zone of necrosis, which penetrates the entire dermis, the subcutaneous tissue, and sometimes the underlying muscle. These cores of necrotic material (sequestra) become separated from the adjacent skin and are called "sit-fasts." Secondary bacterial infections within the necrotic cores are common. Nodules may occur on the muzzle, nares, head, neck, back, legs, scrotum, perineum, udder, eyelids, lower ear, nasal mucosa, oral mucosa, and tail. Nodules can also develop in the gastrointestinal tract, especially the abomasum, as well as the trachea and lungs, resulting in primary and secondary pneumonia.

Additional related signs include depression, anorexia, excessive salivation, rhinitis and conjunctivitis with oculonasal discharge, agalactia, and emaciation. The lymph nodes may become enlarged up to 4 to 10 times normal size from draining the infected skin. Lameness may occur from inflammation and necrosis of the tendons, and severe edema of the brisket and legs. This lameness can be permanent with severe damage to tendons and joints from secondary bacterial infections. Permanent damage may occur to teats and mammary glands due to secondary bacterial infections and mastitis. Abortion, intrauterine infection, and temporary or permanent sterility in both bulls and cows may occur.

Post mortem lesions

The post mortem lesions can be extensive. The characteristic deep nodules with necrotic centers are found in the skin; these nodules often extend into the subcutis and underlying skeletal muscle, and adjacent tissue exhibits congestion, hemorrhage, and edema. Flat or ulcerative lesions may also be found in the mucous membranes of the oral and nasal cavities, pharynx, epiglottis, and trachea, as well as the gastrointestinal tract and urinary bladder, and nodules occasionally occur within the lungs, kidneys, and testes. Pleuritis, edema, and focal lobular atelectasis in the lungs may occur, with enlargement of the mediastinal lymph nodes in severe cases. Enlarged superficial lymph nodes draining affected areas are common with lymphoid proliferation, edema, congestion, and hemorrhage. Synovitis and tendosynovitis may be seen with fibrin in the synovial fluid.

Morbidity and mortality

The morbidity rate can vary from 3% to 85%, depending on the presence of insect vectors and host susceptibility. Mortality is low in most cases (1% to 3%) but can be as high as 20% to 85%.

Diagnosis

Clinical

Lumpy skin disease should be suspected when there are clinical signs of a contagious disease with the characteristic skin nodules (sitfast), fever, emaciation, and low mortality.

Differential diagnosis

Differentials include pseudo–lumpy skin disease (a much milder disease caused by a herpesvirus), bovine herpes mammillitis (a disease with lesions generally confined to the teats and udder), dermatophilosis, ringworm, insect or tick bites, besnoitiosis, rinderpest, demodicosis, *Hypoderma bovis* infestation, photosensitization, bovine papular stomatitis, urticaria, cutaneous tuberculosis, and onchocercosis. Most of these diseases can be distinguished by the clinical signs, including the duration of the disease, histopathology, and other laboratory tests.

Laboratory tests

Confirmation of lumpy skin disease in a new area requires virus isolation and identification. Lamb testicle or fetal bovine lung cell cultures are best for the growth of LSD virus. Microscopic examination of cell cultures will indicate a characteristic cytopathic effect and intracytoplasmic inclusion bodies. Pseudo lumpy skin disease, caused by a herpesvirus, produces syncytia and intranuclear inclusion bodies in cell culture. Antigen testing can be done using direct immunofluorescent staining, virus neutralization, or ELISA.

Typical capripox virions can be seen using transmission electron microscopy of biopsy samples or desiccated crusts. This finding, in combination with a history of generalized nodular skin lesions and lymph node enlargement in cattle, can be diagnostic. The capripoxvirus can be distinguished from the parapoxvirus that causes bovine papular stomatitis and pseudocowpox. Cowpox and vaccinia virus cannot be distinguished morphologically from capripoxvirus, but do not cause generalized infection and are not commonly seen in cattle.

Serological tests include an indirect fluorescent antibody test, virus neutralization, and enzyme–linked immunosorbent assay (ELISA). Cross–reactions may occur with other poxviruses.

Samples to collect

Before collecting or sending any samples from animals with a suspected foreign animal disease, the proper authorities should be contacted. Samples should only be sent under secure conditions and to authorized laboratories to prevent the spread of the disease.

Skin biopsies taken of early lesions without necrosis from at least 3 animals can be used for virus isolation or histopathology. Lung lesions, lymph nodes, or lymph node aspirates are also good samples for virus isolation. Tissue samples should be sent on ice for virus isolation as well as preserved in 10% buffered formalin for histopathology. These samples should not be frozen. Lesions (even dry crusts) removed from the skin, subcutis, or oropharynx of dead animals may be used. Blood samples in anticoagulant (heparin or EDTA) collected early in the disease during the viremic stage can be used for virus isolation. Serum samples from acute and chronic cases with follow–up samples 2 to 3 weeks after the first skin lesions appear should be sent for antigen detection and can be frozen.

Recommended actions if lumpy skin disease is suspected

Notification of authorities

State and federal veterinarians should be immediately informed of any suspected cases of lumpy skin disease.

Federal: Area Veterinarians in Charge (AVICs):
http://www.aphis.usda.gov/vs/area_offices.htm
State Veterinarians:
http://www.aphis.usda.gov/vs/sregs/official.html

Quarantine and disinfection

Quarantine, slaughter and burning of carcasses, disinfection of the premises, and insect control are important in controlling an outbreak of lumpy skin disease. A vaccine is available for use in infected countries. LSD virus is susceptible to ether (20%), chloroform, formalin (1%), and some detergents, as well as phenol (2%/15 min). It can survive for long periods in the environment—up to 35 days in desiccated scabs.

Public health

The lumpy skin disease virus does not infect humans.

For more information

World Organization for Animal Health (OIE)
http://www.oie.int
OIE Manual of Standards
http://www.oie.int/eng/normes/mmanual/a_summry.htm

OIE International Animal Health Code
http://www.oie.int/eng/normes/mcode/A_summry.htm
USAHA Foreign Animal Diseases Book
http://www.vet.uga.edu/vpp/gray_book/FAD/

References

"Lumpy Skin Disease." In *Manual of Standards for Diagnostic Tests and Vaccines*. Paris: World Organization for Animal Health, 2000, pp. 134–143.

"Lumpy Skin Disease." In *The Merck Veterinary Manual*, 8th ed. Edited by S.E. Aiello and A. Mays. Whitehouse Station, NJ: Merck and Co., 1998, pp. 621–622.

House, James A. "Lumpy Skin Disease." In *Foreign Animal Diseases*. Richmond, VA: United States Animal Health Association, 1998, pp. 303–310.

"Lumpy Skin Disease." 30 Aug. 2000. World Organization for Animal Health 16 Oct. 2001 http//www.oie.int/eng/maladies/fiches/a_A070.htm.

Maedi-Visna

Ovine Progressive Pneumonia, Marsh's Progressive Pneumonia, Montana Progressive Pneumonia, Chronic Progressive Pneumonia, Zwoegersiekte, La bouhite, Graff-Reinet Disease

Importance

Maedi–visna is a chronic viral infection of sheep and goats that can cause progressive dyspnea (maedi), progressive neurologic signs (visna), arthritis, or mastitis. Both maedi and visna are fatal. Additional economic costs may include marketing and export restrictions, premature culling, and possible losses from poor milk production. Economic losses can vary considerably between flocks.

Etiology

Maedi–visna results from infection by the maedi–visna virus, a lentivirus in the family Retroviridae. This virus becomes integrated into leukocyte DNA; infected animals become chronic carriers.

Species affected

Maedi–visna affects sheep and, to a lesser extent, goats. Breed susceptibility varies. Texel, Border Leicester, and Finnish Landrace sheep appear to be relatively susceptible to disease; Columbia, Rambouillet, and Suffolk sheep seem to be relatively resistant.

Geographic distribution

Maedi–visna exists in most of continental Europe, the United Kingdom, Canada, the United States, Peru, Kenya, South Africa, Israel, India, Myanmar, and the southern regions of the former U.S.S.R.

Transmission

Most animals become infected from drinking infected colostrum or milk. The virus can also be spread during close contact, probably by the respiratory route. Transmission has been reported from water contaminated with feces, but indirect spread is generally thought to be rare. Intrauterine spread is negligible or very minor. Asymptomatic carriers are common.

Incubation period

The incubation period for maedi is more than 2 years; clinical signs usually develop when animals are 3 to 4 years old. The incubation period for visna is somewhat shorter, and symptoms can appear in sheep as young as 2 years.

Clinical signs

Most infections with the maedi–visna virus are asymptomatic. In animals with clinical signs, the disease can take several forms. Sheep with maedi, the most common form, experience wasting, progressive dyspnea, and sometimes a dry cough. Fever, bronchial exudates, or depression are not usually seen. Maedi is fatal; death results from anoxia or secondary bacterial pneumonia.

Visna is more rare. This form usually begins with hindlimb weakness and loss of condition, and progresses to ataxia, incoordination, muscle tremors, paresis, and paraplegia. The clinical course may be as long as a year.

Maedi–visna infections can also result in a slowly progressive arthritis with severe lameness, or a chronic indurative mastitis with decreased milk production.

Post mortem lesions

In maedi, the lungs are enlarged, abnormally firm and heavy, and fail to collapse when the thoracic cavity is opened. The affected lungs are emphysematous and usually mottled, with pale gray or pale brown areas of consolidation. Nodules may be found around the smaller airways and blood vessels, and the mediastinal and tracheobronchial lymph nodes are usually enlarged and edematous. Secondary bacterial pneumonia may mask the primary lesions. On histological examination, a chronic, diffuse interstitial pneumonia is seen.

No gross lesions are seen in visna, apart from wasting of the carcass. On microscopic examination, the typical lesion is a meningoleukoencephalitis with secondary demyelination.

In other forms, the udder may be diffusely indurated and the associated lymph nodes may be enlarged. Arthritis may also be seen.

Morbidity and mortality

In the United States, antibodies to the maedi–visna virus can be found in 1% to 70% of sheep; the prevalence varies with the region of the country. Infection rates are highest in the Western and Midwestern States. Most infections are asymptomatic, but once clinical signs appear the disease is usually fatal.

No treatment or vaccine is available.

Diagnosis

Clinical

Maedi–visna should be suspected in animals that are at least 2 years old and have a wasting disease with slowly progressive respiratory distress, neurologic signs, or arthritis.

Differential diagnosis

The differential diagnosis includes pulmonary adenomatosis, parasitic lung infections, caseous lymphadenitis with lung involvement, chronic bacterial pneumonias, caprine arthritis–encephalitis, and various plant toxicities. In cases with neurologic symptoms, scrapie, listeriosis, rabies, louping ill, parasitic central nervous system (CNS) infections, and space–occupying lesions of the CNS should also be considered.

Laboratory tests

Maedi–visna is usually diagnosed by serology, clinical evaluation, and histology. Serology can also detect most asymptomatic carriers. However, screening is usually more effective in populations than in individual animals. Seroconversion generally occurs months after infection.

The two most common serologic tests are agar gel immunodiffusion (the prescribed test for international trade) and enzyme–linked immunosorbent assays (ELISAs). Immunoblotting (Western blotting) and immunoprecipitation are used in some laboratories. A milk antibody assay has been used in goat herds.

Virus isolation is not routinely attempted, but can sometimes be successful. Leukocytes from peripheral blood or milk are cultured with ovine or caprine cell cultures. Appropriate cell cultures include choroid plexus (MVV) or synovial membrane (CAEV) cells. Cytopathic effects may take weeks to appear. Post–mortem, virus isolation can be attempted from the lung, alveolar macrophages, choroid plexus, synovial membrane, or udder.

Polymerase chain reaction (PCR) tests, Southern blotting, and in situ hybridization are occasionally used.

Samples to collect

At least 20 ml of serum should be collected from several suspect and in–contact animals.

For virus isolation from live animals, blood samples should be collected into an anticoagulant and antibiotics should be added. Necropsy samples from cases of maedi should include the lung, spleen, and mediastinal lymph nodes. In animals with suspected visna, a sample of the brain should be sent. The samples should be transported on wet ice or with gel packs as soon as possible. If shipping is to be delayed for more than 48 hours, the samples may be frozen and shipped on dry ice.

Samples for histology should include all affected tissues, including lung, mediastinal lymph nodes, spleen, brain, spinal cord, or udder.

Recommended actions if maedi–visna is suspected

Notification of authorities

Maedi–visna is a reportable disease in many states. State guidelines should be consulted for more specific information.

Federal: Area Veterinarians in Charge (AVICs):
http://www.aphis.usda.gov/vs/area_offices.htm
State Veterinarians:
http://www.aphis.usda.gov/vs/sregs/official.html

Quarantine and disinfection

Maedi–visna is a contagious disease. Infections can be controlled by strict separation of seropositive from seronegative animals, with re–testing every 6 months. Newborns can also be separated from their dams at birth and reared artificially with uninfected colostrum and milk.

The maedi–visna virus cannot survive for more than a few days in the environment, particularly under hot, dry conditions. Lentiviruses can be destroyed with most common disinfectants.

Public health

The maedi–visna virus does not appear to affect humans.

For more information

World Organization for Animal Health (OIE)
http://www.oie.int
OIE Manual of Standards
http://www.oie.int/eng/normes/mmanual/a_summry.htm
OIE International Animal Health Code
http://www.oie.int/eng/normes/mcode/A_summry.htm
Animal Health Australia. The National Animal Health Information System (NAHIS)
http://www. aahc.com.au/nahis/disease/dislist.asp

References

"Caprine Arthritis/Encephalitis and Maedi–Visna." In *Manual of Standards for Diagnostic Tests and Vaccines*. Paris: World Organization for Animal Health, 2000, pp. 497–502.

Cutlip, R.C., J. DeMartini, G. Ross, and G. Snowder. "Ovine Progressive Pneumonia." American Sheep Industry Association Feb 2000. 15 Oct 2001. http//www.sheepusa.org/resources/diseases/shopp.html.

"Maedi–Visna." Animal Health Australia. The National Animal Health Information System (NAHIS). 15 Oct 2001. http//www. aahc.com.au/nahis/disease/dislist.asp.

"Progressive Pneumonia." In *The Merck Veterinary Manual*, 8th ed. Edited by S.E. Aiello and A. Mays. Whitehouse Station, NJ: Merck and Co., 1998, pp. 1111–1112.

Malignant Catarrhal Fever

Malignant Catarrh, Malignant Head Catarrh, Gangrenous Coryza, Catarrhal Fever, Snotsiekte

Importance

Malignant catarrhal fever is a highly fatal disease of cattle and other ruminants. This infection occurs sporadically and is difficult to control; the causative viruses are carried inapparently by most or all sheep and wildebeest, as well as other wild animals. The risk of malignant catarrhal fever may increase as wild game animal ranches become increasingly popular in North America and cattle come into close contact with exotic ruminants.

Etiology

Malignant catarrhal fever results from infection by either of two gamma herpesviruses, alcelaphine herpesvirus–1 (AHV–1), and ovine herpesvirus–2 (OvHV–2 or OHV–2). AHV–1 is carried asymptomatically by wildebeest. This virus causes malignant catarrhal fever in Africa and in zoos throughout the world. OHV–2 is carried by sheep and causes the disease in most of the world. OHV–2 has not yet been isolated; evidence for its existence is still indirect. A third virus related to AHV–1, AHV–2, is also carried as a latent infection by wildebeest, hartebeest, and topi. AHV–2 is not thought to be pathogenic.

Species affected

Wildebeest, hartebeest, and topi are carriers of AHV–1. All wildebeest in the wild, and most wildebeest in zoos, appear to be infected by this virus. Several other wild ruminants in Africa, including species of oryx and addax, also have antibodies to AHV–1 and may be reservoir hosts. Sheep and goats (both domestic and wild species) are the carriers for OVH–2. All sheep appear to have antibodies to this virus.

Clinical disease usually affects members of the subfamily Bovinae and family Cervidae. Cattle, water buffalo, bison, and many species of wild ruminants (including gaur, banteng, and deer) can be affected. Susceptibility to disease caused by OVH–2 varies. *Bos taurus* and *B. indicus* are relatively resistant to this infection, water buffalo and many species of deer are more susceptible, and bison, Bali cattle, and Pere David's deer are extremely susceptible. Malignant catarrhal fever has also been seen in domestic pigs, giraffes, and some species of antelope.

Geographic distribution

Disease caused by OVH–2 occurs throughout the world. AHV–1 associated disease is mainly seen in Africa, in areas where wildebeest, hartebeest, and topi are naturally found. Malignant catarrhal fever caused by AHV–1 has also been seen in zoos and wild animal parks that contain wildebeest.

Transmission

AHV–1 in adult wildebeest, hartebeest, and topi is mainly cell–associated. The cell–associated form is rarely transmitted to other animals; however, cell–free virus can be isolated from the nasal secretions of adult wildebeest after the animals are stressed or given corticosteroids. Neonatal wildebeest can spread the infection more readily. Wildebeest calves can be infected in utero, and shed the virus in nasal and ocular secretions and in the feces. Free–living calves are all infected by the time they are six months old. Cell–free AHV–1 can be transmitted to cattle and other susceptible animals by inhalation in aerosol droplets, ingestion of contaminated feed or water, or possibly mechanical transmission by arthropods. This virus is quickly inactivated by sunlight.

OHV–2 has not been isolated as an intact virion, and its means of transmission is not known. OHV–2 is often spread by neonatal lambs, but all ages can be infectious. Fairly close contact between susceptible animals and sheep, especially lambing ewes, is thought to be necessary. The role of goats in spreading OVH–2 is unknown.

Ruminants that develop malignant catarrhal fever appear to be dead end hosts. Cases of cattle–to–cattle transmission have been documented, but this seems to be rare.

Incubation period

The incubation period in experimental infections is 9 to 77 days. In natural infections, the incubation period is unknown. Epidemiological evidence suggests that it may be up to 200 days; some animals appear to become subclinically infected and only develop disease after periods of severe stress.

Clinical signs

A wide variety of symptoms are seen in this disease. Sudden death may occur; this may be preceded by 12 to 24 hours of depression, diarrhea and dysentery, signs of disseminated intravascular coagulation, or dyspnea. In less acute cases, there may be fever (41–41.5°C) and inappetence. Animals often develop bilateral corneal opacity that begins at the corneoscleral junction and progresses inward. Serous discharges from the eyes and nose are typical; later, these discharges become mucopurulent. The muzzle and nares are usually encrusted, and dyspnea, open–mouthed breathing, and salivation may be seen. The oral mucosa is often hyperemic and may contain multifocal or diffuse areas of necrosis. Erosions may be found at the tips of the buccal papillae. The skin is sometimes ulcerated, and hardened scabs may develop on the perineum, udder, and teats. In some animals, the horn and hoof coverings may be loosened or sloughed. The joints may be swollen, milk production may drop, and the superficial lymph nodes may be enlarged. Constipation is common, but diarrhea or hemorrhagic gastroenteritis can also be seen. Occasionally, animals have nervous signs including hyperesthesia, incoordination, nystagmus, or head pressing, either with or without other characteristic symptoms.

Post mortem lesions

Malignant catarrhal fever causes epithelial necrosis in the gastrointestinal, respiratory, and urinary tracts, lymphoproliferation, interstitial infiltration of nonlymphoid tissues by lymphoid cells, and vasculitis. The post–mortem lesions are variable, depending on the severity and course of the disease. After sudden death, there may be few abnormalities other than a hemorrhagic enterocolitis. In a less acute case, the carcass may be dehydrated, emaciated, or normal. The muzzle is often raw and encrusted, with a serous, mucopurulent, or purulent nasal discharge. Hyperemia, edema, and small focal erosions may be found on the nasal mucosa. Generalized exudation, crusting, and matting of the hair is common on the ventral thorax and abdomen, inguinal region, perineum, and sometimes the head. The lymph nodes are usually enlarged and edematous, particularly in the head, neck, and periphery. On cut surface, they may be firm and white, hemorrhagic, or necrotic. The gastrointestinal tract may contain erosions and hemorrhages; in severe cases, the intestinal contents may be hemorrhagic. The respiratory tract often has catarrhal exudate and erosions, and a diphtheritic membrane may be present. Ecchymotic hemorrhages, hyperemia, and edema are common in the mucosa of the urinary bladder, and the renal cortex may contain raised white foci. In more chronic cases, small arteries in the subcutaneous tissues, thorax, abdomen, and central nervous system are very prominent and tortuous, with thickened walls. The feces are usually scant, pasty, dry, or blood stained. Fibrinous polyarthritis is common.

Morbidity and mortality

Malignant catarrhal fever in the United States usually occurs sporadically in one to a few animals; however, in one outbreak in a U.S. feedlot the morbidity was 37%. In AHV–1 outbreaks in Malaysia, the morbidity is 28% to 45% percent. The mortality rate in symptomatic animals is 90% to 100%. Antibiotics to control secondary infections and supportive therapy may occasionally help, but any surviving animals are likely to remain virus carriers. Commercial vaccines are not available.

Diagnosis

Clinical

Malignant catarrhal fever should be suspected in susceptible animals with the characteristic clinical signs, particularly if they have been in contact with sheep, goats, alcelaphine antelope, or wildebeest (especially around the period of parturition). The symptoms of typical infections include sudden death or fever with nasal and lacrimal discharges, erosions of the mucosa, and bilateral corneal opacity, but other syndromes may be seen. Post–mortem lesions that support a diagnosis of malignant catarrhal fever include corneal opacity, enlarged lymph nodes, inflammation and erosions in the nasal passages, gastrointestinal mucosa, and urinary bladder, and prominent tortuous small arteries in the subcutaneous tissue, thorax, and abdomen.

Differential diagnosis

Malignant catarrhal fever must be differentiated from BVD mucosal disease, bluetongue, rinderpest, infectious bovine rhinotracheitis, vesicular diseases such as foot and mouth disease and vesicular stomatitis, ingestion of caustic materials, and some poisonous plants and mycotoxins.

Laboratory tests

In practice, malignant catarrhal fever is often confirmed by histopathologic demonstration of multisystem lymphoid infiltration, disseminated vasculitis, and degenerative epithelial lesions. However, polymerase chain reaction (PCR) tests are becoming the diagnostic method of choice. PCR can detect both AHV–1 and OHV–2 viral DNA. AHV–1 infections can also be confirmed by virus isolation. This virus can be recovered from peripheral blood leukocytes, lymph nodes, or spleen. Viable cells are necessary, as the virus cannot be isolated from dead cells. Virus isolation has not been successful in OHV–2 infections.

Serology can also be helpful. In wildebeest, antibodies to AHV–1 can be detected by virus neutralization, immunoblotting, enzyme–linked immunosorbent assay (ELISA), immunofluorescence, and immunocytochemistry. Ruminants with malignant catarrhal fever rarely develop neutralizing antibodies; in symptomatic cases, immunofluorescence or immunoblotting must be used. In sheep, antibodies to OVH–2 can be found by immunofluorescence or immunoblotting. Immunofluorescence is often useful in cattle infected by OHV–2, but antibodies may not be found in more acute cases, particularly in deer.

Samples to collect

Ten to 20 ml of blood should be collected in EDTA for virus isolation. Pieces of the spleen, lung, lymph nodes, adrenal glands, and thyroid should be collected for virus isolation, fluorescent antibody, or immunoperoxidase tests. The virus quickly becomes inactivated in dead animals, and samples should be collected as soon as possible. The most useful samples are collected immediately after euthanasia of a dying animal. The samples should be refrigerated (not frozen) and shipped on ice.

Samples of lung, liver, lymph nodes, skin (if lesions are present), kidney, adrenals, eyes, oral epithelium, esophagus, Peyer's patches, urinary bladder, carotid rete, thyroid, heart muscle, and whole brain should be submitted for histopathology. These tissues should be fixed as thin pieces in 10% neutral buffered formalin.

PCR can be done on peripheral blood samples, fresh tissues, and paraffin–embedded tissue samples. Serum should be taken 3 to 4 weeks apart for serology if possible. Single samples are of limited value; some asymptomatic cattle in the U.S. carry antibodies to these viruses.

Recommended actions if malignant catarrhal fever is suspected

Notification of authorities

Malignant catarrhal fever is a reportable disease in many states. State authorities should be consulted for more specific information.

Federal: Area Veterinarians in Charge (AVICs):
http://www.aphis.usda.gov/vs/area_offices.htm
State Veterinarians:
http://www.aphis.usda.gov/vs/sregs/official.html

Quarantine and disinfection

In outbreaks, susceptible animals must be immediately separated from sheep and goats (OHV–2), or from alcelaphine or wild ruminants (AHV–1) to contain the disease. OHV–2 and AHV–1 are susceptible to commonly used disinfectants.

Public health

There is no evidence that OVH–2 or AHV–1 can infect humans.

For more information

World Organization for Animal Health (OIE)
http://www.oie.int
OIE Manual of Standards
http://www.oie.int/eng/normes/mmanual/a_summry.htm
OIE International Animal Health Code
http://www.oie.int/eng/normes/mcode/A_summry.htm
USAHA Foreign Animal Diseases Book
http://www.vet.uga.edu/vpp/gray_book/FAD/
USDA Training Manual. Malignant Catarrhal Fever
http://aphisweb.aphis.usda.gov/vs/ep/fad_training/
Malivol5/mal5index.htm

References

H.I. Fraser, B.W.J. Heide, C.D. Hicks, and S.J.G. Otto. Malignant Catarrhal Fever. March 2000. 11 Sept 2001. http//duke. usask.ca/~misra/virology/stud2000/mcf2/mcf.html.

Heuschele, W.P. "Malignant Catarrhal Fever." In *Foreign Animal Diseases*. Richmond, VA: United States Animal Health Association, 1998, pp. 311–321.

"Malignant Catarrhal Fever." In *Manual of Standards for Diagnostic Tests and Vaccines*. Paris: World Organization for Animal Health, 2000, pp. 813–821.

"Malignant Catarrhal Fever." In *The Merck Veterinary Manual*, 8th ed. Edited by S.E. Aiello and A. Mays. Whitehouse Station, NJ: Merck and Co., 1998, pp. 534–36.

"Malignant Catarrhal Fever." Dec 2000. U.S. Department of Agriculture. 10 Sept. 2001. http//aphisweb.aphis.usda.gov/ vs/ep/fad_training/Malivol5/mal5index.htm>

Melioidosis

Pseudoglanders, Whitmore Disease

Importance

Melioidosis is a zoonotic bacterial disease infecting a wide variety of host species. This disease is characterized by abscesses in a variety of organs, and can mimic other diseases. Infections range from asymptomatic to chronic and fatal. Disseminated septicemia may develop, particularly in debilitated or immunocompromised humans, and can be fatal. The agent of this disease is a potential bioterrorist weapon.

Etiology

Melioidosis results from infection by *Burkholderia pseudomallei*, a motile Gram negative bacillus (family Pseudomonadaceae). This organism was formerly known as *Pseudomonas pseudomallei*.

Species affected

Infection with *B. pseudomallei* is seen most often in pigs, goats, and sheep. It occurs less often in cattle, horses, dogs, rodents, birds, dolphins, tropical fish, primates, and various wild animals. Hamsters, guinea pigs, and rabbits can be infected in the laboratory.

Geographic distribution

Melioidosis is endemic in Southeast Asia, Africa, Australia, the Middle East, India, and China. This infection is mainly associated with tropical and subtropical regions; however, the organism has also been isolated from the temperate regions of southwest Australia and France. Isolated cases have occurred in South America and in the states of Hawaii and Georgia in the United States. *B. pseudomallei* is generally found in water or moist soil.

Transmission

New infections are primarily acquired from organisms in the environment. Contaminated swamps, muddy water, and rodents are important sources of infection. Soil–borne infections are generally associated with heavy rainfall or flooding in areas with high humidity or temperatures. Infection can occur by ingestion, inhalation, or through wounds and abrasions. The role of insect bites is uncertain. Direct human–to–human and animal–to–human transmission is rare but can occur after contact with blood or body fluids. Depending on the site of the infection, contaminated body fluids may include urine, nasal secretions, and milk. Shed organisms can survive for months in soil and water.

Incubation period

The incubation period is variable and appears to be longer in pigs than in other animals.

Clinical signs

B. pseudomallei infection results in suppurating or caseous lesions in the lymph nodes or other organs. Infections may be asymptomatic and abscesses may be found in clinically normal goats, sheep, and pigs. Symptomatic melioidosis mimics other diseases; the clinical signs vary with the site of the lesion. They may include fever, loss of appetite, and lymphadenopathy, often involving the submandibular nodes in pigs. Lameness or posterior paresis, nasal discharge, encephalitis, gastrointestinal symptoms, or respiratory signs may also be seen in some species. Extensive abscesses and infections of vital organs can be fatal.

In sheep and goats, lung abscesses and pneumonia are common. Other common symptoms in sheep include high fever, ocular and nasal discharge, and gradual emaciation. Mastitis may be seen in goats and the superficial lymph nodes and udder may contain palpable abscesses. Pulmonary lesions in goats are usually less severe than in sheep and coughing is not prominent. In horses, neurologic disease, respiratory symptoms, or colic and diarrhea have been described. Infections in pigs are usually chronic and asymptomatic. Acute infections in this species may result in septicemia with fever, anorexia, coughing, and nasal and ocular discharges. Abortions and stillbirths may occur but are rare, and orchitis may occur in boars. Cattle are rarely affected, but may develop pneumonia or neurologic signs.

B. pseudomallei is susceptible to various antibiotics, but relapses can occur when treatment is stopped. Vaccines are available in some countries but are not effective against large challenge doses.

Post mortem lesions

At necropsy, the major findings are multiple abscesses containing thick, caseous, greenish–yellow or off–white material. These abscesses are generally not calcified. The regional lymph nodes, spleen, lung, liver, and subcutaneous tissues are most often involved, but abscesses can occur in most organs. In acute cases, pneumonic changes in the lungs, meningoencephalitis, and suppurative polyarthritis may be found. In cases with suppurative arthritis, the joints may contain fluid and large masses of greenish–yellow purulent material.

In sheep, common findings include abscesses and suppuration in the nasal mucosa. Splenic abscesses are often found in pigs at slaughter.

Morbidity and mortality

Mortality varies with the site of the lesions, but can be high in sheep. Extensive abscesses and infections of vital organs can be fatal. Disseminated septicemic infections have a high mortality rate, but are less common in animals than humans.

Diagnosis

Clinical

Melioidosis should be suspected when multiple caseous abscesses are found.

Differential diagnosis

The differential diagnosis varies with the site of the lesions and includes tuberculosis, nonspecific purulent conditions such as pneumonia, and various arthritides. Melioidosis can be confused with caseous lymphadenitis in sheep and goats, or actinobacillosis in sheep. In horses, melioidosis can resemble strangles or glanders.

Laboratory tests

Melioidosis is diagnosed by isolation and identification of *Burkholderia pseudomallei*. This organism has a wrinkled colony form, which may be mixed with smooth colonies. A characteristic odor has been described. (Due to the risk of infection, directly sniffing the plates is not recommended.) Organisms are oval, Gram negative bacilli, with bipolar staining in young cultures. In some species, agglutination tests, indirect hemagglutination, immunofluorescence, and enzyme immunoassays can be used for diagnosis. Cross–reactions may occur in serologic tests with *Burkholderia mallei*, the causative agent of glanders. A polymerase chain reaction can differentiate *B. mallei* DNA from *B. pseudomallei*.

Samples to collect

Before collecting or sending any samples from animals with a suspected foreign animal disease, the proper authorities should be contacted. Samples should only be sent under secure conditions and to authorized laboratories to prevent the spread of the disease.

Swabs of nasal discharges and samples collected from lesions should be submitted for culture. Organisms may be isolated from the sputum, blood, wound exudates or tissues. In some species, serum may also be collected for serologic tests.

Recommended actions if melioidosis is suspected

Notification of authorities

Melioidosis is considered to be a potential bioterrorist weapon by the federal government. In response, it has recently been added to some state lists of reportable diseases. State or federal authorities should be consulted for specific regulations and information.

Federal: Area Veterinarians in Charge (AVICs):

http://www.aphis.usda.gov/vs/area_offices.htm
State Veterinarians:
http://www.aphis.usda.gov/vs/sregs/official.html

Quarantine and disinfection

B. pseudomallei can survive for months to years in the soil and water, but can be readily destroyed by heat. Moist heat of 121°C for at least 15 min or dry heat of 160–170°C for at least 1 hour is recommended for disinfection. The organism is also susceptible to numerous disinfectants, including 1% sodium hypochlorite, 70% ethanol, glutaraldehyde, and formaldehyde.

Public health

B. pseudomallei is pathogenic to humans. Infections may be inapparent or may result in pulmonary infections, disseminated septicemia, acute nondisseminated septicemia, or localized chronic suppurative infections. In humans, the incubation period can vary from two days to months or years.

The most serious form is disseminated septicemic infection. This form is most common in people with pre–existing debilitating diseases such as AIDS, cancer, diabetes, and kidney failure. It is often accompanied by septic shock and may be fatal. Pulmonary infections vary in severity, from mild bronchitis to severe necrotizing pneumonia. Acute nondisseminated septicemic infection involves a single organ. Localized chronic suppurative infections are characterized by abscesses in the skin, lymph nodes, or other organs. Osteomyelitis is relatively common with localized infections.

The mortality rate is usually less than 10%, except in disseminated septicemic infections. Fatal infections are more common in patients who are immunosuppressed or have concurrent disease.

For more information

World Organization for Animal Health (OIE)
http://www.oie.int
Material Safety Data Sheets–Canadian Laboratory Centre
for Disease Control
http://www.phac-aspc.gc.ca/msds-ftss/index.html
Manual for the Recognition of Exotic Diseases of Livestock
http://www.spc.int/rahs/
Centers for Disease Control and Prevention (CDC)
http://www.cdc.gov/ncidod/dbmd/diseaseinfo/melioidosis_g.htm

References

Bauernfeind A., Roller C., Meyer D., Jungwirth R., and Schneider I. "Molecular procedure for rapid detection of *Burkholderia mallei* and *Burkholderia pseudomallei*." *J. Clin. Microbiol.* 36 (1998): 2737–2741.

Bogle, R.B. "Bioterrorism: Hype or Hazard?" Cactus Chronicle (Arizona Society for Clinical Laboratory Science) 23, no. 1 (January/February 2000). 7 Oct 2002. http://pw1.netcom.com/~aguldo/agga/txt/cactusbt.htm.

Gilbert, R.O. "Glanders" In *Foreign Animal Diseases*. Richmond, VA: United States Animal Health Association, 1998, pp. 245–252.

Herenda, D., P.G. Chambers, A. Ettriqui, P. Seneviratna, and T.J.P. da Silva. "Manual on meat inspection for developing countries. FAO Animal Production and Health Paper 119." 1994. Publishing and Multimedia Service, Information Division, FAO. 8 Oct 2002. http://www.fao.org/docrep/003/t0756e/t0756e00.htm.

"Material Safety Data Sheet –*Burkholderia (Pseudomonas) pseudomallei*." January 2001 Canadian Laboratory Centre for Disease Control. 4 October 2002. http://www.phac-aspc.gc.ca/msds-ftss/index.html.

"Melioidosis." Animal Health Australia. The National Animal Health Information System (NAHIS). 4 Oct 2002. http://www.aahc.com.au/nahis/disease/dislist.asp.

"Melioidosis." In *Manual for the Recognition of Exotic Diseases of Livestock: A Reference Guide for Animal Health Staff*. Food and Agriculture Organization of the United Nations, 1998. 8 Oct 2002. http://panis.spc.int/.

"Melioidosis." In *The Merck Manual*, 17th ed. Edited by M.H. Beers and R. Berkow. Whitehouse Station, NJ: Merck and Co., 1999. 7 Oct 2002. http://www.merck.com/pubs/mmanual/section13/chapter157/157d.htm.

"Melioidosis." In *The Merck Veterinary Manual*, 8th ed. Edited by S.E. Aiello and A. Mays. Whitehouse Station, NJ: Merck and Co., 1998, pp. 481–2.

"Melioidosis (*Burkholderia pseudomallei*)" Centers for Disease Control and Prevention (CDC). 8 Oct 2002. http://www.cdc.gov/ncidod/dbmd/diseaseinfo/melioidosis_g.htm.

Menangle
Menangle Virus

Importance

Menangle is a newly emerged disease of swine, currently limited to one outbreak in Menangle, New South Wales, Australia. This viral disease caused mummified and stillborn piglets, reduced farrowing rates and reduced litter number and size, as well as occasional abortions. All postnatal pigs seroconverted to the virus and were unaffected. The disease appears to be maintained and spread by fruit bats (flying foxes); however the route of transmission among swine is currently unknown.

Etiology

Menangle is one of several recently discovered RNA viruses in the family Paramyxoviridae. Molecular characterization of the virus has placed it in the genus *Rubulavirus*. No serological cross–reactivity occurs between Menangle and other known paramyxoviruses (i.e., Hendra or Nipah viruses). The virus does not appear to be highly contagious but tends to spread slowly throughout the population. The virus does not appear able to survive in the environment for any length of time.

Species affected

Menangle virus infections have only been reported in pigs in New South Wales, Australia. Cattle, sheep, birds, rodents, cats and dogs in the vicinity of the outbreak piggery were found to be seronegative for the virus. During the 1997 outbreak, only two of more than 250 humans with potential exposure were clinically affected by and seropositive for the virus. These two people were in prolonged close contact with infected pigs. Fruit bats (*Pteropus* spp.), are the probable reservoir for the virus. They have been found to be seropositive for the virus but are asymptomatic.

Geographic distribution

Menangle virus has only been reported in one outbreak in a 2600–sow intensive piggery in New South Wales, Australia in 1997. Several species of fruit bats (*Pteropus* spp.) are native to this geographic area and have been found to be seropositive for the virus prior to the outbreak.

Transmission

Currently, the route of transmission of Menangle virus between pigs, flying foxes and humans is unknown; a fecal–oral or urinary–oral transmission is suspected. In the two human cases of Menangle, both were closely associated with the infected pigs (i.e., birthing piglets and performing necropsies of infected piglets without wearing protective gloves or eyewear). Menangle virus has been found in the lung, brain and myocardium of fetal pigs.

Pigs between 10 to 16 weeks old are considered to harbor an active infection since this is the period when their maternal antibody protection is waning. These pigs do seroconvert to the virus as their immune system matures. Experimentally, susceptible sentinel pigs were placed into an uncleaned area, which had been recently occupied by infected pigs. The sentinel pigs did not become infected with the virus.

Incubation period

The incubation period for Menangle is not known. However, infection in pigs seems to be of short duration (10 to 14 days) and results in strong immunity. Persistent infection in pigs does not occur.

Clinical signs

Menangle virus is thought to cross the placenta to affect the developing fetuses and reproductive performance of naïve swine. Affected litters consisted of a mixture of mummified, autolysed and fresh stillborn piglets and a few normal live piglets. Many had deformities of the skeletal or nervous systems (i.e., arthrogryposis, brachygnathia, degeneration of spinal cord). Although no disease is observed in postnatal animals of any age, sows will have reduced farrowing rates; smaller litters sizes and possibly abort. Some sows returned to estrus approximately 28 days after mating; however others remain in a state of pseudopregnancy until more then 60 days after mating.

Post mortem lesions

Post mortem examination of the affected piglets revealed severe degeneration of the brain or spinal cord (was almost absent in some), arthrogryposis, brachygnathia, kyphosis, ad occasionally fibrinous body cavity effusions and pulmonary hypoplasia were seen. The cranium of some piglets was slightly domed in some cases.

Histological examination of the brain and spinal cord revealed extensive degeneration and necrosis of the gray and white matter with infiltrations of inflammatory cells. Neurons contain intranuclear and intracytoplasmic inclusion bodies. Nonsuppurative myocarditis was found in some piglets.

Morbidity and mortality

Menangle virus affected the reproductive potential and productivity of swine herds. Once infection was endemic in the herd, no further reproductive failures occur. No disease is observed in postnatal animals of any age.

During the 1997 outbreak, farrowing rates decreased from an expected 82% to as low as 38%. Additionally, the number of live piglets declined in 27% of litters. A total of 45% of sows farrowed litters with a reduced number of live piglets and an increased number of mummified and stillborn piglets. The mummified fetuses were of varying size, ranging upward in gestation age from 30 days.

Diagnosis

Clinical

The most notable clinical signs with Menangle infection would be an increased proportion of mummified and stillborn piglets and reduced litter size.

Differential diagnosis

The differential diagnosis includes classical swine fever, porcine reproductive and respiratory syndrome, porcine parvovirus, Aujesky's disease (pseudorabies), and blue eye (La Piedad Michoacan) paramyxovirus.

Laboratory tests

The most rapid method of testing for Menangle virus is by testing sows for the presence of specific antibody by virus neutralization or ELISA testing. Fetal specimens should be collected for virus isolation, serology and pathology. Virus can be isolated from brain, lung and myocardium of piglets. The virus does not hemagglutinate,

therefore definitive diagnosis depends on election microscopy and neutralization results with specific antiserum.

Samples to collect

Before collecting or sending any samples from animals with a suspected foreign animal disease, the proper authorities should be contacted. Samples should only be sent under secure conditions and to authorized laboratories to prevent the spread of the disease.

Two human infections of Menangle have been documented in persons closely associated with infected pigs. Precautions should be taken while working with this virus.

Menangle virus can be isolated from the brain, lung and myocardium of piglets. Serum from the farrowing sow should also be collected.

Recommended actions if Menangle is suspected

Notification of authorities

Menangle virus infections must be reported to state of federal authorities immediately upon diagnosis or suspicion of the disease.
Federal: Area Veterinarians in Charge (AVICs):
http://www.aphis.usda.gov/vs/area_offices.htm
State Veterinarians:
http://www.aphis.usda.gov/vs/sregs/official.html

Quarantine and disinfection

In areas with native fruit bat populations, prevention of contact between bats and pigs is essential. Flowering or fruiting trees should not be grown near pig farm buildings as they may attract bat activity. In an outbreak situation, infection will most likely have spread through the herd before the first affected litters are farrowed.

To eradicate the disease from an endemic population, pigs ages 10 to 16 weeks should be isolated or removed from the population (most pigs become infected at 12 to 16 weeks of age, after colostral immunity wanes) or the herd should be restocked with unexposed pigs or pigs known to be immune to the virus. Currently there is no vaccine for Menangle available.

Public health

During the 1997 Menangle outbreak, two humans in close contact with infected pigs developed influenza–like illness followed by the development of a macular rash. Both recovered after 10 to 14 days. People in close contact with infected pigs should take proper precautions since the route of transmission for pigs to humans is not know at this time.

For more information

Menangle virus, Australia, Emerging Disease Notice. U.S. Department of Agriculture – Animal and Plant Health Inspection Service – Center for Emerging Issues.
www.aphis.usda.gov/vs/ceah/cei/menangle.htm
Menangle virus. Commonwealth Scientific & Industrial Research Organisation – CSIROnline
www.csiro.au/index.asp?type=faq&id=Menangle
Australian bat Lyssavirus, Hendra virus and Menangle virus information for veterinary practitioners. Communicable Diseases Network Australia
www.health.gov.au/pubhlth/cdi/pubs/pdf/batsgen.pdf

References

Chant K, Chan R, Smith M, Dwyer DE, Kirkland P, et. al. Probable human infection with a newly described virus in the family Paramyxoviridae. *Emerging Infectious Diseases* 1998;4(2):273–275.

Kirkland PD, Daniels PW, Mohd Nor MN, Love RJ, Philbey AW, Ross AD. Menangle and Nipah virus infections of pigs. *Vet Clin of N Amer Prac Food Anim* 2002;18:557–571.

Kirkland PD, Love RJ, Philbey AW, Davis RJ, Hart KG. Epidemiology and control of Menangle virus in pigs. *Aust Vet J* 2001;79(3):199–206.

Love RJ, Philbey AW, Kirkland PD, Ross AD, Davis RJ, Morrissey C, Daniels PW. Reproductive disease and congenital malformations caused by Menangle virus in pigs. *Aust Vet J* 2001;79(3):192–198.

Philbey AW, Kirkland PD, Ross AD, Davis RJ, Gleeson AB, Love RJ, Daniels PW, Gould AR, Hyatt AD. An apparently new virus (Family Paramyxoviridae) infectious for pigs, humans and fruit bats. *Emerging Infectious Diseases* 1998;4(2):269–271.

Monkeypox

Importance

Monkeypox is a contagious viral disease of non-human primates, rodents and rabbits endemic to parts of Africa. The disease causes fever and cutaneous lesions in affected animals, and sometimes death. Monkeypox is zoonotic affecting humans in close contact with infected animals. An outbreak of monkeypox occurred in the United States in 2003 following the importation of exotic rodent species from Africa. This was the first report of the virus ever occurring in the Western Hemisphere. Due to the similarity of lesions to those of smallpox, a potential biological weapon, prompt detection and diagnosis is essential.

Etiology

Monkeypox results from infection by the monkeypox virus, an *Orthopoxvirus* related to the variola (smallpox), vaccinia, cowpox, buffalopox, and camelpox viruses. Some isolates of the monkeypox virus appear to differ in their virulence in non–human primates.

The monkeypox virus is also related to the tanapox virus, which causes Benign Epidermal Monkeypox (BEMP), an antigenically unrelated virus to vaccinia and smallpox.

Species affected

Old and New World monkeys and apes, a variety of rodents (including rats, mice, squirrels, and prairie dogs) and rabbits are susceptible to monkeypox infection. Approximately nine outbreaks have been documented in captive primates, mainly in rhesus macaques and cynomolgus monkeys. Infections have also been reported in languors, baboons, chimpanzees, orangutans, marmosets, gorillas, gibbons, owl–faced monkeys (*Cercopithecus hamlyn*), and squirrel monkeys. No cases have been reported in dogs or cats to date; however, the full host range is still unknown and these and other domestic species may be susceptible. Antibodies to the monkeypox virus have been found in a wide variety of nonhuman primates, rodents, and squirrels in Africa.

The natural reservoir(s) of the monkeypox virus remains to be established but is thought to be mainly rodents. Two species of African squirrels, *Funisciurus anerythrus* and *Heliosciurus rufobrachium*, have been suggested as possible reservoirs or vectors. It is not known whether primates also maintain the infection in the wild, or are only incidental hosts.

During the 2003 outbreak in the U.S., human cases resulted from exposure to infected pet prairie dogs. An imported exotic mammal, the Gambian giant rat, was thought to have transmitted the virus to prairie dogs. The U.S. government embargoed six genera of African rodents, including rope squirrels (*Funisciurus* sp.), tree squirrels (*Heliosciurus* sp.), Gambian giant rats, brushtail porcupines (*Atherurus* sp.), dormice (*Graphiurus* sp.), and striped mice (*Hybomys* sp.).

Geographic distribution

Monkeypox was first reported in the Democratic Republic of the Congo (DRC, formerly known as Zaire) in the 1970s. This disease is currently endemic only in Central and West Africa. In 2003, an outbreak of monkeypox occurred in the Midwestern United States. The U.S. cases occurred in pet prairie dogs and other small exotic mammals in captivity.

Transmission

The routes of transmission for monkeypox in animals are not clearly understood. The virus may be transmitted in aerosols, through skin abrasions, or by the ingestion of infected tissues.

Incubation period

In one study, experimentally infected cynomolgus monkeys developed symptoms 6 to 7 days after aerosol exposure to a lethal dose of virus. The U.S. Centers for Disease Control and Prevention (CDC) recommends that animals that have been exposed to monkeypox be quarantined for 6 weeks after exposure.

Clinical signs

Non–human primates

In non–human primates, monkeypox usually occurs as a self–limiting rash. The initial symptoms are fever and cutaneous papules (1-4 mm), which develop into pustules then crust over. A typical monkeypox lesion has a red, necrotic, depressed center, surrounded by epidermal hyperplasia. These "pocks" can be seen over the entire body, but may be more common on the face, limbs, palms, soles, and tail. The number of lesions varies from a few individual pocks to extensive, coalescing lesions. The crusts over the pustules eventually drop off, leaving small scars. In one outbreak in common marmosets, the skin lesions persisted for 4 to 6 weeks. Some animals have only skin lesions.

In more severe cases, coughing, nasal discharge, dyspnea, anorexia, facial edema, oral ulcers, or lymphadenopathy may also be seen. Disseminated disease, with visceral lesions, is uncommon in natural infections. Pneumonia is common only in monkeys infected experimentally by aerosol.

Most naturally infected animals recover; however, fatalities are sometimes seen, particularly in infant monkeys. Asymptomatic infections also occur.

BEMP, caused by tanapox, is characterized by epidermal pocks on the arms, face, and perineum of monkeys, without generalized illness.

Rabbits and rodents

In rabbits and rodents, including prairie dogs, the initial signs may include fever, conjunctivitis, nasal discharge, cough, lymphadenopathy, anorexia, and lethargy. Animals may then develop a nodular rash, pustules ("pocks"), or patchy alopecia. Pneumonia has also been seen. Monkeypox was fatal in some but not all infected animals during the 2003 outbreak in the U.S. Mild symptoms, with no respiratory signs and limited skin lesions, were seen in an infected Gambian giant rat.

During an outbreak, veterinarians should consider the possibility of monkeypox in sick prairie dogs or Gambian rats, or any animal with a history of fever, conjunctivitis, respiratory signs, and a nodular rash.

Post mortem lesions

Animals should be necropsied only by individuals who have a current smallpox vaccination, and the biological safety guidelines recommended by the CDC should be followed. [See the CDC's "Interim Guidance for Necropsy and Animal Specimen Collection for Laboratory Testing" at http://www.cdc.gov/ncidod/monkeypox/necropsy.htm]

Due to the risk of infection, the CDC recommends that practicing veterinarians avoid doing necropsies or biopsies on suspected cases. Pending necropsy, whole carcasses should be double–bagged and frozen.

At necropsy, the skin may contain papules, umbilicated pustules ("pocks") with central necrosis, or crusts over healing lesions. The skin lesions may vary from barely detectable, single small papules to extensive lesions. In some animals, visceral lesions may be seen, including multifocal necrotizing pneumonitis, orchitis, and peripheral lymphadenopathy.

Necropsy lesions have also been described in cynomolgus monkeys given a fatal aerosol dose of monkeypox. In addition to the typical skin lesions, bronchopneumonia was common. The lungs were heavy, congested, and failed to collapse and a dark red, lobular, mottled pattern of edema, atelectasis, and necrosis was seen throughout all of the lobes. In some cases, fibrinous pleuritis or a clear pericardial effusion was also present. Lymph node congestion, peripheral lymphadenopathy, facial exanthema, ulcerative cheilitis, gingivitis, papulovesicular pharyngitis, or ulcerative stomatitis occurred in some animals. The oral lesions, which were most common on the hard palate and the dorsal surface of the tongue, were described as variably sized, depressed, reddened foci of necrosis, erosion, or ulceration surrounded by pale tan to white, slightly raised margins. Some animals had gastritis or 2 to 3 mm raised lesions with umbilicated necrotic centers on the mucosa of the distal colon or rectum.

Morbidity and mortality

Sporadic cases of monkeypox occur in wild primates in Africa and approximately nine outbreaks have been reported in captive primates. In most of these outbreaks, the morbidity rate tended to be high and the mortality rate low; respiratory disease was uncommon and most animals recovered. More severe infections were seen in cynomolgus macaques, orangutans, and infants of all species, and deaths were seen mainly in infants. Experimental aerosol infections can result in more severe disease, an increased risk of pneumonia, and higher mortality rates in adult primates.

The morbidity and mortality rates are not well documented in rodents. In prairie dogs, some infections have been fatal while other animals recovered. A single known case in a Gambian giant rat during the U.S. outbreak was very mild. Infections may be particularly common among squirrels in Africa; many wild *Funisciurus anerythrus* and *Heliosciurus rufobrachium* squirrels have antibodies to monkeypox.

Diagnosis

Clinical

Monkeypox can be tentatively diagnosed if the characteristic skin lesions are present, or if other symptoms consistent with the disease are seen during an outbreak. These may include history of fever, conjunctivitis, respiratory signs and a nodular rash.

Differential diagnosis

Differentials for monkeypox in animal species may include tularemia and plague for rodents and various herpes viruses or simian varicella in non-human primates.

Laboratory tests

The diagnosis can be confirmed by histopathology and virus isolation. Polymerase chain reaction (PCR) tests can also detect monkeypox DNA in tissues. If the animal has not been exposed to other orthopoxviruses, virions can be detected with electron microscopy or orthopoxvirus antigens can be identified with immunohistochemistry. An ELISA test has been developed. Serology may also be helpful.

Samples to collect

Before collecting or sending any samples from animals with a suspected foreign animals disease, the proper authorities should be contacted. Samples should only be sent under secure conditions and to authorized laboratories to prevent the spread of the disease. Monkeypox is zoonotic; samples should be collected and handled with all appropriate precautions.

Serum, samples of skin lesions, and conjunctival swabs may be collected from live animals. At necropsy, tissues should be collected from all organs that have lesions. Minimally, samples of the lungs, lymph nodes, liver, spleen, kidneys, gonads, and any skin lesions should be collected. The tissues should be divided into two parts; half should be placed in 10% formalin and kept at room temperature, and the other half collected aseptically for virus isolation. Transport medium should not be used. The sample collected for virus isolation should be refrigerated if it will be shipped within 24 hours, or frozen if shipment will be delayed.

Tissues and other specimens must be packaged and shipped under secure conditions to prevent infections in humans and animals, and must comply with all local, state, and federal regulations.

Recommended actions if monkeypox is suspected
Notification of authorities

Cases of monkeypox should be reported immediately to state or federal authorities upon diagnosis or suspicion of the disease.
Federal: Area Veterinarians in Charge (AVICs):
http://www.aphis.usda.gov/vs/area_offices.htm
State Veterinarians:
http://www.aphis.usda.gov/vs/sregs/official.html

Quarantine and disinfection

The CDC recommends disinfection of contaminated surfaces with 0.5% sodium hypochlorite or other EPA–approved high–level disinfectants. Incineration or autoclaving is appropriate for some contaminated materials. Burial without decontamination is not recommended.

Public health

Monkeypox can affect humans in close contact with infected animal species. Transmission may occur from animal bites, aerosols, or by direct contact with lesions, blood, or body fluids. Person-to-person spread is rare but can occur following skin-to-skin contact, by aerosol, or on fomites. Monkeypox is less transmissible than smallpox.

In humans, symptoms may include fever, chills, headache, sore throat, myalgia, backache, fatigue and a nonproductive cough. Swelling of the lymph nodes may occur. Typically a vesicular and pustular rash develops on the skin, 1 to 10 days later, which will scab. In severe cases, respiratory complications or dyspnea may occur.

In Africa, the case-fatality rates ranged from 1% to 10%, however during the outbreak in the U.S. in 2003, no human fatalities were reported. Treatment is mainly supportive. The human smallpox vaccine is thought to help prevent monkeypox as well as decrease the severity of disease symptoms.

For more information

American Veterinary Medical Association Monkeypox Alert
http://www.avma.org/pubhlth/monkeypox/default.asp
Armed Forces Institute of Pathology - Monkeypox
http://www.afip.org/Departments/infectious/mp/index.html
Centers for Disease Control and Prevention (CDC).
Monkeypox Index
http://www.cdc.gov/ncidod/monkeypox/index.htm
Medical Microbiology
http://www.gsbs.utmb.edu/microbook
Center for Infectious Disease Research & Policy (CIDRAP).
University of Minnesota. Monkeypox
http://www.cidrap.umn.edu/cidrap/content/hot/monkeypox/index.html
Pathology of Nonhuman Primates from Primate Info Net.
Wisconsin Primate Research Center
http://www.primate.wisc.edu/pin/pola6–99.html

Primate Info Net. Wisconsin Primate Research Center
http://www.primate.wisc.edu/pin/

References

"Basic information about monkeypox." Centers for Disease Control and Prevention (CDC). June 2003. Accessed 27 June 2003 at http://www.cdc.gov/ncidod/monkeypox/factsheet.htm.

Baskin, G.B. "Pathology of nonhuman primates." Primate Info Net. Feb 2002 Wisconsin Primate Research Center. Accessed 27 June 2003 at http://www.primate.wisc.edu/pin/pola6–99.html.

Baxby, D. "Poxviruses." In *Medical Microbiology*. 4th ed. Edited by Samuel Baron. New York; Churchill Livingstone, 1996. Accessed 27 June 2003 at http://www.gsbs.utmb.edu/microbook/ch069.htm.

"Case I-952287 (AFIP 2554549)." *AFIP* Wednesday Slide Conference No. 14. Armed Forces Institute of Pathology. January 1997. Accessed 30 June 2003 at http://www.afip.org/vetpath/WSC/WSC96/96wsc14.htm.

Cohen, J. "Is an old virus up to new tricks?" *Science* 1997;277(5324):312–313.

"Considerations for selection and prioritization of animal specimens for laboratory testing." Centers for Disease Control and Prevention (CDC). June 2003. Accessed 30 June 2003 at http://www.cdc.gov/ncidod/monkeypox/labsubmissionguid.htm.

Gough A.W., N.J. Barsoum, S.I. Gracon, L. Mitchell and J.M. Sturgess. "Poxvirus infection in a colony of common marmosets (*Callithrix jacchus*). [Abstract]" *Lab. Anim. Sci.* 1982;32(1):87–90.

"Interim case definition for animal cases of monkeypox." Centers for Disease Control and Prevention (CDC). June 2003. Accessed 30 June 2003 at http://www.cdc.gov/ncidod/monkeypox/animalcasedefinition.htm.

"Interim guidance for necropsy and animal specimen collection for laboratory testing." Centers for Disease Control and Prevention (CDC). June 2003. Accessed 30 June 2003 at http://www.cdc.gov/ncidod/monkeypox/necropsy.htm.

Khodakevich L., M. Szczeniowski, J.Z. Manbu–ma–Disu, S. Marennikova, J. Nakano and D. Messinger. "The role of squirrels in sustaining monkeypox virus transmission." *Trop. Geogr. Med.* 1987;39(2): 115–22.

"Monkeypox." Department of Infectious and Parasitic Diseases. Armed Forces Institute of Pathology. July 2003. Accessed 1 July 2003 at http://www.afip.org/Departments/infectious/mp/index.html.

"Monkeypox." Laboratory Primate Newsletter, Brown University. (July 1997: vol 36 iss 3) Accessed 30 June 2003 at http://www.brown.edu/Research/Primate/lpn36–3.html#pox.

"Monkeypox backgrounder." American Veterinary Medical Association. June, 2003. Accessed 30 June 2003 at http://www.avma.org/pubhlth/monkeypox/default.asp.

"Monkeypox infections in animals: updated interim guidance for persons who have frequent contact with animals, including pet owners, pet shop employees, animal handlers, and animal control officers." Centers for Disease Control and Prevention (CDC). June 2003. Accessed 30 June 2003 at http://www.cdc.gov/ncidod/monkeypox/animalhandlers.htm.

"Monkeypox infections in animals: updated interim guidance for veterinarians." Centers for Disease Control and Prevention (CDC). June 2003. Accessed 30 June 2003 at http://www.cdc.gov/ncidod/monkeypox/animalguidance.htm.

"Multistate outbreak of monkeypox - Illinois, Indiana, and Wisconsin, 2003." *Morb. Mortal. Wkly. Rep.* 2003;52(23):537–540. Accessed 30 July 2003 at http://www.cdc.gov/mmwr/preview/mmwrhtml/mm5223a1.htm.

Rand, M.S. "Zoonotic diseases." Institutional Animal Care and Use Committee, University of California, Santa Barbara. Accessed 30 June 2003 at http://www.research.ucsb.edu/connect/pro/disease.html.

Schoeb, T.R. "Diseases of laboratory primates." Accessed 27 June 2003 at http://netvet.wustl.edu/species/primates/primate1.txt.

"Update: Multistate outbreak of monkeypox - Illinois, Indiana, Kansas, Missouri, Ohio, and Wisconsin, 2003." *Morb. Mortal. Wkly. Rep.* 2003;52(24):561–564. Accessed 30 June 2003 at http://www.cdc.gov/mmwr/preview/mmwrhtml/mm5224a1.htm.

"Update: Multistate outbreak of monkeypox - Illinois, Indiana, Kansas, Missouri, Ohio, and Wisconsin, 2003." *Morb. Mortal. Wkly. Rep.* 2003;52(25): 589–590. Accessed 30 June 2003 at http://www.cdc.gov/mmwr/preview/mmwrhtml/mm5225a4.htm.

"Updated interim CDC guidance for use of smallpox vaccine, cidofovir, and vaccinia immune globulin (VIG) for prevention and treatment in the setting of an outbreak of monkeypox infections." Centers for Disease Control and Prevention (CDC). June 2003. Accessed 30 June 2003 at http://www.cdc.gov/ncidod/monkeypox/treatmentguidelines.htm.

Zaucha G.M., P.B. Jahrling, T.W. Geisbert, J.R. Swearengen and L. Hensley. "The pathology of experimental aerosolized monkeypox virus infection in cynomolgus monkeys (*Macaca fascicularis*)." *Lab. Invest.* 2001;81:1581–1600. Accessed 30 June 2003 at http://labinvest.uscapjournals.org/cgi/content/full/81/12/1581.

Mycoplasmosis (Avian) (*Mycoplasma gallisepticum*)

Pleuropneumonia-like Organism (PPLO) Infection, Chronic Respiratory Disease, Infectious Sinusitis

Importance

Mycoplasma gallisepticum infections can cause significant economic losses on poultry farms from chronic respiratory disease, decreased growth, and decreased egg production. The carcasses of birds sent to slaughter may also be downgraded. An eradication program exists for *M. gallisepticum* in breeding flocks in the United States.

Etiology

Avian mycoplasmosis can be caused by several mycoplasmas (class Mollicutes, order Mycoplasmatales, family Mycoplasmataceae), including *Mycoplasma gallisepticum*, *M. synoviae*, *M. meleagridis,* and *M. iowae*. *M. gallisepticum* causes respiratory disease in poultry and game birds and conjunctivitis in house finches.

Species affected

Mycoplasma gallisepticum causes disease in chickens, turkeys, game birds including pheasants, chukar partridges and peafowl, and house finches.

Geographic distribution

M. gallisepticum can be found worldwide. In the United States, this organism is being eradicated from commercial chicken and turkey breeding stock.

Transmission

M. gallisepticum is transmitted by aerosols or close contact between birds and can be spread on fomites. It is also transmitted vertically; in some parts of the world, the organism is often introduced into flocks by infected eggs. Birds can carry *M. gallisepticum* asymptomatically until they are stressed. Infected birds carry the organism for life.

Incubation period

Experimentally infected birds develop symptoms after 6 to 21 days. In natural infections, the incubation period is variable; infected birds may be asymptomatic for days or months until stressed.

Clinical signs

Infected chickens may develop respiratory symptoms, including rales, coughing, sneezing, nasal discharge, frothiness around the eyes, or difficulty breathing. The severity of the symptoms varies; more severe infections are seen when the bird is infected concurrently with Newcastle disease virus, infectious bronchitis virus, *Escherichia coli* or other pathogens. Some chickens are asymptomatic. Turkeys usually experience more severe disease, often with swelling of the paranasal sinus. Production is decreased in turkeys, with lower weight gain, feed efficiency and egg production. Upper respiratory disease is seen in game birds and conjunctivitis in house finches.

Post mortem lesions

In uncomplicated cases in chickens, the lesions typically include mild sinusitis, tracheitis, and airsacculitis. If the chicken is infected concurrently with *Escherichia coli*, thickening and turbidity of the air sacs, exudative accumulations, fibrinopurulent pericarditis, and perihepatitis may be seen. In turkeys, severe mucopurulent sinusitis may be found, with variably severe tracheitis and airsacculitis.

Morbidity and mortality

In chickens with uncomplicated infections, the morbidity rate is high and the mortality rate low. If the birds are concurrently infected with other viruses or bacteria, the disease is more severe. Infections can also result in decreased productivity in the flock. Virus infections, vaccination with live viruses, cold weather, or crowding can trigger clinical disease in infected flocks.

M. gallisepticum infections can be treated with antibiotics, which decrease the clinical signs but do not eliminate the infection. A live vaccine is available; in some states, it can be used only with permission from the state veterinarian.

Diagnosis

Clinical

M. gallisepticum infections should be considered in poultry or game birds with upper respiratory disease and wild house finches with conjunctivitis.

Differential diagnosis

The differential diagnosis includes respiratory diseases such as Newcastle disease, infectious bronchitis, and avian influenza.

Laboratory tests

M. gallisepticum infections can be diagnosed by culturing the organism. The colonies are identified by indirect immunofluorescence, immunoperoxidase staining, a growth inhibition test, or polymerase chain reaction (PCR). Animal inoculation, using mycoplasma–free chicken embryos or chickens, is sometimes necessary to isolate the organism. PCR–based assays can detect *M. gallisepticum* DNA directly in infected tissues or exudates.

Serology can be used for diagnosis and is particularly helpful in screening flocks. Commonly used assays include a rapid serum agglutination (RSA) test, enzyme–linked immunosorbent assays (ELISAs), and hemagglutination inhibition. Other tests, including radioimmunoassay, microimmunofluorescence, and indirect immunoprecipitation assays, may be available. Nonspecific reactions are common in serologic tests.

Samples to collect

Swabs should be collected from affected organs, tissues, and exudates for mycoplasma culture. The samples can be taken from live birds, recently dead animals, or carcasses frozen soon after death. In live animals, swabs can be taken from the choanal cleft, oropharynx, esophagus, trachea, cloaca, and phallus. At necropsy, samples can be collected from the air sacs, trachea, nasal cavity, and infraorbital sinus. *M. gallisepticum* can also be cultured from tissue homogenates, embryos, yolk from the egg, or aspirates from the infraorbital sinuses or joint cavities.

Tissues or swab samples can be transported in mycoplasma broth. Samples should be transported to the laboratory as soon as possible and kept chilled with an ice pack.

Recommended actions if *Mycoplasma gallisepticum* infection is suspected

Notification of authorities

Mycoplasma gallisepticum infections are reportable in some states; state requirements should be consulted for more specific information.

Federal: Area Veterinarians in Charge (AVICs):
http://www.aphis.usda.gov/vs/area_offices.htm
State Veterinarians:
http://www.aphis.usda.gov/vs/sregs/official.html

Quarantine and disinfection

Infections can be eliminated from a farm by depopulation of the flock, followed by thorough cleaning and disinfection of the premises. Recommended disinfectants for buildings and equipment include phenolic or cresylic acid disinfectants, hypochlorite, and 0.1% glutaraldehyde. Birds should not be re–introduced for two weeks.

M. gallisepticum–negative breeding stock can be maintained by serologic testing. Heat treatment or tylosin can eliminate egg transmission from valuable breeding animals.

Public health

Mycoplasma gallisepticum does not appear to be zoonotic.

For more information

World Organization for Animal Health (OIE)
http://www.oie.int
OIE Manual of Standards
http://www.oie.int/eng/normes/mmanual/a_summry.htm
OIE International Animal Health Code
http://www.oie.int/eng/normes/mcode/A_summry.htm
The Merck Veterinary Manual
http://www.merckvetmanual.com/mvm/index.jsp
Mycoplasma gallisepticum Infection and Prevention Avian Research Center, University of Minnesota
http://www.cvm.umn.edu/avian/SFPC/*Mycoplasma*.html

References

Avian Mycoplasmosis (*Mycoplasma gallisepticum*) In *Manual of Standards for Diagnostic Tests and Vaccines*. Paris: Office International des Epizooties, 2000. 10 March 2003. http//www.oie.int/eng/normes/mmanual/A_00089.htm.

Bokhari, S.A. *Mycoplasma gallisepticum* infection and prevention. Avian Research Center, University of Minnesota. 17 March 2003. http://www.cvm.umn.edu/avian/SFPC/Mycoplasma.html.

"*Mycoplasma gallisepticum* infection." In *The Merck Veterinary Manual*, 8th ed. Edited by S.E. Aiello and A. Mays. Whitehouse Station, NJ: Merck and Co., 1998, p. 1928–1929.

Nairobi Sheep Disease

Importance

Nairobi sheep disease is one of the most pathogenic diseases of sheep and goats. In susceptible animals, this virus infection results in a hemorrhagic gastroenteritis with very high morbidity and mortality. There is no effective treatment.

Etiology

Nairobi sheep disease results from infection by a tick–borne virus, Nairobi sheep disease virus (NSDV), in the genus *Nairovirus* (family Bunyaviridae).

Species affected

Among domestic and laboratory animals, only sheep and goats can be readily infected by NSDV. The African field rat (*Arvicathus abysinicus nubilans*) is a potential reservoir host.

Geographic distribution

Nairobi sheep disease is found mainly in east Africa. Infected animals have been reported in Kenya, Uganda, Tanzania, Somalia, and Harar Province of Ethiopia. A similar disease called Kisenyi sheep disease is found in the Republic of the Congo.

Transmission

NSDV is transmitted mainly through the bite of the brown tick, *Rhipicephalus appendiculatus*. The virus can be maintained in this host by transovarial passage, and unfed adult ticks can transmit NDSV for more than two years after infection. *R. pulchellus* in Somalia and the African bont tick *Amblyomma variegatum* in Kenya may also transmit NSDV.

Under natural conditions, this virus is not transmitted by contact with an infected animal. Animals can be infected experimentally with inoculations of infectious blood, serum, and organ suspensions. Experimental infections may also be possible with large oral doses (50 cc) of infected blood or serum.

Incubation period

After transmission through the bite of a tick, the incubation period is 4 to 15 days. Experimental inoculations result in clinical signs after 1 to 3 days.

Clinical signs

NSDV causes an acute hemorrhagic gastroenteritis. The disease begins with a fever of 40° -41°C (104°-106°F), leukopenia, and profound depression, followed by diarrhea and a concomitant drop in body temperature. At the onset, the feces are thin and watery; later, blood and mucus may appear. Other symptoms include an abundant bloodstained mucopurulent nasal discharge, conjunctivitis, hyperventilation, and anorexia. The superficial lymph nodes may be palpable. Animals with less acute signs may be anorexic, weak, and recumbent with signs of diarrhea. Abortions are common. Hyperacute infections are characterized by a sudden fever, followed by a temperature decline and fatal collapse. In some cases, death may occur within 12 hours after the onset of the fever.

Post mortem lesions

Nairobi sheep disease can be difficult to identify from post–mortem lesions. Early in the course of infection, the only abnormalities noted may be lymphadenitis with ecchymotic and petechial hemorrhages on the serosa of the gastrointestinal tract, spleen, heart, and other organs. In animals that survive longer, evidence of hemorrhagic gastroenteritis becomes more apparent. Typically, the intestinal contents are bloodstained. Hyperemia and petechial hemorrhages may be found on the mucosa of the abomasum, cecum, rectum, and around the ileocecal valve. Zebra striping of the rectum may be seen. Generalized hyperplasia of the lymphoid tissue is common. The lymph nodes are enlarged and edematous, and the spleen may be swollen and filled with blood. In groups of pregnant ewes, an aborted fetus with hemorrhages throughout its organs may be found. The genital tract may be hyperemic and the fetal membranes may be swollen, edematous, and hemorrhagic. In addition, nonspecific congestion and petechial and ecchymotic hemorrhages can be found in most organs and tissues.

Morbidity and mortality

Sheep and goats in endemic regions are often immune to NSDV. The most severe infections develop in susceptible animals moved into an endemic area. In non–endemic regions, outbreaks often follow high rainfall and the appearance of ticks.

In animals showing clinical signs, the prognosis is generally poor. Mild infections occur in some susceptible animals, but the mortality rate usually ranges from 40% to 90%. Mortality varies with the breed. The death rate is approximately 40% in Merino and Merino crossbreds, and much higher in Masai sheep. Supportive treatment with good shelter and quality feed may improve survival.

Diagnosis

Clinical

Nairobi sheep disease should be suspected in recently introduced sheep or goats with severe gastroenteritis and nasal discharge in an endemic area. The diagnosis is particularly likely if sheep native to the area do not become ill, and if the incidence of disease is high in sheep, low in goats, and absent in cattle and other animals.

Differential diagnosis

Other diseases that may resemble Nairobi sheep disease include heartwater, Rift Valley fever, anthrax, some types of plant and heavy metal poisoning, peste des petits ruminants, and coccidiosis.

Laboratory tests

The Nairobi sheep disease virus can be isolated by inoculating laboratory animals or cell cultures with organ or plasma samples. The test animals of choice are suckling mice inoculated intracerebrally or laboratory–raised sheep. The recommended cells are lamb kidney cell cultures, hamster kidney cell cultures, or a baby hamster kidney cell line. The virus can also be identified in tissue samples by agar gel immunodiffusion.

Antibodies to NSDV can be identified with an indirect fluorescent antibody test. Other serological tests include immunodiffusion, complement fixation, hemagglutination, and ELISA. Virus neutralization tests are unreliable for NSDV.

Samples to collect

Before collecting or sending any samples from animals with a suspected foreign animal disease, the proper authorities should be contacted. Samples should only be sent under secure conditions and to authorized laboratories to prevent the spread of the disease. Rare cases of an influenza–like disease have been seen in humans; investigators should take precautions against aerosol infections when working with this virus.

Uncoagulated blood should be collected from live animals, and mesenteric lymph nodes and spleen from dead animals. During the initial fever, NSDV can be isolated from heparinized blood; however, little or no virus can be found in the blood after the body temperature falls. During this later stage, virus can be found in the spleen or mesenteric lymph nodes. Serum samples, preferably paired specimens, should also be submitted for serology.

Recommended actions if Nairobi sheep disease is suspected

Notification of authorities

Nairobi sheep disease must be reported to state or federal authorities immediately upon diagnosis or suspicion of the disease.

Federal: Area Veterinarians in Charge (AVICs):
  http://www.aphis.usda.gov/vs/area_offices.htm
State Veterinarians:
  http://www.aphis.usda.gov/vs/sregs/official.html

Quarantine and disinfection

Sheep and goats can be protected from the vector by dipping and spraying with an acaricide. Hypochlorite or phenolic disinfectants are effective decontaminants for the Bunyaviridae.

In endemic areas strict quarantine is not necessary, as the infection is not transmitted by contact. In these regions, dead animals should be disposed of by burial or incineration.

Public health

NSDV appears to cause a rare, mild, influenza–like disease in humans. At least one naturally acquired infection has been reported in Uganda. Investigators should take precautions against aerosol infections when working with this virus.

For more information

World Organization for Animal Health (OIE)
  http://www.oie.int
OIE Manual of Standards
  http://www.oie.int/eng/normes/mmanual/a_summry.htm
OIE International Animal Health Code
  http://www.oie.int/eng/normes/mcode/A_summry.htm
USAHA Foreign Animal Diseases Book
  http://www.vet.uga.edu/vpp/gray_book/FAD/

References

Groocock, C.M. "Nairobi Sheep Disease." In *Foreign Animal Diseases*. Richmond, VA: United States Animal Health Association, 1998, pp. 322–331.

"Medical Management Guidelines. Viral Hemorrhagic Fevers – Medical Management." 22 May 2001. Arizona Department of Health. 29 Aug 2001 http://www.hs.state.az.us/phs/edc/edrp/es/viralhfeversm.htm.

"Nairobi Sheep Disease." In *Manual of Standards for Diagnostic Tests and Vaccines*. Paris: World Organization for Animal Health, 2000, pp. 868–872.

"Nairobi Sheep Disease." In *The Merck Veterinary Manual*, 8th ed. Edited by S.E. Aiello and A. Mays. Whitehouse Station, NJ: Merck and Co., 1998, pp. 536.

Newcastle Disease

Exotic Newcastle Disease, Asiatic Newcastle Disease, Velogenic Newcastle Disease, Avian Pneumoencephalitis

Importance

Newcastle disease viruses produce a wide range of clinical signs in avian species, from mild to severe. Exotic Newcastle disease (END), the most severe form with neurologic and gastrointestinal signs, is not endemic in the United States. Frequent outbreaks do occur in the U.S. due to illegal importation of exotic birds. The disease is highly contagious and can have high mortality rates. Chickens are highly susceptible and economic losses can be significant.

Etiology

Newcastle disease viruses are classified in the serotype group avian paramyxovirus type 1 (APMV–1) in the genus *Rubulavirus*, family Paramyxoviridae. There are 9 avian paramyxovirus serotypes designated APMV–I to APMV–9.

Species affected

Many avian species are affected by Newcastle disease viruses. Of poultry, chickens are the most susceptible, ducks and geese are the least. Inapparent infections and carrier states can occur in psittacine and some wild bird populations.

Geographic distribution

Exotic Newcastle disease is endemic in many parts of the world including countries in Asia, the Middle East, Africa, and Central and South America. Some countries in Europe are free of the disease. The United States and Canada have seen high mortality in wild cormorants caused by END. There was an outbreak of END in the U.S. in southern California in 2002 and parts of Arizona, Nevada, Texas, and New Mexico in 2003.

Transmission

Transmission can occur by direct contact with feces and respiratory discharges or by contamination of the environment including food, water, equipment, and human clothing. Newcastle disease viruses can survive for long periods in the environment, especially in feces. Generally, virus is shed during the incubation period and for a short time during recovery. Some psittacine species can shed the virus intermittently for a year or more. Virus is present in all parts of the carcass of an infected bird.

Incubation period

The incubation period for Newcastle disease can vary from 2 to 15 days depending on the virulence of the strain and the susceptibility of the population. In chickens with the velogenic form, an incubation period of 2 to 6 days is common.

Clinical signs

Newcastle disease virus strains used to be grouped into pathotypes based on their clinical signs and virulence. These pathotypes included: asymptomatic enteric, which is generally subclinical; lentogenic or respiratory, which has mild or subclinical respiratory signs; mesogenic, which has respiratory and occasional neurologic signs with low mortality; and velogenic, which is the most virulent pathotype with high mortality rates. The velogenic pathotype is divided into a neurotropic form, which has respiratory and neurologic signs, and a viscerotropic form with hemorrhagic intestinal lesions. This classification is not always clear–cut and many strains have varied manifestations in different birds. In addition, less pathogenic strains can produce severe clinical signs depending on secondary infections or environmental factors.

The OIE provides a clearer definition for the reporting of any case of Exotic Newcastle as: "Newcastle disease is defined as an infection of birds caused by a virus of avian paramyxovirus serotype 1 (APMV–1) that meets one of the following criteria for virulence:
  a. The virus has an intracerebral pathogenicity index (ICPI) in day–old chicks (*Gallus gallus*) of 0.7 or greater.
  Or,
  b. Multiple basic amino acids have been demonstrated in the virus (either directly or by deduction) at the C–terminus of the F2 protein and phenylalanine at residue 117, which is the N–terminus of the F1 protein. The term 'multiple basic amino acids' refers to at least three arginine or lysine residues between residues 113 and 116. Failure to demonstrate the characteristic pattern of amino acid residues as described above would require characterization of the isolated virus by an ICPI test."

Clinical signs that can be seen with END, particularly in chicken flocks, include an initial drop in egg production followed by numerous deaths within 24 to 43 hours. Deaths in the flock may continue for 7 to 10 days. Birds that survive for 12 to 14 days usually live but may have permanent neurological damage including paralysis, and reproductive damage causing decreased egg production. Viscerotropic strains may cause edema and hemorrhages of the head, especially around the eyes (1, 2), and dark green watery diarrhea. Respiratory and neurological signs can also be seen, though these are not as severe as with the neurotropic form. The neurotropic strains cause respiratory signs of gasping and coughing followed by neurological signs which may include muscle tremors, drooping wings, dragging legs, twisting of the head and neck, circling, depression, inappetence, or complete paralysis. There is generally no diarrhea with the neurotropic form. Clinical signs associated with the various strains can be different in species other than chickens. Psittacines and pigeons may show neurologic signs when infected with the viscerotropic strain. Finches and canaries may show no signs of disease at all. Vaccinated birds will have less severe signs.

Post mortem lesions

There are no specific diagnostic post mortem lesions seen with Newcastle disease. A tentative diagnosis can be made with the examination of several carcasses. Gross lesions can be very similar to those of highly pathogenic avian influenza; therefore, laboratory isolation and identification is important in definitive diagnosis. Lesions may include edema of the interstitial tissue of the neck, especially near the thoracic inlet, and congestion and sometimes hemorrhages on the tracheal mucosa. Petechiae and small ecchymoses and/or foci of necrosis may be found on the mucosa of the proventriculus, especially around the orifices of the mucous glands. Additional lesions may include edema, hemorrhages, necrosis, or ulceration of lymphoid tissue in the intestinal mucosa and submucosa (including Peyer's patches), as well as edema, hemorrhages, or degeneration of the ovaries.

Morbidity and mortality

Morbidity and mortality rates can vary greatly depending on the virulence of the virus strain and susceptibility of the host. Environmental conditions, secondary infections, vaccination history, and host species all affect these rates. In chickens, morbidity can be up to 100% with 90% mortality. In other species such as finches and canaries, clinical signs may not be present.

Diagnosis

Clinical

Newcastle disease may be suspected, especially in chicken flocks, with a sudden decrease in egg production, high morbidity and mortality, and the characteristic signs and gross lesions; however, due to the wide variety of signs and similarities to other avian diseases, particularly fowl cholera and highly pathogenic avian influenza, definitive diagnosis requires virus isolation and identification in the laboratory.

Differential diagnosis

Differentials include fowl cholera, highly pathogenic avian influenza, laryngotracheitis, coryza, fowl pox (diphtheritic form), psittacosis (chlamydiosis in psittacine birds), mycoplasmosis, infectious bronchitis, Pacheco's disease (seen in psittacine birds), as well as management problems such as deprivation of water, feed or poor ventilation.

Laboratory tests

Samples for virus isolation are inoculated into 9–11 day old embryonated chicken eggs. Chorioallantoic fluid of dead embryos can then be tested for hemagglutination activity and hemagglutination–inhibition. Further tests may be performed to determine pathogenicity and virus strain. Tests available for serology include hemagglutination–inhibition and enzyme–linked immunosorbent assay (ELISA). Vaccination and previous exposure to disease may affect serology results.

Samples to collect

Before collecting or sending any samples from animals with a suspected foreign animal disease, the proper authorities should be contacted. Samples should only be sent under secure conditions and to authorized laboratories to prevent the spread of the disease. Newcastle disease is zoonotic; samples should be collected and handled with all appropriate precautions.

Swabs can be taken for virus isolation from the trachea and cloaca of live birds, or tissue samples from dead birds including trachea, lung, spleen, cloaca and brain. Feces can also be used for culture. Cell culture broth such as brain and heart infusion broth with high levels of antibiotics should be used for transport. Samples may be pooled in one broth tube if multiple animals are to be tested. Culture tubes should be kept on ice if they will reach the laboratory within 24 hours; otherwise the samples should be quick–frozen and not allowed to thaw during transport. Clotted blood or serum samples can be submitted for serology.

Recommended actions if Newcastle Disease is suspected
Notification of authorities

State and federal veterinarians should be immediately informed of any suspected cases of Newcastle disease.

Federal: Area Veterinarians in Charge (AVICs):
http://www.aphis.usda.gov/vs/area_offices.htm
State Veterinarians:
http://www.aphis.usda.gov/vs/sregs/official.html

Quarantine and disinfection

Recommendations for the control and eradication of Newcastle disease include strict quarantine, slaughter and disposal of all infected and exposed birds, and disinfection of the premises. The reintroduction of new birds should be delayed for 30 days. Pests such as insects and mice should be controlled, human traffic should be limited, and the introduction of new animals with unknown health status should be avoided. Vaccines are available, though they may interfere with testing. Effective disinfectants include the cresylics and phenolics.

Public health

People can be infected with velogenic Newcastle disease and show signs of conjunctivitis which resolve quickly, with virus shed in the ocular discharges for 4 to 7 days. Infected individuals should avoid direct and indirect contact with avian species during this time. Laboratory workers and vaccination crews are most at risk, with poultry workers rarely being infected. No known infections have occurred from handling or consuming poultry products.

For more information

World Organization for Animal Health (OIE)
http://www.oie.int
OIE Manual of Standards
http://www.oie.int/eng/normes/mmanual/a_summry.htm
OIE International Animal Health Code
http://www.oie.int/eng/normes/mcode/A_summry.htm
USAHA Foreign Animal Diseases Book
http://www.vet.uga.edu/vpp/gray_book/FAD/

References

"Newcastle Disease." In *Manual of Standards for Diagnostic Tests and Vaccines*. Paris: World Organization for Animal Health, 2000, pp. 221–232.

"Newcastle Disease." In *The Merck Veterinary Manual*, 8th ed. Edited by S.E. Aiello and A. Mays. Whitehouse Station, NJ: Merck and Co., 1998, pp. 1941–1942.

Beard, Charles W. "Velogenic Newcastle Disease." In *Foreign Animal Diseases*. Richmond, VA: United States Animal Health Association, 1998, pp. 396–405.

"Newcastle Disease." 30 Aug. 2000. World Organization for Animal Health. 16 Oct. 2001. http//www.oie.int/eng/maladies/fiches/a_A060.htm.

Nipah

Porcine Respiratory and Encephalitis Syndrome (PRES), Porcine Respiratory and Neurologic Syndrome, Barking Pig Syndrome, Hendra-like virus

Importance

Nipah virus infection is an emerging new disease, first described during a 1998–1999 epidemic in Malaysia and Singapore. Outbreaks in Bangladesh in 2001, 2003, 2004 and 2005 affected humans but not domestic animals. Although mortality appears to be low in pigs, the virus can spread readily from pigs to humans and other animals, with serious consequences. Infected humans may develop serious and often fatal encephalitis. Epidemics of Nipah can also result in serious economic losses to pig farmers; the outbreak in Malaysia was only controlled after more than 1 million pigs were culled. The reservoir of the virus appears to exist in asymptomatic fruit bats.

Etiology

Nipah virus is a previously unknown virus. It has been placed in a new genus, Henipavirus, in the family Paramyxoviridae. Antibodies to the Nipah virus cross–react with the Hendra virus.

Species affected

Nipah virus infections or antibodies have been seen in pigs, humans, dogs, cats, horses, and goats. Virus antigens were found in one case of meningitis in a horse. Sheep may also be affected. Fruit bats (flying foxes) are thought to be natural hosts for this virus.

Geographic distribution

Nipah virus infections have been reported in Malaysia, Singapore, Bangladesh and India. In Malaysia, cases occurred in swine and humans in close contact with swine. Cases in Singapore occurred among abattoir workers in contact with pigs imported from Malaysia. In Bangladesh and India only human cases were reported.

On the basis of known infections, this virus should be considered to be endemic in Southeast Asia. The probable reservoir host, the fruit bat of the genus *Pteropus* (also known as the 'flying fox'), is found in Malaysia, Australia, Indonesia, the Philippines, and some of the Pacific Islands. The virus has also been isolated from bats in Cambodia.

Transmission

Most infections are thought to occur after close direct contact with the excretions or secretions from an infected pig. Infections spread readily from infected pigs to other species. Human to human transmission has been suggested following the Bangladesh outbreak. Transmission from horses to humans seem to be rare.

Nipah virus or its antigens have been found in the lungs, upper and lower airways, central nervous system, and kidneys. Virus excretion through oral–nasal routes has been proven. Experimentally, pigs can be infected by oral or parental inoculation. Aerosol spread does not appear to be a major route, although respiratory infection may occur. Transmission may also be possible in the semen and by fomites such as contaminated needles or equipment. Animals are infectious during the incubation period.

Fruit bats are thought to be the reservoir host; infections in this species are common and appear to be asymptomatic.

Incubation period

The incubation period in pigs is estimated to be 7 to 14 days, but may be as short as 4 days.

Clinical signs

In pigs, asymptomatic infections appear to be common. Symptomatic infections are usually acute febrile illnesses, but fulminating infections and sudden death have also been seen. In general, mortality is low except in young piglets.

In pigs from 4 weeks to 6 months old, respiratory symptoms appear to be more common than neurologic signs. In this age group, common symptoms include fever, open mouth breathing, rapid and labored respiration, and a loud barking cough. Neurologic signs are sometimes seen and can include trembling, twitches, muscle spasms, myoclonus, weakness in the hind legs, spastic paresis, lameness, an uncoordinated gait when driven or hurried, and generalized pain that is particularly evident in the hind quarters.

Similar symptoms are seen in sows and boars, but neurologic disease appears to be more common. The neurological signs may include agitation, head pressing, nystagmus, chomping of the mouth, tetanus–like spasms, seizures, and apparent pharyngeal muscle paralysis. Increased salivation and nasal discharge, and possible first trimester abortion have also been reported.

In piglets, common clinical signs include open mouth breathing, leg weakness with muscle tremors, and twitching.

An unproductive cough, poor growth, severe respiratory signs, and death have been seen in goats. The symptoms in dogs are similar to those seen in pigs.

Post mortem lesions

Mild to severe lung lesions can be found in most symptomatic pigs. These lesions may include varying degrees of consolidation, petechial or ecchymotic hemorrhages, and emphysema. On cut surface, the interlobular septa may be distended. The bronchi and trachea may contain frothy, sometimes bloodstained, fluid. In the brain, generalized congestion and edema has been seen. Petechial hemorrhages were noted in one case. The kidneys may be congested, but are often normal. No lesions have been seen in other internal organs.

In dogs, the lesions may include hemorrhages and congestion in the kidneys and exudates in the bronchi and trachea.

Morbidity and mortality

In Malaysia, Nipah virus appeared to be present mainly in pigs. Prior to depopulation, antibodies to the virus were found in approximately 5.6% of all pig farms. In contrast, only 5 horses out of more than 3200 were positive by serology. No signs of current infection were seen in 2 necropsied horses; however, virus antigens were found in a horse that had died with symptoms of meningitis in 1998.

In pigs older than 4 weeks, morbidity appears to be high but mortality low. In the Malaysian outbreak, morbidity in pigs from 4 weeks to 6 months old approached 100% but mortality ranged from less than 1% to 5%. The mortality rate was approximately 40% in piglets; however, neglect by ill sows may have contributed to the high death rate. Infections in swine were not reported during the Bangledesh outbreaks.

Diagnosis

Clinical

The symptoms of Nipah virus infections are not dramatically different from other respiratory and neurologic illnesses of pigs. The unusual loud, barking cough or the presence of human cases of encephalitis may raise the index of suspicion.

Differential diagnosis

Nipah virus infections must be differentiated from Japanese encephalitis. Other respiratory or neurologic syndromes of pigs must also be ruled out.

Laboratory tests

Infections can be diagnosed by a serum neutralization test, a polymerase chain reaction (PCR) assay, and virus isolation. Nipah virus can be isolated in several cell lines including African green monkey kidney (Vero), baby hamster kidney (BHK), and porcine spleen (PS) cells. An enzyme linked immunosorbent assay (ELISA) is available for serologic testing in Malaysia.

All procedures should be carried out in a biosafety level 4 (BSL–4) laboratory

Samples to collect

Before collecting or sending any samples from animals with a suspected foreign animal disease, the proper authorities should be contacted. Samples should only be sent under secure conditions and to authorized laboratories to prevent the spread of the disease. Nipah is a zoonotic disease; samples should be collected and handled with all appropriate precautions.

Nipah virus or its antigens have been found in the lungs, upper and lower airways, central nervous system, and kidneys. In the Malaysian outbreak, samples of the lungs, kidneys, spleen, liver, heart, and brain were collected. Serum should also be collected for serology.

Recommended actions if Nipah virus infection is suspected

Notification of authorities

Nipah virus infections must be reported to state or federal authorities immediately upon diagnosis or suspicion of the disease.

Federal Area Veterinarians in Charge (AVIC)
http://www.aphis.usda.gov/vs/area_offices.htm
State Veterinarians
http://www.aphis.usda.gov/vs/sregs/official.html

Quarantine and disinfection

Nipah virus is contagious and appears to be easily spread by contact from pigs. Infections may also be spread between farms by fomites and possibly infected dogs or cats. The epidemic in Malaysia was controlled by mass culling of seropositive animals. This virus has been classified as a Hazard Group 4 pathogen; infected animals and blood and tissue samples must be handled with appropriate biosecurity precautions.

Nipah virus is readily inactivated by detergents; routine cleaning and disinfection with sodium hypochlorite, Betadine®, Virkon®, or Lysol® is expected to be effective. Sodium hypochlorite has been recommended for disinfection of pig farms in Malaysia. For spills, disinfection with 10,000 ppm chlorine is recommended.

Public health

Human infections range from asymptomatic to fatal infections. Reported symptoms are flu–like and may include fever, severe headaches, myalgia, a sore throat, disorientation, dizziness, drowsiness, or other signs of encephalitis or meningitis. During the 1998–1999 epidemic in Malaysia, 265 cases of suspected Nipah virus infection were seen in humans; 105 cases were fatal. Most cases occurred in pig farmers or others who had contact with swine.

Small outbreaks occurred in Bangladesh in 2001, 2003, 2004 and 2005. There were no links to pigs during these outbreaks, and the source of the virus transmission to humans is unknown. The Bangladesh outbreaks had an overall mortality rate greater than 60%. An outbreak of encephalitis in 2001 in Siliguri, India was suspected, and later confirmed by the Centers for Disease Control and Prevention, as Nipah virus.

Humans in contact with animals from endemic areas should wear protective clothing, including gloves, disposable gowns, and a face visor. Nipah virus is classified as a Hazard Group 4 pathogen.

For more information

World Organization for Animal Health (OIE)
http://www.oie.int
OIE International Animal Health Code
http://www.oie.int/eng/normes/mcode/A_summry.htm
Nipah Virus, Malaysia, May 1999. Emerging Disease Notice. Center for Emerging Issues, Centers for Epidemiology and Animal Health, and Animal and Plant Health Inspection Service, USDA
http://www.aphis.usda.gov:80/vs/ceah/cei/nipah.htm
Emerging Disease Notice Update. Nipah Virus, Malaysia, November 1999. Center for Emerging Issues, Centers for Epidemiology and Animal Health, and Animal and Plant Health Inspection Service, USDA
http://www.aphis.usda.gov:80/vs/ceah/cei/nipahupd.htm
Hendra Virus and Nipah Virus. Management and Control. Department of Health Social Services, and Public Safety U.K. http://www.doh.gov.uk/hendra_nipah
The Henipavirus Ecology Collaborative Research Group http://www.henipavirus.net

References

Chua, K.B., W.J. Bellini, P.A. Rota et al. "Nipah Virus: A Recently Emergent Deadly Paramyxovirus." *Science* 2000;288:1432–1435.

"Emerging Disease Notice Update. Nipah Virus, Malaysia, November 1999." Center for Emerging Issues, Centers for Epidemiology and Animal Health, USDA APHIS. Accessed 12 November 2001 at http://www.aphis.usda.gov:80/vs/ceah/cei/nipahupd.htm.

"Hendra Virus and Nipah Virus. Management and Control." September 2000 Department of Health Social Services, and Public Safety U.K. Accessed 12 November 2001 at http://www.doh.gov.uk/hendra_nipah.

Hooper, P.T. and M.M. Williamson. Hendra and Nipah Virus Infections. *Emerg Inf Dis* 2000;16(3):597–603.

Hsu VP, Hossain MJ, Parashar UD, Ali MM, Ksiazek TG, Kuzmin I, Niezgoda M, Rupprecht C, Bresee J, Breiman RF. "Nipah virus encephalitis reemergence, Bangladesh." *Emerg Infect Dis* 2004;10:2082-2087.

Mackenzie, J.S., K.B. Chua, P.W. Daniels, B.T. Eaton, H.E. Field, R.A. Hall, K. Halpin, C.A. Johansen, P.D. Kirkland, S.K. Lam, P. McMinn, D.J. Nisbet, R. Paru, A.T. Pyke, S.A. Ritchie, P. Siba, D.W. Smith, G.A. Smith, A.F. van den Hurk, L.F. Wang, and D.T. Williams. Emerging viral diseases of Southeast Asia and the Western Pacific. *Emerg Inf Dis* 2001:7(3):Supplement. Accessed 12 November 2001 at http://www.cdc.gov/ncidod/eid/vol7no3_supp/mackenzie.htm.

"Malaysian Outbreak of Nipah virus in people and swine." California Department of Food and Agriculture. Accessed 12 November 2001 at http://www.cdfa.ca.gov/ahfss/ah/pdfs/nipah.pdf.

Mohd Nor M.N, C.H. Gan, and B.L. Ong. "Nipah virus infection of pigs in Peninsular Malaysia." *Rev Sci Tech Off Int Epiz* 2000;19(1):160–165. Accessed 12 November 2001 at http://agrolink.moa.my/jph/dvs/nipah/oie990808.html.

"Nipah-like virus in Bangladesh. 12 February 2004." World Health Organization. Accessed at http://www.who.int/csr/don/2004_02_12/en/index.html.

"Nipah-like virus in Bangladesh-update 26 February 2004." World Health Organization. Accessed at http://www.who.int/csr/don/2004_02_26/en/index.html.

Chadha MS, Comer JA, Lowe L, Rota PA, Rollin PE, Bellini WJ, Ksiazek TG, Mishra AC. "Nipah virus-associated encephalitis outbreak, Siliguri, India." *Emerg Infect Dis* 2006;12(2):235-240.

"Nipah virus in Bangladesh. 20 April 2004." World Health Organization. Accessed at http://www.who.int/csr/don/2004_04_20/en/index.html.

"Nipah virus, Malaysia, May 1999. Emerging Disease Notice." Center for Emerging Issues, Centers for Epidemiology and Animal Health. Accessed 12 November 2001 at http://www.aphis.usda.gov:80/vs/ceah/cei/nipah.htm.

Reynes JM, Counor D, Ong S, Faure C, Seng V, Molia S, Walston J, Georges-Courbot MC, Deubel V, Sarthou JL. "Nipah virus in Lyle's flying foxes, Cambodia." *Emerg Infect Dis* 2005;11:1042-1047.

Uppal, P.K. "Emergence of Nipah virus in Malaysia." *Ann NY Acad Sci* 2000;916:354–357.

Oncorhynchus masou
Virus Disease

Salmonid Herpesvirus Type 2 Disease

Importance

Oncorhynchus masou virus disease (OMVD) is an economically significant disease of salmonid fish (salmon and rainbow trout). In young salmon, OMVD is a systemic disease with high mortality. Surviving fish often develop cutaneous tumors, particularly around the mouth. Symptomatic and asymptomatic carriers can spread the virus to uninfected stocks.

Etiology

OMVD results from infection by the *Oncorhynchus masou* virus (OMV). This virus is also known as Yamame tumor virus (YTV), coho salmon tumor virus (CSTV), *Oncorhynchus kisutch* virus (OKV), coho salmon herpesvirus (CSHV), rainbow trout kidney virus (RKV), rainbow trout herpesvirus (RHV), Nerka tumor virus, and Nerka virus Towada Lake, Akita, and Amori prefecture (NeVTA).

Species affected

Oncorhynchus masou virus disease affects only salmonid fish, including kokanee salmon, masou salmon, chum salmon, coho salmon, and rainbow trout.

Geographic distribution

Oncorhynchus masou virus disease is found in Japan and probably in the coastal rivers of eastern Asia.

Transmission

The reservoirs of virus are diseased fish and asymptomatic carriers. OMV is shed in the feces, urine, sexual products at spawning, and probably the skin mucus. Transmission is by direct contact or through the water. "Egg associated" transmission occurs, and the virus can be spread by living vectors and fomites. Age influences susceptibility; fish are most likely become infected when they are approximately one month old.

Incubation period

The period from infection to neoplasia varies from 120 to 270 days.

Clinical signs

During the initial systemic infection, the clinical signs may include lethargy, anorexia, darkening of the body, and petechiae on the body wall. Infection is often fatal. Four to nine months later, some surviving fish develop epitheliomas (cutaneous carcinomas), mainly on the jaws but also on the fins, operculum, cornea, and body surface. Skin ulcers can also develop. Infected rainbow trout have very few external signs of disease, other than skin ulcers. Fish that recover from OMVD often become carriers.

Post mortem lesions

Infections are characterized by edema and hemorrhages. In Coho salmon, the lesions may include skin ulcers, white spots on the liver, and neoplasia around the mouthparts or on the body surface. Tumors may also be found in the kidney. In rainbow trout, there may be skin ulcers, intestinal hemorrhages, or white spots on the liver.

Morbidity and mortality

Kokanee, masou, and chum salmon are most susceptible; coho salmon and rainbow trout are less likely to develop disease. Low water temperatures (below 14°C) increase the likelihood of infection. The age of the fish is also critical; 1 month old alevins are the most susceptible. High mortality may be seen among young salmon; in some outbreaks, the cumulative mortality among kokanee salmon fry exceeds 80%. Tumors develop on 12% to 100% of surviving chum, coho, and masou salmon and rainbow trout.

Diagnosis

Clinical

Oncorhynchus masou virus disease should be suspected in salmon with epithelial tumors or young salmonids that develop a systemic disease with a high mortality rate. Infected rainbow trout may have few signs of disease other than skin ulcers.

Laboratory tests

Oncorhynchus masou virus disease can be diagnosed by virus isolation in cell cultures; appropriate cell lines include RTG–2 (Rainbow trout gonad) or CHSE–214 (Chinook salmon embryo) cells. Infections can also be diagnosed by co–culturing neoplastic tissues with salmonid cell lines. The identity of the virus is confirmed by virus neutralization, immunofluorescence, or an enzyme–linked immunosorbent assay.

Virus antigens can also be identified directly in tissues with immunofluorescence or an ELISA.

Serology is not currently helpful for routine diagnosis.

Samples to collect

Before collecting or sending any samples from animals with a suspected foreign animal disease, the proper authorities should be contacted. Samples should only be sent under secure conditions and to authorized laboratories to prevent the spread of the disease.

If the fish are symptomatic, the samples to collect depend on the size of the fish. Small fish (less than or equal to 4 cm) should be sent whole. The viscera including the kidney should be collected from fish 4 to 6 cm long. The ulcerative skin lesions, any neoplastic tissues, the kidney, spleen, liver, and encephalon should be sent from larger fish. Samples from asymptomatic animals should include the kidney, spleen, encephalon, and the ovarian fluid at spawning. Samples should be taken from 10 diseased fish and combined to form pools with approximately 1.5 g of material (no more than 5 fish per pool).

The pools of organs or ovarian fluids should be placed in sterile vials. The samples may also be sent in cell culture medium or Hanks' basal salt solution with antibiotics. They should be kept cold (4°C) but not frozen. If the shipping time is expected to be longer than 12 hours, serum or albumen (5–10%) may be added to stabilize the virus. Ideally, virus isolation should be done within 24 hours after fish sampling.

Recommended actions if OMVD is suspected

Notification of authorities

Oncorhynchus masou virus disease should be reported to state or federal authorities immediately upon diagnosis or suspicion of the disease.

Federal: Area Veterinarians in Charge (AVICs):
  http://www.aphis.usda.gov/vs/area_offices.htm
State Veterinarians:
  http://www.aphis.usda.gov/vs/sregs/official.html

Quarantine and disinfection

Quarantine is necessary for the control of outbreaks; OMVD is a contagious disease and asymptomatic carriers occur. Disinfecting eggs with iodine can prevent OMV infection. In endemic areas, the fry and alevins should be reared in virus free water, in separate premises from fish that may be virus carriers. Contact through fomites must also be avoided.

Public health

There is no indication that this disease is a threat to human health.

For more information

World Organization for Animal Health (OIE)
http://www.oie.int
OIE Diagnostic Manual for Aquatic Animal Diseases
http://www.oie.int/eng/normes/fmanual/A_summry.htm
OIE International Aquatic Animal Health Code (2001)
http://www.oie.int/eng/normes/fcode/a_summry.htm

References

"Fish Health Management: Viral Diseases." In *The Merck Veterinary Manual*, 8th ed. Edited by S.E. Aiello and A. Mays. Whitehouse Station, NJ: Merck and Co., 1998, pp. 1291–1293.

"General Information." In *Diagnostic Manual for Aquatic Animal Diseases*. Paris: World Organization for Animal Health, 2000. http//www.oie.int/eng/normes/fmanual/A_00010.htm>.

"Herpesviridae." In *Fish Diseases and Disorders*. Edited by J.F. Leatherland and P.T.K. Woo. Wallingford, UK: CAB International, 1995, pp. 57–58.

"*Oncorhynchus masou* Virus Disease." Animal Health Australia. The National Animal Health Information System (NAHIS). 19 Nov 2001. http//www. aahc.com.au/nahis/disease/dislist.asp.

"*Oncorhynchus masou* Virus Disease." In *Diagnostic Manual for Aquatic Animal Diseases*. Paris: World Organization for Animal Health, 2000. http//www.oie.int/eng/normes/fmanual/A_00014.htm.

Yoshimizu, M., H. Fukuda, T. Sano, and T. Kimura. "Salmonid Herpesvirus 2. Epizootiology and Serological Relationship." *Veterinary Research* 26 (1995):486–492.

Ovine Pulmonary Adenomatosis

Jaagsiekte, Ovine Pulmonary Carcinoma

Importance

Pulmonary adenomatosis is a contagious viral disease that results in pulmonary neoplasia in sheep and occasionally goats. The economic impact can be significant: up to 60% of the flock can be lost upon first exposure to the virus. There is no treatment and no vaccine. Pulmonary adenomatosis exists in the United States.

Etiology

Pulmonary adenomatosis results from infection by the jaagsiekte sheep retrovirus (also known as the pulmonary adenomatosis virus). The virus is a member of the family Retroviridae and appears to most closely resemble the type D oncoviruses. It has not been grown in vitro, but has been isolated in immune complexes from the lungs of infected animals. An infectious molecular clone is able to reproduce the disease in sheep.

Species affected

Pulmonary adenomatosis affects sheep and, to a lesser extent, goats. All breeds of sheep are susceptible.

Geographic distribution

Pulmonary adenomatosis can be found in continental Europe, the United Kingdom, Africa, India, China, the Middle East, North America, and some parts of South America.

Transmission

Pulmonary adenomatosis is spread by the respiratory route, probably by aerosol or droplet infection. Infectious virus can be found in the respiratory exudates of infected sheep. There is no evidence of transmission in utero; however, neonates seem to be particularly susceptible to infection.

Incubation period

The incubation period varies from 9 months to 3 years.

Clinical signs

The clinical signs of pulmonary adenomatosis include progressive emaciation, weight loss, and severe dyspnea. There is usually a thin mucus discharge from the nostrils and, if the head is lowered, copious frothy mucus may pour from the nares. Affected sheep often lag behind the flock. Moist rales may be heard on auscultation, but coughing is not prominent. The symptoms are slowly progressive. Death usually occurs after 2 to 6 months, often from secondary bacterial pneumonia.

Post mortem lesions

The lungs are usually enlarged and, in advanced cases, do not collapse upon opening the chest cavity. Frothy fluid may be seen in the trachea and bronchi, and nodular tumors are found in the lungs. These tumors vary from small nodules to solid masses. They are sharply demarcated, firm, and gray or pinkish–gray. On cut surface, the tumors are glistening and granular; a frothy fluid may be squeezed from them. Most tumors occur in the apical, cardiac, and ventral portions of the diaphragmatic lobes. Metastasis sometimes occurs to the nearby lymph nodes, but the tumors do not usually become more widespread. Secondary pneumonia and fibrinous pleuritis may be found.

Morbidity and mortality

Most cases of pulmonary adenomatosis occur in sheep over 2 years old; the peak incidence is in 3 to 4 year old animals. Upon first exposure, the mortality rate is usually high: up to 60% of the animals in the herd may die during the first 3 years. Eventually, the annual rate of loss drops to approximately 1% to 3%, although the disease usually remains endemic in the herd for a long time.

No treatment or vaccine is available.

Diagnosis

Clinical

Pulmonary adenomatosis should be suspected in sheep with chronic respiratory symptoms, particularly in 3 to 4 year old animals with a frothy mucoid discharge from the nostrils.

Differential diagnosis

The differential diagnosis includes maedi–visna, bacterial pneumonia, and infestation by lungworms.

Laboratory tests

Diagnosis is usually based on clinical signs, postmortem lesions, and histopathology. Occasionally, electron microscopy, immunoblotting (Western blotting), or inter–species competitive radioimmunoassay is used to demonstrate type D retrovirus particles in the lungs.

Recently, a polymerase chain reaction (PCR) method was able to detect the jaagsiekte sheep retrovirus in the blood before symptoms appeared. This technique could also find the virus in the tumors and lymphoid organs of affected sheep.

Samples to collect

Regional lymph nodes and samples of affected lung should be collected aseptically. These samples should be transported cold with wet ice or frozen gel packs. Duplicate samples should also be taken (in neutral buffered formalin) for histopathology.

Recommended actions if pulmonary adenomatosis is suspected

Notification of authorities

Pulmonary adenomatosis is a reportable disease in many states. Specific guidelines should be consulted for each state.

Federal: Area Veterinarians in Charge (AVICs):
http://www.aphis.usda.gov/vs/area_offices.htm
State Veterinarians:
http://www.aphis.usda.gov/vs/sregs/official.html

Quarantine and disinfection

The respiratory secretions of sheep with pulmonary adenomatosis are contagious. Retroviruses are generally fragile in the environment and are susceptible to most common disinfectants.

Public health

There is no definitive evidence that pulmonary adenomatosis affects humans; however, antibodies against the pulmonary adenomatosis virus can recognize some human bronchioalveolar carcinomas.

For more information

World Organization for Animal Health (OIE)
http://www.oie.int
OIE International Animal Health Code
http://www.oie.int/eng/normes/mcode/A_summry.htm
Animal Health Australia. The National Animal Health Information System (NAHIS)
http://www. aahc.com.au/nahis/disease/dislist.asp

References

De las Heras M., S.H. Barsky, P. Hasleton, M. Wagner, E. Larson, J. Egan, A. Ortin, J.A. Gimenez–Mas, M. Palmarini, and J.M. Sharp. Evidence for a protein related immunologically to the jaagsiekte sheep retrovirus in some human lung tumours. *European Respiratory Journal* 16, no. 2 (2000):330–332.

Gonzalez L., M. Garcia–Goti, C. Cousens, P. Dewar, N. Cortabarria, A.B. Extramiana, A. Ortin, M. De Las Heras, and J.M. Sharp. Jaagsiekte sheep retrovirus can be detected in the peripheral blood during the pre–clinical period of sheep pulmonary adenomatosis. *The Journal of General Virology* 82, Pt. 6 (2001):1355–1358.

Palmarini M., J.M. Sharp, M. de las Heras, and H. Fan. Jaagsiekte sheep retrovirus is necessary and sufficient to induce a contagious lung cancer in sheep. *Journal of Virology* 73, no. 8 (1999):6964–6972.

"Pulmonary Adenomatosis." Animal Health Australia. The National Animal Health Information System (NAHIS). 12 Oct 2001 http//www. aahc.com.au/nahis/disease/dislist.asp

"Pulmonary Adenomatosis." In *The Merck Veterinary Manual*, 8th ed. Edited by S.E. Aiello and A. Mays. Whitehouse Station, NJ: Merck and Co., 1998, pp. 1112–1113.

Parafilariasis

Importance

Parafilariasis, a nematode infestation of cattle, is a skin disease characterized by nodules and "bleeding points." The main impact of this disease is economic. The cost of controlling the parasite and its vector, together with economic losses in the slaughterhouse, can be significant. *Musca autumnalis*, a potential vector for the parasite, exists in the United States.

Etiology

Parafilariasis is caused by infestation with the filaroid nematode parasite *Parafilaria bovicola* (family Filariidae, subfamily Filariinae).

Species affected

Parafilariasis affects cattle and buffalo. No age, sex, or breed susceptibility appears to exist.

Geographic distribution

Parafilariasis occurs in the Philippines, Japan, Pakistan, India, and several countries in Africa (Morocco, Tunisia, Rwanda, Burundi, Namibia, South Africa, Zimbabwe, and Botswana). This parasite is also found in Bulgaria, Romania, France, Sweden, and the former U.S.S.R.

Transmission

P. bovicola is transmitted by flies in the genus *Musca*. The licking flies *M. xanthomelas*, *M. lusoria*, and *M. nevilli* are vectors in Africa, and the face fly *M. autumnalis* is a vector in Sweden. *M. vitripennis*, another licking fly, may be able to transmit the parasite in India.

Parafilariasis is spread when flies feed on infected lesions in cattle and ingest parasite eggs. The parasite develops into the infective form inside the fly; this process takes approximately 10 to 12 days in South Africa and 20 days in Sweden. The infective third stage larvae are probably transmitted to susceptible animals when the face fly feeds on wounds or ocular secretions. There is evidence that mature parasites do not survive in lesions from year to year, and infestations are newly acquired each year.

Incubation period

The characteristic skin lesions of parafilariasis appear when the female nematode breaks the skin and begins to lay her eggs. This occurs approximately 240 days after infection

Clinical signs

The clinical signs of parafilariasis are nodules and focal hemorrhages ("bleeding points" or "bleeding spots"), commonly found on the skin of the back and neck. Before the female worm begins to oviposit, the nodules are typically 12-15 mm diameter and 5-7 mm high. Bleeding points appear when the female worm penetrates the skin to lay her eggs. Usually, blood trickles from the small wound for minutes to hours. The skin nodules also become swollen (typically 40 mm diameter and 10 mm deep), painful, and hemorrhagic.

In the northern hemisphere, lesions usually begin to appear in December. Bleeding points are most common in the spring and early summer then gradually disappear. In the southern hemisphere, the seasonal pattern is reversed.

Post mortem lesions

In affected animals, the subcutaneous tissues, fascia, and superficial muscles contain irregular, edematous lesions that resemble bruises. Most of the lesions are superficial, but in more severe cases, the underlying muscles can be extensively involved. Acute lesions are usually opaque and yellow–green, and are a mixture of edematous areas and clearer areas with petechiae. Chronic lesions are usually greenish dirty brown. The lesions of parafilariasis have a characteristic metallic, unpleasant smell.

Morbidity and mortality

In Sweden, morbidity in young cattle raised on pastures is approximately 35%. Parafilariasis is not usually a problem in cattle managed indoors. Mortality is not seen in this disease.

Anthelmintics such as ivermectin can be used to destroy the nematodes and improve the quality of the meat at slaughter. Insecticides and permethrin–impregnated ear tags have been used to control the fly vector.

Diagnosis

Clinical

Parafilariasis should be suspected in cattle with bleeding points along the back and neck.

Differential diagnosis

In live animals, the differential diagnosis includes injuries caused by wire, thorns, biting insects, or ticks. In animals at slaughter, parafilariasis resembles bruises from trauma.

Laboratory tests

Parafilariasis can be diagnosed by finding *Parafilaria microfilaria* at a bleeding point. Blood from a bleeding point is centrifuged at 400G for 10 minutes to concentrate the parasite eggs and microfilaria. Microscopic examination of the sediment should reveal *P. bovicola* eggs containing microfilaria or free microfilaria (200 to 300 mm wide). Affected carcasses usually contain only small numbers of worms; the tissues can be incubated in warm saline to improve the recovery of parasites.

Significant antibody titers to *P. bovicola* appear approximately 3 months after the animal has been exposed. An enzyme–linked immunosorbent assay (ELISA) test is available.

Samples to collect

Before collecting or sending any samples from animals with a suspected foreign animal disease, the proper authorities should be contacted. Samples should only be sent under secure conditions and to authorized laboratories to prevent the spread of the disease.

Either fresh or dried blood from a bleeding point should be collected into 1 ml of 0.85% saline. Serum should also be collected for serology. These samples should be kept cool and sent to a laboratory familiar with parafilariasis. A biopsy of a skin sample may also be taken and shipped in 10% formalin.

Recommended actions if parafilariasis is suspected

Notification of authorities

A diagnosis or suspicion of parafilariasis should be reported immediately to state or federal authorities.

Federal: Area Veterinarians in Charge (AVICs):
http://www.aphis.usda.gov/vs/area_offices.htm
State Veterinarians:
http://www.aphis.usda.gov/vs/sregs/official.html

Quarantine and disinfection

Parafilariasis is not a communicable disease; development to the infectious form occurs inside the fly vector. However, prevention of transmission to potential arthropod vectors is critical. Sodium hypochlorite solutions are effective disinfectants against other species of filarial parasites

Public health

There are no reports of human infections with *P. bovicola*.

For more information

World Organization for Animal Health (OIE)
http://www.oie.int
OIE International Animal Health Code
http://www.oie.int/eng/normes/mcode/A_summry.htm
USAHA Foreign Animal Diseases Book
http://www.vet.uga.edu/vpp/gray_book/FAD/

References

Bech–Nielsen, S. "Parafilariasis in Cattle." In *Foreign Animal Diseases*. Richmond, VA: United States Animal Health Association, 1998, pp. 332–343.

"Parafilaria Infection." In *The Merck Veterinary Manual*, 8th ed. Edited by S.E. Aiello and A. Mays. Whitehouse Station, NJ: Merck and Co., 1998, pp. 660–661.

"Material Safety Data Sheet – *Onchocerca volvulus*." Sept 2001. Canadian Laboratory Centre for Disease Control. 4 Oct 2001. http//www.phac-aspc.gc.ca/msds-ftss/index.html.

Paratuberculosis
Johne's Disease

Importance

Paratuberculosis is a chronic disease of ruminants, characterized by irreversible wasting, diarrhea and death from cachexia. Only a minority of the animals in a herd develops the typical clinical signs; however, economic losses can also result from decreased production in asymptomatically infected animals. Some limited data suggest that the causative agent, *Mycobacterium avium* subsp. *paratuberculosis*, has been implicated as a possible cause of Crohn's disease of humans.

Etiology

Paratuberculosis results from infection by *Mycobacterium avium* subsp. *paratuberculosis*, an acid–fast rod previously known as *Mycobacterium paratuberculosis* and *M. johnei*. Some strains of *M. avium paratuberculosis* appear to preferentially infect certain host species. Other subspecies of *M. avium* have also been isolated from animals with paratuberculosis.

Species affected

Paratuberculosis usually affects domestic and wild ruminants, including cattle, sheep, goats, llamas, alpaca, camels, moose, buffalo, deer, and reindeer. Disease has also been seen in wild rabbits, nonhuman primates, and pigs. Horses and dogs can be infected experimentally.

Geographic distribution

Paratuberculosis can be found worldwide. Sweden and some states in Australia are the only areas proven to be free of this disease.

Transmission

M. avium paratuberculosis is mainly transmitted by the fecal–oral route. Infected animals can shed large numbers of organisms in the feces; this shedding can begin before the onset of clinical signs. Asymptomatic carriers may shed the bacteria intermittently. *M. avium paratuberculosis* has also been isolated from the colostrum, milk, udder, and male and female reproductive tracts. Young animals are most susceptible to infection. Calves usually become infected when they nurse from an udder soiled with contaminated feces or are housed in contaminated pens. Calves may also be infected in the uterus or by drinking infected milk or colostrum.

M. avium paratuberculosis is resistant to environmental conditions and can survive on pastures for more than a year. Sunlight, drying, and alkaline soils help to inactivate the organism.

Incubation period

The incubation period is usually months or years. Calves generally become infected soon after birth but rarely show clinical signs before they are 2 years old.

Clinical signs

In cattle, the main symptoms of paratuberculosis are diarrhea and wasting. Most cases are seen in 2 to 6 year old animals. The initial symptoms can be subtle and may be limited to weight loss, decreased milk production, or roughening of the hair coat. The diarrhea is usually thick, without blood, mucus, or epithelial debris, and may be intermittent at first. Tenesmus is not seen. As the disease progresses, the diarrhea becomes more severe over weeks or months and intermandibular or ventral edema may occur. The temperature and appetite are usually normal and animals are alert. Paratuberculosis is progressive; affected animals become increasingly emaciated and usually die as the result of dehydration and severe cachexia.

The clinical signs are similar in other ruminants. In sheep and goats, the wool is often damaged and easily shed, and diarrhea is uncommon. In deer, paratuberculosis can be rapidly progressive.

Intestinal disease has also been reported in rabbits and non–human primates.

Post mortem lesions

In cattle, the carcass may be thin or emaciated and is sometimes edematous. The characteristic lesion is a thickened, often corrugated, wall in the distal small intestine. In some cases, the lesions can extend to the jejunum or colon. The mucosa is not ulcerated. Discrete plaques may be seen early in the disease; these plaques can sometimes be detected by holding the intestine up to a light source. The mesenteric lymph nodes and other regional nodes are generally enlarged.

Similar lesions are seen in sheep and goats. The mucosa is often only slightly thickened in these species, but caseated or calcified nodules are sometimes found the intestines and associated lymph nodes. Some strains of *M. avium paratuberculosis* produce a pigment that stains the intestinal lesions brownish–yellow.

Morbidity and mortality

In an endemic herd, only a minority of the animals develops clinical signs; most animals either eliminate the infection or become asymptomatic carriers. The mortality rate is approximately 1%, but up to 50% of the animals in the herd can be asymptomatically infected, resulting in losses in production. Once the symptoms appear, paratuberculosis is progressive and affected animals eventually die. The percentage of asymptomatic carriers that develops overt disease is unknown.

Diagnosis

Clinical

A diagnosis of paratuberculosis should be confirmed with laboratory tests, particularly on farms where the disease is not known to exist. In endemically infected herds, paratuberculosis is sometimes diagnosed clinically.

Differential diagnosis

The differential diagnosis includes gastrointestinal parasitism, peritonitis, renal amyloidosis, lymphosarcoma, kidney failure, chronic salmonellosis and other chronic infectious diseases, copper deficiency, and starvation.

Laboratory Tests

Paratuberculosis can be diagnosed with a variety of tests; the choice of test varies with the stage of disease. Early "silent" infections can be detected only by culturing the organisms from postmortem tissues or, rarely, by histopathology. Some subclinical carriers can be identified with serology, delayed–type hypersensitivity (DTH) reactions, or fecal culture. Bacteria are usually shed intermittently by carriers. Clinical cases can be diagnosed by culturing *M. avium paratuberculosis* from the feces or tissues, or by demonstrating the organism with microscopy or DNA probes. Polymerase chain reaction (PCR) tests can detect *M. avium paratuberculosis* and distinguish it from other species and subspecies of mycobacteria. Serology, pathology, and histopathology can also be used in clinical cases.

Microscopy

Ziehl– Neelsen stains are used to detect *M. avium paratuberculosis* in the feces; clumps of small, strongly acid–fast bacilli are diagnostic. Organisms may also be found in smears from the intestinal mucosa or the cut surfaces of lymph nodes.

Culture

Bacteria can be cultured from the feces, thickened areas of the intestinal wall, and mesenteric and ileocecal lymph nodes. Suitable media include Herrold's egg yolk medium, modified Dubos's medium, and Middlebrook 7H9, 7H10 and 7H11 media; mycobactin is necessary for bacterial growth. *M. avium paratuberculosis* grows slowly; colonies may take 5 to 14 weeks to appear. On Herrold's medium, *M. avium paratuberculosis* colonies are initially very small, colorless, hemispherical, and translucent, with round, even margins and a smooth, glistening surface. With time, the colonies become larger, more opaque, rough, and mammilate. Some strains, particularly some sheep strains, can be difficult to grow.

Serology and tests for cell–mediated immunity

A variety of serological tests are available, including complement fixation, enzyme–linked immunosorbent assays (ELISAs), and agar gel immunodiffusion. Animals that have cleared the infection can be seropositive. Intradermal testing with johnin or avian purified protein derivative tuberculin can detect delayed–type hypersensitivity (DTH) reactions to *M. avium paratuberculosis*. DTH reactions may diminish or disappear as the disease progresses. Exposure to other mycobacteria, including environmental saprophytes, can result in false positives. In vitro tests that detect cell–mediated immunity to *M. avium paratuberculosis* include a gamma interferon assay and a lymphocyte transformation test.

Samples to collect

Although the link has not been proven, veterinarians collecting samples should keep in mind that this organism may be linked to Crohn's disease.

M. avium paratuberculosis can be isolated from the feces, mesenteric and ileocecal lymph nodes, and thickened areas of the intestinal wall. Smears may be taken from the intestinal mucosa or cut surfaces of the lymph nodes for microscopic examination. Multiple samples of the intestinal wall and mesenteric lymph nodes should be collected into fixative for histology. Serum samples may be taken for serology.

Recommended actions if paratuberculosis is suspected

Notification of authorities

Paratuberculosis is a reportable disease in some states; state regulations should be consulted for more specific guidelines. Federal regulations prohibit culture–positive or DNA test–positive animals from being moved across state lines except to slaughter.

Federal: Area Veterinarians in Charge (AVICs):
http://www.aphis.usda.gov/vs/area_offices.htm
State Veterinarians:
http://www.aphis.usda.gov/vs/sregs/official.html

Quarantine and disinfection

Paratuberculosis is controlled by farm sanitation and manure management; young animals should be separated from potential sources of infection, including infected milk and colostrum. *M. avium paratuberculosis* is resistant to most disinfectants. Contaminated surfaces should be thoroughly cleaned with soap and water, followed by "tuboricidal" disinfectants if needed. In test–and–cull programs, herds are tested every 6 months to a year, with the removal of serologically positive animals or fecal shedders, until three or more consecutive tests have been negative.

Farms may participate in a voluntary herd status certification program conducted by the U.S. Animal Health Association. Eradication programs are also underway in some states. Culture–positive or DNA test–positive animals cannot be moved across state lines except to slaughter.

Public health

Some data suggest that *M. avium paratuberculosis* may be involved in Crohn's disease, a chronic enteritis of humans. The data are controversial and remain to be confirmed.

For more information

World Organization for Animal Health (OIE)
http://www.oie.int
OIE Manual of Standards
http://www.oie.int/eng/normes/mmanual/a_summry.htm

OIE International Animal Health Code
http://www.oie.int/eng/normes/mcode/A_summry.htm
International Association for Paratuberculosis
http://www.paratuberculosis.org/
Johne's Information Center. University of Wisconsin School of
Veterinary Medicine http://www.johnes.org/
Diagnosis and Control of Johne's Disease. National Academies Press
http://www.nap.edu/books/0309086116/html
The Merck Veterinary Manual
http://www.merckvetmanual.com/mvm/index.jsp

References

Collins M. and E. Manning. "Johne's Information Center." The
University of Wisconsin–School of Veterinary Medicine. 13
March 2003. http//www.johnes.org.

Committee on Diagnosis and Control of Johne's Disease, National Research Council. Diagnosis and Control of Johne's
Disease. National Academies Press, 2003. 13 March 2003.
http//www.nap.edu/books/0309086116/html/.

"Paratuberculosis." In *The Merck Veterinary Manual*, 8th ed. Edited
by S.E. Aiello and A. Mays. Whitehouse Station, NJ: Merck
and Co., 1998, p. 537–539.

"Paratuberculosis." In *Manual of Standards for Diagnostic Tests and
Vaccines*. Paris: Office International des Epizooties, 2000.
10 March 2003. http//www.oie.int/eng/normes/mmanual/
A_00043.htm.

Peste des Petits Ruminants

*Pest of Small Ruminants, Pest of Sheep and Goats,
Stomatitis-Pneumoenteritis Complex or Syndrome,
Pseudorinderpest of Small Ruminants, Kata, Goat
Plauge, Contagious Pustular Stomatitis*

Importance

Peste des petits ruminants (PPR) is an acute contagious disease
of small ruminants, particularly goats. Clinical signs are similar to
rinderpest in cattle and the two organisms are closely related. Clinical signs may include fever, necrotic stomatitis, gastroenteritis, and
bronchopneumonia.

Etiology

Peste des petits ruminants virus (PPRV) is a paramyxovirus of
the genus *Morbillivirus*. It is antigenically very similar to the rinderpest virus.

Species affected

Goats and sheep are the species primarily affected by peste
des petits ruminants. Cattle and pigs can be infected, but show no
clinical signs and do not transmit the disease to other animals. PPR
has also been reported in a few wild ungulates and the American
white–tailed deer is susceptible when experimentally infected.

Geographic distribution

Peste des petits ruminants occurs in Africa, the Middle East,
and India.

Transmission

Transmission of PPRV requires close contact. The virus is
present in ocular, nasal, and oral secretions as well as feces. Most
infections occur through inhalation of aerosols from sneezing and
coughing animals, though fomite transmission can also occur. Animals may be infectious during the incubation period, but there is no
known carrier state.

Incubation period

The incubation period can range from 3 to 10 days, 4 to 5 days
being typical.

Clinical signs

Most cases of PPR are acute, with signs of a sudden fever that
may last for 5 to 8 days before the animal either dies or begins to
recover. Nonspecific signs include restlessness and a decreased
appetite. The characteristic signs begin with a serous nasal discharge that becomes mucopurulent. The nasal discharge may
remain mild or progress to a severe catarrhal exudate that crusts
over, blocking the nostrils and causing respiratory distress. The
nasal mucous membranes may develop small areas of necrosis.
The conjunctiva may be congested with crusting on the medial
canthus, and profuse catarrhal conjunctivitis with matted eyelids is
often seen. Necrotic stomatitis is also common and can be severe.
Concurrently, animals will most likely have profuse, non–hemorrhagic diarrhea resulting in severe dehydration, which may progress
to emaciation, dyspnea, hypothermia, and death within 5 to 10
days. Bronchopneumonia with coughing is common late in the disease. Abortion may be seen in pregnant animals. A peracute form
with higher mortality occurs frequently in goats. Subacute and
chronic forms can occur with inconsistent signs developing over
10 to 15 days.

Post mortem lesions

The post mortem lesions are similar to rinderpest, with inflammatory and necrotic lesions in the oral cavity and throughout the
gastrointestinal tract. The carcass is generally emaciated, with conjunctivitis and erosive stomatitis. Necrotic lesions may be seen on
the inside surface of the lower lip and adjacent gum, commissures,
and tongue. In severe cases, the hard palate, pharynx, and upper
esophagus also have lesions. The rumen, reticulum, and omasum
rarely have lesions, however, the abomasum may have outlined
erosions that may bleed. In the small intestine, small streaks of
hemorrhages and sometimes erosions can occur in the first portion of the duodenum and the terminal ileum. The Peyer's patches
have extensive necrosis and, sometimes, severe ulceration. The
most severe lesions are seen in the large intestine, with congestion
around the ileo–cecal valve, at the ceco–colic junction, and in the
rectum. "Zebra stripes" of congestion are often seen in the posterior part of the colon on the mucosal folds. Erosive lesions may
also occur in the vulva and vaginal mucous membranes. Unlike
rinderpest, the respiratory system is usually also affected. Respiratory lesions include small erosions and petechiae in the nasal
mucosa, turbinates, larynx, and trachea. Bronchopneumonia with
consolidation and atelectasis occurs frequently as well as pleuritis
and sometimes hydrothorax. Congestion and enlargement of the
spleen may be seen. The lymph nodes are generally congested,
enlarged, and edematous.

Morbidity and mortality

The morbidity and mortality rates can be up to 100% in severe
outbreaks. In milder outbreaks, morbidity is still high but the
mortality rate may be closer to 50%. Severity depends upon the
susceptibility of the population. Goats are generally more susceptible to peste des petits ruminants than sheep. Certain breeds of
goats are predisposed to infection.

Diagnosis

Clinical

Peste des petits ruminants should be considered in sheep or
goats with any acutely febrile, highly contagious disease with oral
erosions and/or gastrointestinal signs.

Differential diagnosis

Differentials include rinderpest, contagious caprine pleuro-pneumonia, bluetongue, pasteurellosis, contagious ecthyma, foot and mouth disease, heartwater, coccidiosis, and mineral poisoning. The case history, geographic location, and the combination of clinical signs can help to differentiate some of these diseases. Laboratory testing is important in confirming the diagnosis.

Laboratory tests

Tests used to identify the organism include antigen detection methods such as agar gel immunodiffusion, counter immuno-electrophoresis, indirect immunofluorescence, enzyme–linked immunosorbent assays (ELISA), and immunohistopathology. Virus isolation and identification can be done using primary lamb kidney cells or VERO cell lines, virus neutralization, and electron microscopy. Viral RNA can be detected with PPR–specific cDNA probes or amplification by polymerase chain reaction (PCR). Serological tests include virus neutralization, competitive ELISA, counter immunoelectrophoresis, agar gel immunodiffusion, and immunodiffusion inhibition tests.

Samples to collect

Before collecting or sending any samples from animals with a suspected foreign animal disease, the proper authorities should be contacted. Samples should only be sent under secure conditions and to authorized laboratories to prevent the spread of the disease.

Samples include blood in EDTA, clotted blood or serum (paired serum samples taken two weeks apart if possible), swabs of nasal and lachrymal discharges, mesenteric lymph nodes, spleen, lung, tonsils, and sections of the ileum and large intestine. Samples should be shipped fresh on ice (not frozen) within 12 hours. It is important to collect samples in the acute phase of the disease when clinical signs are still evident.

Recommended actions if peste des petits ruminants is suspected

Notification of authorities

State and federal veterinarians should be immediately informed of any suspected cases of peste des petits ruminants.

Federal: Area Veterinarians in Charge (AVICs):
http://www.aphis.usda.gov/vs/area_offices.htm
State Veterinarians:
http://www.aphis.usda.gov/vs/sregs/official.html

Quarantine and disinfection

The affected area should be quarantined and exposed or infected animals should be slaughtered and the carcasses burned or buried. The peste des petits ruminants virus can be killed by most common disinfectants (phenol, or sodium hydroxide 2% for 24 hours) as well as alcohol, ether, and detergents. It can survive for long periods of time in chilled or frozen tissues.

Public health

The peste des petits ruminants virus does not infect humans.

For more information

World Organization for Animal Health (OIE)
http://www.oie.int
OIE Manual of Standards
http://www.oie.int/eng/normes/mmanual/a_summry.htm
OIE International Animal Health Code
http://www.oie.int/eng/normes/mcode/A_summry.htm
USAHA Foreign Animal Diseases Book
http://www.vet.uga.edu/vpp/gray_book/FAD/

References

"Peste des Petits Ruminants." In *Manual of Standards for Diagnostic Tests and Vaccines*. Paris: World Organization for Animal Health, 2000, pp. 114–122.

"Peste des Petits Ruminants." In *The Merck Veterinary Manual*, 8th ed. Edited by S.E. Aiello and A. Mays. Whitehouse Station, NJ: Merck and Co., 1998, pp. 539–541.

Saliki, J. T. "Peste des Petits Ruminants." In *Foreign Animal Diseases*. Richmond, VA: United States Animal Health Association, 1998, pp. 344–352.

"Peste des Petits Ruminants." 30 Aug. 2000 World Organization for Animal Health 16 Oct. 2001. http//www.oie.int/eng/maladies/fiches/a_A040.htm.

Plague

Pestis, Peste, Black Death, Bubonic Plague, Pneumonic Plague, Septicemic Plague, Pestis Minor

Importance

Plague is a zoonotic disease spread by flea bites, direct contact with infected animals, and sometimes aerosols. The mortality rate can be high if this disease is not recognized and treated early. Aerosols, the most likely method of bioterrorist attack with the plague bacteria, result in a rapidly fatal pneumonia.

Etiology

Plague is caused by *Yersinia pestis*, a Gram–negative, bipolar–staining bacillus in the bacterial family Enterobacteriaceae.

Species affected

More than 200 species of mammals can be infected with *Y. pestis*. Rodents, including rats, squirrels, prairie dogs, voles, and field mice, are the main animal hosts and the reservoir hosts. Infections are also seen occasionally in humans, rabbits, cats, and other carnivores.

Geographic distribution

Plague is endemic in the southwestern and western United States, Asia, the Middle East, South America, and some areas of Africa. It is not found in Europe, Canada, Australia, or Japan.

Transmission

Plague is usually spread by the bites of infected fleas. The vectors include a variety of rodent fleas, as well as human fleas (*Pulex irritans*). *Y. pestis* is also present in the tissues and body fluids of infected animals; these bacteria can be transmitted directly through mucous membranes and broken skin. Aerosols from people or animals with the pneumonic form are infectious and animals may transmit bacteria in bites. Carnivores often become infected when they eat diseased rodents.

In the wild, *Y. pestis* is maintained in cycles between wild rodents and fleas; sporadic cases occur in humans and domestic animals when they come into contact with infected animals or fleas. Infection of rodents in urban areas, particularly house rats, can result in epidemic plague in humans.

Incubation period

Clinical signs develop can develop within 24 to 48 hours in experimentally infected cats. In humans, the incubation period is 1 to 8 days.

Clinical signs

The symptoms of plague may include fever, lymphadenitis, abscessed internal organs, pneumonia, or sudden death from sepsis. Four forms of plague have been described: the bubonic form, which is characterized by enlarged lymph nodes, the more severe pneumonic and septicemic forms, and a rare meningeal form that is usually seen in humans.

The bubonic form is the most common form in naturally infected cats, but pneumonia and septicemia also occur. In this species, the symptoms of plague may include fever, anorexia, dehydration, and depression. Infected cats may develop enlarged lymph nodes near the site of infection; the submandibular or cervical lymph nodes are most often involved. The infected lymph nodes can become abscessed, ulcerate and drain. Swellings may also be seen around the head, neck and eyes. Sneezing, hemoptysis, incoordination, quadriplegia, necrotic tonsillitis, and symptoms of pneumonia can also be seen.

Dogs seem to be relatively resistant to plague and animals may seroconvert without symptoms. High fevers and lymphadenopathy, with occasional deaths, have also been reported. Ten experimentally infected dogs developed a fever and other signs of illness but recovered spontaneously during the following week.

Asymptomatic infections and mild illness are typical in some rodent reservoir hosts, although periodic die–offs of rodents also occur in endemic areas. Wild carnivores including coyotes, skunks, and raccoons sometimes seroconvert without clinical disease.

Post mortem lesions

Post mortem lesions vary with the type of infection. The lesions can include lymphadenopathy, necrosis in the internal organs especially the liver and spleen, and bacterial pneumonia with lung hemorrhage.

Morbidity and mortality

In endemic areas, many rodents – including chipmunks, wood rats, ground squirrels, deer mice, and voles – suffer occasional epidemics. Mortality in some rodent species can be high; infections are fatal in nearly 100% of prairie dogs. Between outbreaks, bacteria seem to cycle in reservoir populations without causing many deaths.

The mortality rate is 50% in cats fed plague–infected mice; sick cats may die within 1 to 2 days or after several weeks. Dogs, coyotes, raccoons, skunks, and other carnivores often seroconvert without symptoms; clinical infections and deaths are relatively rare in these species. Ten experimentally infected dogs recovered spontaneously.

Diagnosis

Clinical

In endemic areas, plague should always be considered with signs of fever, lymph node enlargement, or pneumonia.

Differential diagnosis

The differentials can be numerous with the vague signs of fever, sepsis, pneumonia, and lymph node enlargement. They can include abscesses, neoplasia, and other causes of pneumonia and sepsis. The diagnosis can be missed in animals not in plague endemic areas.

Laboratory tests

A tentative diagnosis may be made with a Gram's stain of aspirated infected material; *Y. pestis* is Gram–negative and has a bipolar "safety–pin" appearance. The diagnosis can be confirmed by culture and identification. Fluorescent antibody and antigen–capture ELISA tests are often used for identification, as well as a polymerase chain reaction (PCR) test. Serology should reveal at least a 4–fold increase in antibody titer with paired samples 2 weeks apart. The passive hemagglutination (PHA) test is often used for serology.

Samples to collect

Before collecting or sending any samples, the proper authorities should be contacted. Samples should only be sent under secure conditions and to authorized laboratories to prevent the spread of the disease. Plague is a zoonotic disease; samples should be collected and handled with all appropriate precautions.

Samples may include aspirates from enlarged lymph nodes, infected tissue samples, cerebrospinal fluid, sputum, blood, and serum. Care should be taken to avoid contact with purulent material and respiratory secretions. The state veterinarian should be contacted prior to shipment of samples to ensure proper handling. Due to the rapid progression of disease, antimicrobial treatment should be begun prior to the confirmation of plague.

Recommended actions if plague is suspected

Notification of authorities

The state veterinarian should be contacted prior to sample shipment from animals. State authorities should be consulted for additional guidelines. All suspected human plague cases should be reported to the Public Health Department and the World Health Organization.

Federal: Area Veterinarians in Charge (AVICs):
http://www.aphis.usda.gov/vs/area_offices.htm
State Veterinarians:
http://www.aphis.usda.gov/vs/sregs/official.html

Quarantine and disinfection

All forms of plague can be infectious for humans and other animals. Animals and humans with the pneumonic form excrete the bacteria in aerosols. Appropriate precautions should be taken to prevent infections. Cases of pneumonic plague should be quarantined for at least 48 hours after antibiotic treatment is initiated. Flea and rodent control are important in containing the spread of disease.

Public health

Plague is highly infectious to humans. Bubonic, septicemic, pneumonic, and meningeal forms occur, as well as a mild infection termed "pestis minor." The most common form is bubonic plague. Bubonic plague is characterized by acute fever, weakness, and headache followed by the development of "buboes" – painful, enlarged lymph nodes. Buboes are generally found in the groin, axilla, or neck regions. In this form, death can occur within 2 to 4 days after the initial clinical signs. Septicemic plague occurs when there are large amounts of bacteria in the bloodstream, but no buboes. The septicemic form can be rapidly fatal without prompt treatment. The pneumonic form occurs after inhalation of *Y. pestis* or hematogenous spread of the bacteria to the lungs. This form is severe, often fatal, and highly contagious by aerosol. Meningitis is much more rare and can occur a week or more after inadequate treatment of bubonic plague. Pestis minor is a benign form of bubonic plague, usually seen only in regions where plague is endemic. Pestis minor is characterized by fever, lymphadenitis, headache, and prostration that resolve spontaneously within a week.

Early detection and treatment is critical to survival. The mortality rate is high in untreated cases, with a 50% to 60% case fatality rate for bubonic plague and nearly 100% mortality for the pneumonic and septicemic forms. Antibiotic treatment early in the course of disease greatly reduces mortality. Treatment for pneumonic plague should begin within 18 hours of the onset of respiratory signs to be successful. A vaccine may be available to those with increased exposure to the disease.

For more information

World Organization for Animal Health (OIE)
http://www.oie.int
OIE International Animal Health Code
http://www.oie.int/eng/normes/mcode/A_summry.htm
Centers for Disease Control and Prevention (CDC). Plague.
http://www.bt.cdc.gov/agent/plague/index.asp

Material Safety Data Sheets–Canadian Laboratory Centre
for Disease Control
http://www.phac-aspc.gc.ca/msds-ftss/index.html
Medical Microbiology
http://www.gsbs.utmb.edu/microbook
The Merck Manual
http://www.merck.com/pubs/mmanual/
USAMRIID's Medical Management of Biological
Casualties Handbook
http://www.vnh.org/BIOCASU/toc.html

References

Biberstein, E.L. and J. Holzworth. "Bacterial Diseases. Plague." In *Diseases of the Cat*. Edited by J. Holzworth. Philadelphia, PA: W.B. Saunders, 1987, p. 294; 660.

Collins, F.M. "Pasteurella, Yersinia, and Francisella." In *Medical Microbiology*. 4th ed. Edited by Samuel Baron. New York; Churchill Livingstone, 1996. 20 November 2002. http//www.gsbs.utmb.edu/microbook/ch029.htm.

"Bacterial infections caused by Gram–negative bacilli. Enterobacteriaceae." In *The Merck Manual*, 17th ed. Edited by M.H. Beers and R. Berkow. Whitehouse Station, NJ: Merck and Co., 1999. 8 Nov 2002. http//www.merck.com/pubs/mmanual/section13/chapter157/157d.htm.

Butler, T. In *Zoonoses*. Edited by S.R. Palmer, E.J.L. Soulsby and D.I.H Simpson. New York: Oxford University Press, 1998, pp. 286–292.

Control of Communicable Diseases. Edited by J. Chin. American Public Health Association, 2000, pp.532–535.

"Information on plague." Centers for Disease Control and Prevention (CDC), June 2001. 19 Nov 2002. http://www.cdc.gov/ncidod/dvbid/plague/info.htm.

Macy, D.W. "Plague." In *Infectious Diseases of the Dog and Cat*. Edited by C.E. Greene. Philadelphia: W.B. Saunders, 1998, pp. 295–300.

Macy, D.W. "Plague." In *Current Veterinary Therapy X*. Small Animal Practice. Edited by R.W. Kirk and J.D. Bonagura. Philadelphia: W.B. Saunders, 1989, pp. 1088–1091.

"Material Safety Data Sheet –Yersinia pestis." Canadian Laboratory Centre for Disease Control, March 2001. 20 November 2002. http//www.phac-aspc.gc.ca/msds-ftss/index.html.

"Plague." In *Medical Management of Biological Casualties Handbook*, 4th ed. Edited by M. Kortepeter, G. Christopher, T. Cieslak, R. Culpepper, R. Darling J. Pavlin, J. Rowe, K. McKee, Jr., E. Eitzen, Jr. Department of Defense, 2001. 19 Nov 2002. http//www.vnh.org/BIOCASU/9.html.

"Plague." In *The Merck Veterinary Manual*, 8th ed. Edited by S.E. Aiello and A. Mays. Whitehouse Station, NJ: Merck and Co., 1998, pp. 485–486.

Psoroptes ovis

Sheep Scab Mite

Importance

Psoroptes ovis causes psoroptic mange in sheep and cattle. In cattle, psoroptic mange is characterized by intense pruritis, papules, and sticky yellowish crusts. Excoriation and lichenification may be seen. The lesions usually begin on the shoulders and rump, but can spread to involve almost the entire body. The economic impact can include weight loss, decreased milk production, and increased susceptibility to other diseases. Infestations may be fatal in untreated calves.

Sheep with psoroptic mange develop large, yellowish, scaly, crusted lesions, mainly on the wooly areas of the body. These lesions are intensely pruritic. Anemia and emaciation may be seen in untreated animals.

Species affected

Psoroptes ovis infests sheep and cattle. This mite has also been found on goats, llamas, and alpacas.

Geographic distribution

Psoroptes infestations are found worldwide. In the United States, *P. ovis* infections are seen in beef cattle from the central and western states; most cases occur in Texas, New Mexico, Kansas, Nebraska, Colorado, and Oklahoma. Infestations have not been seen in sheep in the U.S. since 1970.

Life cycle

P. ovis spends its entire life cycle on one host; all stages – larvae, nymphs, and adults – feed on the host. The life cycle is approximately 12 days from egg to egg. This mite is usually spread by direct contact between animals, but it can also be transmitted on fomites such as fences, chutes, and trucks. It can survive in the environment from 10 days to 6 weeks. All infested animals do not necessarily develop symptoms; asymptomatic sheep can spread the infestation to other animals. Sheep may also be able to transmit *P. ovis* to cattle.

Identification

P. ovis infestations are diagnosed by microscopic examination of skin scrapings. The scrapings should be made with a sharp curette or scalpel and taken from the edges of active lesions. The specimens are placed in closed glass tubes. Mites may be visible with a magnifying glass or the naked eye when the tube is warmed between the hands. Scrapings can be enriched for mites by adding a 10% solution of caustic potash (KOH) and carefully heating the tube; the sediment is placed on a slide and examined microscopically. *P. ovis* adults are oval and about 0.25 to 0.4 mm long, with eight long legs. The pretarsi have long segmented pedicels and the mouthparts are pointed.

Recommended actions if *Psoroptes ovis* is suspected

Notification of authorities

P. ovis infestations are reportable in both cattle and sheep in most states. State authorities should be consulted for specific details.

Federal: Area Veterinarians in Charge (AVICs):
http://www.aphis.usda.gov/vs/area_offices.htm
State Veterinarians:
http://www.aphis.usda.gov/vs/sregs/official.html

Control measures

Ivermectin injections or several types of dips can eliminate *P. ovis* infestations. Animals must be quarantined to prevent the spread of the mites. Houseflies may be capable of transmitting the mite and should be controlled.

Public health

Psoroptes ovis does not infest humans.

For more information

World Organization for Animal Health (OIE)
http://www.oie.int
OIE International Animal Health Code
http://www.oie.int/eng/normes/mcode/A_summry.htm
USAHA Foreign Animal Diseases Book
http://www.vet.uga.edu/vpp/gray_book/FAD/

References

Corwin, R.M. and J. Nahm. "*Psoroptes* spp." 1997 University of Missouri College of Veterinary Medicine. 3 December 2001. http://www.missouri.edu/~vmicrorc/Arthropods/Arachnida/Psoropte.htm.

"Mange in Cattle. Psoroptic Mange." In *The Merck Veterinary Manual*, 8th ed. Edited by S.E. Aiello and A. Mays. Whitehouse Station, NJ: Merck and Co., 1998, pp. 665–666.

"Mange in Sheep and Goats. Psoroptic Mange (Sheep Scab)." In *The Merck Veterinary Manual*, 8th ed. Edited by S.E. Aiello and A. Mays. Whitehouse Station, NJ: Merck and Co., 1998, pp. 666.

"Mites." Bayer Animal Health. 3 December 2001. http// www.bayeranimalhealth.com/ah/en/farmanimal.nsf/ ActiveBySubject/C1256AAF0021EBFDC1256AAF00724B0 3?OpenDocument&nav=HZUE–4ZVHUD.

Wilson, D.D. and R.A. Bram. "Foreign Pests and Vectors of Arthropod–Borne Diseases." In *Foreign Animal Diseases*. Richmond, VA: United States Animal Health Association, 1998, pp. 225–239.

Q Fever

Query Fever

Importance

Q fever is a zoonotic disease that causes influenza–like signs and occasional cases of chronic endocarditis in humans. The symptoms are often minimal in animals, with abortion the most common sign. The causative organism is highly stable in the environment and is extremely contagious to people. Infections are usually spread in aerosols, which could also be used in a bioterrorist attack.

Etiology

Q fever is caused by *Coxiella burnetii*, a rickettsial organism. The organism has two distinct antigenic phases, I and II. In humans, serological tests for both phases can be helpful in determining if a case is acute or chronic.

Species affected

Humans show the most severe signs of infection. Sheep, goats, and cattle are the most common domestic animal reservoirs. Dogs, cats, horses, pigs, camels, buffalo, pigeons, geese, and fowl can also carry the disease. Many wild species can harbor *C. burnetii*; infections are particularly common in rodents and rabbits, and also occur in birds and many arthropod species.

Geographic distribution

Q fever has been found worldwide.

Transmission

C. burnetii can be transmitted by aerosols or direct contact; it is also spread by ingestion of an infected placenta, other reproductive discharges, or milk. In infected mammals, the organism is localized in the endometrium and mammary glands. It multiplies during pregnancy and is shed in high numbers in the placenta and reproductive discharges during parturition. *C. burnetii* can also be found in the milk, feces and urine. Ticks seem to spread infections among ruminants and sometimes people. Transmission has occurred in blood transfusions and by sexual contact in humans. Organisms have also been found in the semen of bulls. Vertical transmission is possible but rare.

C. burnetii is highly resistant to environmental conditions and is easily spread by aerosols; infectious airborne particles can travel a half–mile or more. Viable organisms can be found for weeks to years in the environment.

Incubation period

The incubation period is variable; reproductive failure is usually the only symptom in animals. Abortions generally occur late in pregnancy.

Clinical signs

Subclinical infections are common in animals. Abortion, stillbirth, retained placenta, endometritis, and infertility can occur. Several abortions followed by uncomplicated recovery may occur in a group of animals. Bronchopneumonia and fever have also been seen.

Post mortem lesions

Placentitis is the most characteristic sign in ruminants. The placenta is typically leathery and thickened and may contain large quantities of white–yellow, creamy exudate at the edges of the cotyledons and in the intercotyledonary areas. In some cases, the exudate may be reddish–brown and fluid. Severe vasculitis is uncommon, but thrombi and some degree of vascular inflammation may be noted. Fetal pneumonia has been seen in goats and cattle and may occur in sheep; however, the lesions in aborted fetuses are usually non–specific.

Morbidity and mortality

Information on the prevalence of infection is limited. In an endemic region in California, 18% to 55% of sheep had antibodies to *C. burnetii*; the number of seropositive sheep varied seasonally and was highest soon after lambing. In other surveys, 82% of cows in some California dairies were seropositive, as well as 78% of coyotes, 55% of foxes, 53% of brush rabbits, and 22% of deer in Northern California. In Ontario, Canada, infections were found in 33% to 82% of cattle herds and 0% to 35% of sheep flocks. Close contact with sheep appears to increase the risk of infection in dogs.

Significant morbidity can be seen in some species. In sheep, abortions can affect 5% to 50% of the flock. In one California study, Q fever may have been responsible for 9% of all abortions in goats. Deaths are rare in natural infections.

Diagnosis

Clinical

Q fever may be suspected when abortions or infertility are seen in otherwise asymptomatic animals.

Differential diagnosis

The differentials for animals, especially sheep, goats, and cattle, should include diseases and other agents that cause abortion.

Laboratory tests

Stained slides of infected tissues may be used to identify the organism along with serology. Staining is usually done with a modified Ziehl–Neelsen or Gimenez stain, as *C. burnetii* is not usually detected by Gram stains. Serological tests include complement fixation, indirect immunofluorescence, and enzyme–linked immunosorbent assays (ELISA). Polymerase chain reaction techniques may be available in some laboratories.

C. burnetii can be isolated in cell cultures, embryonated chicken eggs, or laboratory animals including mice, hamsters and guinea pigs; however, isolation is dangerous to laboratory personnel and is rarely used for diagnosis.

Samples to collect

Q fever is highly infectious to humans; samples should be collected and handled with all appropriate precautions.

The placenta, vaginal discharges, and stomach contents of the aborted fetus are useful samples. Milk and colostrum can be tested, but the agent is generally only found in small amounts if at all. Serum can be taken for antibody testing.

Recommended actions if Q fever is suspected

Notification of authorities

Q fever has recently become a notifiable disease in the United States. State authorities should be consulted for more specific guidelines.

Federal: Area Veterinarians in Charge (AVICs):
http://www.aphis.usda.gov/vs/area_offices.htm
State Veterinarians:
http://www.aphis.usda.gov/vs/sregs/official.html

Quarantine and disinfection

Separation of pregnant animals and burning or burying reproductive discharges including placentas helps reduce transmission of the disease.

C. burnetii is highly resistant to physical and chemical agents; 0.05% hypochlorite (household bleach), 5% peroxide, or a 1:100 solution of Lysol can be used as disinfectants.

Public health

C. burnetii is highly infectious to humans. Most cases of Q fever occur in people occupationally exposed to farm animals or their products; farmers, abattoir workers, researchers, laboratory personnel, dairy workers, and woolsorters have an increased risk of infection. Approximately 60% of cases are thought to be asymptomatic. An additional 38% of infected people experience mild illness, while 2% develop severe disease and require hospitalization.

Humans usually become infected by aerosols, but cases also occur from unpasteurized milk or by other routes. The incubation period varies with the infecting dose, but is generally 2 to 3 weeks. The symptoms appear acutely and can include fever, chills, a severe headache, fatigue, malaise, myalgia, and chest pains. The illness usually lasts from a week to more than 3 weeks. A nonproductive cough, with pneumonitis on X–ray, sometimes develops during the second week. In severe cases, lobar consolidation and pneumonia may occur; severe infections are particularly common in elderly or debilitated patients. Hepatitis is seen in approximately one third of patients with prolonged disease. In pregnant women, infections may result in premature delivery, abortion and placentitis. Complications are not common but may include chronic hepatitis, aseptic meningitis, encephalitis, osteomyelitis, vasculitis and endocarditis.

Q fever is usually a self–limiting illness; most cases resolve spontaneously within 2 days to 2 weeks. In acute cases, the case–fatality rate is minimal with treatment and 1% to 2.4% if untreated. With antibiotic treatment, the acute form generally resolves quickly. The chronic form requires antibiotic treatment for two or more years with regular serological monitoring. Chronic cases of endocarditis have a higher mortality rate even with treatment and often require cardiac valve replacement surgery. A vaccine is available for those with increased exposure to the disease.

For more information

World Organization for Animal Health (OIE)
http://www.oie.int
OIE Manual of Standards
http://www.oie.int/eng/normes/mmanual/a_summry.htm
Animal Health Australia. The National Animal Health
Information System (NAHIS)
http://www. aahc.com.au/nahis/disease/dislist.asp
Material Safety Data Sheets–Canadian Laboratory Centre
for Disease Control
http://www.phac-aspc.gc.ca/msds-ftss/index.html
Q Fever: An Overview. United States Animal Health Association
http://www.usaha.org/speeches/speech01/s01conch.html
USAMRIID's Medical Management of Biological
Casualties Handbook
http://www.vnh.org/BIOCASU/toc.html

References

Control of Communicable Diseases. Edited by J. Chin. American Public Health Association, 2000, pp.407–411.

De la Concha–Bermejillo, A., E.M. Kasari, K.E. Russell, L.E. Cron, E.J. Browder, R. Callicott and R.W. Ermel1. "Q Fever: An Overview. United States Animal Health Association. 4 Dec 2002. http//www.usaha.org/speeches/speech01/s01conch.html.

Marrie, T.J. *Q Fever.* Edited by S.R. Palmer, E.J.L. Soulsby and D.I.H Simpson. New York: Oxford University Press, 1998, pp. 171–185.

Martin J. and P. Innes. "Q Fever." Ontario Ministry of Agriculture and Food, Sept 2002. 4 Dec 2002. http//www.gov.on.ca/OMAFRA/english/livestock/vet/facts/info_qfever.htm.

"Material Safety Data Sheet–*Coxiella burnetii*." Canadian Laboratory Centre for Disease Control. January 2001. 2 Dec 2002. http//www.phac-aspc.gc.ca/msds-ftss/index.html.

"Q Fever." In *Manual of Standards for Diagnostic Tests and Vaccines.* Paris: World Organization for Animal Health, 2000, pp. 822–831.

"Q Fever." In *Medical Management of Biological Casualties Handbook,* 4th ed. Edited by M. Kortepeter, G. Christopher, T. Cieslak, R. Culpepper, R. Darling J. Pavlin, J. Rowe, K. McKee, Jr., E. Eitzen, Jr. Department of Defense, 2001. 2 Dec 2002. http//www.vnh.org/BIOCASU/10.html.

"Q Fever." In *The Merck Manual,* 17th ed. Edited by M.H. Beers and R. Berkow. Whitehouse Station, NJ: Merck and Co., 1999. 7 Oct 2002. http://www.merck.com/pubs/mmanual/section13/chapter159/159i.htm.

"Q Fever." In *The Merck Veterinary Manual,* 8th ed. Edited by S.E. Aiello and A. Mays. Whitehouse Station, NJ: Merck and Co., 1998, pp. 486–7.

Van der Lugt, J, B. van der Lugt and E. Lane. "An approach to the diagnosis of bovine abortion." Paper presented at the mini–congress of the Mpumalanga branch of the SAVA, 11 March 2000. Pathology for the practicing veterinarian, Large Animal Section, no. 1 (April 2000). 2 December 2002. http//vetpath.vetspecialists.co.za/large1.htm.

Walker, D.H. "Rickettsiae." In *Medical Microbiology.* 4th ed. Edited by Samuel Baron. New York; Churchill Livingstone, 1996. 3 December 2002. http//www.gsbs.utmb.edu/microbook/ch038.htm.

Rabbit Hemorrhagic Disease

Viral Hemorrhagic Disease of Rabbits, Necrotic Hepatitis of Rabbits, Rabbit Hemorrhagic Disease Syndrome, Rabbit Calicivirus Disease, X Disease

Importance

Rabbit hemorrhagic disease (RHD) is an extremely contagious and often fatal disease of domestic and European rabbits. The mortality rate in a colony may be as high as 90%. The causative virus is very resistant to inactivation; it can persist in the environment, as well as in refrigerated or frozen carcasses, for months.

Etiology

Rabbit hemorrhagic disease results from infection by a calicivirus. Only a single serotype of the rabbit hemorrhagic disease virus (RHDV) has been identified.

A similar disease, known as European brown hare syndrome, is seen in continental Europe. This disease seems to affect only hares; the causative virus is closely related to RHDV.

Species affected

RHD affects only domestic and European rabbits (*Oryctolagus cuniculus*). Eastern cottontails, black–tailed jackrabbits, and volcano rabbits can be infected experimentally, but remain asymptomatic. European brown hares and varying hares do not seem to be affected by RHDV but are susceptible to European brown hare syndrome.

Geographic distribution

Rabbit hemorrhagic disease is endemic in China, Korea, most of continental Europe, Morocco, Cuba, Australia, and New Zealand. Rabbit hemorrhagic disease once existed in Mexico, but was eradicated by 1992. RHD was diagnosed in the U.S. in 2000 (Iowa), 2001 (Utah, Illinois, New York) and 2005 (Indiana). However, no massive outbreaks have occurred outside of small groups of affected rabbits.

Transmission

Rabbit hemorrhagic disease is transmitted by direct contact with infected animals and on fomites. Rabbits can acquire this disease through the oral, nasal, or conjunctival routes. Animals can shed RHDV in the urine or feces for as long as 4 weeks after infection. The virus may also be acquired by exposure to an infected carcass or hair from an infected animal. In addition, RHDV can be spread on contaminated food, bedding, and water. Mechanical transmission over short distances by biting insects, birds, rodents, wild animals, or vehicles may be possible.

Experimentally, rabbits can be infected by oral, nasal, subcutaneous, intramuscular, and intravenous inoculation

RHDV is very resistant to inactivation in the environment. The virus can survive for more than 9 months in blood stored at 4°C, or more than 3 months at room temperature in dried organ homogenates. RHDV can also survive exposure to pH 3.0, heat of 50°C for an hour, or freeze–thaw cycles.

Incubation period

The incubation period is 1 to 3 days.

Clinical signs

All rabbits can become infected with RHDV, but clinical signs are usually seen only in animals that are more than 40–50 days old. Typically, infected rabbits develop a fever and die suddenly within 12 to 36 hours of its onset. In some cases, the only symptoms are terminal squeals followed rapidly by collapse and death. Dullness, anorexia, congestion of the palpebral conjunctiva, or prostration may also be seen. Occasionally, animals develop neurologic signs, including incoordination, excitement, opisthotonos, and paddling. Some rabbits turn and flip quickly in their cages; this can resemble convulsions or mania. Respiratory symptoms, including dyspnea and a terminal, blood–stained, frothy nasal discharge, are sometimes seen. Approximately 5% to 10% of the animals experience a more chronic course with severe jaundice, lethargy, and weight loss, and death within 1 to 2 weeks.

Post mortem lesions

Rabbits found dead of rabbit hemorrhagic fever are usually in good condition. The most consistent post–mortem lesions are hepatic necrosis and splenomegaly. The liver is usually pale, and has a fine reticular pattern of necrosis outlining each lobule. In cases with extensive necrosis, the liver may be diffusely pale. The spleen is usually black and thickened, with rounded edges. The kidneys may be very dark brown. Hemorrhages in the lungs, trachea, and thymus are common, and petechiae may be found on the serosal membranes or viscera. Infarcts may be seen in most organs. Catarrhal enteritis and congestion of the meninges have also been reported.

Morbidity and mortality

Morbidity occurs in 30% to 80% of animals, and mortality ranges from 40% to 90%. Vaccines have been used in some countries where rabbit hemorrhagic disease is endemic. No treatment is available.

Diagnosis

Clinical

Rabbit hemorrhagic fever should be suspected when several animals die suddenly after a brief period of lethargy and fever. Hepatic necrosis and hemorrhages at necropsy support the diagnosis. This disease can be more difficult to diagnose when it occurs in an isolated rabbit.

Differential diagnosis

Rabbit hemorrhagic disease should be differentiated from acute pasteurellosis, atypical myxomatosis, poisoning, heat exhaustion, and enterotoxemia due to *E. coli* or *Clostridium perfringens* Type E.

Laboratory tests

The rabbit hemorrhagic disease virus has not been grown in cell cultures. However, viruses can be concentrated from the liver, blood, spleen, or other organs and identified by a hemagglutination test, a polymerase chain reaction (PCR) test, immunoblotting (Western blotting), negative–staining immunoelectron microscopy, immunostaining, or a sandwich enzyme–linked immunosorbent assay (ELISA).

Antibodies can also be detected in convalescent rabbits by hemagglutination inhibition, an indirect ELISA, or a competitive ELISA.

Where the disease is not endemic, inoculation into rabbits can confirm the first diagnosis. Animal inoculations can also help to identify cases that have not been definitively diagnosed by other tests.

Samples to collect

Before collecting or sending any samples from animals with a suspected foreign animal disease, the proper authorities should be contacted. Samples should only be sent under secure conditions and to authorized laboratories to prevent the spread of the disease.

Samples from suspect cases should include heparinized blood, serum, unfixed liver, fixed liver, spleen, kidney, lung, small intestine, and brain. The liver contains the highest titers of virus and is the best organ to submit for virus identification. Serum and spleen may also contain high levels of virus.

Recommended actions if rabbit hemorrhagic disease is suspected

Notification of authorities

Rabbit hemorrhagic disease must be reported to state or federal authorities immediately upon diagnosis or suspicion of the disease.

Federal: Area Veterinarians in Charge (AVICs):
　http://www.aphis.usda.gov/vs/area_offices.htm
State Veterinarians:
　http://www.aphis.usda.gov/vs/sregs/official.html

Quarantine and disinfection

RHDV can be inactivated by 10% sodium hydroxide or 1% to 1.4% formalin. Other suggested disinfectants include 2% One–stroke Environ® (Vestal Lab Inc., St. Louis, MO) and 0.5% sodium hypochlorite (10% household bleach). This virus resists degradation by ether or chloroform.

RHDV is extremely contagious and can be transmitted on fomites. Strict quarantine is very important.

Public health

There is no indication that the rabbit hemorrhagic disease virus infects humans.

For more information

World Organization for Animal Health (OIE)
　http://www.oie.int

OIE Manual of Standards
    http://www.oie.int/eng/normes/mmanual/a_summry.htm
OIE International Animal Health Code
    http://www.oie.int/eng/normes/mcode/A_summry.htm
USAHA Foreign Animal Diseases Book
    http://www.vet.uga.edu/vpp/gray_book/FAD/

References

"Rabbit Haemorrhagic Disease." In *Manual of Standards for Diagnostic Tests and Vaccines*. Paris: World Organization for Animal Health, 2000, pp. 762–776.

"Viral Hemorrhagic Disease." In *The Merck Veterinary Manual*, 8th ed. Edited by S.E. Aiello and A. Mays. Whitehouse Station, NJ: Merck and Co., 1998, pp. 1398–1399.

Gregg, D.A. "Viral Hemorrhagic Disease of Rabbits." In *Foreign Animal Diseases*. Richmond, VA: United States Animal Health Association, 1998, pp. 424–431.

Rabbit Calicivirus Disease, Iowa, April 2000 Impact Worksheet. Center for Emerging Issues. http://www.aphis.usda.gov:80/vs/ceah/cei/rabbitcal.htm.

Rabbit Hemorrhagic Disease, Indiana, June 15, 2005. Impact Worksheet. Center for Emerging Issues. Accessed 25 Jan 2006 at http://www.aphis.usda.gov/vs/ceah/cei/IW_2005_files/RHD_Indiana_061505_files/RHD_Indiana_061505.htm.

Rabies

Hydrophobia, Lyssa

Importance

Rabies is a fatal central nervous system (CNS) disease that can affect all mammals. This disease is an important human zoonosis. Infection results in a wide variety of neurologic signs; in some cases, the disease may be difficult to diagnose. Although post–exposure prophylaxis in humans is usually successful, there is no effective treatment once the clinical signs appear.

Etiology

Rabies results from infection by the rabies virus, a *Lyssavirus* in the family Rhabdoviridae. Other members of the *Lyssavirus* genus are the Lagos bat virus, Mokola virus, Duvenhage virus, the European bat viruses, and the Australian bat virus. These rabies–related viruses cause a disease indistinguishable from classical rabies.

Species affected

The rabies virus can infect all warm–blooded animals, including humans. The major reservoir hosts are members of the Mustelidae (skunks, weasels, stoats, and martens), Canidae (dogs, wolves, and jackals), Procyonidae (raccoons), Vivveridae (mongooses and meerkats), and Order Chiroptera (bats).

Geographic distribution

Rabies is present in North, Central, and South America, Africa, the Middle East, and most of Asia. This disease can also be found in most of Europe, except the United Kingdom, Ireland, and areas of Scandinavia. Rabies is not present in Japan, Australia, New Zealand, Singapore, most of Malaysia, some islands of Indonesia, Papua New Guinea, or the Pacific Islands.

Transmission

Rabies is usually spread by the contamination of a wound or mucus membrane with infectious saliva. Most often, the disease is transmitted by the bite from a rabid animal; however, the virus can also enter the body through abraded skin. Oral transmission is possible, but rare. Respiratory spread is also rare, but may occur in bat caves or laboratory settings when high concentrations of virus are found in the air. Hematogenous spread is extremely uncommon.

The rabies virus is excreted in the saliva in 50% to 90% of cases. In dogs and cats, the saliva may be infectious for 3 to 5 days before the symptoms appear. This stage can be as long as 8 days in skunks and 2 weeks in bats.

Urban transmission cycles occur in Africa, Asia, and Central and South America. In these cycles, the virus is maintained mainly in the dog population. Sylvatic transmission cycles occur in many countries; foxes, skunks, raccoons, Arctic foxes, raccoon–dogs, meerkats, mongooses, jackals, wolves, vampire bats, or insectivorous bats are the host species.

Incubation period

The incubation period is variable. In dogs, symptoms most often appear within 21 to 80 days. In humans, the incubation period is usually 2 to 8 weeks, but cases have been seen years after exposure.

Clinical signs

Rabies results in CNS signs. The most reliable symptoms are unexplained paralysis or behavioral signs such as anorexia, apprehension, nervousness, irritability, or hyperexcitability. Ataxia, altered temperament, and changes in phonation may be seen. Some animals seek solitude or become uncharacteristically aggressive. Rabid carnivores often roam extensively or swallow foreign objects. Abnormal bellowing is common in cattle. In horses, distress and extreme agitation may resemble colic. Wild animals often lose their fear of humans and nocturnal animals may be seen in the daylight.

The clinical course is divided into prodromal, excitative, and paralytic phases; however, the length and prominence of these phases varies. The prodromal stage usually lasts 1 to 3 days and is characterized by vague but rapidly intensifying neurologic signs. In the furious form of rabies, this is followed by extreme aggression and unpredictable behavior, then muscular incoordination, seizures, and death from progressive paralysis. In the paralytic form, animals have minimal behavioral changes and are not usually aggressive. In this form, the throat and masseter muscles become paralyzed; the animal may be unable to swallow and may salivate profusely. In dogs, the lower jaw may drop. The paralysis spreads rapidly and is followed by coma and death. Some animals with rabies exhibit only minimal clinical signs and die quickly.

Post mortem lesions

There are no characteristic gross lesions. Occasionally, abnormal objects such as sticks and stones may be found in the stomach. Microscopic lesions are seen mainly in the CNS and consist of nonsuppurative encephalomyelitis and ganglioneuritis.

Morbidity and mortality

Rabies is highly infectious, and is fatal once the clinical signs appear. Death usually occurs within 10 days.

Rabies vaccines are available for dogs, cats, ferrets, horses, cattle, sheep, and humans. Wildlife vaccines have been used in foxes and are being tested in raccoons and coyotes. There is no treatment once the clinical signs appear; however, in humans, post–exposure prophylaxis is usually effective if started early.

Diagnosis

Clinical

Rabies should be suspected in animals with behavioral signs or unexplained paralysis. However, the clinical signs are highly variable and not always characteristic; therefore, laboratory diagnosis is essential.

Differential diagnosis

The differential diagnosis includes canine distemper, infectious canine hepatitis, Aujeszky's disease, Borna disease, equine viral encephalomyelitis, equine encephalosis, acute psychosis in dogs and cats, and foreign bodies or other traumatic injuries in the oropharynx or esophagus. Bacterial and mycotic diseases of the CNS such as listeriosis and cryptococcosis, and various poisonings (e.g. heavy metals, chlorinated hydrocarbons, organophosphate pesticides, and sodium fluoroacetate "1080") must also be considered.

Laboratory tests

Rabies is usually diagnosed by the identification of the virus in tissue samples. The recommended test is the fluorescent antibody test (FAT) on a fixed brain tissue smear. The rapid rabies enzyme immunodiagnosis (RREID) test, an enzyme linked immunosorbent assay (ELISA), can be used for large numbers of samples. In 98% to 100% of cases, either test will provide a reliable diagnosis. Histological tests can detect aggregates of viral material (Negri bodies) in neurons, but are less sensitive than the FAT or RREID; up to 40% of samples may give false–negative results with this test.

As a backup, virus isolation is carried out concurrently in mice or cell culture. Results from intracerebral inoculation of mice are available after 5 to 28 days. Cell culture gives more rapid results, is as sensitive as animal inoculation, and is the preferred test for virus isolation.

Other tests that may be used are monoclonal antibody assays, specific nucleic acid probes, polymerase chain reaction (PCR) tests, and DNA sequencing. These techniques can distinguish vaccine strains from field strains.

Serology is rarely useful, as few animals survive long enough to develop antibodies to the virus. Available tests include virus neutralization assays in cell cultures and ELISAs. The fluorescent antibody virus neutralization test and rapid fluorescent focus inhibition test (RFFIT) are the prescribed tests for international trade.

Samples to collect

Rabies is a highly fatal zoonotic disease; samples should be collected and handled with all appropriate precautions. The collection and shipment of samples should conform to all state and federal regulations.

The organ of choice for testing is the brain, and the tissues of choice are the hippocampus, cerebellum and medulla oblongata. Normally, to minimize human exposure, the entire carcass or the head is shipped to the laboratory without opening the skull. Occasionally, brain samples are collected with a disposable plastic pipette through the occipital foramen or the posterior wall of the eye socket. Exposure to brain tissue is hazardous if the operator is not fully trained.

The rabies virus becomes inactivated quickly; samples must be sent as soon as possible and under cold conditions. For shipment, animal heads or carcasses should be wrapped in absorbent material and sealed securely in plastic bags. Brains must be sent in a rigid, leak–proof container. These samples should be placed in insulated boxes that contain a refrigerant. Transport must comply with all regulations for the shipping of dangerous materials and the prevention of human exposure.

If prompt shipping is impossible, the samples may be preserved. Samples preserved in formalin are not appropriate for virus isolation, but can be tested with the modified direct fluorescent antibody test (FAT), immunohistochemistry, or histology. Small pieces of brain placed in 50% glycerol in phosphate buffered saline (PBS) will remain infective for a prolonged period. Such samples may be used in all available tests. Acetone will reduce the intensity of fluorescence in the FAT.

Recommended actions if rabies is suspected

Notification of authorities

Rabies must be reported to state officials upon diagnosis or suspicion of the disease. State authorities should be consulted for more specific information.

Federal: Area Veterinarians in Charge (AVICs):
http://www.aphis.usda.gov/vs/area_offices.htm

State Veterinarians:
http://www.aphis.usda.gov/vs/sregs/official.html

Quarantine and disinfection

Animals with suspected rabies should be destroyed and the brain submitted for rabies testing. Any unvaccinated dog, cat, or livestock animal that has been exposed to rabies should be killed immediately. If the owner is not willing to destroy the animal, it should be placed in strict quarantine for 6 months and observed. One month before release, it should be vaccinated for rabies. Some authorities recommend vaccination at the beginning of the quarantine period. Exposed animals with current vaccinations should be revaccinated and closely watched for 45 days.

The rabies virus does not remain infective for long periods in the environment. This virus can be inactivated by lipid solvents, 45–75% ethanol, 1% sodium hypochlorite, 2% glutaraldehyde, 70% ethanol, formaldehyde, quaternary ammonium compounds, iodine preparations, heat, and ultraviolet light.

Public health

Rabies can be spread to humans by inoculation of skin wounds or mucus membranes and, under some circumstances, by respiratory or oral spread. Appropriate safety precautions must be taken when handling potentially rabid animals or material from possible cases of rabies. Cases of human exposure must be treated immediately.

Laboratories that work with suspect material must follow national biocontainment and biosafety regulations and the staff should be vaccinated against lyssaviruses.

For more information

World Organization for Animal Health (OIE)
http://www.oie.int
OIE Manual of Standards
http://www.oie.int/eng/normes/mmanual/a_summry.htm
OIE International Animal Health Code
http://www.oie.int/eng/normes/mcode/A_summry.htm
Animal Health Australia. The National Animal Health Information System (NAHIS)
http://www. aahc.com.au/nahis/disease/dislist.asp
Compendium of Animal Rabies Prevention and Control. National Association of State Public Health Veterinarians. (ASPHV). http://www.avma.org/pubhlth/rabcont.asp
Canadian Laboratory Centre for Disease Control
http://www.phac-aspc.gc.ca/msds-ftss/index.html

References

"Compendium of Animal Rabies Prevention and Control, 2001." National Association of State Public Health Veterinarians. 25 October 2001. http//www.avma.org/pubhlth/rabcont.asp.

"Material Safety Data Sheet–Rabies." January 2001. Canadian Laboratory Centre for Disease Control. 25 October 2001. http//www.phac-aspc.gc.ca/msds-ftss/index.html.

"Rabies." In *Manual of Standards for Diagnostic Tests and Vaccines*. Paris: World Organization for Animal Health, 2000, pp. 276–291.

"Rabies." In *The Merck Veterinary Manual*, 8th ed. Edited by S.E. Aiello and A. Mays. Whitehouse Station, NJ: Merck and Co., 1998, pp. 966–970.

"Rabies." Animal Health Australia. The National Animal Health Information System (NAHIS). 24 Oct 2001. http//www.aahc.com.au/nahis/disease/dislist.asp.

Rhipicephalus appendiculatus
Brown Ear Tick

Importance

Rhipicephalus appendiculatus is a hard tick found in the ears of cattle, other livestock, and antelope. This tick is considered to be a major pest in areas where it is endemic. Heavy infestations on cattle can result in severe damage to the ears, a potentially fatal toxemia, or the loss of resistance to some infections. R. appendiculatus can transmit a number of diseases, including East Coast fever, corridor disease, Zimbabwe malignant theileriosis, Nairobi sheep disease, and Kisenly sheep disease. It can also spread Theileria taurotragi, Ehrlichia bovis, Rickettsia conorii, Babesia bigemina, and Thogoto virus.

Species affected

R. appendiculatus mainly infests cattle, but can also be found on other species including sheep, goats, and antelope. Immature ticks may also be seen on carnivores and occasionally rodents.

Geographic distribution

R. appendiculatus prefers cool, shaded shrubby or woody savannas with at least 24 inches of annual rainfall. It is endemic from southern Sudan and eastern Zaire to South Africa and Kenya and can be found from sea level to 7400 feet (2300 meters).

Life cycle

R. appendiculatus is a 3–host tick. Both immature and adult ticks feed in the ears of cattle and other livestock. During massive infestations, they may also be found on other parts of the body. The immature ticks also feed on small antelope, carnivores, and sometimes rodents. Cattle must be present to sustain significant populations of this tick.

Identification

R. appendiculatus is a member of the family Ixodidae (hard ticks). Hard ticks have a dorsal shield (scutum) and their mouthparts (capitulum) protrude forward when they are seen from above Rhipicephalus ticks are brown ticks with short palps. The basis capitulum is usually hexagonal and generally inornate. Eyes and festoons are both present and Coxa I is deeply cleft. The spiracular plates are comma–shaped. The males of this genus have adanal shields and usually have accessory shields.

The male R. appendiculatus is brownish, reddish–brown, or very dark, with reddish–brown legs. They vary from 1.8 to 4.4 mm in length. The basis capitulum is variable; the lateral margins may be more or less angled. The scutal punctuations are scattered and of moderate size; they are evenly dispersed in the center, but few or none may be found beyond the lateral grooves and in the lateral fields. The cervical grooves are moderately reticulate or non–reticulate. The posteromedian and para–median grooves are narrow and distinct. The adanal shields are long and have slightly rounded angles, but can be somewhat variable. Coxa I has a distinctly pointed dorsal projection.

The female R. appendiculatus is also brown, reddish brown, or very dark. The punctuations are small to moderate sized and are similar to those found in the male. The scutum is approximately equal in length and width; its posterior margin is slightly tapering or abruptly rounded. The lateral grooves are short, poorly defined, or absent. The cervical grooves are long and shallow and almost reach the posterolateral margins.

Recommended actions if R. appendiculatus is suspected
Notification of authorities

Known or suspected R. appendiculatus infestations should be reported immediately to state or federal authorities.

Federal: Area Veterinarians in Charge (AVICs):

http://www.aphis.usda.gov/vs/area_offices.htm
State Veterinarians:
http://www.aphis.usda.gov/vs/sregs/official.html

Control measures

Acaricides can eliminate these ticks from the animal, but do not prevent reinfestation. Three–host ticks spend at least 90% of their life cycle in the environment rather than on the host animal; ticks must also be controlled in the environment to prevent their spread.

Public health

R. appendiculatus can transmit tick typhus (infection by Rickettsia conorii) to humans.

For more information

World Organization for Animal Health (OIE)
http://www.oie.int
OIE International Animal Health Code
http://www.oie.int/eng/normes/mcode/A_summry.htm
USAHA Foreign Animal Diseases Book
http://www.vet.uga.edu/vpp/gray_book/FAD/
Identification of the Paralysis Tick I. holocyclus and Related Ticks
http://members.ozemail.com.au/~norbertf/identification.htm
Hard Ticks (photographs) from the University of Edinburgh
http://www.nhc.ed.ac.uk/collections/ticks/hard.htm#Amblyomma

References

Arthur, D.R. "Diagnosis of Rhipicephalus appendiculatus." In Ticks and Disease. New York: Pergamon Press, 1961, pp. 70–73.

"Disease Information." 2001 Merial. 3 December 2001. http//nz.merial.com/farmers/sheep/disease/haema.html.

"Identification of the Paralysis Tick I. holocyclus and Related Ticks." February 2001 New South Wales Department of Agriculture. 29 November 2001. http//members.ozemail.com.au/~norbertf/identification.htm.

Kettle, D.S. "Rhipicephalus appendiculatus." In Medical and Veterinary Entomology. Tucson, AZ: C.A.B International, 1990, pp. 472–475.

"Rhipicephalus spp." In The Merck Veterinary Manual, 8th ed. Edited by S.E. Aiello and A. Mays. Whitehouse Station, NJ: Merck and Co., 1998, pp. 680–682.

Wilson, D.D. and R.A. Bram. "Foreign Pests and Vectors of Arthropod–Borne Diseases." In Foreign Animal Diseases. Richmond, VA: United States Animal Health Association, 1998, pp. 225–239.

Rift Valley Fever
Infectious Enzootic Hepatitis of Sheep and Cattle

Importance

Rift Valley fever (RVF) is an arthropod–borne, acute, febrile, viral disease of sheep, cattle, and goats. RVF is highly contagious to humans producing fever and flu–like symptoms. Severe hemorrhages, meningoencephalitis, and retinopathy occasionally occur and may be fatal in humans. The mortality rate is high in young animals, as is the abortion rate in infected animals.

Etiology

Rift Valley Fever virus (RVFV) is a single–stranded RNA virus in the Phlebovirus genus of the family Bunyaviridae.

Species affected

Many species can be infected by RVFV, including humans. Sheep and cattle are the primary hosts and amplifiers of this virus. Goats and dogs are also highly susceptible. Horses and pigs are resistant to this disease.

Geographic distribution

Rift Valley fever is found throughout most of Africa. Recent outbreaks have occurred in Saudi Arabia and Yemen.

Transmission

Rift Valley fever is spread between hosts by mosquito vectors. *Aedes* mosquitoes are the reservoir for the virus. In endemic regions, outbreaks often occur in 5 to 15 year cycles, and are typically seen after periods of heavy rainfall in normally dry areas. Between outbreaks, the virus may be present in dormant eggs of the mosquito *Aedes lineatopinnus* in the dry soil of grasslands. Heavy rainfall allows water to pool and gives the eggs a place to hatch. These infected mosquitoes develop, and transmit the virus to a ruminant amplifying host. Other genera and species of mosquitoes can then become infected and rapidly spread the disease. If susceptible animal species are present, there are many clinical cases. In many areas of Africa, the disease is enzootic and sentinel animals are used to monitor its presence.

The Rift Valley fever virus can also spread, by aerosols, to humans who handle infected tissues (as when performing field necropsies). This virus can survive up to 4 months at 4°C, and 8 years at temperatures below 0°C. It can also survive for over 1 hour in aerosols.

Incubation period

The incubation period for Rift Valley fever is up to 3 days in sheep, cattle, goats, and dogs. In newborn animals, it can be as short as 12 hours.

Clinical signs

The clinical signs of Rift Valley fever vary with species and age. They can include fever, anorexia, weakness, and death within 36 hours in lambs. Adult sheep will have a fever, mucopurulent nasal discharge, and possibly vomiting. Fever and depression are seen in calves, and fever, weakness, anorexia, excessive salivation, and possibly fetid diarrhea in adult cattle. Abortion is the most common sign when pregnant animals are present.

Post mortem lesions

Hepatic necrosis is the primary lesion, and is especially extensive in younger animals and fetuses. The liver will appear enlarged, yellow, and friable with petechial hemorrhages. In older animals, hepatic necrosis can be more focal and may only be visible microscopically. Cutaneous hemorrhages, hemorrhages on serosal membranes, and hemorrhagic enteritis may also be seen.

Morbidity and mortality

Rift Valley fever is often fatal in young lambs, calves, and kids. In lambs less than 1 week of age, the mortality rate can be 90% or higher. In calves it is 10% to 70%. The mortality rate is about 20% in adult sheep, especially ewes that have aborted, and 10% in adult cattle. Abortion rates are high; up to 100% of infected sheep, cattle, and dogs may abort.

Diagnosis

Clinical

Rift Valley fever should be considered when the following group of conditions occur: high abortion rates, especially in sheep, cattle and dogs; high mortality in young ruminants; severe hepatic necrosis on necropsy of young animals and fetuses; flu–like symptoms in humans; high numbers of mosquitoes; and rapid spread of disease.

Differential diagnosis

The clinical signs of Rift Valley fever in animals can be similar to those of bluetongue, Wesselsbron, ephemeral fever, enterotoxemia of sheep, brucellosis, vibriosis, trichomoniasis, Nairobi sheep disease, heartwater, ovine enzootic abortion, *Campylobacter* or *Salmonella* infection, listeriosis, toxoplasmosis, or any other cause of abortion.

Laboratory tests

The Rift Valley fever virus can be isolated in mice or hamsters, 1 to 2 day old lambs, embryonated chicken eggs, or tissue culture. Viral antigen is identified by immunofluorescence, complement fixation, and immunodiffusion. Antigens can be detected in the blood with immunodiffusion or enzyme immunoassays. Serological tests include enzyme–linked immunosorbent assay (ELISA), virus neutralization, immunofluorescence, hemagglutination inhibition, plaque reduction neutralization, complement fixation, and immunodiffusion.

Samples to collect

Before collecting or sending any samples from Rift Valley fever suspects, the proper authorities should be contacted. Samples should only be sent under secure conditions and to authorized laboratories to prevent spread of the disease. Rift Valley fever is a zoonotic disease. Care should be taken to avoid exposure to aerosols and infected tissues. At the minimum, a face mask or shield and rubber gloves should be worn.

For virus isolation, heparinized blood or serum should be collected from febrile animals, and tissue samples of the liver, spleen, kidney, lymph node, heart blood, and brain from dead animals or aborted fetuses. Specimens should be submitted preserved in 10% buffered formalin and in glycerol/saline and transported at 4°C.

Recommended actions if Rift Valley fever is suspected

Notification of authorities

State and federal veterinarians should be immediately informed of any suspected cases of Rift Valley fever.

Federal: Area Veterinarians in Charge (AVICs):
http://www.aphis.usda.gov/vs/area_offices.htm
State Veterinarians:
http://www.aphis.usda.gov/vs/sregs/official.html

Quarantine and disinfection

Sanitation and vector control should be attempted, but often do not control the spread of disease. RVFV is inactivated by ether, chloroform, and strong solutions of sodium or calcium hypochlorite (residual chlorine should exceed 5000 ppm). It is also destroyed by low pH (<6.8) and detergents. Carcasses should be buried or burned.

Public health

Humans are highly susceptible to infection by mosquitoes or by exposure to aerosols when handling infected tissues during slaughter, necropsy of aborted fetuses, or laboratory procedures. In humans, the incubation period is 4 to 6 days. The symptoms are flu–like and may include fever, weakness, muscle pain, headache, nausea, and photophobia. Recovery generally occurs after 4 to 7 days. Occasionally, a hemorrhagic condition may develop 2 to 4 days after the fever appears. The signs include jaundice, hematemesis, melena, petechiae, and death. Some patients may have meningoencephalitis and others a retinopathy that develops 5 to 15 days after the onset of fever. Vaccination is available for those at risk of exposure.

For more information

World Organization for Animal Health (OIE)
http://www.oie.int
OIE Manual of Standards
http://www.oie.int/eng/normes/mmanual/a_summry.htm
OIE International Animal Health Code
http://www.oie.int/eng/normes/mcode/A_summry.htm
USAHA Foreign Animal Diseases Book
http://www.vet.uga.edu/vpp/gray_book/FAD/

References

Mebus, C.A. "Rift Valley Fever." In *Foreign Animal Diseases*. Richmond, VA: United States Animal Health Association, 1998, pp. 353–361.

"Rift Valley Fever." In *Manual of Standards for Diagnostic Tests and Vaccines*. Paris: World Organization for Animal Health, 2000, pp. 144–152.

Rift Valley Fever. Disease Lists and Cards. World Organization for Animal Health. http//www.oie.int.

Rinderpest

Cattle Plague

Importance

Rinderpest is an acute, contagious disease of cattle, domestic buffalo, and some species of wildlife. It is characterized by fever, oral erosions, diarrhea, lymphoid necrosis, and high mortality.

Etiology

Rinderpest virus (RPV) is a single–stranded RNA virus in the family Paramyxoviridae, genus *Morbillivirus*. Although there is just one serotype of RPV, individual strains vary in their virulence.

Species affected

Most cloven–hooved animals are susceptible to rinderpest virus to varying degrees. Domestic cattle, buffalo, and yaks are particularly susceptible. Sheep, goats, pigs, and wild ungulates can also be affected.

Geographic distribution

In the past, rinderpest was found throughout Europe, Africa, Asia, and West Asia. It is still found in a few areas of Africa, and perhaps of central Asia, its original ancestral home. A Global Rinderpest Eradication Programme (GREP) has been managed by the Food and Agriculture Organization of the United Nations (FAO) with the goal of completing the global eradication of rinderpest by 2010.

Transmission

Transmission of the rinderpest virus occurs through direct or close indirect contact with infected animals. The virus is shed in nasal and ocular secretions and feces. The most infectious period is from 1 to 2 days prior to the onset of clinical signs, to 8 to 9 days after the clinical signs are apparent.

Incubation period

The incubation period for rinderpest ranges from 3 to 15 days; 4 to 5 days is typical. Virulence, dosage, and route of exposure all affect the incubation period.

Clinical signs

Rinderpest infections can be peracute, acute, or subacute depending on the virulence of the strain and resistance of the infected animal. In the peracute form, seen in highly susceptible and young animals, the typical signs are high fever, congested mucous membranes, and death within 2 to 3 days. Animals with the acute or classic form begin with signs of fever, depression, anorexia, and increased respiration and heart rate, which then progress to include mucous membrane congestion, serous to mucopurulent ocular and nasal discharge, and oral erosions with salivation. After 2 to 3 days, the fever subsides and gastrointestinal signs appear. Animals may have profuse watery or hemorrhagic diarrhea containing mucus and necrotic debris, severe tenesmus, dehydration, abdominal pain, abdominal respiration, weakness, and recumbency. Death may occur within 8 to 12 days. Occasionally, in the acute form, the clinical signs will regress by the tenth day and animals may recover within another 10 to 15 days. The subacute or mild form has a low mortality rate and only a few of the classic signs are present.

In sheep, goats and pigs, signs may include fever, anorexia, and sometimes diarrhea. Pigs may also have conjunctivitis and oral erosions, followed by death.

Post mortem lesions

Depending on the strain of virus, rinderpest will sometimes cause oral lesions that initially appear as small necrotic foci, which then slough leaving red erosions. These lesions may be present on the gums, lips, hard and soft palate, cheeks, and base of the tongue. These erosions and areas of necrosis as well as congestion, hemorrhage, and edema can extend into the gastrointestinal and upper respiratory tracts. The abomasum may be particularly affected. "Tiger" or "zebra" striping is often seen in the large intestines due to congestion in the colonic mucosal ridges probably caused by tenesmus. The Peyer's patches may have necrotic foci and the lymph nodes may be enlarged and edematous. The carcass will most likely be emaciated and dehydrated.

Morbidity and mortality

The morbidity rate for rinderpest is high. The mortality rate can be high with virulent strains but varies with milder strains.

Diagnosis

Clinical

Rinderpest should be considered in cattle with any acutely febrile, highly contagious disease with oral erosions and/or gastrointestinal signs.

Differential diagnosis

Differentials for rinderpest include bovine virus diarrhea (mucosal disease), infectious bovine rhinotracheitis, malignant catarrhal fever, foot–and–mouth disease, vesicular stomatitis, salmonellosis, necrobacillosis, paratuberculosis, and arsenic poisoning. Bovine virus diarrhea–mucosal disease primarily affects animals from 4 to 24 months of age, whereas rinderpest can affect cattle of any age. In sheep and goats, peste des petits ruminants is a differential.

Laboratory tests

Virus isolation and identification is necessary to confirm a diagnosis of rinderpest.

Peste des petits ruminants virus (also a *Morbillivirus*) has common antigens with rinderpest virus. When both diseases are present, the diagnosis must be confirmed using an enzyme–linked immunosorbent assay (ELISA test) following specific antigen capture. The diagnosis can also be confirmed with viral–specific RNA detection methods such as nucleic acid probe hybridization and reverse–transcription polymerase chain reaction (RT–PCR).

Samples to collect

Before collecting or sending any samples from animals with a suspected foreign animal disease, the proper authorities should be contacted. Samples should only be sent under secure conditions and to authorized laboratories to prevent the spread of the disease.

The best time to collect samples for rinderpest is when a high fever and oral lesions are present but before the onset of diarrhea. This is when viral titers are highest. Ideally, an animal should be necropsied and the following samples collected: blood in EDTA or heparin, blood for serum, swabs of lacrimal fluid, necrotic tissue from oral lesions, lymph nodes (aspiration biopsy may be helpful from a live animal), spleen, and tonsil. Samples should be transported on wet ice, not frozen. If a necropsy is performed, a complete set of all tissues and lesions should also be sent in 10% formalin.

Recommended actions if this rinderpest is suspected

Notification of authorities

State and federal veterinarians should be immediately informed of any suspected cases of Rinderpest.

Federal: Area Veterinarians in Charge (AVICs):
http://www.aphis.usda.gov/vs/area_offices.htm

State Veterinarians:
http://www.aphis.usda.gov/vs/sregs/official.html

Quarantine and disinfection

The affected area should be quarantined, exposed or infected animals should be slaughtered and the carcasses burned or buried. The rinderpest virus can be killed by most common disinfectants (phenol, cresol, sodium hydroxide 2%/24 hours used at a rate of 1 liter/m2), but can survive for long periods of time in chilled or frozen tissues.

Public health

Rinderpest has not been reported to affect humans.

For more information

World Organization for Animal Health (OIE)
http://www.oie.int

OIE Manual of Standards
http://www.oie.int/eng/normes/mmanual/a_summry.htm

OIE International Animal Health Code
http://www.oie.int/eng/normes/mcode/A_summry.htm

USAHA Foreign Animal Diseases Book
http://www.vet.uga.edu/vpp/gray_book/FAD/

References

"Rinderpest." In *Manual of Standards for Diagnostic Tests and Vaccines*. Paris: World Organization for Animal Health, 2000, pp. 105–113.

"Rinderpest." In *The Merck Veterinary Manual*, 8th ed. Edited by S.E. Aiello and A. Mays. Whitehouse Station, NJ: Merck and Co., 1998, pp. 542–544.

Mebus, C.A. "Rinderpest." In *Foreign Animal Diseases*. Richmond, VA: United States Animal Health Association, 1998, pp. 362–371.

"Rinderpest." 30 Aug. 2000 World Organization for Animal Health. 16 Oct. 2001. http//www.oie.int/eng/maladies/fiches/a_A040.htm.

Salmonella Abortusovis

Paratyphoid Abortion

Importance

Salmonella Abortusovis primarily infects sheep. Infections can cause abortion storms when the organism is newly introduced into a flock; where this organism is endemic, sporadic abortions occur in young and newly introduced animals. Economic losses result mainly from abortions, stillbirths, and illness in lambs infected at birth. Occasionally, ewes develop metritis and septicemia.

Etiology

This disease is caused by *Salmonella enterica* subspecies *enterica* serovar (serotype) Abortusovis. *Salmonella* Abortusovis, a member of the Enterobacteriaceae, is a short, aerobic, Gram–negative rod.

Species affected

Salmonella Abortusovis is adapted to sheep and considered to be host specific; however, it has occasionally been isolated from other animals, including goats and rabbits. Mice and rabbits can be experimentally infected. Antibodies have been found in red deer.

Geographic distribution

Salmonella Abortusovis infections can be found worldwide, but are particularly common in Europe and Western Asia. Infections have been reported in France, Spain, Germany, Cyprus, Italy, Switzerland, Russia, and Bulgaria. This disease was once very common in southwest England and Wales, but it is now rare in the United Kingdom.

Transmission

Salmonella Abortusovis is almost always introduced into a flock by an infected sheep; unlike other *Salmonella* species, spread by feed, water, other mammals, or birds is negligible. Sheep may become infected by the oral, conjunctival, or respiratory routes. Venereal spread appears to be possible, but of minor importance. Sheep can be asymptomatic carriers.

Infectious organisms are mainly found in vaginal discharges, the placenta, aborted fetuses, and infected newborns. Vaginal discharges are highly infectious during the first week after an abortion; in some cases, they may be infectious up to a month. The feces may contain organisms in animals with septicemia, and a few sheep excrete the bacteria in the colostrum or milk. It is possible that the respiratory secretions are infectious in young lambs.

Incubation period

Animals infected at 1 month of gestation may abort after a 2–month incubation period. If the ewes are infected during the third month of gestation, abortions occur after approximately 20 days. Animals infected 1 month before mating do not abort.

Clinical signs

The major clinical sign is abortion, primarily during the second half or last third of gestation. Lambs may also be stillborn or die within a few hours of birth from septicemia. Occasionally, lambs appear to be healthy but die within 3 weeks; some have diarrhea or symptoms of pulmonary infections.

Most ewes appear to be otherwise healthy, although some animals have a transient fever. A vaginal discharge may be apparent for a few days before and after the abortion. Diarrhea is rare. Occasional ewes may develop post–parturient metritis and peritonitis from secondary bacterial invaders.

Post mortem lesions

The aborted fetus and the placenta may be grossly normal or autolyzed. Sometimes, signs of septicemia are apparent in the placenta; they can include edema and hemorrhages in the chorio-allantois and necrosis or swelling of the cotyledons. Multifocal suppurative inflammation, necrosis, edema, or hemorrhages may be seen in the fetal tissues. The liver and spleen may be swollen and contain pale foci.

In young lambs or ewes with diarrhea, there may be enteritis and abomasitis, with swelling of the regional lymph nodes. Ewes that die with septicemia generally have acute metritis; the uterus is usually swollen and contains necrotic tissue, serous exudate, and a retained placenta.

Morbidity and mortality

During an outbreak in a naïve flock, *Salmonella* Abortusovis usually affects large numbers of animals. As many as 60% of all ewes may abort and mortality in ewes and newborn lambs may be significant. If the disease becomes endemic in a flock, abortions are usually sporadic; only young animals and new sheep introduced into the flock tend to be affected. Most ewes develop good immunity after infection but some may become carriers.

Antibiotics appear to stop the abortions during an outbreak. Vaccines may be available in some areas.

Diagnosis

Clinical

Salmonella Abortusovis infections should be suspected in sheep that abort or give birth to stillborn lambs. Usually, there are few signs of disease in the ewe, unless the placenta is retained and metritis develops.

Differential diagnosis

The differential diagnosis includes chlamydiosis, brucellosis, campylobacteriosis, listeriosis, Q fever, and toxoplasmosis. Other *Salmonella* species must also be ruled out.

Laboratory tests

A diagnosis of *Salmonella* Abortusovis infection is supported by finding short, Gram–negative rods in direct smears, but isolation of the organism is necessary for a definitive diagnosis. *Salmonella* Abortusovis will grow on MacConkey, desoxycholate citrate (DCA), or *Salmonella–Shigella* agar. Colonies on nonselective media are grayish, smooth, moist, and translucent to opaque. *Salmonella* Abortusovis grows relatively slowly in culture; colonies can be usually be found in 36 to 48 hours at 35–37°C, but occasionally reach a significant size only after 72 hours of incubation. Pure cultures are identified by biochemical tests, which must be read after 36 to 48 hours. Some authors feel that conventional identification systems for Gram–negative bacteria, such as the AP120E system, are unreliable.

Serology can be helpful for diagnosis. Serologic tests include a serum agglutination test (SAT), hemagglutination inhibition, complement fixation, indirect immunofluorescence, gel immunodiffusion, and enzyme–linked immunosorbent assay (ELISA). Antibodies may become undetectable in some animals 2 to 3 months after abortion. An allergic skin test has also been reported; this test may detect infections longer than other assays.

Samples to collect

Direct smears may be made from the vaginal discharge, placenta, and the stomach contents of the aborted fetus. Isolation of *Salmonella* Abortusovis can be attempted from the vaginal discharge of aborted ewes, the placenta, and fetal tissues. Vaginal swabs are most likely to be diagnostic if they are collected during the first week after the abortion. Fetal tissues for bacterial isolation should include the liver and contents of the gastrointestinal tract.

Recommended actions if *Salmonella* Abortusovis infection is suspected

Notification of authorities

Salmonella Abortusovis is a reportable infection in many states. State authorities should be consulted for specific details.

Federal: Area Veterinarians in Charge (AVICs):
http://www.aphis.usda.gov/vs/area_offices.htm
State Veterinarians:
http://www.aphis.usda.gov/vs/sregs/official.html

Quarantine and disinfection

Salmonella Abortusovis is a contagious disease; to prevent its spread, sheep must be quarantined, aborted animals must be isolated, and the abortion products must be destroyed. Affected farms, with all potential fomites, should be disinfected with an agent effective against *Salmonella*. Effective disinfectants include 1% sodium hypochlorite, 70% ethanol, 2% glutaraldehyde, iodine compounds, phenolics, and formaldehyde, as well as other agents. *Salmonellae* are also susceptible to moist heat (121°C for 15 min or longer) and dry heat (160–170°C for 1 hour or longer).

Public health

Unlike other *Salmonella* species, *Salmonella* Abortusovis does not appear to be a significant threat to human health. Human infections with this species appear to be very rare.

For more information

World Organization for Animal Health (OIE)
http://www.oie.int
OIE International Animal Health Code
http://www.oie.int/eng/normes/mcode/A_summry.htm
Animal Health Australia. The National Animal Health Information System (NAHIS)
http://www. aahc.com.au/nahis/disease/dislist.asp

References

Euzéby, J.P. "List of bacterial names with standing in nomenclature. *Salmonella* nomenclature." July 2000. 26 November 2001. http://www.bacterio.cict.fr/salmonellanom.html.

Gonzales, L. "*Salmonella* Abortusovis infection." In *Diseases of Sheep*, 3rd ed. Edited by W.B. Martin and I.D. Aitken. Malden, MA : Blackwell Science, 2000, pp. 102–107.

"Material Safety Data Sheet–*Salmonella choleraesuis*." January 2001. Canadian Laboratory Centre for Disease Control. 27 November 2001. http//www.phac-aspc.gc.ca/msds-ftss/index.html.

Pardon, P., R. Sanchis, J. Marly, F. Lantier, L. Guilloteau, D. Buzoni–Gatel, I.P. Oswald, M. Pepin, B. Kaeffer, P. Berthon, and M.Y. Popoff. "Experimental Ovine Salmonellosis (*Salmonella* Abortusovis): Pathogenesis and Vaccination." *Res. Microbiol.* 141 (1990): 945–953.

"*Salmonella*." Animal Health Australia. The National Animal Health Information System (NAHIS). 24 Oct 2001. http//www. aahc.com.au/nahis/disease/dislist.asp.

"*Salmonella*." In *Schnierson's Atlas of Diagnostic Microbiology*, 9th ed. Abbott Park, IL: Abbott Laboratories, p. 24.

"*Salmonella* Abortion." Organic Livestock Research Group, VEERU, The University of Reading March 2000. 19 November 2001. http//www.organic–vet.reading.ac.uk/Sheepweb/disease/salmon/salmon1.htm.

"*Salmonella* Abortion." In *Jensen and Swift's Diseases of Sheep*, 3rd ed. Edited by C.V. Kimberling. Philadelphia: Lea & Febiger, 1988, pp. 54–57.

"Salmonellosis." Animal Health Australia. The National Animal Health Information System (NAHIS). 19 Nov 2001. http//www. aahc.com.au/nahis/disease/dislist.asp.

Screwworm Myiasis

Gusanos, Mosca Verde, Gusano barrendor, Gusaneras

Importance

Screwworms are fly larvae (maggots) that feed on living flesh. These parasites can infect any mammal or bird and can enter wounds as small as a tick bite. Left untreated, screwworm infestation can be fatal. Screwworms have been eradicated in the United States, Mexico, and all countries in Central America; however, they could become re–established from larvae carried on infested animals.

Etiology

New World screwworm myiasis is caused by the larvae of *Cochliomyia hominivorax* (Coquerel). Old World screwworm myiasis is caused by the larvae of *Chrysomya bezziana* (Villeneuve). These fly larvae are obligate parasites of live animals and feed on the living tissues and fluids inside wounds.

Species affected

All warm–blooded animals can be infested by screwworms; however, these parasites are much more common in mammals than in birds.

Geographic distribution

Screwworms are very susceptible to freezing temperatures and to long periods of near–freezing temperatures. These organisms are seasonal in some areas, and can spread into colder climates during the summer.

New World screwworms are found only in the western hemisphere, primarily in the tropical and semitropical regions of South America, but are rare above 7,000 feet. These parasites were once widespread, but eradication programs (through the release of sterile male flies) have eliminated them from the United States, Mexico, Puerto Rico, the Virgin Islands, Curacao, and all of Central America and most of Panama, leaving only a small zone at the border with Colombia. The New World screwworm still exists in some countries of South America and on some Caribbean islands. Eradication programs are ongoing in Jamaica. In 1988, New World screwworms were detected in Libya, but have since been eradicated.

C. bezziana, the Old World screwworm, can be found in Southeast Asia, Kuwait, the Indian subcontinent, the main island of Papua New Guinea, tropical and sub–Saharan Africa, Oman, Muscat, and Fujaira. This fly has never become established in Europe, North Africa, Australia, the Middle East, or the Western Hemisphere.

Transmission

Screwworm infestations are transmitted when a female fly lays her eggs on a superficial wound. Occasionally, Old World screwworms also lay their eggs on unbroken soft skin, particularly if it has blood or mucous discharges on its surface. The larvae hatch and burrow into the wound or into the flesh. Wounds infested by screwworms often attract other female screwworms, and multiple infestations are common. After feeding for 5 to 7 days, the screwworm larvae leave the wound and fall to the ground, then burrow into the soil to pupate. The adults that emerge feed on wound fluids and mate after 3 to 5 days. The lifespan of a male fly is approximately 14 days; 30 days is common for a female.

Female screwworms are attracted to all warm–blooded animals. The distance a fly will travel can range from 10 to 20 km in tropical environments with a high density of animals to as far as 300 km in arid environments. Outbreaks in non–endemic areas often occur when animals with screwworm myiasis are introduced or when adult flies are carried in vehicles.

Incubation period

Screwworm larvae emerge from the eggs in 8 to 12 hours. They mature in 5 to 7 days and leave the wound to pupate.

Clinical signs

Screwworms can infest a wide variety of wounds, from tick bites to cuts, dehorning or branding wounds, and other injuries. Infestations are very common in the navels of newborns.

In the first day or two, screwworm infestations are difficult to detect. Often, all that can be seen is slight motion inside the wound. As the larvae feed, the wound gradually enlarges and deepens. Infested wounds often have a serosanguineous discharge and sometimes a distinctive odor. By the third day, the larvae may be easily found; as many as 200 vertically oriented parasites can be packed deep inside the wound. However, screwworm larvae do not generally crawl on the surface, and tend to burrow deeper when disturbed. Sometimes, there may be large pockets of larvae with only small openings in the skin. Screwworms may be particularly difficult to find inside the nasal, anal, and vaginal openings. In dogs, the larvae often tunnel under the skin. Larvae from other species of flies, which feed on dead and decaying tissues, may also infest the wound.

Infested animals usually separate from the herd and lie down in shady areas. Discomfort, decreased appetite, and lower milk production are common. Untreated animals may die in 7 to 14 days from toxemia and dehydration and/or secondary infections.

Post mortem lesions

Screwworms may be found post–mortem in any wound.

Morbidity and mortality

The morbidity from screwworms varies, but can be very high when the ecological conditions are favorable. In some areas, screwworms may infest the navel of nearly every newborn animal.

A single deposition of eggs, or a treated infestation, is not usually fatal; however, deaths may occur in smaller animals or from secondary infections. Untreated wounds usually develop multiple infestations and are often fatal within 7 to 10 days. Deaths seem to be more common with the New World screwworm than with the Old World screwworm.

Screwworm infestations can be successfully treated with topical larvicides or some drugs. No vaccine is available.

Diagnosis

Clinical

Screwworm myiasis should be suspected in animals with draining or enlarging wounds with symptoms of infestation. New World screwworm eggs are creamy and white, and are deposited in a shingle–like array on or near the edges of superficial wounds. The egg masses of Old World screwworms are similar but larger. The eggs from other species of flies are usually not well organized.

The second and third instar larvae of screwworms resemble a wood screw. They are cylindrical, with one pointed end and one blunt end, and have complete rings of dark brown spines around the body. In third stage larvae, dark tracheal tubes can be found on the dorsum of the posterior end. Field diagnosis, even with a microscope or magnifying glass, is difficult.

Female screwworm flies are larger than a housefly. The thorax of a New World screwworm is dark blue to blue–green and the head is reddish–orange. On the back of the thorax, there are three longitudinal dark stripes; the center stripe is incomplete. The Old World screwworm is green to bluish–black, with two transverse stripes on the thorax. Adult screwworms are difficult to distinguish from other flies.

Differential diagnosis

The differential diagnosis includes all other blowfly larvae that may infest wounds.

Laboratory tests

Laboratory diagnosis is by identification of the parasites under the microscope. Serology is not used.

Samples to collect

Before collecting or sending any samples from animals with a suspected foreign animal disease, the proper authorities should be contacted. Samples should only be sent under secure conditions and to authorized laboratories to prevent the spread of the disease. Screwworms can infest humans; samples should be collected and handled with all appropriate precautions.

Larvae should be removed from the wound with forceps before the wound is treated. The larvae should be collected from the deepest parts of the wound. Any eggs on the edge of the wound should be carefully removed with a scalpel. The samples of eggs, larvae, or flies should be placed in 80% alcohol and transported to the laboratory. Formalin should not be used.

Recommended actions
if screwworm is suspected
Notification of authorities

Screwworm infestations should be reported to state or federal authorities immediately upon diagnosis or suspicion of the disease.
Federal: Area Veterinarians in Charge (AVICs):
http://www.aphis.usda.gov/vs/area_offices.htm
State Veterinarians:
http://www.aphis.usda.gov/vs/sregs/official.html

Quarantine and disinfection

Organophosphate insecticides are effective against newly hatched larvae, immature forms, and adult flies. Larvae inside wounds must be treated with a suitable larvacide. Spraying or dipping animals with an approved insecticide and treating infested wounds can protect against new infestations for 7 to 10 days. Larvae that are removed from the wound must be placed in alcohol preservative or destroyed. If any larvae leave an infested wound and mature into adults, screwworm can become established in an area.

Public health

Humans can be hosts for screwworm larvae.

For more information

World Organization for Animal Health (OIE)
http://www.oie.int
OIE Manual of Standards
http://www.oie.int/eng/normes/mmanual/a_summry.htm
OIE International Animal Health Code
http://www.oie.int/eng/normes/mcode/A_summry.htm
USAHA Foreign Animal Diseases Book
http://www.vet.uga.edu/vpp/gray_book/FAD/

References

"New World Screwworm (*Cochliomyia hominivorax*) and Old World Screwworm (*Chrysomya bezziana*)." In *Manual of Standards for Diagnostic Tests and Vaccines*. Paris: World Organization for Animal Health, 2000, pp. 313–321.

"Obligatory Myiasis–Producing Flies." In *The Merck Veterinary Manual*, 8th ed. Edited by S.E. Aiello and A. Mays. Whitehouse Station, NJ: Merck and Co., 1998, pp. 652–654.

Novy, J. E. "Screwworm Myiasis." In *Foreign Animal Diseases*. Richmond, VA: United States Animal Health Association, 1998, pp. 372–383.

Sheep Pox and Goat Pox

Importance

Sheep and goat pox are contagious viral skin diseases. These diseases may be mild in indigenous breeds from endemic areas, but are often fatal in newly introduced animals. Sheep and goat pox infections can limit trade, export, and the development of intensive livestock production. They may also prevent new breeds of sheep or goats from being imported into endemic regions.

Etiology

Sheep pox and goat pox result from infection by members of the *Capripox* genus in the family Poxviridae. Most isolates cause disease mainly in sheep or mainly in goats; some isolates can cause serious disease in both species. The causative viruses cannot be distinguished from each other with current techniques. Only 1 serotype exists.

Species affected

Sheep and goat poxviruses cause disease only in these 2 species. Infections have not been seen in wild ungulates.

Geographic distribution

Sheep pox and goat pox are found in central and north Africa, central Asia, the Middle East, and parts of the Indian subcontinent.

Transmission

Sheep and goat poxviruses are usually transmitted by the respiratory route, but may also enter the body through abraded skin. Most animals become infected while they are in close contact with infected sheep or goats. Infectious virus is found in all secretions, excretions, and the scabs from skin lesions. Contagious aerosols may also be generated from dust that contains pox scabs. These viruses can be spread on fomites and are probably transmitted mechanically by insects. Chronically infected carriers are not seen.

Sheep and goat poxviruses can remain infectious for up to 6 months in sheep pens. These viruses may also be found on the wool or hair for as long as 3 months after infection.

Incubation period

The incubation period is 8 to 13 days in most natural infections, but may be as short as 4 days.

Clinical signs

The first sign of infection is a fever, followed 2 to 5 days later by erythematous macules that develop into 0.5 to 1.5 cm hard papules. The centers of the papules are initially edematous but become depressed (umbilicated vesicles), gray, and necrotic, and surrounded by an area of hyperemia. Large fluid–filled vesicles have been seen over the lesions but are rare. Dark, hard, sharply demarcated scabs eventually form over pustules and may take up to 6 weeks to heal. Skin lesions have a predilection for sparsely wooled/haired skin such as the axilla, perineum, and groin but may cover the body. In animals with heavy wool, the lesions can be easier to find by palpation than visual inspection. Mild infections can easily be missed; only a few lesions may be present, often around the ears or the tail.

Systemic signs may include conjunctivitis, rhinitis, lymphadenopathy, depression, and a variable degree of blepharitis. Anorexia is sometimes present if the mucous membranes are involved. Lung lesions can cause dyspnea. The mucous membranes can become necrotic and animals may develop a mucopurulent nasal or ocular discharge. Secondary bacterial infections are common and death can occur at any stage of the disease. Some European breeds of sheep die before the characteristic skin lesions appear.

Post mortem lesions

The skin usually contains macules and papules, with surrounding areas of edema, hemorrhage, and congestion. The papules penetrate through both the dermis and epidermis; in severe cases, they may extend into the musculature. The lungs often contain discrete congested or edematous lesions or firm white nodules. Papules or ulcerated papules are common on the abomasal mucosa. They may also be found on the rumen, large intestine, trachea, esophagus, tongue, and hard or soft palate. Pale foci are sometimes present on the surface of the kidney, liver, and testicles. The lymph nodes are usually swollen and the mucous membranes may be necrotic.

Morbidity and mortality

Morbidity and mortality vary with the breed of the host and the strain of the virus. Disease is usually more severe in young animals. Mild infections are common in indigenous breeds; however, symptoms may be more severe in kids or lambs, stressed animals, animals that have concurrent infections, or animals from areas where pox has not occurred for some time. Imported breeds of sheep and goats usually develop severe disease when they are moved into an endemic area. Mortality may be up to 50% in a fully susceptible flock and as high as 100% in young animals.

Infection results in good immunity. Vaccines are available in some areas.

Diagnosis

Clinical

Sheep or goat pox should be suspected in animals with the characteristic full–thickness skin lesions, fever, and lymphadenitis. Dyspnea may also be seen.

Differential diagnosis

The differential diagnosis includes contagious ecthyma (contagious pustular dermatitis), bluetongue, mycotic dermatitis, sheep scab, mange, photosensitization, peste des petits ruminants, parasitic pneumonia, and caseous lymphadenitis.

Laboratory tests

Sheep or goat pox can be tentatively diagnosed by electron microscopy; the morphology of the virus particle is characteristic. The causative viruses can be isolated in lamb testis or kidney cell cultures or in other sheep, goat, or bovine cell lines. Identification is by immunofluorescence or immunoperoxidase staining.

An agar gel immunodiffusion (AGID) test or enzyme–linked immunosorbent assay (ELISA) can detect virus antigens. Cross–reactions occur in the AGID test with parapoxvirus. A polymerase chain reaction (PCR) technique has also been reported.

Antibodies can be found 1 week after the skin lesions appear. Serologic tests include virus neutralization, agar gel immunodiffusion, indirect immunofluorescence, ELISA, and immunoblotting (Western blotting). Virus neutralization is the most specific serological test, but is not sensitive enough to detect infections in all animals. Cross–reactions with other viruses are seen in the AGID and indirect immunofluorescence tests.

Samples to collect

Before collecting or sending any samples from animals with a suspected foreign animal disease, the proper authorities should be contacted. Samples should only be sent under secure conditions and to authorized laboratories to prevent the spread of the disease.

Skin biopsies should be taken for virus isolation and antigen detection. In live animals, virus can also be isolated from blood samples or lymph nodes. Samples taken at necropsy should include the skin, lymph nodes and lung lesions. Neutralizing antibodies can interfere with virus isolation or antigen–detection ELISAs; samples for these tests must be collected during the early stages of infection. Blood samples must be sent to the laboratory within two days and, ideally, as soon as possible. They should be shipped on wet ice or gel packs. Tissues for virus isolation, antigen detection, or PCR should be kept at 4°C or –20°C. Glycerol (10%) can be added to tissue samples that must be shipped long distances without refrigeration; these samples must be large enough that the medium does not penetrate into the center of the tissue.

Serum should be collected for serology. Samples for histology should include skin (with a wide range of lesions) from live animals and a full set of tissues at necropsy. Lesions from the skin, rumen, lungs, and trachea are particularly useful.

Recommended actions if sheep or goat pox is suspected

Notification of authorities

Sheep or goat pox must be reported immediately to state or federal authorities.

Federal: Area Veterinarians in Charge (AVICs):
http://www.aphis.usda.gov/vs/area_offices.htm
State Veterinarians:
http://www.aphis.usda.gov/vs/sregs/official.html

Quarantine and disinfection

A limited outbreak of sheep or goat pox can sometimes be controlled by depopulating infected and exposed animals, cleaning and disinfecting affected farms and equipment, and imposing a quarantine on animal movement. Sodium hypochlorite is an effective disinfectant. When the disease has spread more widely, vaccination may also be required.

Public health

Sheep and goat pox viruses do not appear to infect humans.

For more information

World Organization for Animal Health (OIE)
http://www.oie.int
OIE Manual of Standards
http://www.oie.int/eng/normes/mmanual/a_summry.htm
OIE International Animal Health Code
http://www.oie.int/eng/normes/mcode/A_summry.htm
USAHA Foreign Animal Diseases Book
http://www.vet.uga.edu/vpp/gray_book/FAD/
Animal Health Australia. The National Animal Health Information System (NAHIS)
http://www. aahc.com.au/nahis/disease/dislist.asp

References

Blackwell, J.H. "Cleaning and Disinfection." In *Foreign Animal Diseases*. Richmond, VA: United States Animal Health Association, 1998, pp. 445–448.

House, J.A. "Sheep and Goat Pox." In *Foreign Animal Diseases*. Richmond, VA: United States Animal Health Association, 1998, pp. 384–391.

"Sheep Pox and Goat Pox." Animal Health Australia. The National Animal Health Information System (NAHIS). 11 December 2001. http//www. aahc.com.au/nahis/disease/dislist.asp.

"Sheep Pox and Goat Pox." In *Manual of Standards for Diagnostic Tests and Vaccines*. Paris: World Organization for Animal Health, 2000, pp. 168–177.

"Sheeppox and Goatpox." In *The Merck Veterinary Manual*, 8th ed. Edited by S.E. Aiello and A. Mays. Whitehouse Station, NJ: Merck and Co., 1998, pp. 622–623.

Spring Viremia of Carp

Infectious Dropsy of Carp, Hydrops, Rubella, Hemorrhagic Septicemia

Importance

Spring viremia of carp (SVC) is a contagious viral disease that mainly affects species of carp. This disease is often fatal; mortality up to 90% may be seen in outbreaks. The causative virus can be spread by fomites and parasitic invertebrates; once it is established in a pond, eradication is difficult unless all aquatic life is destroyed.

Etiology

Spring viremia of carp is caused by the virion, *Rhabdovirus carpio*, a member of the family Rhabdoviridae. Virus strains vary in their pathogenicity.

Species affected

SVC affects common carp, koi carp, grass carp, silver carp, bighead carp, crucian carp, goldfish, tench, and sheatfish. Common carp are the most susceptible species and are considered to be the principal host. Very young fish of various pond species, including pike and perch, are also susceptible.

Geographic distribution

Spring viremia of carp is found in Europe, the Middle East and Asia. More recently, it has been reported in North and South

America. SVC was found in the U.S. in 2002 (North Carolina, Wisconsin, Illinois) and in 2004 (Washington, Missouri).

Transmission

The virus is shed in the feces, urine, and gill and skin mucus of infected fish. It is also found in the exudate of skin blisters and edematous scale pockets. Reservoirs of virus include diseased fish and asymptomatic carriers. Transmission is by direct contact or through the water. The virus may enter through the gills, but oral infection is not thought to be likely. SVC can also spread by fomites or living vectors, including the parasitic invertebrates *Argulus foliaceus* and *Piscicola piscicola*. "Egg–associated" transmission has not been ruled out.

Incubation period

Incubation periods varying from 7 to 15 days have been reported in experimental infections.

Clinical signs

The clinical signs may include darkening of the body, sluggish breathing, tilting to one side, abdominal distension, exophthalmia, anemia, hemorrhagic spots on the gills, and reddening and swelling of the anus. Diseased fish tend to gather at the water inlet. Some recovered fish may become virus carriers.

Post mortem lesions

The abdominal cavity often contains serous fluid, sometimes mixed with blood or necrotic material. The muscles may be reddened from hemorrhages. Hemorrhagic spots are also common on the internal organs, particularly on the walls of the air bladder. The intestines may be severely inflamed and dilated, and may contain necrotic material. The spleen is often very swollen, with a coarse surface texture. Other lesions may include jaundice, edema and swelling of other internal organs, hepatic necrosis, cardiac inflammation, and pericarditis.

Morbidity and mortality

High fish mortality can occur when water temperatures are between 10-17°C. When water temperatures reach 20-22°C, clinical signs may no longer be seen even though fish can still be infected. Susceptibility to SVC is highest in younger fish; it is uncommon in fry and juvenile fish, since the water is usually warm during their growth period. Mortality rates can range from 30% to 90% and varies depending on the water temperature, fish species and fish age. Recovery from infection usually results in strong immunity.

Diagnosis

Clinical

SVC should be suspected in species of carp with systemic infection.

Laboratory tests

Spring viremia of carp can be diagnosed by virus isolation in cell cultures; appropriate cell lines include EPC (*Epithelioma papulosum cyprini*) or FHM cells. The identity of the virus is confirmed by virus neutralization. Rapid, presumptive identification can be made by immunofluorescence or an enzyme–linked immunosorbent assay (ELISA). Virus antigens can also be identified directly in tissues by immunofluorescence or ELISA. Ideally, the diagnosis should be confirmed by virus isolation, but this may not always be possible. Serology may become effective in screening fish populations, but has not yet been validated for routine diagnosis.

Samples to collect

Before collecting or sending any samples from animals with a suspected foreign animal disease, the proper authorities should be contacted. Samples should only be sent under secure conditions and to authorized laboratories to prevent the spread of the disease.

If the fish are symptomatic, the samples to collect depend on the size of the fish. Small fish (less than or equal to 4 cm) should be sent whole. The viscera including the kidney and encephalon should be collected from fish 4 to 6 cm long. The kidney, spleen, liver, and encephalon should be sent from larger fish. Samples from asymptomatic animals should include the kidney, spleen, gill, and encephalon. Samples should be taken from 10 diseased fish and combined to form pools with approximately 1.5 g of material (no more than 5 fish per pool).

The pools of organs or ovarian fluids should be placed in sterile vials. The samples may also be sent in cell culture medium or Hanks' basal salt solution with antibiotics. They should be kept cold (4°C) but not frozen. If the shipping time is expected to be longer than 12 hours, serum or albumen (5–10%) may be added to stabilize the virus. Ideally, virus isolation should be done within 24 hours after fish sampling.

Recommended actions if spring viremia of carp is suspected

Notification of authorities

Spring viremia of carp should be reported to state or federal authorities immediately upon diagnosis or suspicion of the disease.

Federal Area Veterinarians in Charge (AVIC):
http://www.aphis.usda.gov/vs/area_offices.htm
State Veterinarians:
http://www.aphis.usda.gov/vs/sregs/official.html

Quarantine and disinfection

Quarantine is necessary for the control of outbreaks; spring viremia of carp is a contagious disease and asymptomatic carriers occur. Once this disease is established in a pond, it can be very difficult to eradicate unless all forms of aquatic life at the site are destroyed. The virus is heat labile.

Public health

There is no indication that this disease is a threat to human health.

For more information

World Organization for Animal Health (OIE)
http://www.oie.int
OIE Diagnostic Manual for Aquatic Animal Diseases
http://www.oie.int/eng/normes/fmanual/A_summry.htm
OIE International Aquatic Animal Health Code (2001)
http://www.oie.int/eng/normes/fcode/a_summry.htm

References

"Fish Health Management: Viral Diseases." In *The Merck Veterinary Manual*, 8th ed. Edited by S.E. Aiello and A. Mays. Whitehouse Station, NJ: Merck and Co., 1998, pp. 1291–1293.

"General Information." In *Diagnostic Manual for Aquatic Animal Diseases*. Paris: World Organization for Animal Health, 2000. http://www.oie.int/eng/normes/fmanual/A_00010.htm.

"Spring Viremia of Carp." In *Diagnostic Manual for Aquatic Animal Diseases*. Paris: World Organization for Animal Health, 2000. http://www.oie.int/eng/normes/fmanual/A_00015.htm.

"Spring Viremia of Carp (SVC)." In *Infectious Diseases of Fish*. Edited by Shuzo Egusa. New Delhi, India: Amerind Pub. Co., 1992, pp. 35–44.

"Spring Viremia of Carp." U.S. Department of Agriculture, Animal and Plant Health Inspection Service. Tech Note. April 2003. Accessed 10 December 2005 at http://www.aphis.usda.gov/lpa/pubs/tn_ahspringcarp.pdf.

"Spring Viremia, United States, June 17, 2004, Impact Worksheet". USDA APHIS VS Center for Emerging Issues. Accessed 10 December 2005 at http://www.aphis.usda.gov/vs/ceah/cei/IW_2004_files/svc_wa_06172004_files/SVCWA06172004.htm.

"Spring Viremia, United States, July 20, 2004, Impact Worksheet". USDA APHIS VS Center for Emerging Issues. Accessed 10 December 2005 at http://www.aphis.usda.

gov/vs/ceah/cei/IW_2004_files/svc_mo_070804_files/
SVCMO070804final.htm.

Staphylococcal Enterotoxin B

Staph enterotoxicosis

Importance

Staphylococcal enterotoxins are the most common cause of food poisoning. They can cause severe immunological reactions and are especially dangerous if inhaled. Inhalation of high doses of these toxins can be fatal, lower doses can also be incapacitating, making them potential biological weapons.

Etiology

Staphylococcal enterotoxin B (SEB) is produced by *Staphylococcus aureus*. There are 6 other enterotoxins produced by various strains of this bacteria, but SEB has been studied the most. These enterotoxins are known as "superantigens" due to the severe immune reactions they cause. These and other similar toxins activate immune system receptors by binding with T-cell antigen receptors and class II molecules of the major histocompatibility complex (MHC) which stimulates t-cells resulting in the release of large amounts of cytokines such as interferon-gamma, interleukin-6 and tumor necrosis factor-alpha.

Species affected

Humans are of primary concern with SEB intoxications, though most animal species can be affected. Primates show an increased sensitivity to pyrogenic toxins due to an increased binding affinity of their MHC class II molecules. Rhesus macaques, rabbits and mice have been used in laboratory studies.

Geographic distribution

Staphylococcus aureus and its toxins are found in all parts of the world.

Transmission

Staphylococcal enterotoxins are generally produced by bacteria growing in food that has been improperly handled, however, SEB has been extensively studied for use as a biological weapon and can be aerosolized.

Incubation period

The incubation period for inhalation SEB appears to be very short (3 to 4 hours). As a foodborne illness, incubation can be from 30 minutes to 8 hours, usually 2 to 4 hours.

Clinical signs

In the case of foodborne enterotoxin exposure, signs are generally a rapid onset of acute gastrointestinal illness including nausea, vomiting, cramps, weakness, and sometimes diarrhea, hypotension and decreased body temperature. Fever which is seen after aerosol SEB exposure is not generally seen in foodborne cases.

Information on clinical signs in humans of inhalational exposure to SEB comes from a few accidental laboratory exposures. These signs included fever, myalgia, nonproductive cough, headache, nausea, anorexia and vomiting in some. More severe cases had dyspnea, rales, and chest pain with radiographic evidence of pulmonary edema. The extreme hypotension sometimes seen in foodborne illness and toxic shock syndrome is not seen with inhalational exposure.

Post mortem lesions

Post mortem lesions from rhesus monkeys with inhalational SEB intoxication included pulmonary fluid, edema, and fibrin, petechial hemorrhages and areas of atelectasis in the lungs as well as petechial hemorrhages and mucosal erosions in the intestines. Mild lymphadenopathy was also generally present.

Morbidity and mortality

Deaths due to foodborne staphylococcal enterotoxins are rare. The possibility of mortality from inhalational exposure is dependent upon the dose of toxin. The inhalational dose of SEB that is incapacitating for 50% of the exposed human population (effective dose [ED_{50}]) is 0.0004 ug/kg and the lethal dose for 50% of the exposed human population (LD_{50}) is 0.02 ug/kg.

Diagnosis

Clinical

The circumstances and epidemiology should be taken into account in determining the cause of illness. Foodborne outbreaks often occur in clusters and aerosol exposure would generally affect a group of people. SEB may be highly suspected in a battlefield situation.

Differential diagnosis

The differential list for these clinical signs can be long. Epidemiology of an outbreak may be helpful in the preliminary diagnosis, though laboratory testing is necessary for confirmation. Some differentials include other staphylococcal and streptococcal toxins, toxic shock syndrome-1, other causes of foodborne illness or intoxication, heavy metal intoxication, viral, and parasitic diseases.

Laboratory tests

Serum antibody testing is not generally helpful as most people have antibodies to several pyrogenic toxins including SEB. Bacterial culture can be attempted if a source is suspected. Polymerase chain reaction (PCR) amplification and toxin gene-specific oligonucleotide primers may be used to identify small quantities of toxigenic bacteria from cultures. Toxins can be identified from nasal swabs in cases of respiratory exposure and may be present for 12 to 24 hours after exposure. Immunoassays of environmental samples may be able to identify the toxin.

Samples to collect

Samples for bacterial culture can be taken if a source is suspected. Nasal swabs for toxin identification may be the most helpful in cases of aerosol exposure.

Recommended actions if Staphylococcal enterotoxin is suspected

Notification of authorities

Suspected cases of Staphylococcal enterotoxin intoxication should be immediately reported to local health authorities. This may be important in the rapid identification of further cases.

Quarantine and disinfection

Proper hygiene and cooking temperatures when handling food are most important in avoiding foodborne illness. There is no necessary quarantine or disinfection.

Public health

Currently no vaccine is available. A toxoid vaccine has been developed, but is not yet approved for human use. A second type of vaccine is also being studied in which the toxins are genetically inactivated, this may provide more effective protection from these enterotoxins.

For more information

http://ccc.apgea.army.mil/reference_materials/textbook/HTML_Restricted/index_2.htm

References

"Staphylococcal Enterotoxin B and Related Pyrogenic Toxins." In *Textbook of Military Medicine -Medical Aspects of Chemical and Biological Warfare*, Specialty editors Frederick R. Sidell, Ernest T. Takafuji, David R. Franz. Office of the Surgeon General at TMM Publications, Borden Institute, Walter Reed Army Medical Center, Washington D.C., 1997, pp. 621-630. "Foodborne Intoxications." In *Control of Communicable Diseases Manual*, 17th ed., edited by James Chin. Washington, D.C.: American Public Health Association, 2000, pp. 202-206.

Surra

Murrina, Mal de Caderas, Derrengadera

Importance

Surra is a protozoal disease that can affect most mammals but is generally more severe in horses. In endemic areas, the economic cost of this disease can be considerable; in Africa, Asia, and South America, surra causes the death of thousands of animals each year.

Etiology

Surra is caused by infection with the protozoal parasite *Trypanosoma evansi*.

Species affected

T. evansi is pathogenic in most domesticated animals and some wild animals. Horses, mules, donkeys, camels, llamas, deer, cattle, buffalo, cats, and dogs are commonly affected. Asymptomatic, mild, or chronic disease has been seen in sheep, goats, elephants, and pigs. Outbreaks have also been reported in captive tigers and jaguars in India.

The main host species varies with the geographic region: camels are most often affected in the Middle East and Africa, horses in South America, and horses, mules, buffalo, and deer in China. In Southeast Asia, surra is seen mainly in horses, cattle, and buffalo. Capybara are reservoir hosts and vampire bats are both reservoir hosts and vectors in South and Central America.

Geographic distribution

Surra is endemic in China, the Indian subcontinent, Southeast Asia, northern Africa, the Middle East, South America, the Philippines, Bulgaria, parts of the former U.S.S.R., and parts of Indonesia.

Transmission

T. evansi is transmitted mechanically by biting flies in the genera *Tabanus*, *Lyperosia*, *Stomoxys*, and *Atylotus*. Species of *Tabanus* appear to be the most significant vectors. There is no intermediate host. Vampire bats can spread infections in South and Central America. Carnivores may become infected after feeding on infected meat. Transmission in milk and during coitus has also been documented.

Incubation period

In the Equidae, the incubation period varies from 5 to 60 days.

Clinical signs

Surra may be a subacute, acute, or chronic disease. In horses, donkeys, and mules, typical clinical signs include an intermittent fever, lethargy, weakness, weight loss, petechiae on the mucus membranes, and extravasation of blood at the mucocutaneous junctions of the nostrils, eyelids, and anus. Urticaria, jaundice, or anemia may be apparent, and there may be edema in the legs, abdomen, and brisket. Exudation, alopecia, necrosis, or ulceration may be seen at the coronary bands and the lymph nodes may be enlarged. In South America, horses with Mal de Caderas have anemia, emaciation, gradually progressive paresis of the hindquarters, and sometimes urticaria. In the Equidae, surra is often fatal within two weeks to four months.

In cattle and buffalo, surra is typically chronic, but may also be mild or asymptomatic. In chronic infections, the clinical signs may include an intermittent fever, anemia, emaciation, edema of the brisket, and paresis in the hind legs. Abortions may be seen in buffalo. Some animals die during the first 6 months, but most recover and become carriers.

Infections in cats and dogs are usually acute and fatal. Common symptoms in dogs include an intermittent fever and edema of the head, legs, and abdominal wall. Dogs may also have nervous signs that resemble rabies.

In deer, surra is usually chronic and is characterized by edema, anemia, emaciation, and nervous signs. Camels experience symptoms similar to those seen in horses, but chronic infections with wasting and anemia are more common. Infections are usually asymptomatic or mild in pigs and chronic in goats.

Post mortem lesions

The post–mortem lesions may include emaciation of the carcass, anemia, and petechiae on some internal organs. Hydrothorax and ascites are sometimes seen. The spleen and lymph nodes may be enlarged.

Morbidity and mortality

The severity of disease can vary with the strain of trypanosome and with host factors, including stress, concurrent infections, and general health. Outbreaks of surra may be associated with the movement of infected animals into disease–free areas or susceptible animals into endemic areas. In some outbreaks, morbidity up to 50% to 70% and comparable mortality can be seen. In China, the average mortality rate in horses is 41%, and the average mortality rate in camel and buffalo 28%. In general, mortality is high in horses, dogs, and cats and lower in cattle, buffalo, and other species.

In endemic areas, surra can be treated with anti–protozoal drugs.

Diagnosis

Clinical

Typical symptoms of surra include fever, anemia, weight loss, edema, and enlargement of the lymph nodes and spleen.

Differential diagnosis

In horses, the differential diagnosis includes African horse sickness, equine viral arteritis, equine infectious anemia, and chronic parasitism. In dogs, rabies must also be considered.

Laboratory tests

Surra can be diagnosed by finding *T. evansi* in the blood, lymph nodes, skin exudates, liver, lungs, or kidney. For microscopic examination, thin films and smears are stained with Giemsa or another Romanowsky–type stain, and thick films by Field's method. The parasites are often difficult to find by direct examination; detection may be improved by the hematocrit tube centrifugation technique or mini anion–exchange chromatography. Morphologically, *T. evansi* cannot be distinguished from *T. equiperdum* or some forms of *T. brucei*.

T. evansi antigens can be detected with a latex agglutination test or enzyme–linked immunosorbent assays (ELISAs). A polymerase chain reaction (PCR) test has also been published and a reverse indirect hemagglutination test is being tested in China.

Serology can be valuable, but may not distinguish between current and past infections. Published serological techniques include ELISAs, fluorescent antibody tests, and a modified card–agglutination test. Animal inoculation studies in rats or mice are occasionally used; they are very sensitive but time–consuming.

Samples to collect

Before collecting or sending any samples from animals with a suspected foreign animal disease, the proper authorities should be contacted. Samples should only be sent under secure conditions and to authorized laboratories to prevent the spread of the disease.

To detect trypanosomes, several thick and thin blood films should be made during the febrile phase and air–dried. Thick and thin slides may be also made from needle biopsies of the prescapular or precrural lymph nodes, and smears from any skin exudates. Post–mortem, impression smears should be collected from the lungs, liver, and kidney.

In live animals, repeated sampling may be necessary to detect the organism.

Approximately 10 ml blood should also be collected into heparin or EDTA, with antibiotics added. Another 25 ml of blood should be taken for serology. These samples should be transported cold, with wet ice or gel packs.

Recommended actions if surra is suspected
Notification of authorities
Surra should be reported to state or federal authorities immediately upon diagnosis or suspicion of the disease.
Federal: Area Veterinarians in Charge (AVICs):
http://www.aphis.usda.gov/vs/area_offices.htm
State Veterinarians:
http://www.aphis.usda.gov/vs/sregs/official.html

Quarantine and disinfection
Trypanosomes cannot survive for long outside the host, and *T. evansi* disappears quickly from the carcass after death. Controlling arthropod vectors and preventing their access to host species is important in preventing new infections. Flies are most infective during the first few minutes after feeding on an infected host; after eight hours, they no longer transmit the parasites. The movement of potentially infected animals must also be restricted.

Public health
There is no evidence that *T. evansi* is a hazard to human health.

For more information
World Organization for Animal Health (OIE)
http://www.oie.int
OIE International Animal Health Code
http://www.oie.int/eng/normes/mcode/A_summry.htm
Animal Health Australia. The National Animal Health
Information System (NAHIS)
http://www. aahc.com.au/nahis/disease/dislist.asp

References
Brun R., H. Hecker, and Z.R. Lun. "*Trypanosoma evansi* and *T. equiperdum*: distribution, biology, treatment and phylogenetic relationship (a review)." *Veterinary Parasitology* 79, no. 2 (1988):95–107.

Corwin, R.M. and J. Nahm. "*Trypanosoma evansi, equinum, equiperdum*." 1997 University of Missouri College of Veterinary Medicine. 1 November 2001. http//www.missouri.edu/~vmicrorc/Protozoa/Mastigophorans/Tevansi.htm.

Losos, G.J. "Diseases Caused by *Trypanosoma evansi*, a review." *Veterinary Research Communications* 4(1980):165–181.

Lun, Z.–R., Y. Fang, C.–J. Wang, and R. Brun. "Trypanosomiasis of Domestic Animals in China." *Parasitology Today* 9, no. 2 (1993):41–45.

"Surra." Animal Health Australia. The National Animal Health Information System (NAHIS). 31 Oct 2001. http//www.aahc.com.au/nahis/disease/dislist.asp.

"Surra." In *The Merck Veterinary Manual*, 8th ed. Edited by S.E. Aiello and A. Mays. Whitehouse Station, NJ: Merck and Co., 1998, pp. 35.

T.W. Jones, R. C. Payne, I.P. Sukanto and S. Partoutomo. "*Trypanosoma evansi* in the republic of Indonesia." 31 October 2001. http//www.fao.org/docrep/W5781E/w5781e05.htm.

Swine Vesicular Disease

Importance
Swine vesicular disease (SVD) has almost identical clinical signs to foot and mouth disease, but is only seen in pigs. Neither disease is present in North America. Differentiation of these two vesicular diseases is important, as the introduction of foot and mouth disease could cause severe economic losses.

Etiology
Swine vesicular disease virus (SVDV) is a porcine enterovirus in the family Picornaviridae. It is antigenically related to the human enterovirus Coxsackie B–5 and unrelated to other known porcine enteroviruses.

Species affected
Pigs are the only species that are naturally infected. Humans have been infected while working in a laboratory setting. Baby mice can be experimentally infected.

Geographic distribution
While SVD has been seen in Italy, England, Scotland, Wales, Malta, Austria, Belgium, France, the Netherlands, Germany, Poland, Switzerland, Greece, and Spain, the disease has been eradicated from all European countries. SVD still remains in many countries in the Far East.

Transmission
Transmission can occur by ingestion of contaminated meat scraps and contact with infected animals or infected feces. Pigs can excrete the virus from the nose, mouth, and feces up to 48 hours before clinical signs are seen. Virus can be shed in the feces for up to 3 months following infection.

SVDV can survive for long periods of time in the environment. This virus is resistant to heat up to 157°F (69°C) and pH ranging from 2.5–12. It can also survive up to 2 years in lymphoid tissue contained in dried, salted, or smoked meat.

Incubation period
The incubation period is 2 to 7 days following exposure to infected pigs and 2 to 3 days after the ingestion of contaminated feed.

Clinical signs
The clinical signs of swine vesicular disease are very similar to foot and mouth disease, and include fever, salivation, and lameness. Vesicles and erosions can be seen on the snout, mammary glands, coronary band, and interdigital areas. Vesicles in the oral cavity are relatively rare. The infection may be subclinical, mild, or severe depending on the virulence of the strain. Severe signs are generally seen only in pigs housed on damp concrete. Younger animals can be more severely affected. Neurological signs due to encephalitis are rare. These include shivering, unsteady gait, and chorea (rhythmic jerking) of the legs. Abortion is not typically seen. Recovery occurs within 2 to 3 weeks with little permanent damage.

Post mortem lesions
The only post–mortem lesions are the vesicles that can be seen in live pigs. These lesions are similar to those of other vesicular diseases, including foot and mouth disease.

Morbidity and mortality
Swine vesicular disease is considered to be moderately contagious. Compared to foot and mouth disease, morbidity is lower and the lesions are less severe. Mortality is not generally a concern with swine vesicular disease.

Diagnosis

Clinical
Swine vesicular disease or other vesicular diseases should be suspected when vesicles or erosions are found on the mouth and/

or feet of pigs. In swine vesicular disease outbreaks, pigs will be the only species affected, the lesions will be mild, and there will be no mortality. Other vesicular diseases must be ruled out with laboratory tests.

Differential diagnosis

Differentials for swine vesicular disease include foot and mouth disease, vesicular stomatitis, vesicular exanthema of swine, and chemical or thermal burns.

Laboratory tests

SVDV can be identified using enzyme–linked immunosorbent assay (ELISA), the direct complement fixation test, and virus isolation in pig–derived cell cultures. Virus neutralization and ELISA can be used for serological diagnosis.

Samples to collect

Before collecting or sending any samples from vesicular disease suspects, the proper authorities should be contacted. Samples should only be sent under secure conditions and to authorized laboratories to prevent spread of the disease. Since vesicular diseases can not be distinguished clinically, and some are zoonotic, samples should be collected and handled with all appropriate precautions.

Samples include vesicular fluid, the epithelium covering vesicles, esophageal–pharyngeal fluid, unclotted whole blood collected from febrile animals, and fecal and serum samples from infected and non–infected animals.

Recommended actions if swine vesicular disease is suspected

Notification of authorities

State and federal veterinarians should be immediately informed of any suspected vesicular disease.

Federal: Area Veterinarians in Charge (AVICs):
http://www.aphis.usda.gov/vs/area_offices.htm
State Veterinarians:
http://www.aphis.usda.gov/vs/sregs/official.html

Quarantine and disinfection

Infected farms or areas should be quarantined. Infected pigs and those in contact with them should be slaughtered and disposed of. The premises should be thoroughly cleaned and disinfected. In the presence of organic matter, sodium hydroxide (1% combined with detergent) can be used. Oxidizing agents and iodophors used with detergents work well for personal disinfection in the absence of gross organic matter.

Public health

Seroconversion and mild clinical disease with one case of meningitis has been seen in laboratory workers.

For more information

World Organization for Animal Health (OIE)
http://www.oie.int
OIE Manual of Standards
http://www.oie.int/eng/normes/mmanual/a_summry.htm
OIE International Animal Health Code
http://www.oie.int/eng/normes/mcode/A_summry.htm
USAHA Foreign Animal Diseases Book
http://www.vet.uga.edu/vpp/gray_book/FAD/
Manual for the Recognition of Exotic Diseases of Livestock
http://www.spc.int/rahs/

References

Mebus C.A. "Swine Vesicular Disease." In *Foreign Animal Diseases.* Richmond, VA: United States Animal Health Association, 1998, pp. 392–395.

"Swine Vesicular Disease." In *Manual of Standards for Diagnostic Tests and Vaccines.* Paris: World Organization for Animal Health, 2000, pp. 100–104.

Swine Vesicular Disease. Disease Lists and Cards. World Organization for Animal Health. http://www.oie.int.

"Swine Vesicular Disease." In *Manual for the Recognition of Exotic Diseases of Livestock: A Reference Guide for Animal Health Staff.* Food and Agriculture Organization of the United Nations, 2002. 21 April 2003. http//www.spc.int/rahs/Manual/Porcine/SVDE.HTM.

Theileriosis -*Theileria parva* and *Theileria annulata*

Theileriasis, East Coast Fever, Corridor Disease

Importance

Infection by *Theileria* parasites limits the movement of cattle between countries and can result in production losses and high mortality in susceptible animals. The two diseases with the greatest economic impact are East Coast fever (infection with *Theileria parva*) and tropical theileriosis (infection with *Theileria annulata*). These tick–borne infections are difficult to control where their vectors are readily available.

Etiology

Theileriosis results from infection with obligate intracellular protozoa in the genus *Theileria*. The two most important species are *T. parva*, which causes East Coast fever, Corridor disease, and Zimbabwean theileriosis, and *T. annulata*, which causes tropical theileriosis (Mediterranean theileriosis). A number of other *Theileria* species can infect ruminants; many of them cause mild or asymptomatic infections.

Species affected

T. parva infects cattle, African buffalo, Indian water buffalo, and waterbucks. Symptomatic infections are common only in cattle and Indian water buffalo. African buffalo and waterbucks are reservoirs for this infection. *T. annulata* infects cattle, yak, and buffalo, with milder infections usually seen in buffalo.

Geographic distribution

East Coast fever is found from southern Sudan to South Africa and west to Zaire. The tick vectors can be found from sea level to over 8,000 feet, in any area where the annual rainfall exceeds 20 inches.

Tropical theileriosis is seen in North Africa, southern Europe, the southern republics of the former U.S.S.R., the Indian subcontinent, China, and the Middle East.

Transmission

Both *T. parva* and *T. annulata* are spread by ticks. The most important vector for *T. parva* is *Rhipicephalus appendiculatus*. *R. zembeziensis* in southern Africa and *R. duttoni* in Angola can also spread East Coast fever. *T. annulata* is transmitted by ticks in the genus *Hyalomma*.

Theileria sporozoites are transmitted to susceptible animals in the saliva of the feeding tick. Ordinarily, *T. parva* and *T. annulata* only mature and enter the saliva after the tick attaches to a host; usually, a tick must be attached for 48 to 72 hours before it becomes infective. However, if environmental temperatures are high, infective sporozoites can develop in ticks on the ground and may enter the host within hours of attachment. Transovarial transmission does not occur with either *T. parva* or *T. annulata*.

Inside the host, *Theileria* sporozoites undergo a complex life cycle involving the replication of schizonts in leukocytes and piroplasms in erythrocytes. Cattle that recover from *Theileria* infections usually become carriers.

Incubation period

The incubation period for theileriosis is 10 to 25 days.

Clinical signs

The typical clinical signs of East Coast fever are swelling of the draining lymph node followed by generalized lymphadenopathy, fever, anorexia, and a rapid loss of condition. Other symptoms can include lacrimation, nasal discharge, corneal opacity, an increased respiratory rate, and diarrhea. Death is common in fully susceptible cattle, but more rare in cattle in endemic areas. Terminally, animals often develop pulmonary edema, severe dyspnea, and a frothy nasal discharge. Cattle with East Coast may also develop a fatal condition called "turning sickness." In this form of the disease, infected cells block capillaries in the central nervous system and cause neurologic signs. Some animals recover from East Coast fever and become asymptomatic carriers; others may have poor productivity and stunted growth.

Tropical theileriosis resembles East Coast fever, but jaundice and anemia may also occur. Common clinical signs in tropical theileriosis include fever, enlarged lymph nodes, pale mucous membranes, a rapid loss of condition, and sometimes hemoglobinuria.

Post mortem lesions

In peracute *T. parva* and *T. annulata* infections, only lymphoid hyperplasia and widespread hemorrhages are usually found post–mortem. In more typical, acute cases, the subcutaneous tissues contain numerous hemorrhages and petechiae; such hemorrhages are particularly common in tropical theileriosis. The lymph nodes are usually enlarged, but may be shrunken in chronic cases. The liver and spleen are typically enlarged, and white foci of lymphoid infiltration (pseudoinfarcts) may be present in the liver and kidney. Myocardial degeneration with hemorrhages is common. The gastrointestinal tract can contain hemorrhages and ulceration, particularly in the small intestine and the abomasum. Petechial and ecchymotic hemorrhages may also be found on the serosal surfaces of internal organs.

Pulmonary signs are common in East Coast fever but not tropical theileriosis. Animals that die from East Coast fever often have a frothy exudate around the nostrils. Interlobular emphysema and severe pulmonary edema are usually apparent. The lungs are reddened and full of fluid, and the trachea and bronchi often contain fluid and froth.

Morbidity and mortality

Morbidity and mortality vary with the host's susceptibility and the strain of the parasite. The mortality rate from East Coast fever can be up to 100% in cattle from non–endemic areas. However, in indigenous zebu cattle in endemic areas, mortality is usually low even with a morbidity of approximately 100%. The mortality rate for tropical theileriosis can also vary from 3% to nearly 90%, depending on the strain of parasite and the susceptibility of the animals.

Theileriosis can be treated with drugs, and vaccines are available for both East Coast fever and tropical theileriosis. Recovery from one strain of *T. annulata* confers cross–protection against other strains. Cross–protection does not occur with *T. parva*.

Diagnosis

Clinical

Theileriosis should be suspected in tick–infested animals with a fever and enlarged lymph nodes. In endemic areas, the mortality rate may be high only in calves.

Differential diagnosis

The differential diagnosis includes heartwater, trypanosomiasis, babesiosis, anaplasmosis, and malignant catarrhal fever. The parasites must also be differentiated from other species of *Theileria*.

Laboratory tests

In live animals, theileriosis is diagnosed by the identification of schizonts in thin smears from blood, lymph node, or liver biopsies. At necropsy, schizonts may be found in impression smears from most internal organs. Piroplasms can sometimes be found in the blood of carrier animals.

Polymerase chain reaction (PCR) tests and DNA probes are sometimes used to detect and identify Theileria species.

Antibodies to *T. parva* and *T. annulata* can be detected with an enzyme–linked immunosorbent assay (ELISA) or an indirect fluorescent antibody test. Serologic tests may not be sensitive enough to detect all infected cattle, and cross–reactions can occur with other species of *Theileria*.

Samples to collect

Before collecting or sending any samples from animals with a suspected foreign animal disease, the proper authorities should be contacted. Samples should only be sent under secure conditions and to authorized laboratories to prevent the spread of the disease.

Blood and lymph node or liver biopsies should be submitted for the detection of Theileria schizonts. Blood or buffy coat smears and lymph node impressions should be air dried and fixed in methanol. Lymph node, lung, spleen, liver, and kidney samples should be collected for histopathology. Serum should also be taken.

Recommended actions if theileriosis is suspected

Notification of authorities

Theileriosis must be reported to state or federal authorities immediately upon diagnosis or suspicion of the disease.

Federal: Area Veterinarians in Charge (AVICs):
   http://www.aphis.usda.gov/vs/area_offices.htm
State Veterinarians:
   http://www.aphis.usda.gov/vs/sregs/official.html

Quarantine and disinfection

Sanitation and disinfection measures are not generally effective in preventing transmission of theileriosis. Tick infestations should be prevented with acaricides and other methods of tick control. The transfer of blood between animals must also be avoided, particularly with *T. annulata* infections.

Public health

There is no evidence that *T. parva* or *T. annulata* are hazards to humans.

For more information

World Organization for Animal Health (OIE)
   http://www.oie.int
OIE Manual of Standards
   http://www.oie.int/eng/normes/mmanual/a_summry.htm
OIE International Animal Health Code
   http://www.oie.int/eng/normes/mcode/A_summry.htm
USAHA Foreign Animal Diseases Book
   http://www.vet.uga.edu/vpp/gray_book/FAD/

References

Pipano, E. and V. Shkap. "Vaccination against Tropical Theileriosis." *Ann N Y Acad Sci* 916 (2000):484–500.
"*Theileria parva*." May 1999 University of Missouri College of Veterinary Medicine. 3 Oct 2001. http//www.missouri.edu/~vmicrorc/Protozoa/Hemosporidians/*Theileria*.htm.

"Theileriases." In *The Merck Veterinary Manual*, 8th ed. Edited by S.E. Aiello and A. Mays. Whitehouse Station, NJ: Merck and Co., 1998, pp. 31–32.

"Theileriosis." In *Manual of Standards for Diagnostic Tests and Vaccines*. Paris: World Organization for Animal Health, 2000, pp. 433–445.

Young, A.S., and C.M. Groocock. "East Coast Fever." In *Foreign Animal Diseases*. Richmond, VA: United States Animal Health Association, 1998, pp. 191–200.

Transmissible Spongiform Encephalopathies

Importance

Transmissible spongiform encephalopathies (TSEs) are progressive and fatal neurodegenerative diseases. TSEs affecting animals include scrapie (tremblante de mouton, rida), bovine spongiform encephalopathy (BSE, "mad cow disease"), transmissible mink encephalopathy (TME, mink scrapie), feline spongiform encephalopathy (FSE), chronic wasting disease (CWD), and a spongiform encephalopathy of exotic ruminants. These diseases were once thought to be entirely species specific, but it now appears that some agents can cross species barriers. In the United Kingdom, a BSE epidemic may have been responsible for concurrent outbreaks of FSE in cats and spongiform encephalopathy in exotic ruminants. The same epidemic has also been linked to a variant of Creutzfeldt-Jakob disease (vCJD) in humans.

Etiology

Transmissible spongiform encephalopathies are caused by unconventional disease agents. These agents are resistant to the treatments that ordinarily destroy bacteria, spores, viruses, and fungi. They are generally thought to be prions; a minority opinion is that they may be virinos or retroviruses. Strain variations have been seen in the scrapie agent, but not the agent of BSE.

Species affected

Scrapie

Scrapie affects sheep, goats, and moufflon. Rats, mice, hamsters, monkeys, and a variety of other laboratory and wild animals can be infected experimentally.

Bovine spongiform encephalopathy

BSE is seen in cattle and can be experimentally transmitted to cats, mink, mice, pigs, sheep, goats, marmosets and cynomolgus monkeys.

Spongiform encephalopathy of exotic ruminants

A spongiform encephalopathy of exotic ruminants has been seen in captive nyala, gemsbok, Arabian oryx, eland, kudu, scimitar-horned oryx, ankole, and bison.

Feline spongiform encephalopathy

FSE has been found in domestic cats and captive wild cats, including tigers, a puma, an ocelot, and a cheetah.

Transmissible mink encephalopathy

TME is seen in ranched mink and has been experimentally transmitted to cattle.

Chronic wasting disease

CWD affects mule deer, white-tailed deer, black-tailed deer, and elk.

Geographic distribution

Scrapie

Scrapie is widespread throughout the world. This disease can be found in the United Kingdom, Ireland, France, Belgium, Iceland, Norway, Cyprus, Israel, Japan, Canada, the United States and parts of Asia. Outbreaks have occurred in Australia and New Zealand but the disease was eradicated.

Bovine spongiform encephalopathy

BSE appears to have originated in the United Kingdom in 1986. Infected indigenous cattle have since been found in Austria, Belgium, Canada, Czech Republic, Denmark, Finland, France, Germany, Greece, Ireland, Israel, Italy, Japan, Lichtenstein, Luxembourg, Netherlands, Poland, Portugal, Slovakia, Slovenia, Spain, and Switzerland and the United States in addition to the United Kingdom. Cases have also been seen in imported cattle in Oman and the Falkland Islands. BSE has never been detected in Australia, New Zealand, Central America or South America.

Feline spongiform encephalopathy and spongiform encephalopathy of exotic ruminants

FSE has been found almost exclusively in the United Kingdom, with a single isolated case in a cat in Norway. Spongiform encephalopathy of exotic ruminants has been detected only in captive ruminants in the United Kingdom. These two diseases have been declining in parallel with the BSE epidemic.

Transmissible mink encephalopathy

Outbreaks of TME have been seen in the United States, Canada, Finland, Germany, and Russia.

Chronic wasting disease

CWD is endemic in the United States. It is found in wild deer and elk in Colorado, Wyoming, Wisconsin, Illinois, South Dakota, Utah, New Mexico and Nebraska. CSD has also been found in captive cervid herds in the previously listed states as well as Minnesota, Kansas, Oklahoma and Montana.

Transmission

Scrapie

Transmission of scrapie is usually oral. Most animals become infected from their dam, either at or soon after birth. The placenta is infectious; in confined lambing areas, the disease can spread to the offspring of uninfected sheep. The scrapie agent can also be detected in the tonsils, lymph nodes, spleen, distal ileum, proximal colon, and nervous system. Scrapie can spread laterally between animals by direct contact, contamination of fomites such as knives or vaccines, or possibly by environmental contamination. Vertical transmission may be possible, but has not been established. Sheep genetics seem to play a major role in whether or not a sheep will become infected with scrapie.

Bovine spongiform encephalopathy

BSE seems to be transmitted orally. The BSE agent is found mainly in nervous tissues. In naturally infected cattle, it has been detected only in the brain, spinal cord, and retina. In experimentally infected calves, it is also seen in the distal ileum. This agent has never been found in muscle, blood, or milk, and natural infections do not seem to spread laterally between cattle. The offspring of BSE-infected cattle have an increased risk of developing BSE, but it is not known whether this is due to vertical transmission or another mode of transmission.

BSE emerged into cattle in the 1980s. This epidemic has been linked to changes in the rendering practices for meat-and-bone-meal (MBM) used in livestock feed; these changes may have allowed TSE agents to survive the rendering process. The BSE agent was probably amplified when BSE-contaminated cattle carcasses and wastes were used to make MBM, which was then fed to cattle.

There are several hypotheses on the actual origins of the BSE agent. Some sources suggest that this agent has been present in cattle since the 1970s, and may have resulted from a genetic mutation in cattle. An alternative hypothesis is that it mutated from the agent that causes scrapie, and crossed species when sheep tissues were fed to cattle in MBM. A recently published report suggests that the BSE agent may have been a mutant of a human TSE agent. This agent is thought to have been present in raw mammalian materials imported from the Indian subcontinent and used to make MBM.

Spongiform encephalopathy of exotic ruminants

The outbreak of spongiform encephalopathy of exotic ruminants paralleled the BSE epidemic, and may have been due to the same agent. Experimentally, this TSE can be transmitted both orally and parenterally. Vertical transmission is uncertain: two offspring of affected animals developed the disease, but vertical transmission has not been seen in experimental infections.

Feline spongiform encephalopathy

The BSE agent or a related agent may also have been the source of feline spongiform encephalopathy. In domestic cats, the source of infection was thought to be pet food that contained cattle offal. Wild cats in zoos may have been infected when they were fed cattle carcasses.

Transmissible mink encephalopathy

TME is thought to be transmitted orally. Outbreaks are thought to begin when mink are fed infectious feed. In some cases, the proposed source was carcasses from scrapie-infected sheep. During an outbreak, the disease probably spreads between animals by fighting and cannibalism. Experimental transmission of scrapie to mink has been unsuccessful; however, mink can be infected by BSE and develop a disease very similar to TME. Brain tissue from mink with TME can also transmit a fatal spongiform encephalopathy to cows and then be back-passaged into mink.

Chronic wasting disease

The method of transmission for CWD is completely unknown. Direct spread may occur between animals, as the disease has a high prevalence in some areas. Vertical transmission and oral transmission have also been suggested.

Incubation period

All transmissible spongiform encephalopathies have incubation periods of months or years. The incubation period of scrapie in sheep is usually 2 to 5 years; cases are rare in sheep less than a year old. In goats, the incubation period is less than 3 years. The incubation period of BSE is more than a year and often several years. The peak incidence of disease occurs in 4 to 5 year old cattle. The incubation period for mink spongiform encephalopathy is 7 to 12 months.

Clinical signs

Transmissible spongiform encephalopathies are usually insidious in onset and tend to progress slowly. In most of these diseases, the symptoms primarily involve the nervous system; however, in CWD, the most prominent symptom is wasting. Once clinical signs appear, these diseases are relentlessly progressive and fatal.

Scrapie

The first symptoms of scrapie are usually behavioral: affected sheep tend to stand apart from the flock and may either trail or lead when the flock is driven. As the disease progresses, animals usually become hyperexcitable and have a high-stepping or hopping gait, fixed stare, and head held high. Other symptoms may include ataxia, incoordination, and trembling or convulsions when being handled. Intense pruritus is common and may lead to rubbing, scraping, or chewing. Most animals die 2 to 6 weeks after the onset of symptoms, but deaths may occur up to 6 months later.

Bovine spongiform encephalopathy

The clinical signs of BSE may include hyperesthesia, hindlimb ataxia, pelvic swaying, hypermetria, tremors, falling, recumbency, and behavioral changes such as apprehension, nervousness, and occasionally frenzy. Intense pruritus is not usually seen. Nonspecific symptoms include loss of condition, weight loss, and decreased milk production. Decreased rumination, bradycardia, and altered heart rhythms have also been reported. The disease progresses to recumbency and coma, and death occurs from weeks to months later. Rare cases may develop acutely and progress rapidly within days.

Spongiform encephalopathy of exotic ruminants

The clinical signs of this disease include loss of condition, unsteadiness, incoordination, and self-mutilation by biting. Asymptomatic cases have been described. This disease appears to progress more rapidly than most TSEs; the mean period from the onset of symptoms to euthanasia is 13.5 days.

Feline spongiform encephalopathy

The clinical signs of FSE may include behavioral changes, tremors, and ataxia. Cats may become aggressive or tend to creep aimlessly around their home and hide. In later stages, somnolence is common and convulsions may occur. Excessive salivation, hyper-responsiveness to loud noises, and dilated pupils have also been seen. Death occurs after 6 to 8 weeks.

Transmissible mink encephalopathy

The early clinical signs of TME include difficulty eating and swallowing, and changes in normal grooming habits. Later, animals may become hyperexcitable and bite compulsively. Affected mink often carry their tails arched over their backs like squirrels. Other symptoms include incoordination, somnolence, and sometimes convulsions. Death occurs after 3 to 8 weeks.

Chronic wasting disease

The clinical signs of CWD include progressive weight loss and lassitude over several weeks to months, with eventual severe emaciation and death. Affected animals may carry their head low and have a fixed gaze; this may alternate with more normal alertness. In elk, excessive salivation and teeth grinding are also common. Nervousness and hyperexcitability may occur, but are much less common than in BSE. Pruritus has not been seen.

Post mortem lesions

No gross lesions are found in transmissible spongiform encephalopathies, other than emaciation or wasting of the carcass in some cases.

The typical histopathologic lesions are confined to the central nervous system. Neuronal vacuolation and non-inflammatory spongiform changes in the gray matter are pathognomonic. Astrocytosis is prominent in some diseases but not others. Amyloid plaques are seen in scrapie and CWD, but are rare in BSE and not found in TME or FSE. Lesions are usually but not always bilaterally symmetrical.

Morbidity and mortality

In sheep, the genetics of the host and the strain of the agent influence the onset and severity of the disease. Theoretically, some combinations result in an incubation period longer than the life expectancy of the sheep. In scrapie the typical mortality rate is 3% to 5% of the flock. In severely affected flocks, up to 20% of the animals may die annually.

Transmissible spongiform encephalopathies are always fatal once the symptoms appear. In scrapie, the typical mortality rate is 3% to 5% of the flock. In severely affected flocks, up to 20% of the animals may die annually. In outbreaks of TME, the mortality rate may be as high as 60% to 80%. In 1992, the annual incidence of BSE in United Kingdom cattle was 1%; however, the number of cases has been decreasing in recent years. The incidence of FSE is unknown. This disease was seen in a total of 81 domestic cats (as well as a few wild felids) in the United Kingdom, but many cases may have been missed. The prevalence of chronic wasting disease varies with the geographic region. In Colorado and Wyoming, 4.7% of mule deer, 2% of white-tailed deer, and 0.5% of elk are positive overall, although there are "hot spots" where up to 15% of the mule deer and up to 16% of the white-tailed deer are infected.

Diagnosis

Clinical

Transmissible spongiform encephalopathies should be suspected in animals that develop a slowly progressive, fatal neurologic disease, and in elk and mule deer with chronic wasting.

Differential diagnosis

Other neurologic diseases must be ruled out. The differential diagnosis of scrapie includes external parasitism (lice, mange, or itch mites), sheep scab, Aujeszky's disease, maedi-visna, cerebral listeriosis, pregnancy toxemia, rabies, cerebrocortical necrosis (polioencephalomalacia), abscesses or tumors in the brain, louping ill and other tick-borne encephalitides, toxins, focal symmetrical encephalomalacia (chronic enterotoxemia), and other degenerative central nervous system diseases. The differential diagnosis of BSE includes nervous ketosis, hypomagnesemia, listeriosis, rabies, tumors, trauma to the spinal cord, and poisonings such as lead.

Laboratory tests

Transmissible spongiform encephalopathies have traditionally been diagnosed by histopathology. A diagnosis can also be made by detecting PrP^{Sc}, a disease-specific isoform of the membrane protein PrP, in the central nervous system. Accumulations of PrP^{Sc} can be found in unfixed brain extracts by immunoblotting and in fixed brains by immunohistochemistry. The diagnosis can also be confirmed by finding characteristic fibrils of PrP^{Sc} (scrapie-associated fibrils) with electron microscopy in brain extracts. Some of these tests can be used on frozen or autolyzed brains.

Scrapie can also be diagnosed by transmission tests in sheep, goats, or mice and BSE by transmission studies in mice. However, an incubation period of several months often makes this technique impractical for diagnosis.

New commercial tests to detect BSE (PrP^{Sc}) in cattle brain samples include a modified immunoblot, a chemiluminescent ELISA test, a sandwich immunoassay, and a two-site noncompetitive immunometric procedure.

A new test to diagnose scrapie in live sheep, the third eyelid test, has recently been approved. Other live animal tests in development include immunohistochemical staining of tonsil biopsies, capillary electrophoresis and fluorescent labeled peptides to detect PrP^{Sc} in the blood, and immunoblotting to detect PrP^{Sc} in blood, cerebrospinal fluid, or tissues.

Serology is not useful for diagnosis, as antibodies are not made against the TSE agents.

Samples to collect

Before collecting or sending any samples from animals with a suspected foreign animal disease, the proper authorities should be contacted. Samples should only be sent under secure conditions and to authorized laboratories to prevent the spread of the disease. A fatal human encephalopathy has been linked to BSE; samples should be collected and handled with all appropriate precautions.

An animal suspected of having a transmissible spongiform encephalopathy should be killed and the brain removed for testing. In sheep, the cerebral spinal cord with the dorsal root ganglia should be included if possible. Half of the longitudinally split brain is kept fresh to test for PrPSc. This portion should be kept cold and sent to the laboratory as soon as possible on wet ice or gel packs. The other half should be placed in 10% formo saline. In sheep, the spleen and a variety of lymph nodes should also be collected and sent to the laboratory unpreserved. During epidemics of BSE, it may be possible to remove only the hindbrain via the foramen magnum for disease monitoring.

During necropsy, a standard neuropathologic approach should be followed to rule out other causes of disease.

Recommended actions if a transmissible spongiform encephalopathy is suspected

Notification of authorities

BSE, FSE, TME, and spongiform encephalopathy of exotic ruminants are exotic diseases and must be reported promptly to state or federal officials. Scrapie and CWD are endemic to the United States, but are reportable diseases in many states. The U.S. has established a scrapie eradication program, with the goal of disease eradication by 2010, and a flock certification program. A herd certification program is also planned for chronic wasting disease; the program will apply to farmed cervids.

Federal: Area Veterinarians in Charge (AVICs):
  http://www.aphis.usda.gov/vs/area_offices.htm
State Veterinarians:
  http://www.aphis.usda.gov/vs/sregs/official.html

Quarantine and disinfection

Scrapie and TME can be contagious; quarantine may be necessary for their control. BSE and some other transmissible spongiform encephalopathies do not appear to spread laterally.

The prototype agent, scrapie, is highly resistant to disinfectants, heat, ultraviolet radiation, ionizing radiation, and formalin. Effective disinfection is possible with a single porous load autoclave cycle of 134-138°C for 18 minutes. Infectious tissues should either be autoclaved under the same conditions or incinerated. Sodium hypochlorite and sodium hydroxide are effective chemical disinfectants; sodium hypochlorite containing 2% available chlorine or 2 N sodium hydroxide should be applied for more than one hour at 20°C. Overnight disinfection is recommended for equipment.

Public health

There is no evidence that scrapie can be transmitted to humans; however, variant Creutzfeldt-Jakob disease (vCJD) appears to be linked to the agent of BSE. This human encephalopathy is progressive and fatal. There is no treatment. The BSE agent is classified in containment category three.

For more information

World Organization for Animal Health (OIE)
    http://www.oie.int
OIE Manual of Standards
    http://www.oie.int/eng/normes/mmanual/a_summry.htm
OIE International Animal Health Code
    http://www.oie.int/eng/normes/mcode/A_summry.htm
Animal Health Australia. The National Animal Health
    Information System
    http://www. aahc.com.au/nahis/disease/dislist.asp
United States Department of Agriculture Animal and
    Plant Health Inspection Service
    http://www.aphis.usda.gov/

References

"Bovine spongiform encephalopathy." Animal Health Australia. The National Animal Health Information System (NAHIS). 7 November 2001. http//www. aahc.com.au/nahis/disease/dislist.asp.

"Bovine Spongiform Encephalopathy." In *Manual of Standards for Diagnostic Tests and Vaccines*. Paris: World Organization for Animal Health, 2000, pp. 457-466.

"Bovine Spongiform Encephalopathy." In *The Merck Veterinary Manual*, 8th ed. Edited by S.E. Aiello and A. Mays. Whitehouse Station, NJ: Merck and Co., 1998, pp. 897-898.

Fischer J.R., Nettles V.F. College of Veterinary Medicine, The University of Georgia. National chronic wasting disease surveillance in free-ranging cervids: accomplishments and needs. In *USAHA 2002 Proceedings*; 2002 Oct 20-23; St. Louis, MO. 2 Dec 2003. http//www.usaha.org/speeches/speech02/s02cwdss.html

Irani, D.N. "Bovine Spongiform Encephalopathy." Johns Hopkins Department of Neurology. Resource on Prion Diseases. 7 November 2001. http//www.jhu-prion.org/animal/ani-bse-hist.shtml.

Irani, D.N. "Chronic Wasting Disease." Johns Hopkins Department of Neurology. Resource on Prion Diseases. 7 November 2001. http//www.jhu-prion.org/animal/ani-cwd-hist.shtml.

Irani, D.N. "Feline Spongiform Encephalopathy." Johns Hopkins Department of Neurology. Resource on Prion Diseases. 7 November 2001. http//www.jhu-prion.org/animal/ani-fse-hist.shtml.

Irani, D.N. "Scrapie." Johns Hopkins Department of Neurology. Resource on Prion Diseases. 7 November 2001. http//www.jhu-prion.org/animal/ani-scrapie2-hist.shtml.

Irani, D.N. "Spongiform Encephalopathy of Exotic Ruminants." Johns Hopkins Department of Neurology. Resource on Prion Diseases. 7 November 2001. http//www.jhu-prion.org/animal/ani-seoer-hist.shtml.

Irani, D.N. "Transmissible Mink Encephalopathy." Johns Hopkins Department of Neurology. Resource on Prion Diseases. 7 November 2001. http//www.jhu-prion.org/animal/ani-tme-hist.shtml.

Kreeger T. Distribution and status of chronic wasting disease in Wyoming [abstract]. In: *National Chronic Wasting Disease Symposium.* 2002 Aug 6-7; Denver, CO. 22 Nov 2003. http://www.cwd-info.org/index.p

"Scrapie." Animal Health Australia. The National Animal Health Information System (NAHIS). 7 November 2001 http//www. aahc.com.au/nahis/disease/dislist.asp.

"Scrapie." In *The Merck Veterinary Manual*, 8th ed. Edited by S.E. Aiello and A. Mays. Whitehouse Station, NJ: Merck and Co., 1998, pp. 970-1.

"Transmissible Mink Encephalopathy." In *The Merck Veterinary Manual*, 8th ed. Edited by S.E. Aiello and A. Mays. Whitehouse Station, NJ: Merck and Co., 1998, pp. 1364.

"Transmissible Spongiform Encephalopathies." July 2000 United States Department of Agriculture Animal and Plant Health Inspection Service. 7 November 2001. http//www.aphis.usda.gov/oa/pubs/fstse.html>.

Trypanosomiasis

Nagana, Tsetse Disease,
Tsetse Fly Disease, Trypanosomosis

Importance

Trypanosomiasis causes serious economic losses in cattle from anemia, loss of condition, and emaciation. This chronic infection often ends in the death of the animal. Because trypanosomes are transmitted by tsetse flies and other vectors, trypanosomiasis is difficult to control. No vaccine is available, and the organisms quickly develop resistance to drugs.

Etiology

Trypanosomiasis is caused by infection with the protozoal parasites *Trypanosoma congolense*, *T. vivax*, or *T. brucei brucei*. Concurrent infections can occur with more than one species.

Species affected

Trypanosomes can infect a wide variety of domestic animals and more than 30 species in the wild. *Trypanosoma congolense* infects cattle, pigs, goats, sheep, and horses. Dogs sometimes become chronically infected carriers of this species. *T. vivax* is predomi-nantly found in cattle, sheep, and goats, and *T. brucei brucei* in cattle, horses, dogs, cats, camels, sheep, goats, and pigs. Monkeys, rats, mice, guinea pigs, and rabbits can also be infected by trypanosomes. Ruminants, wild Equidae, lions, leopards, and wild pigs can serve as carriers.

Geographic distribution

Trypanosomes can be found wherever the tsetse fly vector exists. Tsetse flies are endemic in Africa between latitude 15° N and 20° S, from the southern edge of the Sahara desert to Zimbabwe, Angola, and Mozambique. *T. vivax* and *T. brucei brucei* have spread beyond the "tsetse fly belt" by transmission through mechanical vectors. *T. vivax* is also found in South and Central America and the Caribbean, areas free of the tsetse fly. Its vector there is unknown.

Transmission

Trypanosomes replicate in tsetse flies, primarily *Glossina morsitans*, *G. palpalis*, and *G. fusca*. When an infected fly bites an animal, the parasites are transmitted in the saliva. Trypanosomes can also be spread by fomites and mechanical vectors, including surgical instruments, needles, syringes, and biting flies. The primary mechanical vectors are flies of the genus *Tabanus*. *Haematopota*, *Liperosia*, *Stomoxys*, and *Chrysops* may also transmit trypanosomes. Several species of hematophagous (especially *tabanid* and *hippoboscid*) flies are thought to be mechanical vectors for *T. vivax* in the Western hemisphere; however, the primary vector is unknown.

Incubation period

T. congolense infections usually become apparent 4 to 24 days after infection and *T. vivax* in 4 to 40 days. The incubation period for *T. brucei brucei* is 5 to 10 days.

Clinical signs

Trypanosomiasis in cattle is usually a chronic infection. The major symptoms are anemia, intermittent fever, edema, and weight loss. Infertility (male and female) and abortion may be seen. Poor nutrition, concurrent diseases, and other stressors result in more significant clinical signs. Some cattle may slowly recover, but usually relapse when stressed.

Infection with trypanosomes causes significant immunosuppression; concurrent infections may complicate this disease.

Post mortem lesions

The post–mortem lesions of trypanosomiasis are nonspecific. Typical abnormalities include anemia, serous atrophy of fat, edema (particularly subcutaneous edema), excessive fluid in the body cavities, emaciation, petechial hemorrhages, and an enlarged liver. The spleen may be enlarged, normal, or atrophied. The lymph nodes are often edematous and swollen in acute cases, but may be normal or atrophied. Gastroenteritis and necrosis of the kidneys and heart muscle are common. Focal polioencephalomalacia is sometimes seen, and a chancre (sore) may be detected at the site of entry.

T. brucei brucei causes inflammation, degeneration, and necrosis of various organs. Marked proliferative responses can be seen in most tissues.

Morbidity and mortality

Morbidity and mortality depend on the breed and age of the animal, as well as the virulence and dose of infecting organisms. Genetic resistance to trypanosomiasis is found in some breeds of African cattle, particularly Muturu, Baoule, Laguna, Samba, Dahomey, and N'Dama. In susceptible cattle, the infection is often fatal, particularly under conditions of stress or poor nutrition. Mortality of over 50% can be seen with some strains of *T. vivax*.

Numerous drug treatments are available; however, resistance is common. No vaccine is available.

Diagnosis

Clinical

Trypanosomiasis should be a consideration in endemic areas when an animal is anemic and in poor condition.

Differential diagnosis

Other infections that cause anemia and weight loss, including babesiosis, anaplasmosis, and theileriosis, should be ruled out.

Laboratory tests

Trypanosomiasis is usually diagnosed by finding the organisms in blood or lymph node smears. Both wet–mount blood films and thick films stained with 4% Giemsa for 30 minutes are used. Thin films are helpful in species identification, but the parasites may be difficult to find. Parasite concentration techniques include the microhematocrit centrifugation technique (Woo method), the dark ground/ phase contrast buffy coat technique, and anion exchange chromatography. An enzyme–linked immunosorbent assay (ELISA), for trypanosome antigens, in vitro cultivation, animal inoculation into rodents, and DNA amplification have also been used.

ELISA and indirect fluorescent antibody tests can detect antibodies to trypanosomes. Sensitivity and specificity are high, but the diagnosis is presumptive.

Samples to collect

Before collecting or sending any samples from animals with a suspected foreign animal disease, the proper authorities should be contacted. Samples should only be sent under secure conditions and to authorized laboratories to prevent the spread of the disease. Trypanosomes related to T. brucei brucei infect humans, and precautions are recommended when handling blood and infected animals.

Serum, blood anticoagulated with EDTA, dried thin and thick blood smears, and smears of needle lymph node biopsies should be submitted from several affected animals. During the chronic phase, *T. congolense* can be found in lymph node smears and capillary blood from the ear, but blood smears are preferred during earlier stages. *T. vivax* and *T. brucei brucei* can also be found in lymph node smears.

Recommended actions if trypanosomiasis is suspected

Notification of authorities

Trypanosomiasis must be reported to state or federal authorities immediately upon diagnosis or suspicion of the disease.

Federal: Area Veterinarians in Charge (AVICs):
http://www.aphis.usda.gov/vs/area_offices.htm
State Veterinarians:
http://www.aphis.usda.gov/vs/sregs/official.html

Quarantine and disinfection

Disinfection and sanitation are not generally effective against the spread of this disease. Preventing the transfer of blood from one animal to another is critical. Controlling the arthropod vectors is important in preventing new infections.

Public health

T. congolense, *T. vivax*, and *T. brucei brucei* are not considered to be pathogenic for humans. However, trypanosomes related to *T. brucei brucei* infect humans, and precautions are recommended when handling blood and infected animals.

For more information

World Organization for Animal Health (OIE)
http://www.oie.int
OIE Manual of Standards
http://www.oie.int/eng/normes/mmanual/a_summry.htm
OIE International Animal Health Code
http://www.oie.int/eng/normes/mcode/A_summry.htm

USAHA Foreign Animal Diseases Book
http://www.vet.uga.edu/vpp/gray_book/FAD/

References

"Trypanosomosis." In *Manual of Standards for Diagnostic Tests and Vaccines*. Paris: World Organization for Animal Health, 2000, pp. 855–862.

"Trypanosomiasis." In *The Merck Veterinary Manual*, 8th ed. Edited by S.E. Aiello and A. Mays. Whitehouse Station, NJ: Merck and Co., 1998, pp. 33–35.

Mare, C.J. "Trypanosomiasis." In *Foreign Animal Diseases*. Richmond, VA: United States Animal Health Association, 1998, pp. 29–40.

Tularemia

Rabbit Fever, Deer-fly Fever, Ohara Disease, Francis Disease

Importance

Francisella tularensis subtype *tularensis* is the most important agent of tularemia. It occurs only in North America, is highly virulent for humans and domestic rabbits, and is considered to be a potential biological warfare weapon.

Etiology

Francisella tularensis (formerly *Pasteurella tularensis*), a small gram–negative non–motile coccobacillus, has several subspecies with varying degrees of virulence. The most important of those is *F. tularensis tularensis* (Type A), which is found in lagomorphs in North America and is highly virulent for humans and domestic rabbits. *F. tularensis palaearctica* (Type B) occurs mainly in aquatic rodents (beavers, muskrats) in northern North America and in hares and small rodents in northern Eurasia. It is less virulent for humans and rabbits.

Species affected

Tularemia occurs naturally in lagomorphs (rabbits and hares), rodents (voles, vole rats, and muskrats), and beavers. Infection in a wide variety of other mammals, birds, reptiles, and fish has been reported. In domestic animals sheep, dogs, cats, pigs, and horses are known to be susceptible while cattle seem to be relatively resistant. *F. tularensis* can also infect humans.

Geographic distribution

F. tularensis tularensis is only found naturally in North America. Other *Francisella* species are found throughout the northern hemisphere, most notably in Europe, Asia, and Japan.

Transmission

The most common mode of transmission is via arthropod vectors. Vectors include the wood tick *Dermacentor andersoni*, the dog tick *D. variabilis*, and the lone star tick *Amblyomma americanum*. Tularemia can also be transmitted by biting flies, particularly the deer fly *Chrysops discalis*. Individual flies can remain infective for 14 days and ticks for over 2 years (throughout their lifetime). Tularemia may also be spread by direct contact with contaminated animals or material (especially through direct inoculation into the skin), by ingestion of poorly cooked flesh of infected animals or contaminated water, or by inhalation. The most likely method for bioterrorist transmission is through an aerosol.

Incubation period

The incubation period for tularemia is 1 to 14 days; most human infections become apparent after 3 to 5 days. The incubation period depends on the virulence of the infecting strain and the amount of bacteria present.

Clinical signs

In most susceptible mammals, the clinical signs include fever, lethargy, anorexia, signs of septicemia, and possibly death. Animals rarely develop the skin lesions seen in people. Subclinical infections are common and animals often develop specific antibodies to the organism.

Post mortem lesions

Lesions consistent with septicemia are generally seen on post–mortem examination and may include caseous necrosis of lymph nodes and multiple greyish–white foci of necrosis in the spleen, liver, bone marrow, and lungs. These necrotic foci may only be visible microscopically. The spleen is commonly hypertrophied. In rabbits, the white necrotic foci on a dark, congested liver and spleen have been compared to the Milky Way. The lungs are generally congested and edematous, and there may be areas of consolidation and fibrinous pneumonia or pleuritis. Fibrin may be present in the abdominal cavity. In less susceptible species, the disease may appear more chronic with granulomas present in the liver, spleen, lungs, and kidneys.

Morbidity and mortality

Morbidity is variable depending on the infecting strain and the susceptibility of the species. The case–fatality rate for untreated *F. tularensis tularensis* infections is 5% to 15%; death is usually the result of septicemia or pulmonary disease. With treatment, deaths are rare.

Diagnosis

Clinical

In endemic areas, tularemia should always be considered with signs of fever, lymph node enlargement and pain, pneumonia, or septicemia.

Differential diagnosis

Differentials include plague, staphylococcal and streptococcal infections, cat scratch fever, sporotrichosis, and many other infectious diseases. With heavy tick infestations, tick paralysis may also be a consideration.

Laboratory tests

Laboratory tests include culture and identification of the organism and fluorescent antibody testing. Serological testing of paired antibody titers 2 weeks apart shows a 4–fold increase.

Samples to collect

F. tularensis is highly infectious to humans; samples should be collected and handled with all appropriate precautions. Gloves, masks, and eyeshields should be worn when samples are taken.

Samples may include aspirates from enlarged lymph nodes, infected tissue samples, or serum. If transportation is necessary, samples should be inoculated into sterile nutrient broth and stored at 4–10°C for a few hours, or at –70°C if transit is likely to be prolonged.

Recommended actions
if tularemia is suspected

Notification of authorities

Cases of tularemia should be reported to the local health authority. Due to the possible use of aerosolized *F. tularensis* as a biological weapon, any human case of tularemia pneumonia should be reported to the local FBI and health department.

Federal: Area Veterinarians in Charge (AVICs):
http://www.aphis.usda.gov/vs/area_offices.htm
State Veterinarians:
http://www.aphis.usda.gov/vs/sregs/official.html

Quarantine and disinfection

Tick control and precautions to avoid exposure to infected materials are the best ways to prevent spread of the disease.

Public health

There is a high risk of human infection with *F. tularensis*. Outdoor activity and hunting in endemic areas may predispose people to infection through tick bites and the handling of infected carcasses. Laboratory workers most frequently develop pneumonia or septicemia.

In humans, the most common presentation is fever with ulcers or abscesses at the site of inoculation and painful swelling of the regional lymph nodes. This form is known as the ulceroglandular type. Ingestion may lead to painful pharyngitis, abdominal pain, diarrhea, and vomiting (the oropharyngeal type). The pneumonic type, caused by inhalation of infectious particles, may lead to septicemia, also known as the typhoidal type. The pulmonary and septicemic forms are the most serious and can be fatal without antibiotic treatment. A rare oculoglandular type, caused by infection of the conjunctival sac, is characterized by painful purulent conjunctivitis and regional lymphadenitis. Any localized form can lead to septicemia or pneumonia.

For more information

World Organization for Animal Health (OIE)
http://www.oie.int
OIE Manual of Standards
http://www.oie.int/eng/normes/mmanual/a_summry.htm

References

Control of Communicable Diseases. Edited by J. Chin. American Public Health Association, 2000, pp.532–535.

Pearson, A. In *Zoonoses*. Edited by S.R. Palmer, E.J.L. Soulsby and D.I.H Simpson. New York: Oxford University Press, 1998, pp. 267–279.

"Tularemia." In *Manual of Standards for Diagnostic Tests and Vaccines*. Paris: World Organization for Animal Health, 2000, pp. 756–761.

"Tularemia." In *The Merck Veterinary Manual*, 8th ed. Edited by S.E. Aiello and A. Mays. Whitehouse Station, NJ: Merck and Co., 1998, pp. 494–5; 1394.

Vesicular Stomatitis

Importance

Vesicular stomatitis is an important livestock disease in the Americas. Occasional outbreaks of this zoonotic vesicular disease occurs in limited areas of the United States. Affected herds are quarantined until the disease has run its course. Vesicular stomatitis closely resembles three foreign animal diseases: foot and mouth disease, swine vesicular disease, and vesicular exanthema of swine. Differentiation of these diseases is important, as a wrong diagnosis could mask the spread of an exotic disease. Prompt diagnosis is also important in containing outbreaks of vesicular stomatitis. The spread of this disease within the U.S. could restrict the exportation of animals and animal products to vesicular stomatitis-free countries.

Etiology

Vesicular stomatitis virus (VSV) is a member of the genus *Vesiculovirus* in the family Rhabdoviridae. It is a large bullet-shaped RNA virus. Two strains of VSV that have been found in outbreaks in the United States are New Jersey and Indiana-1. Three strains are found in South America – Indiana-2 (Cocal), Indiana-3 (Alagoas) and Piry – are considered to be exotic.

Species affected

Horses, donkeys, mules, cattle, swine, South American camelids, and humans can be affected by VSV. Sheep and goats are relatively resistant and rarely show clinical signs. Experimentally, a wide host range has been found including deer, raccoons, bobcats, and monkeys.

Geographic distribution

Vesicular stomatitis is endemic in some of the warmer regions of North, Central and South America. Outbreaks have occurred in parts of the United States and in the more temperate regions of the Western Hemisphere.

Transmission

The transmission of vesicular stomatitis is incompletely understood. VSV is thought to be transmitted by insect vectors, particularly sand flies (*Lutzomyia shannoni*) and blackflies (family Simuliidae). Recently, experimental transmission of VSV (New Jersey serotype) from blackflies to swine was shown to be followed by clinical disease. Transovarial transmission has been demonstrated in both sandflies and blackflies. VSV has also been isolated from mosquitoes. In addition, grasshoppers (*Melanoplus sanguinipes*) can be infected experimentally, and cattle that ingest infected grasshoppers can develop disease. There is also some speculation that VSV could be a plant virus found in pastures, with animals at the end of an epidemiological chain.

Once it has been introduced into a herd, vesicular stomatitis can spread from animal to animal by direct contact. Animals can also be infected by exposure to fomites contaminated with saliva or fluid from ruptured vesicles.

Humans may be infected by contact with the vesicular fluid or saliva from infected animals. Aerosol transmission occurs in laboratories. In addition, some people are probably infected through insect bites.

Incubation period

The incubation period is 2 to 8 days; most often, animals become symptomatic in 3 to 5 days. Occasionally, vesicles can develop within 24 hours. The incubation period in humans is usually 3 to 4 days, but can be as short as 24 hours or as long as 6 days.

Clinical signs

Excessive salivation is often the first symptom. Closer examination may reveal the characteristic lesions - blanched, raised vesicles (blisters) that may be found on the lips, nostrils, hooves or teats, and in the mouth. The vesicle size is highly variable; while some are as small as a pea, others can cover the entire surface of the tongue. A fever usually develops at the time the lesions appear, or just before.

In horses, the vesicles occur most often on the upper surface of the tongue, the gums, the lips, and around the nostrils and corners of the mouth. In some horses, the vesicles may go unnoticed and the disease may appear as crusting scabs on the muzzle, lips, or ventral abdomen. In cattle, the vesicles are usually found on the hard palate, lips and gums, and may extend to the nostrils and muzzle. In both horses and cattle, the hooves may have secondary lesions. In pigs, vesicles usually appear first on the feet, and the first symptom may be lameness. The muzzle is also frequently affected in swine.

Eventually, the vesicles swell and break; the resulting painful ulcers and erosions can cause anorexia, refusal to drink, and lameness. Dairy cattle with lesions on the teats may develop mastitis from secondary infections. Animals can have severe weight loss and, in dairy cows, a drop in milk production. Some cattle may appear to be normal, but eat approximately half of their feed. Unless secondary bacterial infections or other complications develop, the animals recover in approximately 2 weeks.

Post mortem lesions

The necropsy lesions are similar to those in live animals, and may include vesicles, ulcers, erosions, and crusting on the lips, nostrils, hooves, or teats, and in the mouth. Heart and rumen lesions, which may be seen in foot and mouth disease, do not occur in cases of vesicular stomatitis.

Morbidity and mortality

In Central and South America, vesicular stomatitis occurs throughout the year, but it is particularly common at the end of the rainy season. In the southwestern U.S., outbreaks of vesicular stomatitis are common during the warmer months, and are often seen along riverways and in valleys.

The morbidity rate is highly variable, and ranges from 5% to 90%. Most cases occur in adults; young cattle and horses under a year of age are uncommonly affected. Deaths are very rare in cattle and horses, but higher mortality rates have been seen in some pigs infected with the New Jersey strain.

Diagnosis

Clinical

Laboratory diagnosis is essential, as vesicular stomatitis cannot be reliably distinguished from other vesicular diseases including foot and mouth disease, vesicular exanthema, and swine vesicular disease. However, the presence of symptoms in horses suggests vesicular stomatitis.

Differential diagnosis

In cattle, the differential diagnosis includes foot and mouth disease, foot rot, and chemical or thermal burns. The oral lesions can be similar to those of rinderpest, infectious bovine rhinopneumonitis, bovine virus diarrhea, malignant catarrhal fever, and epizootic hemorrhagic disease. In pigs, differentials include foot and mouth disease, swine vesicular disease, vesicular exanthema of swine, foot rot, and chemical and thermal burns should be considered.

Laboratory tests

Detection of the virus or viral antigens is the preferred method of diagnosis. VSV can be isolated in tissue culture, embryonated chicken eggs, or unweaned mice. It can also be isolated by intracerebral inoculation of 3-week old mice. Many cell lines are susceptible to VSV; however, this virus can be differentiated from some other vesicular diseases in African green monkey kidney (Vero), baby hamster kidney (BHK-21) or IB-RS-2 cells. Viral identification in cultures is by immunofluorescence, complement fixation, enzyme-linked immunosorbent assays (ELISAs) and other tests.

In tissue samples, viral antigens can be detected with ELISA, complement fixation or virus neutralization tests. Polymerase chain reaction assays (RT-PCR) may also be used.

The most commonly used serological tests are ELISAs and virus neutralization. Complement fixation, agar gel immunodiffusion, and counter immunoelectrophoresis techniques may also be used.

Samples to collect

Before collecting or sending any samples from vesicular disease suspects, the proper authorities should be contacted. Samples should only be sent under secure conditions and to authorized laboratories to prevent spread of the disease. Vesicular stomatitis is zoonotic; samples should be collected and handled with all appropriate precautions.

Vesicle fluid, the epithelium covering unruptured vesicles, epithelial flaps from freshly ruptured vesicles, or swabs of the ruptured vesicles are the preferred diagnostic samples; APHIS recommends collecting swabs from vesicles. Samples may be collected from any site including the mouth or feet. Sedation is often recommended before sample collection, as the lesions are highly painful. If epithelial tissue is not available, samples of esophageal/pharyngeal fluid can be collected from cattle, or throat swabs may be taken from pigs. Samples should be sent refrigerated unless shipping will take longer than two days; in this case, they may be sent frozen.

Serum samples, or paired serum samples taken 1 to 2 weeks apart, may also be collected. In the U.S., paired serum samples are used only for the index case of the nation and index case for each state. Once an outbreak of vesicular stomatitis has been diagnosed in a state, an animal can be declared positive after a single positive complement fixation test.

Recommended actions
if vesicular stomatitis is suspected
Notification of authorities
State and federal veterinarians should be immediately informed of any suspected vesicular disease.

Federal Area Veterinarians in Charge (AVIC):
http://www.aphis.usda.gov/vs/area_offices.htm
State Veterinarians:
http://www.aphis.usda.gov/vs/sregs/official.html

Quarantine and disinfection
During an outbreak, state or federal regulations restrict animal movements, and quarantines are placed on facilities with infected animals. Isolation of symptomatic animals helps control the spread of vesicular stomatitis within a herd. If possible, stabling is the preferred means of isolation, as animals on pastures are infected more often with VSV. There should be no movement of animals from an infected property for at least 21 days after all lesions are healed, unless the animals are going directly to slaughter. Insect control may help prevent disease spread. Insect breeding areas should be eliminated or reduced, and insecticide sprays or insecticide-treated eartags can be used on animals. Vesicular stomatitis vaccines are also being tested.

VSV, which is inactivated in sunlight, does not survive for long periods in the environment except in cool, dark places. However, good sanitation and disinfection are necessary to control the spread of the virus on fomites. VSV is susceptible to various disinfectants including 1% sodium hypochlorite, 70% ethanol, 2% glutaraldehyde, 2% sodium carbonate, 4% sodium hydroxide, 2% iodophore disinfectants, formaldehyde and chlorine dioxide. It is also susceptible to UV light, lipid solvents, or heat.

Public health
Humans may become infected when handling affected animals, contaminated fomites, tissues, blood, and virus cultures. Aerosol transmission occurs, particularly in laboratories. In humans, vesicular stomatitis is an acute illness that resembles influenza. The symptoms may include fever, muscle aches, headache and malaise. Vesicles are rare, but can occasionally be found on the mouth, lips or hands. Deaths have not been reported, and most people recover in 4 to 7 days.

The incidence of vesicular stomatitis in humans is unknown. Although some sources suggest this disease is rare, others point out that human infections may be underreported as they may easily be misdiagnosed as influenza. Approximately 40-46 laboratory-associated infections were documented before 1980, and seroconversion is common.

For more information
OIE International Animal Health Code
http://www.oie.int/eng/normes/mcode/A_summry.htm
OIE Manual of Standards
http://www.oie.int/eng/normes/mmanual/a_summry.htm
USAHA Foreign Animal Diseases Book
http://www.vet.uga.edu/vpp/gray_book/FAD/
U.S. Department of Agriculture, Animal and Plant Inspection Service. Domestic Animal Disease Surveillance Information.Vesicular Stomatitis
http://www.aphis.usda.gov/vs/ceah/ncahs/nsu/surveillance/vsv/vsv.htm
World Organization for Animal Health (OIE)
http://www.oie.int

References
Aiello, S.E., Mays, A., editors. *The Merck Veterinary Manual*. 8th ed. Whitehouse Station, NJ: Merck and Co; 1998. Vesicular stomatitis; p. 495-496.

House, J.A., House, C., Dubourget, P., Lombard, M. Protective immunity in cattle vaccinated with a commercial scale, inactivated, bivalent vesicular stomatitis vaccine. *Vaccine*. 2003 May 16;21(17-18):1932-1937.

Mead, D.G., Gray, E.W., Noblet, R., Murphy, M.D., Howerth EW, Stallknecht DE. Biological transmission of vesicular stomatitis virus (New Jersey serotype) by *Simulium vittatum* (Diptera: Simuliidae) to domestic swine (*Sus scrofa*). *J Med Entomol*. 2004 Jan;41(1):78-82.

Mead, D.G., Howerth, E.W., Murphy, M.D., Gray, E.W., Noblet R, Stallknecht DE. Black fly involvement in the epidemic transmission of vesicular stomatitis New Jersey virus (Rhabdoviridae: Vesiculovirus). *Vector Borne Zoonotic Dis*. 2004 Winter;4(4):351-359.

Mebus, C.A. Vesicular stomatitis. In *Foreign Animal Diseases*. Richmond, VA: United States Animal Health Association, 1998, pp. 419–423.

Nunamaker, R.A., Lockwood, J.A., Stith, C.E., Campbell, C.L., Schell, S.P., Drolet, B.S., Wilson, W.C., White, D.M., Letchworth, G.J. Grasshoppers (Orthoptera: Acrididae) could serve as reservoirs and vectors of vesicular stomatitis virus. *J Med Entomol*. 2003 Nov;40(6):957-963.

Personal communication, Sabrina L. Swenson, DVM, PhD. Bovine and Porcine Viruses Section, Diagnostic Virology Laboratory. National Veterinary Services Laboratories, Ames, Iowa.

Public Health Agency of Canada, Office of Laboratory Security. Material Safety Data Sheet: Vesicular stomatitis virus [online]. Office of Laboratory Security; 2001 Feb. Available at: http://www.phac-aspc.gc.ca/msds-ftss/msds163e.html. Accessed 26 Jan 2006.

U.S. Department of Agriculture, Animal and Plant Health Inspection Service, Veterinary Services [USDA APHIS, VS]. Vesicular stomatitis [online]. Available at: http://www.aphis.usda.gov/lpa/pubs/fsheet_faq_notice/fs_ahvs.html. Accessed 26 Jan 2006.

U.S. Department of Agriculture, Animal and Plant Health Inspection Service, Veterinary Services [USDA APHIS, VS]. Vesicular stomatitis: Questions and answers [online]. USDA APHIS, VS; 2005 June. Available at: http://www.aphis.usda.gov/lpa/pubs/fsheet_faq_notice/faq_ahvs.html. Accessed 26 Jan 2006.

World Organization for Animal Health [OIE]. Manual of diagnostic tests and vaccines for terrestrial animals. Vesicular stomatitis. Available at: http://www.oie.int/eng/normes/mmanual/A_00025.htm. Accessed 26 Jan 2006.

Viral Hemorrhagic Septicemia
Egtved Disease, Infectious Nephrotic Swelling and Liver Degeneration, Abdominal Ascites of Trout, Infectious Anemia of Trout, Pernicious Anemia of Trout

Importance
Viral hemorrhagic septicemia is economically important in rainbow trout and turbot farming. Significant mortality has also been seen in Pacific herring and pilchard along the Pacific coast of North America.

Etiology

Viral hemorrhagic septicemia (VHS) is caused by the viral hemorrhagic septicemia virus (VHSV or Egtved virus). This virus is a member of the genus *Novirhabdovirus* and family Rhabdoviridae. Both marine and freshwater isolates occur.

Species affected

Viral hemorrhagic septicemia affects rainbow trout, brown trout, brook trout, grayling, white fish (*Coregonus* sp.), pike, and turbot. A number of marine species are also susceptible, including Pacific herring, Pacific salmon (*Oncorhynchus* spp.), Pacific cod, Pacific sandlance, and pilchard. In the Atlantic Ocean, susceptible species include Atlantic Cod, haddock, poor cod, rockling, sprat, herring, whiting, blue whiting, lesser argentine, Norway pout, shiner perch, Dab, English sole, flounder, and plaice. Most warm–water fish are resistant to this disease.

Geographic distribution

Viral hemorrhagic septicemia affects farmed rainbow trout and a few other freshwater species in continental Europe and Japan. VHSV has also been isolated from a variety of wild marine fish in North Atlantic, the Baltic sea, and the North American part of the Pacific Ocean.

Transmission

VHSV is shed in the urine, feces, and sexual fluids. Reservoirs include clinically ill fish and asymptomatic carriers. Transmission can occur through the water or by contact. The virus is thought to enter the body through the gills or possibly through wounds. Oral infection probably does not occur. Virus maintenance in invertebrates or transmission by parasitic flagellates may be possible but is unproven.

The virus is unstable in pond water, particularly when it is warm. Infectivity is lost after 24 hours at 20°C but can persist for 5 days at 4°C.

Incubation period

The incubation period varies with water temperature, but is usually 7 to 15 days.

Clinical signs

Viral hemorrhagic septicemia has been divided into acute, chronic, and nervous forms of the disease. These syndromes overlap and characteristics of all 3 forms may be seen during outbreaks.

In the acute form, clinical signs include darkening of the body, anemia, and protrusion of the eyes. Hemorrhages may be seen in the gills and eyes, and sometimes at the base of the pectoral fins and the body surface. The course of acute disease is brief and mortality is high. In the chronic form, infected fish blacken and the gills lose color. Protrusion of the eyes, anemia, and fluid accumulations in the abdomen are often seen. Hemorrhages are less common than in the acute form and mortality is usually low. In the nervous form, the body becomes twisted and fish swim in circles or on their sides, but few other symptoms are typically present.

Post mortem lesions

Scattered hemorrhages may be seen in the skeletal muscles, perivisceral adipose tissue in the abdomen, air bladder, intestines, and other organs. In chronic disease, the body cavity may be filled with fluid. The spleen may be enlarged and in some forms is very dark red. The liver is usually dark red in the acute form; in the chronic form, it often contains petechiae. The kidneys are reddened in the acute form and rarely swollen; in the chronic form, they are often grayish, swollen, and undulating. Fish with the nervous form may have no significant gross lesions. In some cases, muscle degeneration may occur with few other signs.

Morbidity and Mortality

Viral hemorrhagic septicemia can occur at any age, but younger fish appear to be most susceptible. Water temperature influences the likelihood of infection; this disease usually develops at temperatures between 4°C and 14°C. Outbreaks occur most often in the spring, when the temperature of the water is either rising or fluctuating.

The mortality rate varies from 20% to 80% and is influenced by environmental conditions. Mortality of up to 100% has been seen in trout fry.

Diagnosis

Clinical

Viral hemorrhagic septicemia should be suspected in trout, a few other freshwater fish, and marine species with hemorrhages or nervous signs.

Laboratory tests

Viral hemorrhagic septicemia can be diagnosed by virus isolation in cell cultures; appropriate cell lines include BF–2 (Bluegill fry) and RTG–2 (Rainbow trout gonad) cells. EPC (*Epithelioma papulosum cyprini*) cells can also be used, but are less susceptible to infection. Virus identity is confirmed by virus neutralization, immunofluorescence, an enzyme–linked immunosorbent assay, immunoperoxidase staining, or a polymerase chain reaction (PCR)–based assay.

Viral antigens can also be identified directly in tissues by immunofluorescence, immunohistochemistry, or ELISA. A PCR technique is in development.

Serology by virus neutralization or ELISA may be effective in detecting carriers, but has not yet been validated for routine diagnosis.

Samples to collect

The samples to collect depend on the size of the fish. Small fish (less than or equal to 4 cm) should be sent whole. The viscera including the kidney should be collected from fish that are 4 to 6 cm long. The kidney, spleen, heart, and encephalon should be sent from larger fish. Samples of ovarian fluid should also be collected from broodfish at spawning. Samples should be taken from 10 diseased fish and combined to form pools with approximately 1.5 g of material (no more than 5 fish per pool).

The pools of organs or ovarian fluids should be placed in sterile vials. The samples may also be sent in cell culture medium or Hanks' basal salt solution with antibiotics. They should be kept cold (4°C) but not frozen. If the shipping time is expected to be longer than 12 hours, serum or albumen (5–10%) may be added to stabilize the virus. Ideally, virus isolation should be done within 24 hours after fish sampling.

Recommended actions if viral hemorrhagic septicemia is suspected

Notification of authorities

Viral hemorrhagic septicemia should be reported to state or federal authorities immediately upon diagnosis or suspicion of the disease.

Federal: Area Veterinarians in Charge (AVICs):
  http://www.aphis.usda.gov/vs/area_offices.htm
State Veterinarians:
  http://www.aphis.usda.gov/vs/sregs/official.html

Quarantine and disinfection

Viral hemorrhagic septicemia is a highly contagious disease; quarantines are necessary to control outbreaks. VHSV can survive for long periods in the bottom of farm ponds, possibly in protozoans or metazoans, if the ponds are not dried and disinfected.

VHSV can be inactivated by formalin, drying, iodophor disinfectants, sodium hydroxide, sodium hypochlorite, and pH 2.5 or 12.2. The virus is also highly thermolabile. The effectiveness of lime disinfection is suspect.

Public health

There is no indication that this disease is a threat to human health.

For More Information

World Organization for Animal Health (OIE)
http://www.oie.int
OIE Diagnostic Manual for Aquatic Animal Diseases (2000)
http://www.oie.int/eng/normes/fmanual/A_summry.htm
OIE International Aquatic Animal Health Code (2001)
http://www.oie.int/eng/normes/fcode/a_summry.htm

References

"Fish Health Management: Viral Diseases." In *The Merck Veterinary Manual*, 8th ed. Edited by S.E. Aiello and A. Mays. Whitehouse Station, NJ: Merck and Co., 1998, pp. 1291–1293.

"General Information." In *Diagnostic Manual for Aquatic Animal Diseases*. Paris: World Organization for Animal Health, 2000. http//www.oie.int/eng/normes/fmanual/A_00010.htm.

"Viral Haemorrhagic Septicemia." In *Diagnostic Manual for Aquatic Animal Diseases*. Paris: World Organization for Animal Health, 2000. http://www.oie.int/eng/normes/fmanual/A_00016.htm.

"Viral Hemorrhagic Septicemia (VHS)." In *Infectious Diseases of Fish*. Edited by Shuzo Egusa. New Delhi, India: Amerind Pub. Co., 1992, pp. 8–20.

"Viral Hemorrhagic Septicemia (VHS), Infectious Nephrotic Swelling, and Liver Degeneration (INLD)." In *Fish Diseases*, 5th ed. Edited by W. Schäperclaus, H. Kulow, and K. Schreckenbach. Rotterdam: A.A. Balkema, 1992, pp. 349–64.

West Nile Encephalitis

Importance

West Nile encephalitis is an arthropod–borne disease of humans, horses, birds and occasionally other animals caused by West Nile virus (WNV). Signs of WNV infection can range from asymptomatic or very mild flu–like illness to severe meningoencephalitis and death. The West Nile virus (WNV) has recently become established in the United States.

Etiology

West Nile encephalatis is caused by West Nile virus, a mosquito–borne arbovirus in the genus *Flavivirus*, family Flaviviridae. Other flaviviruses are antigenically similar and include St. Louis encephalitis virus, which is found in the United States.

Species affected

West Nile virus primarily infects birds, but can also be found in bats, horses, cats, chipmunks, skunks, squirrels, domestic rabbits, and humans.

Geographic distribution

West Nile fever has been seen in Africa, Europe, the Middle East, west and central Asia, and North America. Outbreaks have occurred in Egypt, Israel, India, France, Romania, the Czech Republic, and the United States.

Transmission

Transmission is by the bite of an infected mosquito, primarily *Culex* species. Ticks and other arthropods may also be able to transmit the disease, but play a minor role. Direct animal–to–animal transmission has been seen only in experimentally infected geese. Birds are the primary reservoir host for West Nile virus, and bird migration facilitates the spread of this virus.

Incubation period

The incubation period is generally 3 to 12 days.

Clinical signs

Most animal species naturally infected with West Nile virus are asymptomatic, although experimental infection can cause signs in a variety of species. Horses can become infected with West Nile virus and most recover. Occasionally horses may exhibit signs of encephalitis such as lethargy, weakness, ataxia, partial paralysis, or death. Fever is seen in less than a quarter of affected horses.

Death is sometimes seen in naturally infected birds, particularly crows in the United States. Domestic geese can also show clinical signs; in natural and experimental infections, the symptoms may include weight loss, decreased activity, depression, myocarditis, and neurologic signs. Infections in geese can be fatal. Naturally or experimentally infected chickens and turkeys are asymptomatic.

Post mortem lesions

Post mortem lesions are not diagnostic. In cases of meningo-encephalitis, generalized lesions of the brain and spinal cord may be seen, including inflammation, small hemorrhages, perivascular cuffing, and neuronal degeneration.

Morbidity and mortality

In endemic areas, the prevalence of infection in wild birds ranges from 10% to 53%. Antibodies have also been found in normal dogs, horses, donkeys, and mules in endemic regions. Estimates of the morbidity rates in horses vary. During outbreaks, 20% to 43% of infected horses appear to develop acute neurologic signs. Experimental studies have been equivocal. In 1 recent study, only 1 of 12 horses experimentally infected by mosquito vectors developed encephalitis. The other 11 horses seroconverted but remained asymptomatic. Higher rates of encephalitis and fever have been seen when foals and horses were infected subcutaneously and intravenously; 4 of 9 animals in 2 studies became ill.

Diagnosis

Clinical

The clinical signs may be vague depending on the severity of the disease, and are indistinguishable from other viral fevers.

Differential diagnosis

In horses, the differential diagnosis includes other neurologic diseases, including rabies, equine herpesvirus–1 infection, equine protozoal myeloencephalitis, and eastern, western, or Venezuelan equine encephalomyelitis.

Laboratory tests

Definitive diagnosis requires isolation and identification of the virus or specific antibody testing. Complement fixation, virus neutralization, hemagglutination inhibition, and enzyme–linked immunosorbent assays (ELISAs) can be used to detect antibodies to the virus. Cross–reactions can occur with other flaviviruses.

Samples to collect

In some areas of the United States, a West Nile virus infection may be treated as foreign animal disease; state or federal authorities may need to be notified before collecting or sending any samples.

Blood or serum samples collected late in the incubation period or up to 5 days after clinical signs are present may be useful for virus isolation. In the presence of meningoencephalitis, blood or cerebrospinal fluid may be used to isolate the virus. Single or paired serum samples are needed for antibody testing.

Recommended actions if
West Nile encephalitis is suspected

Notification of authorities

Health authorities should be notified of any suspected cases of West Nile fever in the United States.

Federal: Area Veterinarians in Charge (AVICs):
http://www.aphis.usda.gov/vs/area_offices.htm
State Veterinarians:
http://www.aphis.usda.gov/vs/sregs/official.html

Quarantine and disinfection

In horses, humans, and most birds, direct transmission does not occur and no quarantine is necessary. Direct animal–to–animal transmission has been documented only in experimentally infected geese. Mosquito control and prevention of exposure to mosquitoes by the use of insect repellants and protective clothing is important in disease control.

Public health

In humans, West Nile fever can range from very mild fever to meningoencephalitis and sometimes death. Less than 1% of people infected with West Nile virus will develop signs of serious illness; of these, the case–fatality rate is 3% to 15%. The elderly are most severely affected. Young adults and children generally have mild disease and recover quickly. The clinical signs generally last less than a week and can include fever, headache, malaise, arthralgia, myalgia, lymphadenopathy, conjunctivitis, photophobia, rash, and occasionally nausea and vomiting. In the more severe cases, the signs may include neck stiffness, stupor, disorientation, coma, tremors, convulsions, muscle weakness, paralysis, and rarely death. In severe cases, recovery can be prolonged, particularly in the elderly.

A vaccine for humans is not currently available for West Nile virus. Natural immunity general develops after infection.

For more information

Centers for Disease Control and Prevention (CDC)
    http://www.cdc.gov/ncidod/dvbid/westnile/index.htm
Articles on West Nile Virus. Emerging Infectious Diseases Vol. 7, No. 4 (Jul–Aug 2001)
    http://www.cdc.gov/ncidod/eid/vol7no4/contents.htm
U.S. Department of Agriculture, Animal and Plant Health Inspection Service. West Nile Index
    http://www.aphis.usda.gov/lpa/issues/wnv/wnv.html
West Nile Virus Guidelines for Horse Owners.
    Nebraska Cooperative Extension
    http://www.ianr.unl.edu/pubs/animaldisease/nf542.htm
What You Should Know About West Nile Virus.
    American Veterinary Medical Association
    http://www.avma.org/communications/brochures/wnv/wnv_faq.asp

References

"Arthropod–Borne Viral Fevers." In *Control of Communicable Diseases Manual*, 17th ed., edited by James Chin. Washington, D.C.: American Public Health Association, 2000, pp. 48–50.

Bunning M.L., R.A. Bowen, C.B. Cropp, K.G. Sullivan, B.S. Davis, N. Komar, M.S. Godsey, D. Baker, D.L. Hettler, D.A. Holmes, B.J. Biggerstaff, C.J. Mitchell. "Experimental infection of horses with West Nile virus." *Emerg Infect Dis* 8, no. 4 (2002): 380–6. 8 Dec 2002. http://www.medscape.com/viewarticle/432142_print.

"Guidelines for Investigating Suspect West Nile Virus Cases in Equine." April 2003 USDA Animal and Plant Health Inspection Service. 22 April 2003. http://www.aphis.usda.gov/lpa/issues/wnv/wnvguide.html.

Komar N., N.A. Panella and E. Boyce. "Exposure of domestic mammals to West Nile virus during an outbreak of human encephalitis, New York City, 1999." *Emerg Infect Dis* 7, no. 4 (Jul–Aug 2001):736–8. 5 Dec 2002. http://www.cdc.gov/ncidod/eid/vol7no4/komar1.htm.

Langevin S.A., M. Bunning, B. Davis and N. Komar. "Experimental infection of chickens as candidate sentinels for West Nile virus." *Emerg Infect Dis* 7, no. 4 (Jul–Aug 2001):726–9. 5 Dec 2002. http://www.cdc.gov/ncidod/eid/vol7no4/langevin.htm.

Leake, C.J. "Mosquito–Borne Arboviruses." In *Zoonoses*. Edited by S.R. Palmer, E.J.L. Soulsby and D.I.H Simpson. New York: Oxford University Press, 1998, pp. 401–413.

Murgue B., S. Murri, S. Zientara, B. Durand, J.–P. Durand and H. Zeller. "West Nile outbreak in horses in southern France, 2000: The return after 35 years." *Emerg Infect Dis* 7, no. 4 (Jul–Aug 2001):692–6. 5 Dec 2002. http://www.cdc.gov/ncidod/eid/vol7no4/murgue.htm.

Ostlund E.N., R.L. Crom, D.D. Pedersen, D.J. Johnson, W.O. Williams and B.J. Schmit. "Equine West Nile encephalitis, United States." *Emerg Infect Dis* 7, no. 4 (Jul–Aug 2001):665–9. 5 Dec 2002. http://www.cdc.gov/ncidod/eid/vol7no4/ostlund.htm.

Peiris, J.S. Malik and F.P. Amerasinghe. "West Nile Fever." In *Handbook of Zoonoses*, 2nd ed. Edited by G.W. Beran. Boca Raton, Florida: CRC Press, 1994, pp. 139–148.

Perl S., L. Fiette, D. Lahav, N. Sheichat, C.Banet, U. Orgad, Y. Stram and M. Malkinson. "West Nile encephalitis in horses in Israel." *Israeli Veterinary Medical Association* 57, no. 2 (2002). 8 Dec 2002 http://www.isrvma.org/article/57_2_2.htm.

Swayne D.E., J.R. Beck, C.S. Smith, W.–J. Shieh and S.R. Zaki. "Fatal encephalitis and myocarditis in young domestic geese (*Anser anser domesticus*) caused by West Nile virus." *Emerg. Infect. Dis.* 7, no. 4 (Jul–Aug 2001):751–3. 5 Dec 2002. http://www.cdc.gov/ncidod/eid/vol7no4/swayne.htm.

Trock S.C. B.J. Meade, A.L. Glaser, E.N. Ostlund, R.S. Lanciotti, B.C. Cropp, V. Kulasekera, L.D. Kramer and N. Komar. "West Nile virus outbreak among horses in New York State, 1999 and 2000." *Emerg Infect Dis* 7, no. 4 (Jul–Aug 2001):745–7. 5 Dec 2002. http://www.cdc.gov/ncidod/eid/vol7no4/trock.htm.

"West Nile Virus." 14 Aug. 2001 Centers for Disease Control and Prevention 10 Jan. 2002. http://www.cdc.gov/ncidod/dvbid/westnile/index.htm.

"West Nile Virus." United States Department of Agriculture 10 Jan. 2002 http://www.aphis.gov/oa/wnv/>.

Section 3
• Images of Emerging and Exotic Diseases of Animals •

Authored by:
Steven D. Sorden, DVM, PhD, Diplomate ACVP
Claire B. Andreasen, DVM, PhD, Diplomate ACVP
Department of Veterinary Pathology
College of Veterinary Medicine
Iowa State University
Ames, IA 50011

Acknowledgments

We are grateful to the many institutions and individuals that made this project possible by contributing images, technical assistance, editing, and feedback. Project directors include: Dr. Steve Sorden, who had primary responsibility for annotation of images, with collection of images assisted by Dr. Claire Andreasen, Department of Veterinary Pathology (VPTH), College of Veterinary Medicine (CVM), Iowa State University (ISU); and Dr. James Roth, Director of the Center for Food Security and Public Health (CFSPH) CVM ISU. Additional collaborators include: Dr. Terrell Blanchard and Dr. Dale Dunn, Armed Forces Institute of Pathology (AFIP); Dr. Samia Metwally (USDA-APHIS), Dr. Thomas McKenna (USDA-APHIS), and Dr. Beth Lautner, Director (DHS), Plum Island Animal Disease Center, N.Y. For technical assistance: Mr. Travis Engelhaupt (CFSPH), Ms. Sara Hall (CFSPH) Ms. Deb Hoyt (VPTH), the staff of the CFSPH, and student assistants. For assessment assistance: Dr. Jared Danielson (VPTH) and the collaborators at AFIP. Image acquisition was funded by a USDA Cooperative State Research, Education, and Extension Service (CSREES) Higher Education Challenge Grant "A Digital Image Database to Enhance Foreign Animal Disease Education" (grant number 2005-38411-15859).

We are grateful to the following institutions for contributing images. In the subsequent pages, each institution is acknowledged for image contribution (abbreviations listed below). Where appropriate, the individual who contributed the image also is acknowledged.

Armed Forces Institute of Pathology (AFIP),
    Education Branch, Division of Research and Education,
    Department of Veterinary Pathology, Washington, D.C.
Canadian Cooperative Wildlife Health Centre (CCWHC), University of Saskatchewan, Saskatoon, Saskatchewan, Canada
California Animal Health and Food Safety
    Laboratory System (CAHFSLS), CA
Central Livestock Hygiene Service Center,
    Saitama pref., Japan
Commonwealth Scientific and Industrial Research Organisation
    (CSIRO), Australia Animal Health Laboratory, East Geelong,
    Victoria, Australia
Elizabeth Macarthur Agricultural Institute (EMAI), NSW, Australia
Federal Research Institute for Animal Health,
    Riems, Germany
Kasetsart University, Department of Pathology,
    Faculty of Veterinary Medicine, Bangkok, Thailand
Kansas State University, Department of Diagnostic Medicine and
    Pathobiology, College of Veterinary Medicine (KSU CVM),
    Manhattan, KS
Iowa State University, College of Veterinary Medicine (ISU
    CVM), Ames, IA
    Department of Veterinary Pathology (VPTH), ISU CVM, Ames, IA
    Veterinary Diagnostic Laboratory (VDL), ISU CVM, Ames, IA
National Institute of Animal Health, Aomori, Japan
Noah's Arkive, University of Georgia, Athens, GA
Plum Island Animal Disease Center (PIADC),
    Greenport, NY
USDA-ARS Southeast Poultry Research Laboratory, Athens, GA
University of Melbourne, Australia

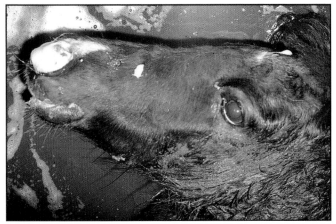

African Horse Sickness
Horse. Abundant froth draining from the nostrils reflects severe pulmonary edema.
Source: PIADC

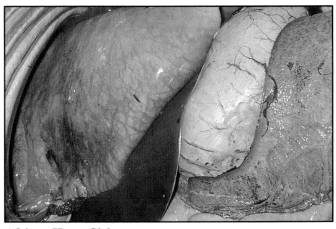

African Horse Sickness
Horse. The lung exhibits severe interlobular edema. There are petechiae on the pulmonary pleura and the splenic capsule.
Source: PIADC

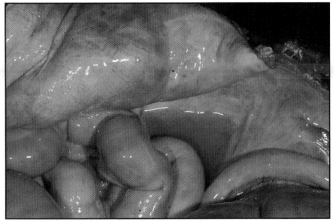

African Horse Sickness
Horse, peritoneal cavity. There is excessive straw-colored fluid (hydroperitoneum).
Source: PIADC

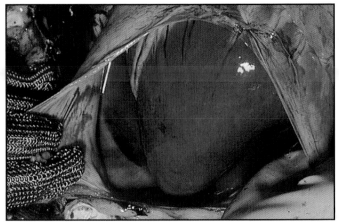

African Horse Sickness
Horse, heart. The pericardial sac contains excessive, slightly turbid straw-colored fluid (hydropericardium).
Source: PIADC

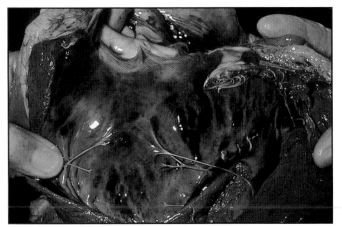

African Horse Sickness
Horse, heart. There are many subendocardial hemorrhages.
Source: PIADC

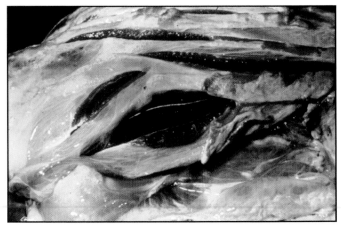

African Horse Sickness
Horse, skeletal muscle. There is marked intermuscular edema.
Source: Noah's Arkive , PIADC

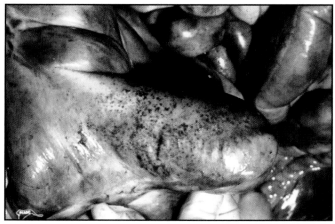

African Horse Sickness
Horse, cecum. There are serosal petechiae on the apex of the cecum.
Source: Noah's Arkive, PIADC

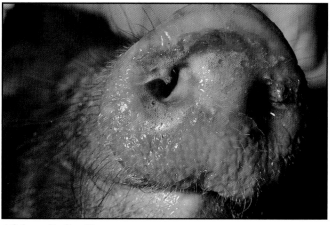

African Swine Fever
Pig. There is bloody, mucoid, foamy nasal discharge.
Source: PIADC

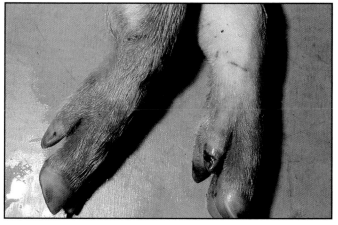

African Swine Fever
Pig, limbs. There is marked hyperemia of the distal limbs.
Source: PIADC

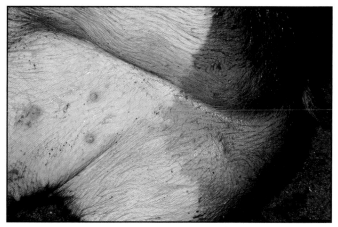

African Swine Fever
Pig, perineal skin. There is a large sharply demarcated zone of hyperemia.
Source: PIADC

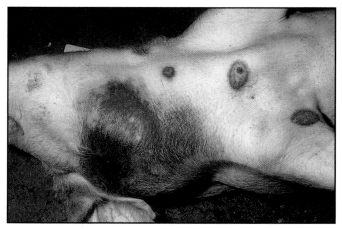

African Swine Fever
Pig. There are multiple sharply demarcated foci of cutaneous hemorrhage and/or necrosis; hemorrhagic lesions may contain dark red (necrotic) centers.
Source: PIADC

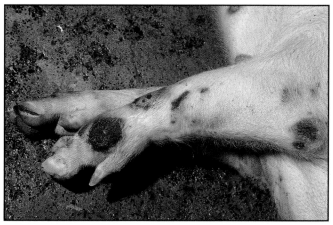

African Swine Fever
Pig. There are multiple sharply demarcated foci of cutaneous hemorrhage and/or necrosis; hemorrhagic lesions may contain dark red (necrotic) centers.
Source: PIADC

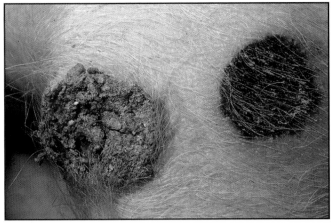

African Swine Fever
Pig, skin. Necrotic exudate is sloughing from the lesion on the left. There is a rim of hyperemia around the focus of hemorrhage and necrosis (infarct) on the right.
Source: PIADC

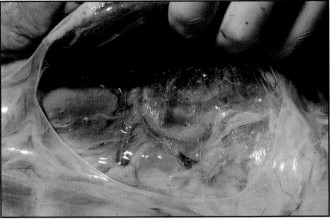

African Swine Fever
Pig, kidney. There is moderate perirenal (retroperitoneal) edema.
Source: PIADC

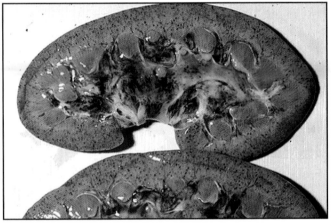

African Swine Fever
Pig, kidney. Petechiae are disseminated throughout the cortex, and there are larger coalescing pelvic hemorrhages.
Source: PIADC

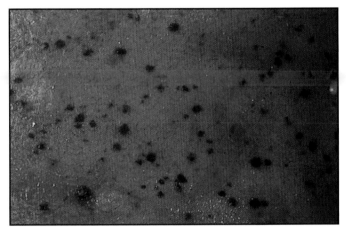

African Swine Fever
Pig, kidney. Close-up of cortical petechiae.
Source: PIADC

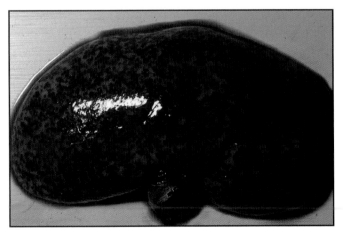

African Swine Fever
Pig, kidney. The cortex contains numerous coalescing petechiae and ecchymoses.
Source: PIADC

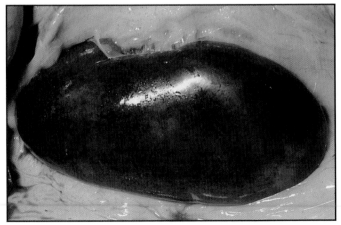

African Swine Fever
Pig, kidney. There is severe disseminated cortical petechiation; the pale foci are infarcts.
Source: PIADC

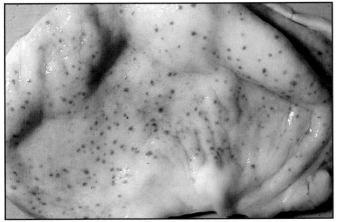

African Swine Fever
Pig, urinary bladder. There are disseminated mucosal petechiae.
Source: PIADC

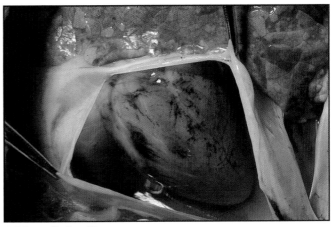

African Swine Fever
Pig, heart. There is abundant straw-colored pericardial fluid (hydropericardium), and multifocal epicardial hemorrhage.
Source: PIADC

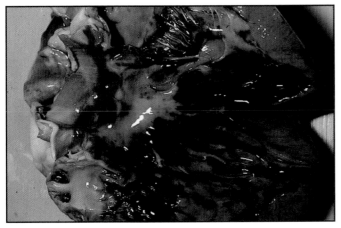

African Swine Fever
Pig, heart. Subendocardial hemorrhage.
Source: PIADC

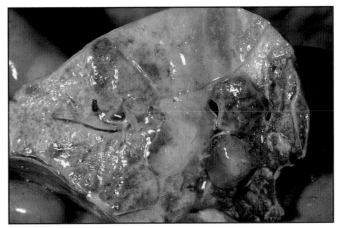

African Swine Fever
Pig, lung. The lung is noncollapsed and edematous; there is dorsal hemorrhage and ventral tan consolidation.
Source: PIADC

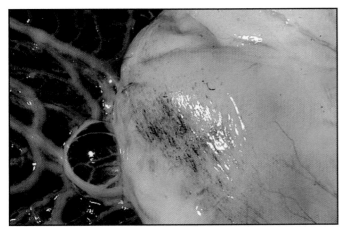

African Swine Fever
Pig, stomach. There is "paintbrush" hemorrhage on the serosa.
Source: PIADC

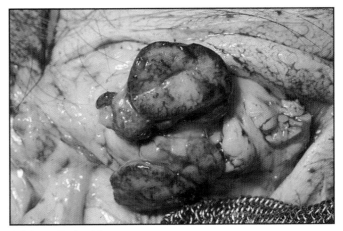

African Swine Fever
Pig, mandibular lymph node. There is moderate peripheral (medullary) hemorrhage.
Source: PIADC

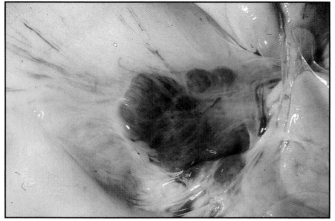

African Swine Fever
Pig, stomach. The hepatogastric lymph node is markedly
enlarged and hemorrhagic, and the adjacent lesser omentum
is edematous.
Source: PIADC

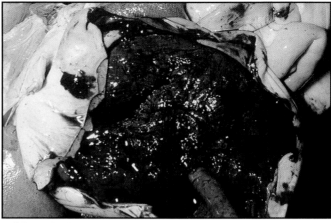

African Swine Fever
Pig, stomach. The stomach is filled with clotted blood, and
the wall is markedly edematous.
Source: PIADC

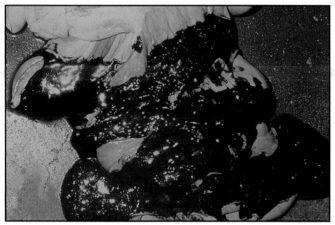

African Swine Fever
Pig, spiral colon. The colon is distended with bloody contents
(due to a hemorrhagic gastric ulcer).
Source: PIADC

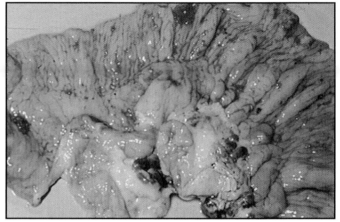

African Swine Fever
Pig, cecum. Mucosa is markedly edematous and hyperemic,
and lymph nodes are hemorrhagic.
Source: PIADC

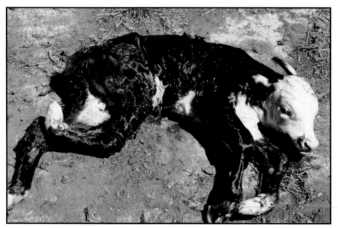

Akabane
Bovine neonate. This live calf cannot stand due to severe
arthrogryposis, primarily affecting the hindlimbs.
Source: Dr. P. Mansell, University of Melbourne

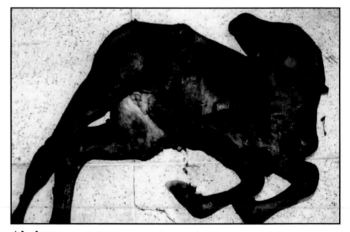

Akabane
Bovine neonate (Aino). This stillborn calf exhibits torticollis
and arthrogryposis.
Source: Dr. K. Kawashima, National Institute of Animal Health, Japan

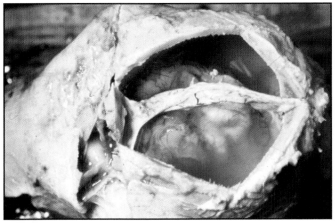

Akabane
Bovine neonate, brain. The entire brain is reduced in size (microencephaly), and surrounded by cerebrospinal fluid.
Source: Dr. K. Kawashima, National Institute for Animal Health, Japan

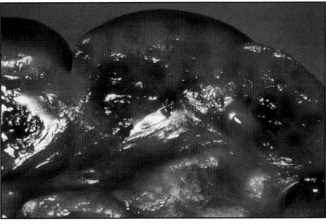

Anthrax
Bovine, lymph node. The node is hyperemic and contains multiple dark foci of hemorrhage.
Source: AFIP

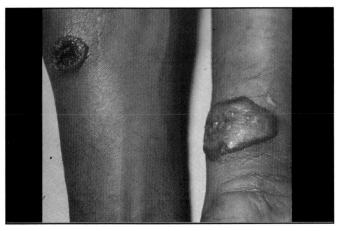

Anthrax
Human, skin. Lesions are raised and have necrotic centers.
Source: AFIP

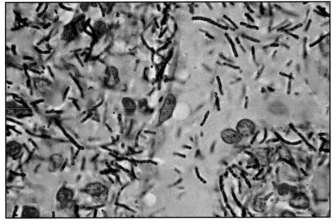

Anthrax
Bacillus anthracis is a large, blunt- to square-ended bacterial rod that forms short chains.
Source: ISU CVM

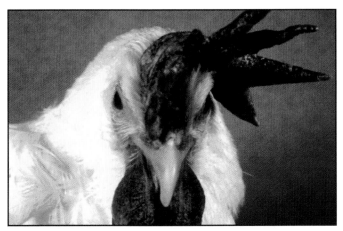

Avian Influenza
Chicken, head. The comb and wattles are congested and markedly edematous.
Source: Dr. D. Swayne, USDA

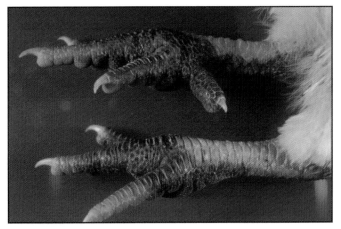

Avian Influenza
Chicken, shanks. The shanks are swollen (edema) and extensively reddened (hemorrhage).
Source: Dr. D. Swayne, USDA

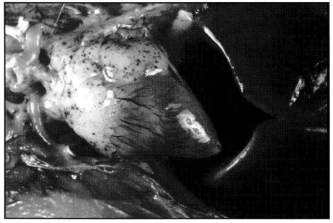

Avian Influenza
Chicken, heart. There are numerous epicardial petechiae.
Source: Dr. D. Swayne, USDA

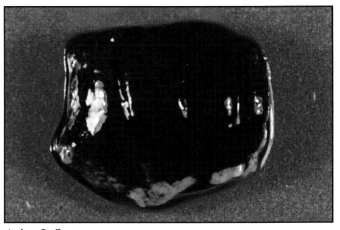

Avian Influenza
Chicken, lung. The lung is diffusely reddened, wet, and swollen (congestion and edema).
Source: Dr. D. Swayne, USDA

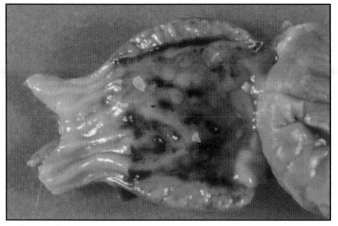

Avian Influenza
Chicken, proventriculus. There are multiple hemorrhages on the mucosal surface of the proventriculus.
Source: Dr. D. Swayne, USDA

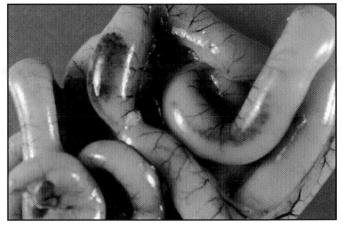

Avian Influenza
Chicken, intestine. There are serosal hemorrhages over the Peyer's patches.
Source: Dr. D. Swayne, USDA

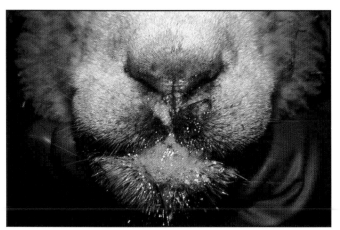

Bluetongue
Sheep. There is bilateral nasal exudate, erosion of the nasal planum, and excessive salivation.
Source: PIADC

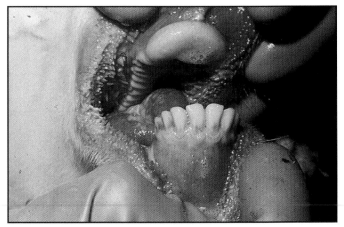

Bluetongue
Sheep, mouth. There is linear erosion and reddening of the right buccal mucosa.
Source: PIADC

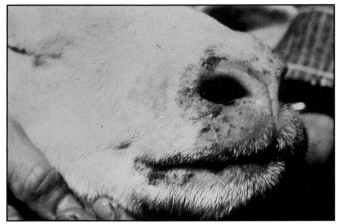

Bluetongue
Sheep. There are multiple erosions and crusts on the muzzle and lips.
Source: PIADC

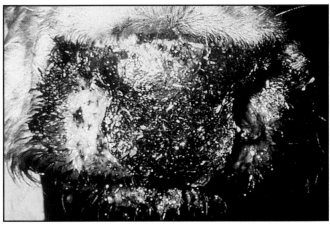

Bluetongue
Bovine. The muzzle is covered by an adherent crust, and the underlying (eroded) tissue is hyperemic.
Source: PIADC

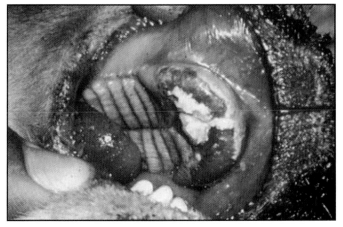

Bluetongue
Sheep, mouth. Most of the dental pad is eroded; the remaining pale mucosa is necrotic.
Source: AFIP

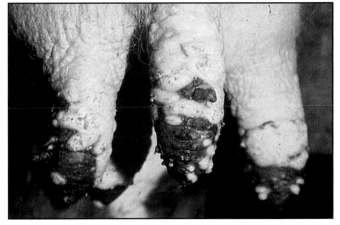

Bluetongue
Bovine, mammary gland. There is extensive coalescing ulceration of the teat skin.
Source: PIADC

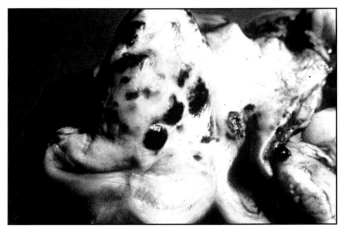

Bluetongue
Sheep, pulmonary artery. There are multiple ecchymoses on the intimal surface.
Source: AFIP

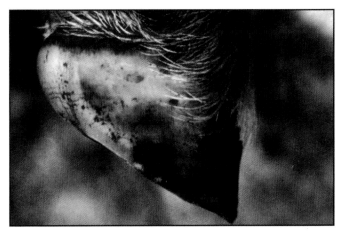

Bluetongue
Sheep, foot. There are multiple petechiae in the hoof wall, and there is marked hyperemia of the coronary band.
Source: AFIP

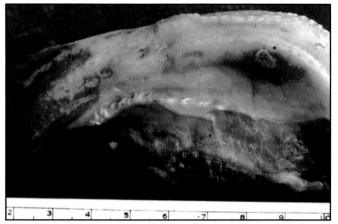

Bluetongue
Sheep, tongue. There are multiple erosions.
Source: PIADC

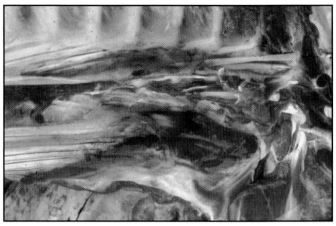

Bluetongue
Sheep, skeletal muscle. There is a focus of hemorrhage on the tendons. Pale areas are consistent with myodegeneration.
Source: AFIP

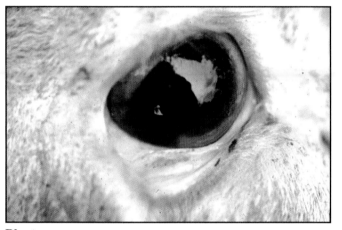

Bluetongue
Sheep, eye. There are foci of bulbar and palpebral conjunctival hemorrhage.
Source: AFIP

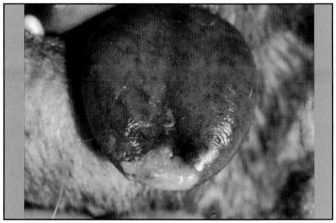

Bluetongue
Sheep, tongue. There are disseminated mucosal petechiae, and a single large vesicle on the tip.
Source: AFIP

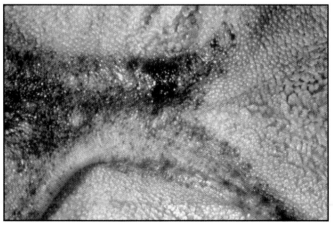

Bluetongue
Sheep, rumen. There are multiple mucosal hemorrhages centered on the pillars.
Source: AFIP

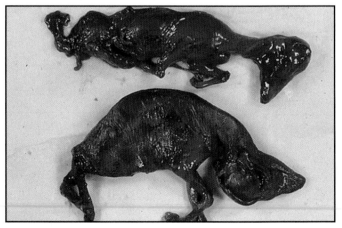

Bluetongue
Aborted, macerated, ovine fetuses. The larger fetus exhibits torticollis.
Source: PIADC

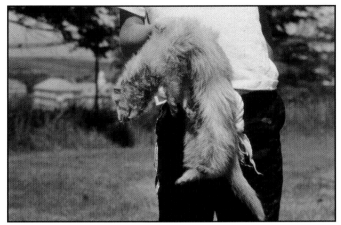

Botulism
Mink. Flaccid paralysis characteristic of botulism.
Source: AFIP

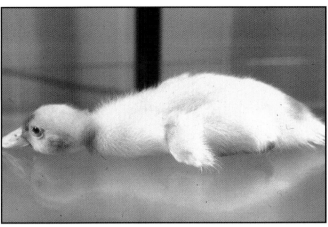

Botulism
Duck. Flaccid paralysis characteristic of botulism.
Source: AFIP

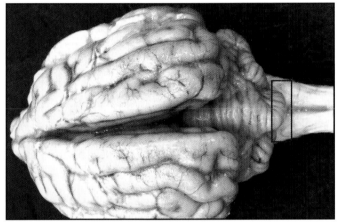

Bovine Spongiform Encephalopathy
Brain. The red box indicates the region of the obex, the portion of the brainstem that is required for BSE diagnosis.
Source: Dr. S. Sorden, ISU CVM, VPTH

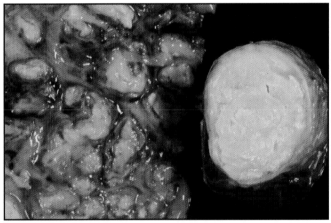

Bovine Tuberculosis
Elk, lung and lymph node. Lung contains multiple coalescing foci of caseous necrosis surrounded by thin pale fibrous tissue capsules (tubercles).
Source: Dr. G. Wobeser, CCWHC

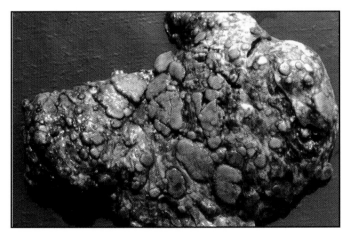

Bovine Tuberculosis
Bovine, lung. Lung parenchyma is almost entirely replaced by variably-sized, coalescing, raised pale nodules.
Source: AFIP

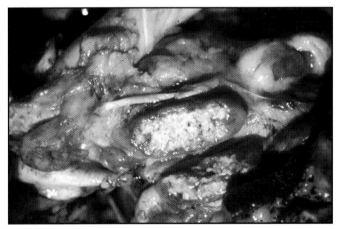

Bovine Tuberculosis
Porcine, tracheobronchial lymph nodes. The center of the sectioned node is replaced by caseous, mineralized debris.
Source: AFIP

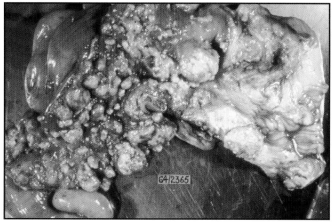

Bovine Tuberculosis
Bovine, uterus. The endometrium contains numerous raised tubercles.
Source: AFIP

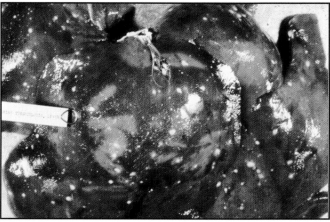

Bovine Tuberculosis
Porcine, liver. Pale, slightly raised granulomas are disseminated throughout all liver lobes.
Source: AFIP

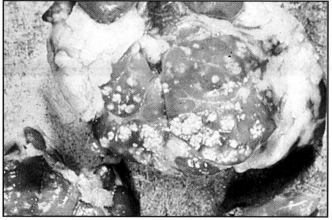

Bovine Tuberculosis
Porcine, lymph nodes. Pale, mineralized granulomas are scattered throughout these cervical lymph nodes.
Source: AFIP

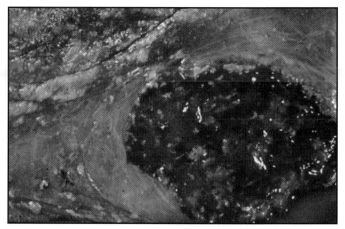

Brucellosis
Bovine, placenta. Numerous pale clumps of exudate are scattered over the cotyledon and adjacent chorion.
Source: AFIP

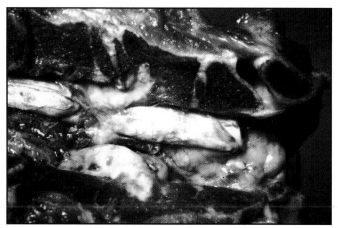

Brucellosis
Bovine, vertebrae. Purulent exudate within a vertebra extends into the adjacent spinal canal.
Source: AFIP

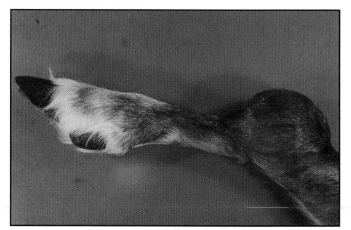

Brucellosis
Caribou, carpus, *B. suis* biovar 4. The carpal bursa is markedly swollen and fluctuant.
Source: Dr. G. Wobeser, CCWHC

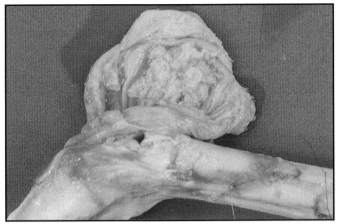

Brucellosis
Caribou, carpus, *B. suis* biovar 4. The carpal bursa contains purulent exudate.
Source: Dr. G. Wobeser, CCWHC

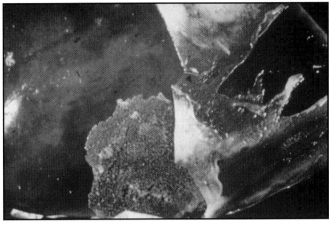

Chlamydiosis (Avian)
Avian, liver. Sheets of fibrinous exudate partially cover the capsular surface of the liver.
Source: AFIP

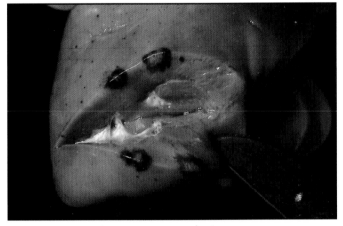

Classical Swine Fever
Pig, kidney. The cortex contains multiple petechiae and pale infarcts surrounded by hemorrhage.
Source: PIADC

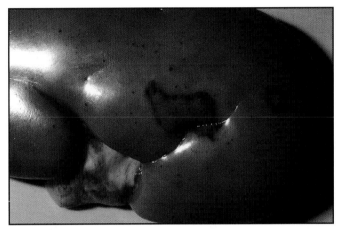

Classical Swine Fever
Pig, kidney. The cortex contains multiple petechiae and pale infarcts surrounded by hemorrhage.
Source: PIADC

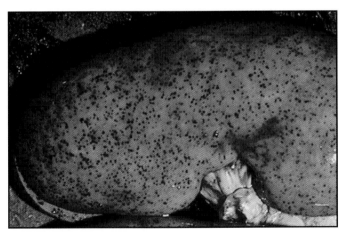

Classical Swine Fever
Pig, kidney. There are numerous disseminated cortical petechiae ("turkey egg kidney").
Source: PIADC

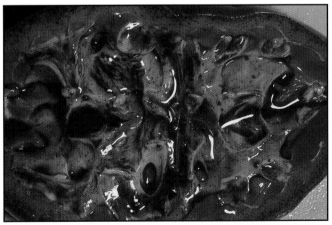

Classical Swine Fever
Pig, kidney. The cortex contains disseminated petechiae. Calyces are moderately dilated (hydronephrosis) and also contain hemorrhages.
Source: PIADC

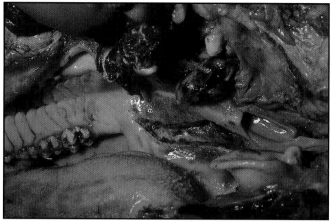

Classical Swine Fever
Pig, retropharyngeal lymph node. The lymph node is markedly enlarged and hemorrhagic; the tonsil contains multiple poorly demarcated hemorrhages.
Source: PIADC

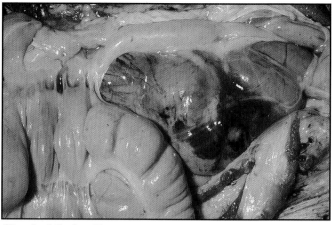

Classical Swine Fever
Pig, kidney. There is extensive hemorrhage on the cortical surface.
Source: PIADC

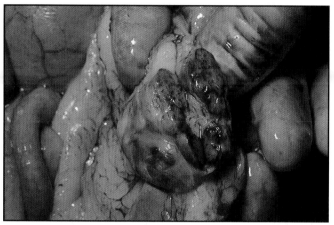

Classical Swine Fever
Pig, inguinal lymph node. There are petechial and peripheral (medullary sinus) hemorrhages.
Source: PIADC

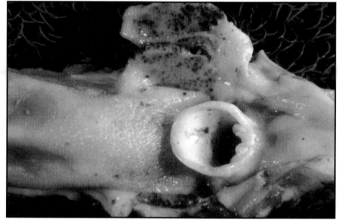

Classical Swine Fever
Pig, pharynx and larynx. There are coalescing foci of petechial hemorrhage (and necrosis) in the palatine tonsils and adjacent pharyngeal and laryngeal mucosa.
Source: Dr. W. Wajjwalku, Kasetsart University, Thailand

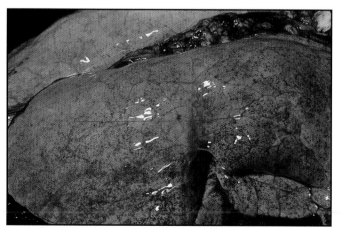

Classical Swine Fever
Pig, lungs. There are numerous disseminated pleural petechiae, and there is mild interlobular edema.
Source: PIADC

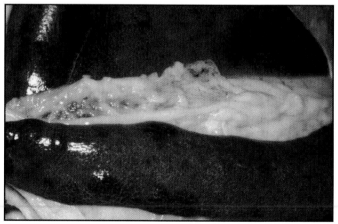

Classical Swine Fever
Pig, spleen. There are multiple coalescing, swollen dark red infarcts along the margins.
Source: Dr. D. Gregg, Noah's Arkive, PIADC

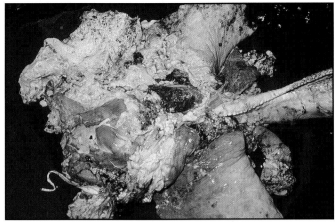

Contagious Bovine Pleuropneumonia
Bovine, lung. Most of the pleural surface is covered by abundant fibrin and fibrous tissue.
Source: PIADC

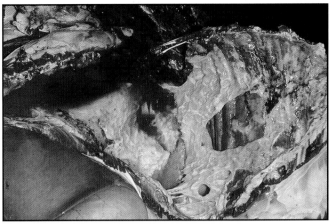

Contagious Bovine Pleuropneumonia
Bovine pleural cavity. Large sheets of fibrin cover the costal and diaphragmatic pleura, and form pockets containing straw-colored fluid.
Source: PIADC

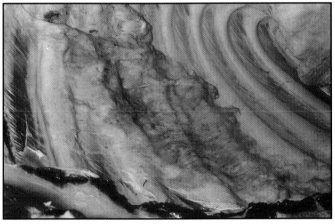

Contagious Bovine Pleuropneumonia
Bovine, pleural cavity. There is a thick plaque (adhesion) of fibrous tissue on the costal pleura.
Source: PIADC

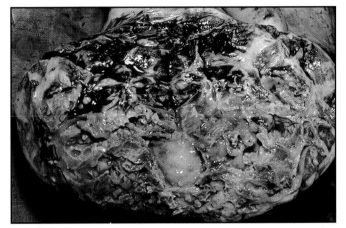

Contagious Bovine Pleuropneumonia
Bovine, lung. Most of the parenchyma is dull and tan (necrotic); partially surrounded by a fibrous capsule, this necrotic zone is termed a sequestrum.
Source: PIADC

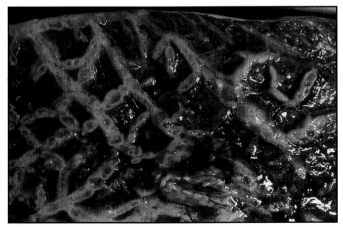

Contagious Bovine Pleuropneumonia
Bovine, lung. Interlobular septa are markedly thickened by fibrous tissue, and also contain small depressions (air pockets = emphysema).
Source: PIADC

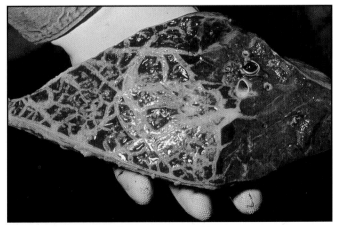

Contagious Bovine Pleuropneumonia
Bovine, lung. In the ventral portion of this lung (left side of the image), interlobular septa and the pleura are markedly thickened with fibrous tissue.
Source: PIADC

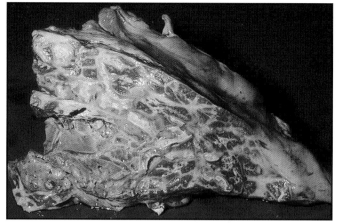

Contagious Bovine Pleuropneumonia
Bovine, lung. The pleura and underlying interlobular septa are severely thickened by fibrous tissue. Lung parenchyma at the lower left is dull and tan (sequestrum).
Source: PIADC

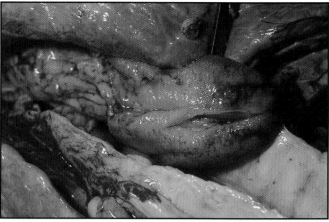

Contagious Bovine Pleuropneumonia
Bovine, tracheobronchial lymph node. This bisected node is enlarged (hyperplasia) and contains a focal area of hemorrhage.
Source: PIADC

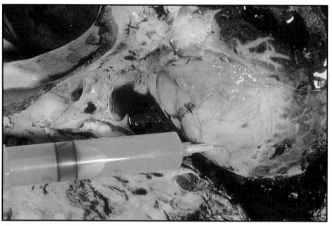

Contagious Bovine Pleuropneumonia
Bovine, heart. The pericardial sac contains abundant pale turbid fluid.
Source: PIADC

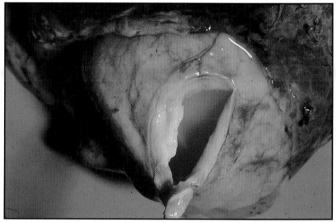

Contagious Bovine Pleuropneumonia
Bovine, heart. The pericardial wall is markedly thickened and the pericardial sac contains abundant pale tan, turbid fluid.
Source: PIADC

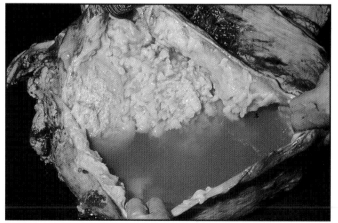

Contagious Bovine Pleuropneumonia
Bovine, incised pericardium. The sac is distended with abundant turbid, tan fluid, and abundant fibrin coats the pericardial surfaces.
Source: PIADC

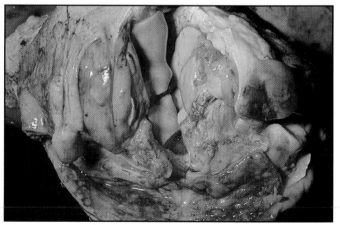

Contagious Bovine Pleuropneumonia
Bovine carpus. The joint capsule and extensor tendon sheath are thickened and contain excessive fluid.
Source: PIADC

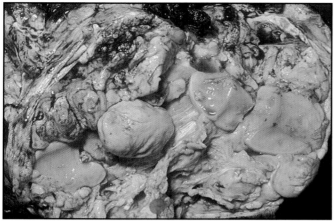

Contagious Bovine Pleuropneumonia
Bovine, carpus. There is abundant fibrin within the synovial space and on the synovium, and articular cartilages contain a few small erosions.
Source: PIADC

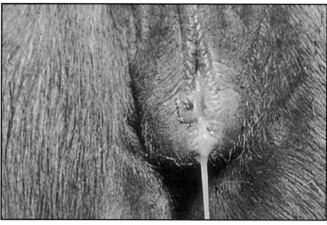

Contagious Equine Metritis
Horse, vulva. Mucopurulent exudate drains from the vulva.
Source: PIADC

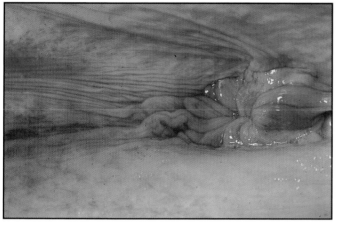

Contagious Equine Metritis
Horse, vagina. There is straw-colored fluid within the cranial vagina.
Source: PIADC

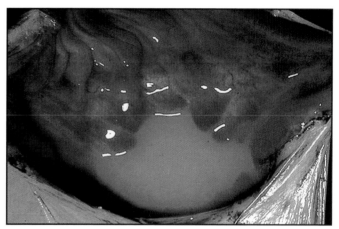

Contagious Equine Metritis
Horse, uterus. The uterine body contains mucopurulent exudate.
Source: PIADC

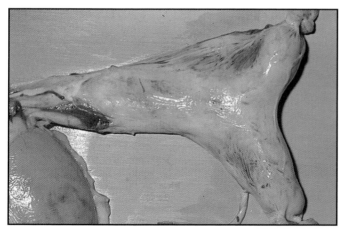

Contagious Equine Metritis
Horse, uterus. The uterine horns and body are mildly distended (with mucopurulent exudate).
Source: PIADC

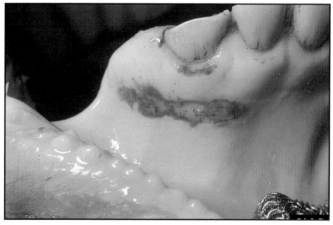

Foot and Mouth Disease
Bovine, gingiva. There is an elongate erosion (ruptured vesicle) ventral to the incisors.
Source: PIADC

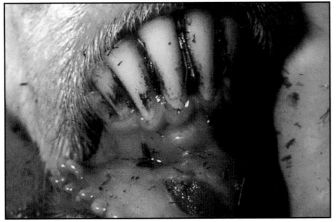

Foot and Mouth Disease
Goat, oral mucosa. There is a large erosion (ruptured vesicle) on the rostral mandibular buccal mucosa.
Source: PIADC

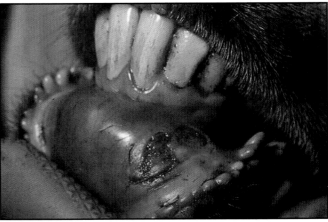

Foot and Mouth Disease
Goat, oral mucosa. There is a large, partially re-epithelialized (healing) erosion on the rostral mandibular buccal mucosa.
Source: PIADC

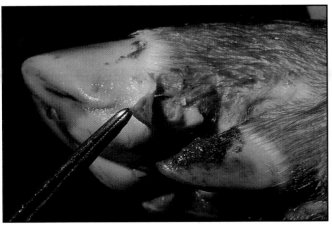

Foot and Mouth Disease
Pig, foot. There is a ruptured vesicle on the caudal-lateral coronary band, with undermining of the heel.
Source: PIADC

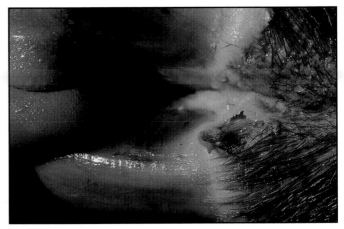

Foot and Mouth Disease
Pig, foot. A ruptured vesicle of the coronary band extends into the interdigital skin.
Source: PIADC

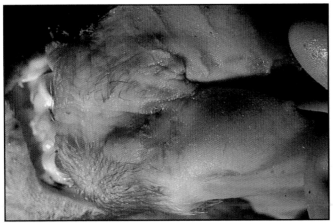

Foot and Mouth Disease
Pig, foot. There is an intact vesicle on the caudal coronary band of the left claw, and a cleft (ruptured vesicle) on the heel bulb of the right claw.
Source: PIADC

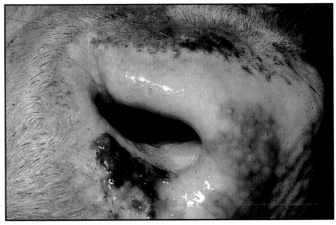

Foot and Mouth Disease
Bovine, muzzle. Within the naris, the ventromedial mucosa contains an intact vesicle.
Source: PIADC

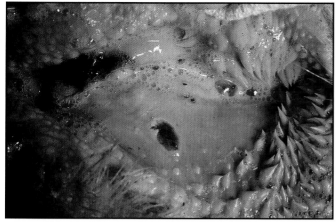

Foot and Mouth Disease
Bovine, lip. The buccal mucosa contains an erosion
(ruptured vesicle).
Source: PIADC

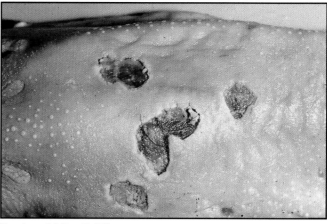

Foot and Mouth Disease
Tongue. There are multiple large mucosal erosions and ulcers.
Source: PIADC

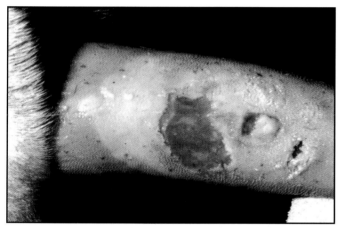

Foot and Mouth Disease
Bovine, tongue. A large area of undermined epithelium
(bulla) is centrally eroded; this lesion probably resulted from
coalescence of several smaller lesions.
Source: Dr. D. Gregg, Noah's Arkive, PIADC

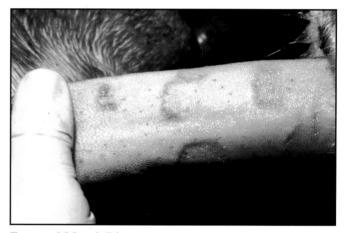

Foot and Mouth Disease
Bovine, tongue. Several healing vesicles have
yellow-tan margins.
Source: Dr. D. Gregg, Noah's Arkive, PIADC

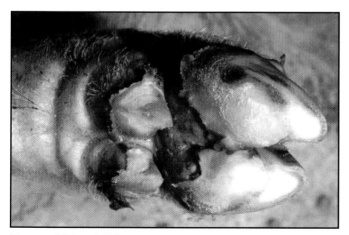

Foot and Mouth Disease
Porcine, foot. Large clefts at the coronary bands precede
sloughing of the claws.
Source: Dr. D. Gregg, Noah's Arkive, PIADC

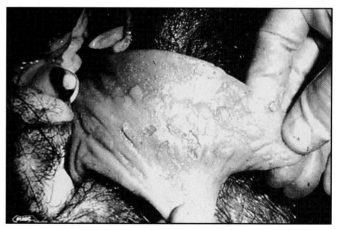

Foot and Mouth Disease
Porcine, tongue. Many ("dry") vesicles are ruptured and
lack fluid.
Source: Foreign Animal Diseases "The Grey Book" USAHA

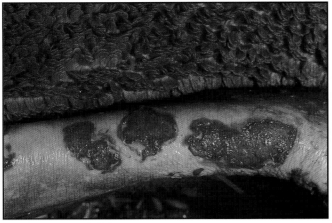

Foot and Mouth Disease
Rumen mucosa, higher magnification. There are several irregularly shaped erosions (ruptured vesicles) on the pillar.
Source: PIADC

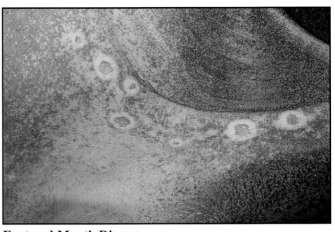

Foot and Mouth Disease
Rumen mucosa, dorsal sac, low magnification. There are several erosions (ruptured vesicles) on the pillars. The pale margins are undermined epithelium.
Source: PIADC

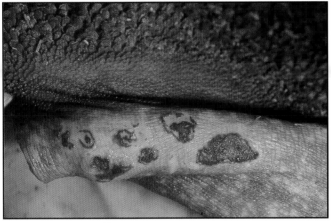

Foot and Mouth Disease
Rumen mucosa, higher magnification. There are several irregularly shaped erosions (ruptured vesicles) on the pillar.
Source: PIADC

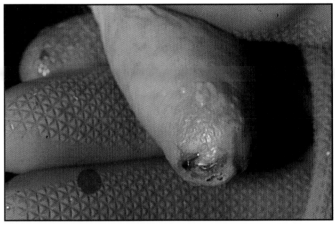

Foot and Mouth Disease
Bovine, teat. There is a ruptured vesicle on the end of the teat.
Source: PIADC

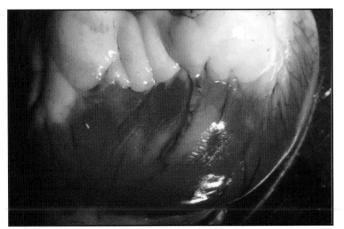

Foot and Mouth Disease
Ovine, heart. There is a pale area of myocardial necrosis visible from the epicardial surface.
Source: Dr. D. Gregg, Noah's Arkive, PIADC

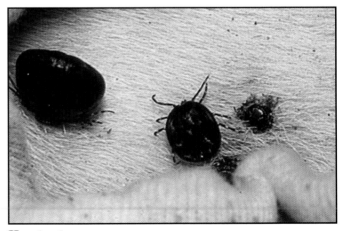

Heartwater
Amblyomma variegatum ticks feeding.
Source: PIADC

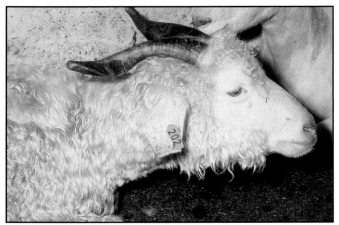

Heartwater
Goat. The neck is extended, consistent with dyspnea.
Source: PIADC

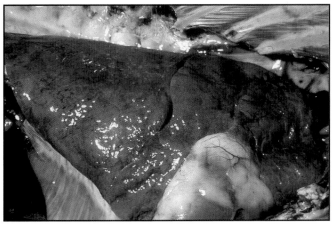

Heartwater
Thoracic viscera. There are many pleural hemorrhages, and the lung is moderately noncollapsed (edema).
Source: PIADC

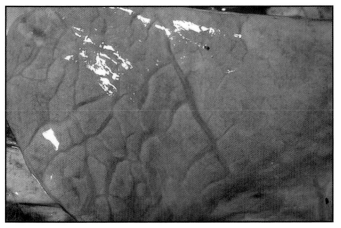

Heartwater
Sheep, lung. There is severe interlobular edema.
Source: PIADC

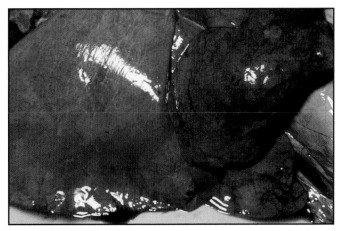

Heartwater
Sheep, lung. Interlobular septa are distended with edema fluid.
Source: PIADC

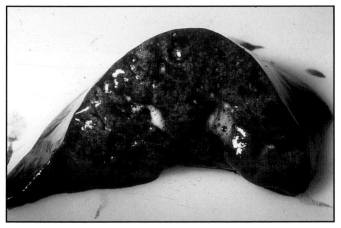

Heartwater
Sheep, lung. The lung is noncollapsed and hyperemic, and the bronchi contain frothy fluid (pulmonary edema).
Source: PIADC

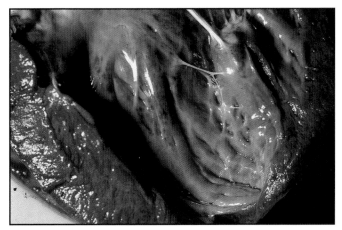

Heartwater
Heart. There are many small hemorrhages on the endocardial surface.
Source: PIADC

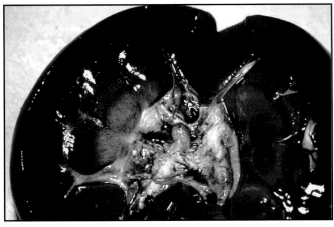

Heartwater
Sheep, kidney. There are multiple petechiae on the cortical surface.
Source: PIADC

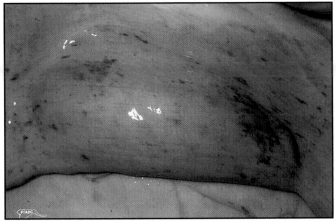

Heartwater
Sheep, kidney. Section reveals numerous fine linear radial hemorrhages; hemorrhages coalesce in the papillae.
Source: PIADC

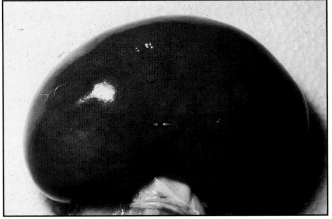

Heartwater
Precapsular lymph node. There are multiple barely discernable petechiae in the cortex.
Source: PIADC

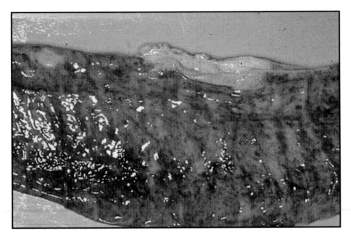

Heartwater
Abomasum. There are multiple petechial and paintbrush serosal hemorrhages.
Source: PIADC

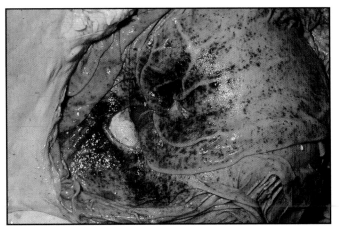

Heartwater
Abomasum. The mucosa contains disseminated petechial and coalescing ecchymotic hemorrhages.
Source: PIADC

Heartwater
Small intestine. The mucosa contains numerous petechiae and ecchymoses.
Source: PIADC

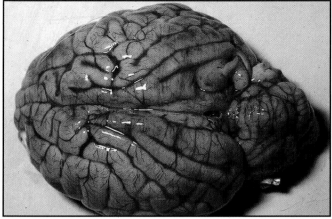

Heartwater
Sheep, brain. The leptomeninges are congested and contain many small hemorrhages. Gyri are flattened (cerebral edema).
Source: PIADC

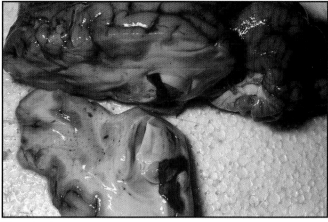

Heartwater
Brain. Section of the cerebrum reveals multiple petechiae and a few ecchymoses, as well as a blood clot in the lateral ventricle.
Source: PIADC

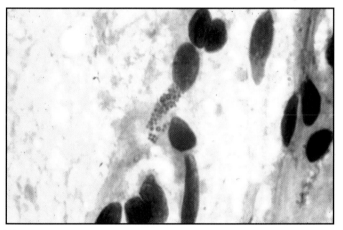

Heartwater
Brain smear. An endothelial cell contains a morula (cluster) of *Ehrlichia ruminantium*.
Source: PIADC

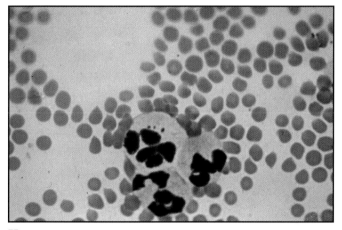

Heartwater
Peripheral blood smear. A neutrophil contains a few *Ehrlichia ruminantium*.
Source: PIADC

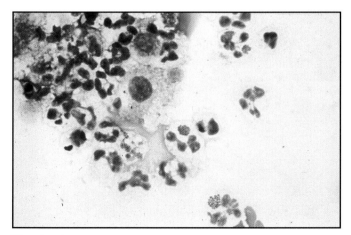

Heartwater
Buffy coat smear. Several neutrophils contain *E. ruminantium* morulae.
Source: PIADC

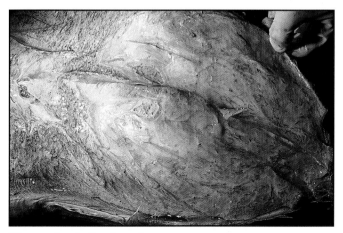

Hemorrhagic Septicemia
Bovine, head and neck. Marked subcutaneous edema.
Source: PIADC

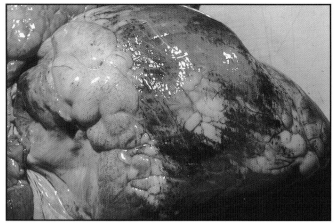

Hemorrhagic Septicemia
Bovine, heart. There are numerous often coalescing petechiae on the epicardium.
Source: PIADC

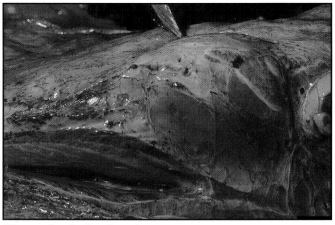

Hemorrhagic Septicemia
Bovine, submandibular region. There is severe subcutaneous/fascial edema and multifocal hemorrhage. The parotid gland exhibits interlobular edema.
Source: PIADC

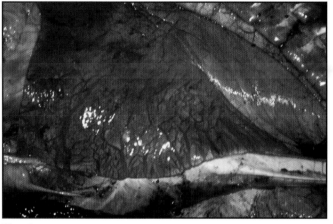

Hendra
Equine, lung. There is severe interlobular edema.
Source: Dr. M. Williamson, CSIRO, Australia

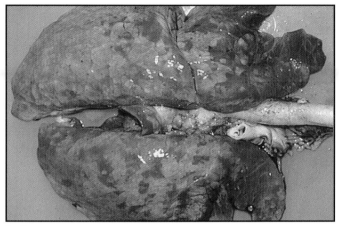

Influenza
Porcine, lungs. There is diffuse tan consolidation of cranial lobes, and multifocal lobular consolidation of the caudal lobes.
Source: Dr. B. Janke, ISU CVM, VDL

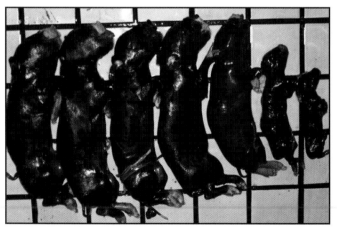

Japanese Encephalitis
Porcine, fetuses. The litter consists of five large (full-term) stillborn fetuses and two small mummified fetuses.
Source: Dr. K. Kawashima, Central Livestock Hygiene Service Center Saitama pref., Japan

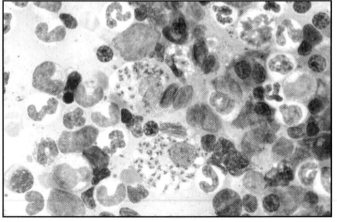

Leishmaniasis
Canine, bone marrow. The bone marrow contains hematopoietic precursors and macrophages with numerous intracytoplasmic Leishmania.
Source: Dr. C. Andreasen, ISU CVM, VPTH

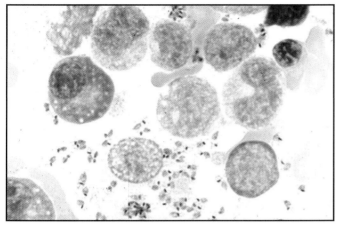

Leishmaniasis
Canine, bone marrow. Higher magnification of bone marrow demonstrating intracellular and extracellular Leishmania organisms.
Source: Dr. C. Andreasen, ISU CVM, VPTH

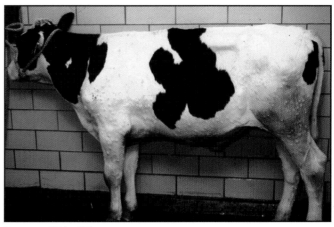

Lumpy Skin Disease
Bovine, skin. There are disseminated cutaneous papules.
Source: Noah's Arkive, PIADC

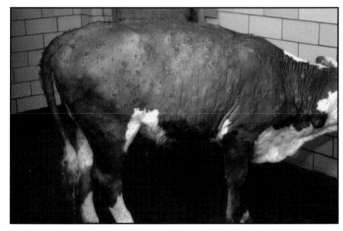

Lumpy Skin Disease
Bovine, skin. There are disseminated cutaneous papules with necrotic centers (sitfasts).
Source: Noah's Arkive, PIADC

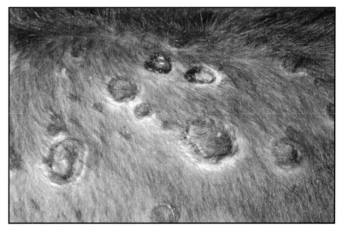

Lumpy Skin Disease
Bovine, skin. Necrotic centers (sitfasts) of two of these papules have sloughed.
Source: Noah's Arkive, PIADC

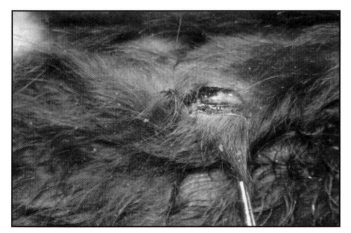

Lumpy Skin Disease
Bovine, skin. Removal of the necrotic center (sitfast) of a papule.
Source: Noah's Arkive, PIADC

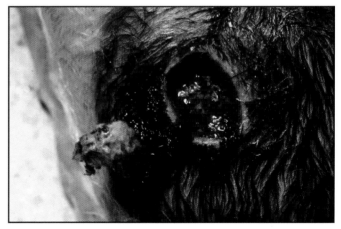

Lumpy Skin Disease
Bovine, skin. There is hemorrhagic exudate subjacent to the necrotic center (sitfast) of a papule.
Source: Noah's Arkive, PIADC

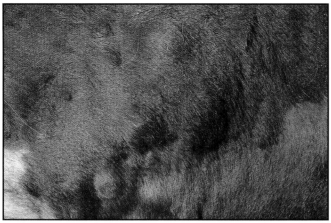

Lumpy Skin Disease
Bovine, skin. Multiple subcutaneous nodules elevate the skin.
Source: PIADC

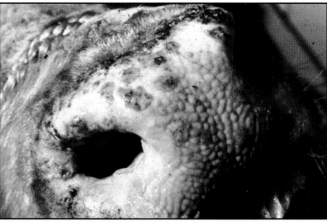

Lumpy Skin Disease
Bovine, muzzle. There are multiple sharply-demarcated slightly raised papules, often with eroded surfaces, that extend into the nares.
Source: Noah's Arkive, PIADC

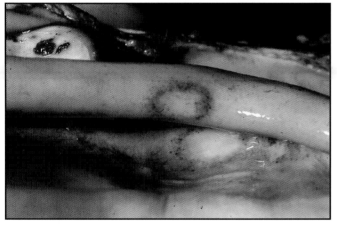

Lumpy Skin Disease
Bovine, nasal turbinate. Early pox lesions are slightly pale round foci rimmed by petechiae.
Source: PIADC

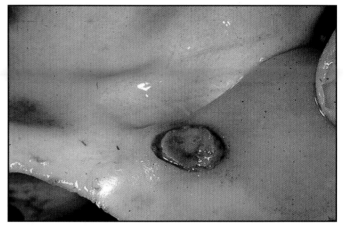

Lumpy Skin Disease
Bovine, nasal turbinate. The centers of well-developed pox are necrotic.
Source: PIADC

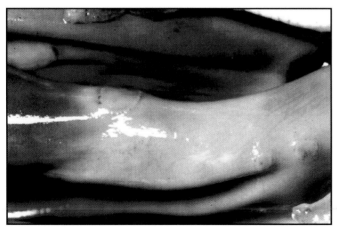

Lumpy Skin Disease
Bovine, nasal turbinate. Nasal mucosa contains several macules with hyperemic margins.
Source: Noah's Arkive, PIADC

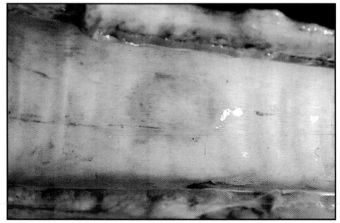

Lumpy Skin Disease
Bovine, trachea. The mucosa contains a poorly demarcated round focus rimmed by mild hemorrhage (early pox lesion).
Source: PIADC

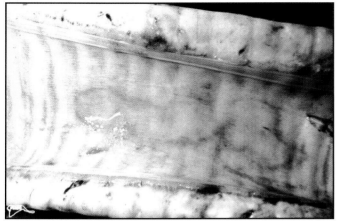

Lumpy Skin Disease
Bovine, trachea. Two coalescing mucosal macules have hyperemic margins.
Source: Noah's Arkive, PIADC

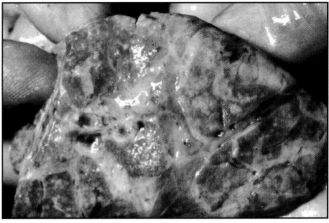

Lumpy Skin Disease
Bovine, lung. There is marked generalized interlobular edema, and there is a small cluster of red nodules on the left side of the specimen.
Source: Noah's Arkive, PIADC

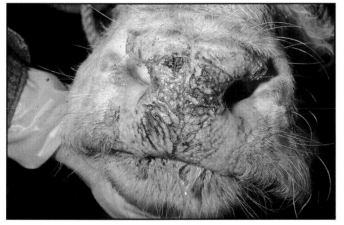

Malignant Catarrhal Fever
Bovine, muzzle. Multiple shallow erosions are filled with dried nasal exudate.
Source: PIADC

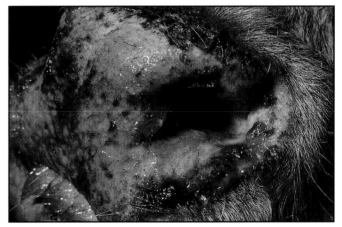

Malignant Catarrhal Fever
Bovine, muzzle. The muzzle is hyperemic, multifocally covered by adherent mucopurulent exudate, and contains many shallow erosions.
Source: PIADC

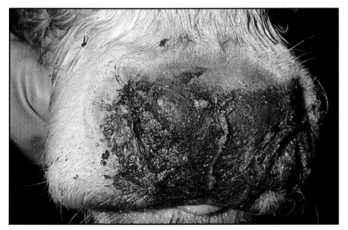

Malignant Catarrhal Fever
Bovine. There is diffuse superficial necrosis of the muzzle.
Source: PIADC

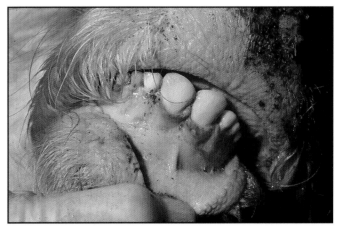

Malignant Catarrhal Fever
Bovine, oral mucosa. There is gingival hyperemia and focal erosion.
Source: PIADC

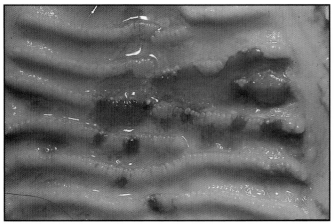

Malignant Catarrhal Fever
Bovine, hard palate. There are multiple coalescing
mucosal erosions.
Source: PIADC

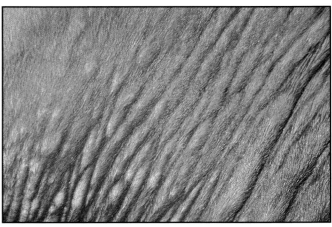

Malignant Catarrhal Fever
Bovine, skin. There are numerous raised plaques
(multifocal dermatitis).
Source: PIADC

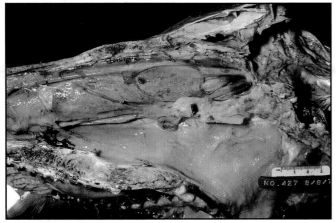

Malignant Catarrhal Fever
Bovine, head, sagittal section. Mucoid exudate multifocally
covers the nasal and pharyngeal mucosa.
Source: PIADC

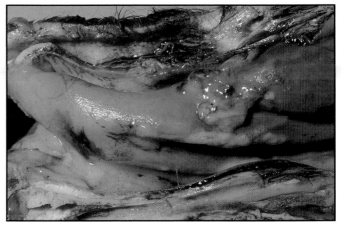

Malignant Catarrhal Fever
Bovine, nasal turbinate. There is a small amount of
mucoid exudate.
Source: PIADC

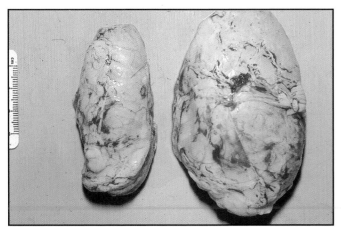

Malignant Catarrhal Fever
Bovine, prescapular lymph nodes: Moderately (left) to mark-
edly enlarged (right) due to MCF.
Source: PIADC

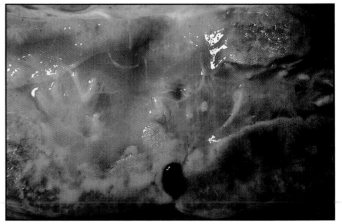

Malignant Catarrhal Fever
Bovine, prescapular lymph node. There are foci of hemorrhage
(and necrosis) in the cortex, and the medulla is edematous.
Source: PIADC

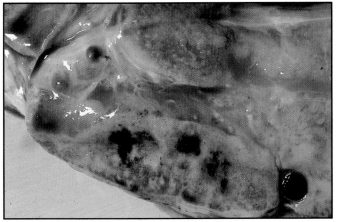

Malignant Catarrhal Fever
Bovine, prescapular lymph node. There are foci of hemorrhage (and necrosis) in the cortex, and the medulla is edematous.
Source: PIADC

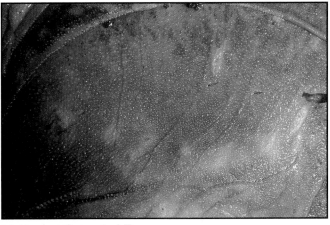

Malignant Catarrhal Fever
Bovine, omasum. Omasal leaves contain multiple pale foci of necrosis; on the right there are several ulcers.
Source: PIADC

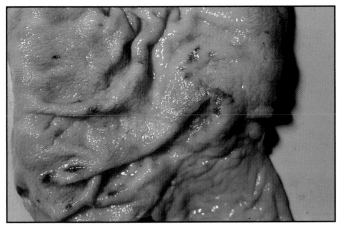

Malignant Catarrhal Fever
Bovine cecum and ileum. There are scattered small foci of mucosal hemorrhage and erosion.
Source: PIADC

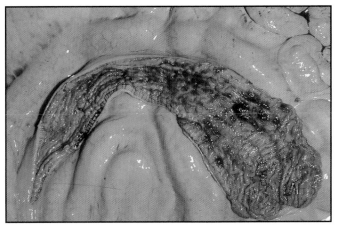

Malignant Catarrhal Fever
Bovine spiral colon. There are multiple mucosal hemorrhages.
Source: PIADC

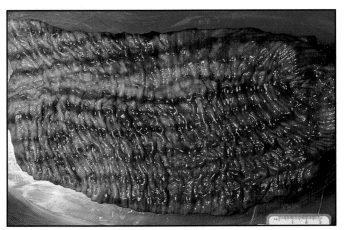

Malignant Catarrhal Fever
Bovine, colon. There is severe longitudinal linear congestion of the mucosa.
Source: PIADC

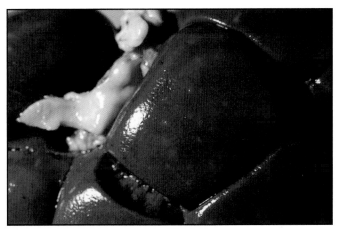

Malignant Catarrhal Fever
Bovine, kidney. Multiple pale foci in the cortex are foci of interstitial nephritis.
Source: PIADC

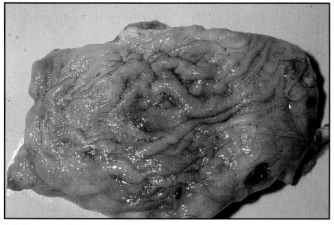

Malignant Catarrhal Fever
Bovine, urinary bladder. The mucosal surface contains several small erosions and one large hemorrhagic ulcer.
Source: PIADC

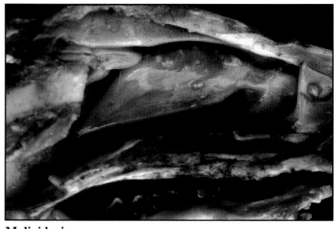

Melioidosis
Caprine, nasal turbinates. There are multiple raised pale nodules (abscesses) on the nasal mucosa.
Source: Dr. K. Kawashima, National Institute of Animal Health, Japan

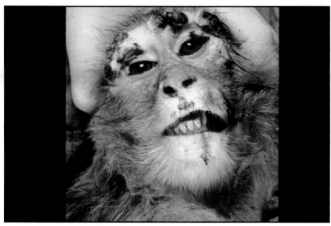

Monkeypox
Rhesus macaque, monkeypox. There are multiple hemorrhagic papules on the forehead and eyelids.
Source: AFIP

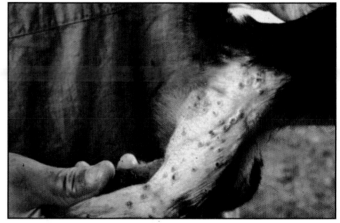

Monkeypox
Primate, hindlimb, monkeypox. There are numerous discrete papules with red, depressed centers.
Source: AFIP

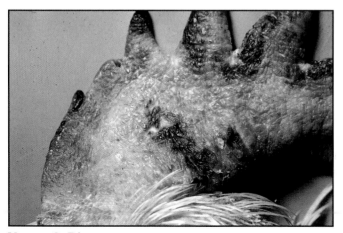

Newcastle Disease
Chicken. The comb is markedly edematous and contains multiple foci of hemorrhage.
Source: PIADC

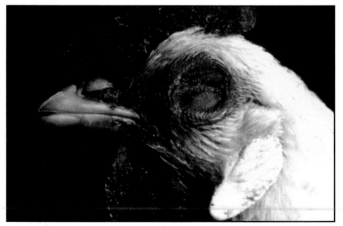

Newcastle Disease
Avian, skin. There is a marked hemorrhage of the comb, wattle, and adjacent skin.
Source: AFIP

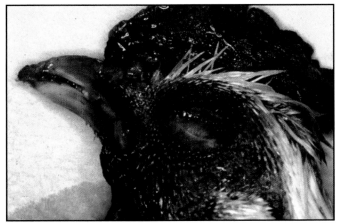

Newcastle Disease
Avian, skin. There is marked hemorrhage of the comb and head, with cyanosis of the margin of the comb.
Source: Dr. R. Moeller, CAHFSLS

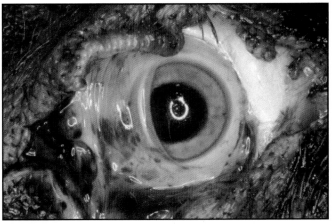

Newcastle Disease
Avian, eye. Conjunctival hemorrhage is most severe in the nictitans.
Source: Dr. R. Moeller, CAHFSLS

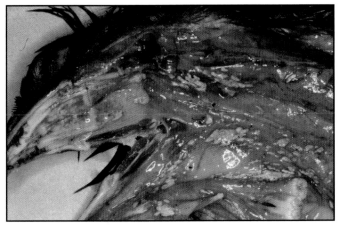

Newcastle Disease
Avian, oral cavity. Numerous clumps of fibrinonecrotic exudate adhere to foci of necrosis in the oral, pharyngeal, and esophageal mucosa.
Source: Dr. R. Moeller, CAHFSLS

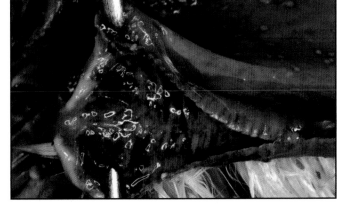

Newcastle Disease
Avian, trachea. Tracheal and laryngeal mucosa contain many foci of hemorrhage and small clumps of fibrinonecrotic exudate.
Source: Dr. R. Moeller, CAHFSLS

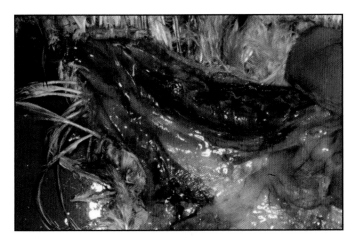

Newcastle Disease
Avian, skin. There is marked subcutaneous edema in the neck, extending to the thoracic inlet.
Source: Dr. R. Moeller, CAHFSLS

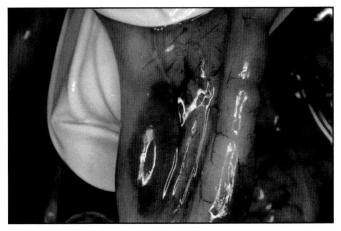

Newcastle Disease
Avian, ceca. Hyperemic, necrotic cecal tonsils are visible from the serosal surface.
Source: Dr. R. Moeller, CAHFSLS

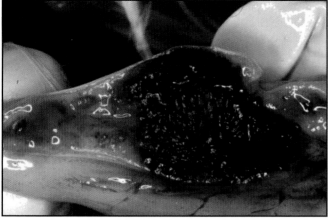

Newcastle Disease
Avian, ceca. The cecal tonsil is red-brown, thickened, and friable (necrotic).
Source: Dr. R. Moeller, CAHFSLS

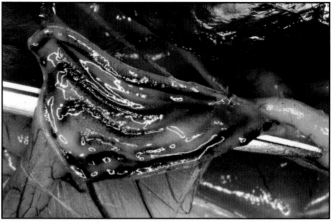

Newcastle Disease
Avian, rectum. There are multiple linear mucosal hemorrhages.
Source: Dr. R. Moeller, CAHFSLS

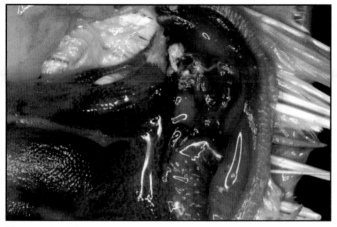

Newcastle Disease
Avian, cloaca. The mucosa is hyperemic and contains foci of hemorrhage.
Source: Dr. R. Moeller, CAHFSLS

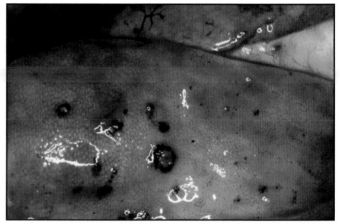

Newcastle Disease
Avian, colon. The mucosa contains multiple sharply demarcated foci of hemorrhage and necrosis.
Source: Dr. R. Moeller, CAHFSLS

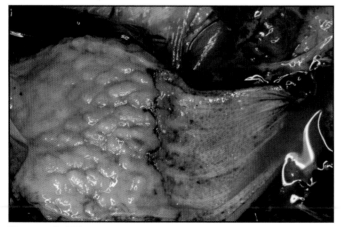

Newcastle Disease
Avian, proventriculus. The proximal mucosa is eroded and covered by a fibrinonecrotic (diptheritic) membrane.
Source: Dr. R. Moeller, CAHFSLS

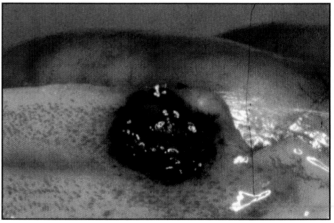

Newcastle Disease
Avian, cecal tonsil necrosis.
Source: Dr. R. Moeller, CAHFSLS

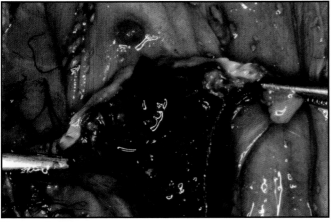

Newcastle Disease
Avian, diphtheritic laryngo-tracheitis.
Source: Dr. R. Moeller, CAHFSLS

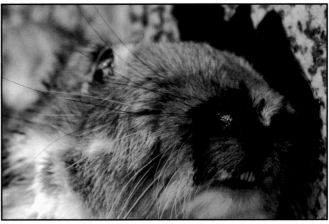

Rabbit Hemorrhagic Disease
Rabbit. Severe epistaxis.
Source: Dr. J.P. Teifke, Federal Research Institute for Animal Health
Riems, Germany

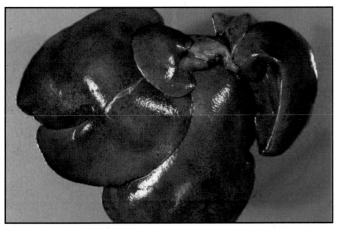

Rabbit Hemorrhagic Disease
Rabbit, liver. All liver lobes are swollen, pale and have a
reticular pattern.
Source: Dr. J.P. Teifke, Federal Research Institute for Animal Health
Riems, Germany

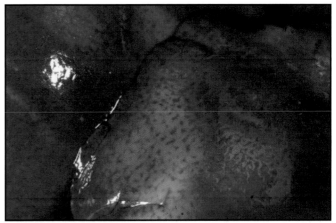

Rabbit Hemorrhagic Disease
Rabbit, liver. There is a large area of pallor (necrosis) with a
prominent reticular pattern.
Source: Dr. J.P. Teifke, Federal Research Institute for Animal Health
Riems, Germany

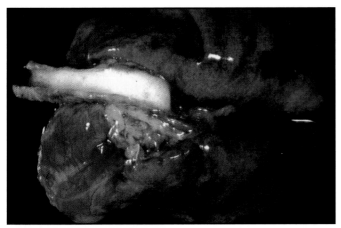

Rabbit Hemorrhagic Disease
Rabbit, lungs. The trachea is filled with foam, and the lungs
are mottled and noncollapsed (severe pulmonary edema).
Source: Dr. J.P. Teifke, Federal Research Institute for Animal Health
Riems, Germany

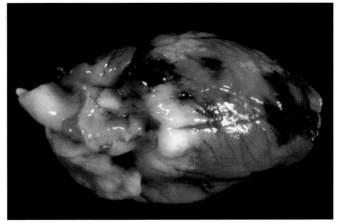

Rabbit Hemorrhagic Disease
Rabbit, heart. There are multiple epicardial hemorrhages.
Source: Dr. J.P. Teifke, Federal Research Institute for Animal Health
Riems, Germany

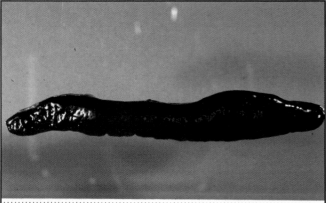

Rabbit Hemorrhagic Disease
Rabbit, spleen. The spleen is markedly enlarged and congested.
Source: Dr. J.P. Teifke, Federal Research Institute for Animal Health Riems, Germany

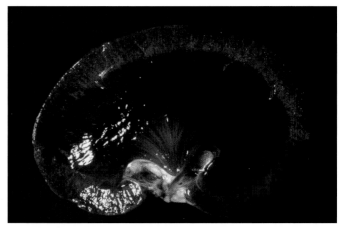

Rabbit Hemorrhagic Disease
Rabbit, kidney. There are petechiae throughout the cortex, and the medulla is severely congested.
Source: Dr. J.P. Teifke, Federal Research Institute for Animal Health Riems, Germany

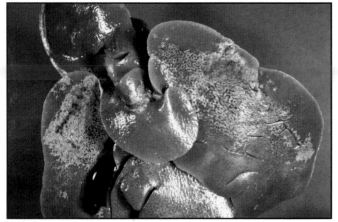

Rabbit Hemorrhagic Disease
Rabbit. This chronically affected liver contains pale areas of postnecrotic scarring.
Source: Dr. J.P. Teifke, Federal Research Institute for Animal Health Riems, Germany

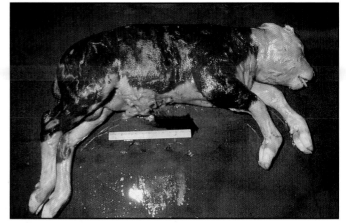

Rift Valley Fever
Bovine fetus. The skin of this emphysematous fetus is stained with meconium.
Source: PIADC

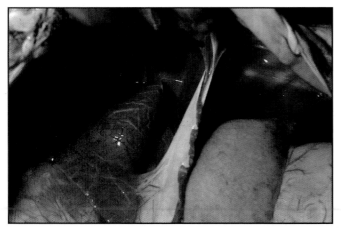

Rift Valley Fever
Sheep, fetus. Both the pleural and peritoneal cavities contain excessive clear, straw-colored fluid.
Source: PIADC

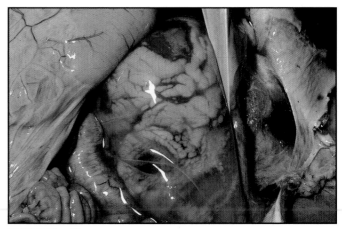

Rift Valley Fever
Sheep, fetus, kidney. There is severe perirenal edema.
Source: PIADC

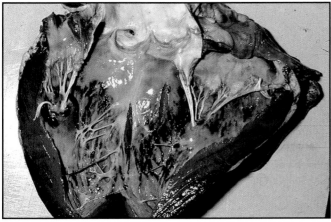

Rift Valley Fever
Sheep, heart. The ventricular endocardium contains many hemorrhages.
Source: PIADC

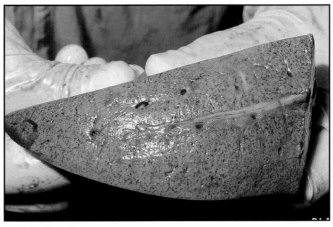

Rift Valley Fever
Sheep, liver. The cut surface of this swollen liver is pale and contains many petechiae.
Source: PIADC

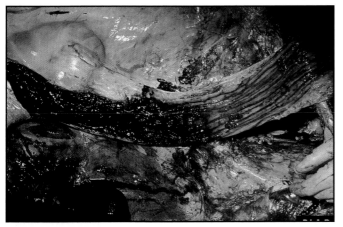

Rift Valley Fever
Sheep, colon. Severe hemorrhagic colitis.
Source: PIADC

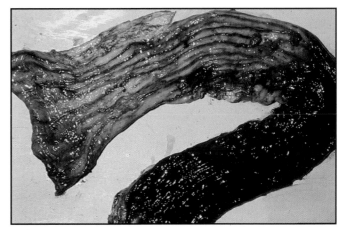

Rift Valley Fever
Sheep, colon. There is severe locally extensive mucosal hemorrhage.
Source: PIADC

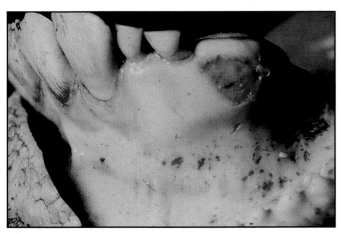

Rinderpest
Bovine, oral mucosa. There are numerous small gingival erosions.
Source: PIADC

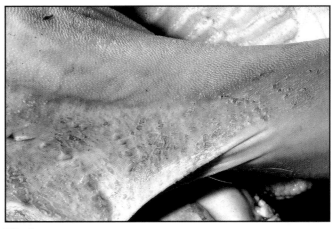

Rinderpest
Bovine, oral mucosa. There are numerous coalescing erosions on the ventrolateral lingual mucosa.
Source: PIADC

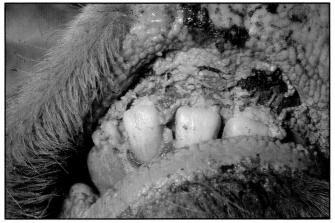

Rinderpest
Bovine, oral mucosa. There is severe diffuse necrosis/
coalescing ulceration of the dental pad; mandibular mucosa
contains smaller erosions.
Source: PIADC

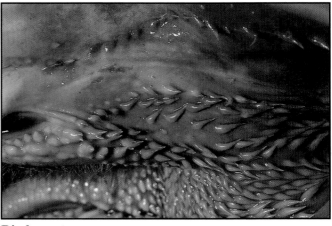

Rinderpest
Bovine, gingiva. There are a few small erosions.
Source: PIADC

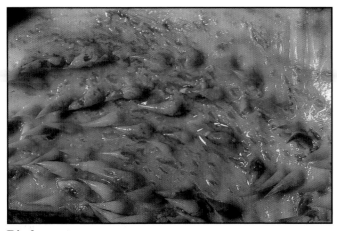

Rinderpest
Bovine, oral mucosa. There are numerous erosions on and
between the buccal papillae.
Source: PIADC

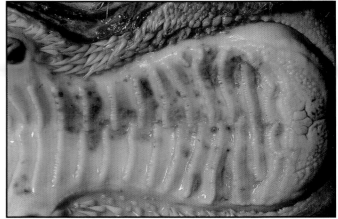

Rinderpest
Bovine, hard palate. The mucosa contains many small,
coalescing, pale to dark red erosions or foci of necrosis.
Source: PIADC

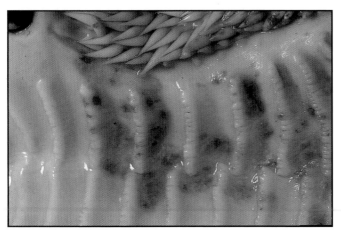

Rinderpest
Bovine, hard palate. Palate erosion.
Source: PIADC

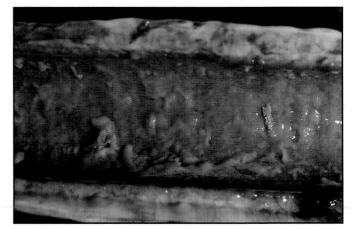

Rinderpest
Bovine, trachea. The mucosa is hyperemic and covered by
abundant mucopurulent exudate.
Source: PIADC

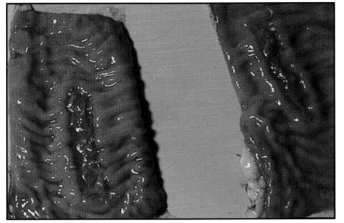

Rinderpest
Bovine, ileum. Peyer's patches are depressed and covered by fibronecrotic exudate.
Source: PIADC

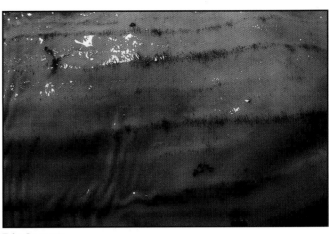

Rinderpest
Bovine, colon. There are many petechiae on the crests of the mucosal folds, and there are several small blood clots on the mucosal surface.
Source: PIADC

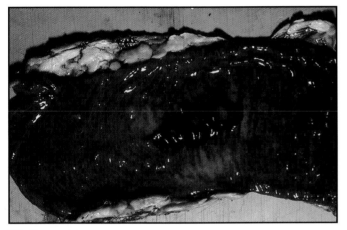

Rinderpest
Bovine, ileum. The mucosa is hemorrhagic and edematous, and the Peyer's patch is depressed (necrosis).
Source: PIADC

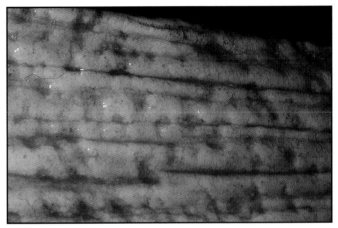

Rinderpest
Bovine, colon. The mucosa is edematous and contains many small hemorrhages and shallow erosions.
Source: PIADC

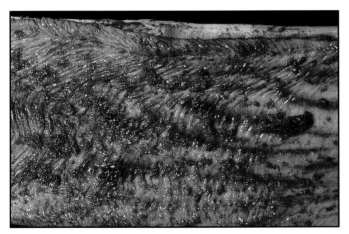

Rinderpest
Bovine, colon. The mucosa contains multiple longitudinal linear hemorrhages.
Source: PIADC

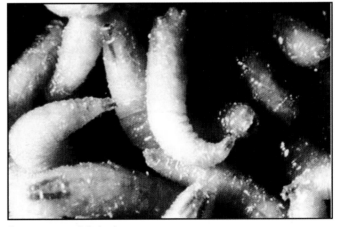

Screwworm Myiasis
Screwworm. Third instar screwworm larvae have dark tracheal tubes.
Source: Foreign Animal Diseases "The Grey Book" USAHA

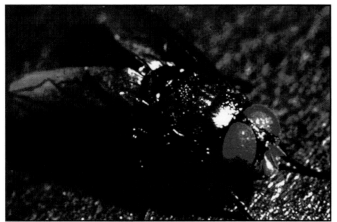

Screwworm Myiasis
Screwworm fly. The head of the adult fly is red-orange.
Source: Foreign Animal Diseases "The Grey Book" USAHA

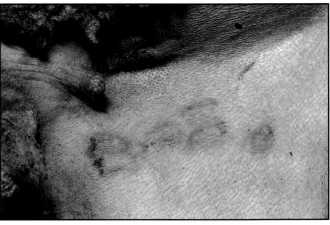

Sheep Pox and Goat Pox
Sheep, inguinal skin. Several coalescing macules
contain petechiae.
Source: PIADC

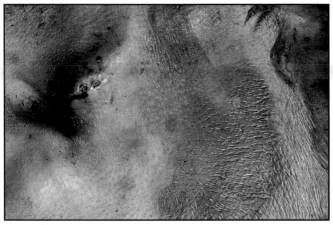

Sheep Pox and Goat Pox
Sheep, inguinal skin. There are several coalescing macules.
Source: PIADC

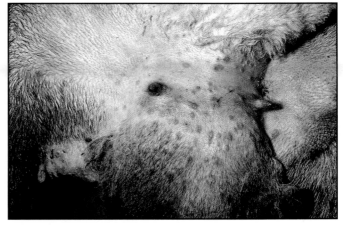

Sheep Pox and Goat Pox
Sheep, scrotum. There are multiple papules on the scrotum
and adjacent inguinal skin.
Source: PIADC

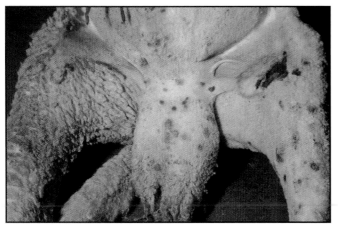

Sheep Pox and Goat Pox
Sheep, scrotum and inguinal skin. There are multiple red
brown papules. There are two hemorrhagic ulcers on the
medial aspect of the stifle.
Source: PIADC

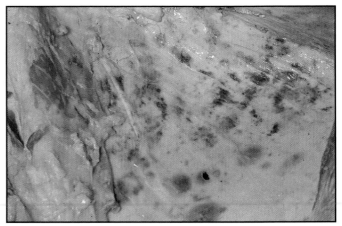

Sheep Pox and Goat Pox
Sheep, subcutis. There are numerous hemorrhages, and several dark red round foci of hemorrhage and necrosis (beneath
cutaneous pox).
Source: PIADC

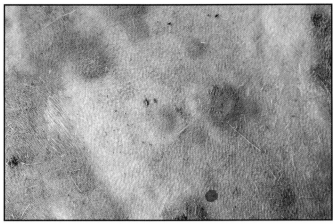

Sheep Pox and Goat Pox
Goat, skin. Pox are coalescing red papules with central, slightly depressed, pale (necrotic) areas.
Source: PIADC

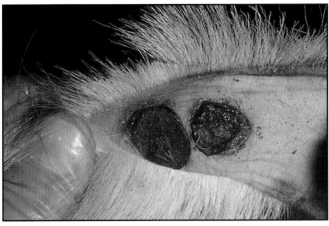

Sheep Pox and Goat Pox
Goat. Two pox on the ventral tail have dessicated, dark red, undermined (necrotic and sloughing) centers.
Source: PIADC

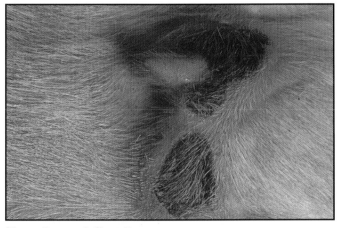

Sheep Pox and Goat Pox
Goat, udder. The skin contains two sharply demarcated necrotic foci (subacute pox).
Source: PIADC

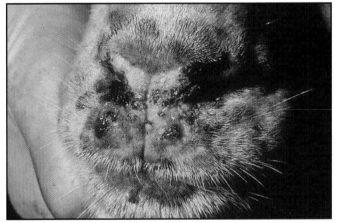

Sheep Pox and Goat Pox
Goat, muzzle. The muzzle contains several papules and is partially covered by hemorrhagic nasal exudate.
Source: PIADC

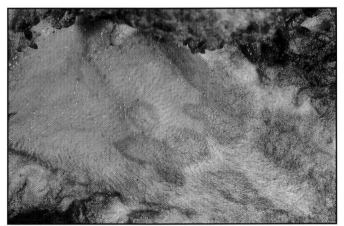

Sheep Pox and Goat Pox
Sheep, skin. Several coalescing pox have pale tan (necrotic) centers.
Source: PIADC

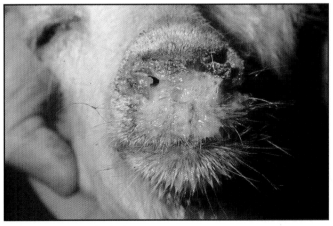

Sheep Pox and Goat Pox
Goat. Abundant thick nasal exudate covers the muzzle and partially occludes the nares.
Source: PIADC

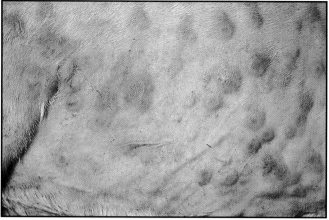

Sheep Pox and Goat Pox
Goat, skin. There are multiple coalescing papules (pox) that often have tan, dry (necrotic) centers.
Source: PIADC

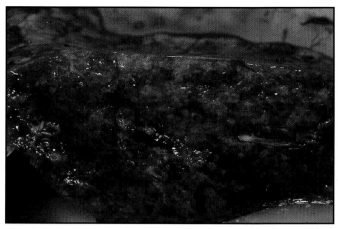

Sheep Pox and Goat Pox
Lung. There are numerous, small, coalescing, red-tan, consolidated foci (pneumonia).
Source: PIADC

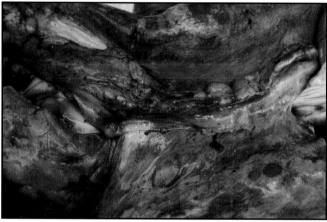

Sheep Pox and Goat Pox
Lungs. The lungs contain multiple discrete tan to red-brown nodules (multifocal interstitial pneumonia). Mediastinal lymph nodes are enlarged.
Source: PIADC

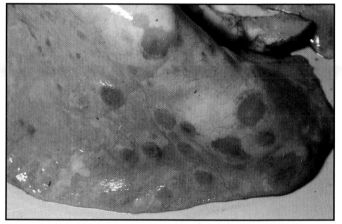

Sheep Pox and Goat Pox
Lung. There are multiple red-brown consolidated foci (multifocal pneumonia).
Source: PIADC

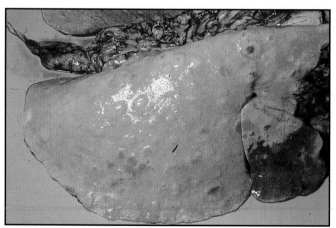

Sheep Pox and Goat Pox
Lung. Numerous nodules are scattered throughout the lung; the cranioventral red-brown consolidation is likely secondary bacterial pneumonia.
Source: PIADC

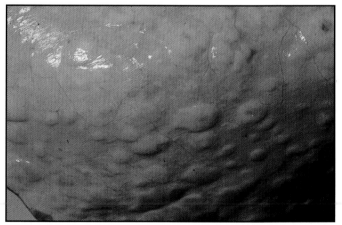

Sheep Pox and Goat Pox
Lung. There are numerous raised pale nodules (multifocal pneumonia).
Source: PIADC

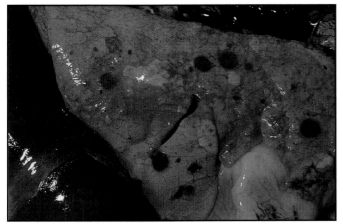

Sheep Pox and Goat Pox
Lung. There are multiple discrete, round, red-brown foci of consolidation (pneumonia).
Source: PIADC

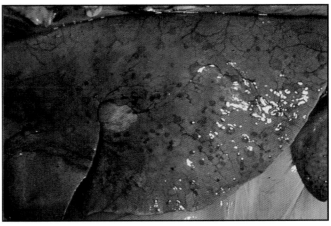

Sheep Pox and Goat Pox
Sheep, lung. The numerous widely disseminated discrete round tan foci are foci of pneumonia; a few have pale (necrotic) centers.
Source: PIADC

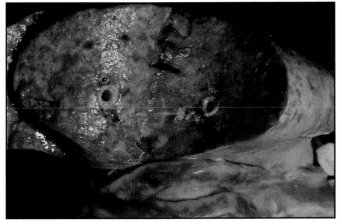

Sheep Pox and Goat Pox
Goat, lung. There are multiple coalescing tan foci of consolidation (pneumonia), and the adjacent lymph node is markedly enlarged.
Source: PIADC

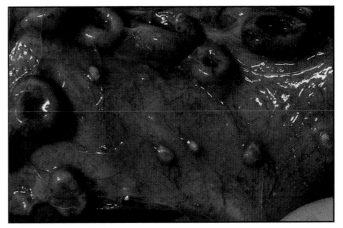

Sheep Pox and Goat Pox
Uterus. The endometrium contains several tan papules (pox) among the caruncles.
Source: PIADC

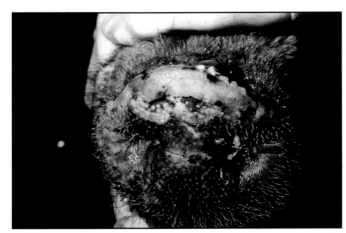

Swine Vesicular Disease
Porcine, skin. There is a deep ulcer on the dorsum of the snout.
Source: ISU CVM

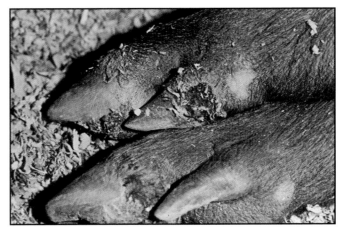

Swine Vesicular Disease
Pig, feet. There are multiple large erosions/ulcers of the coronary bands.
Source: PIADC

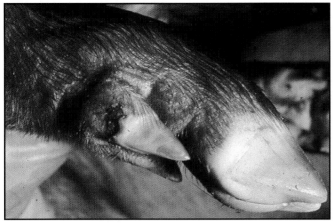

Swine Vesicular Disease
Pig, foot. The wall of the dewclaw is undermined adjacent to an ulcer at the coronary band.
Source: PIADC

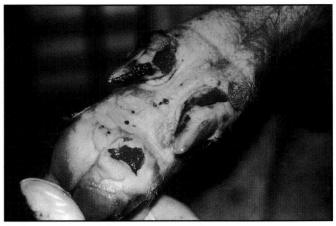

Swine Vesicular Disease
Pig, foot. A claw and both dewclaws have ulcers at the coronary bands.
Source: ISU CVM

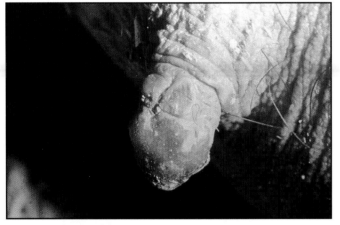

Swine Vesicular Disease
Pig, skin. There are coalescing erosions on the teat.
Source: ISU CVM

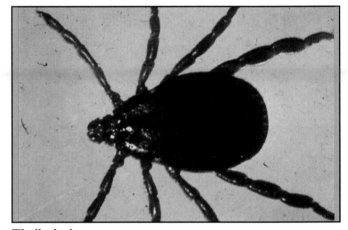

Theileriosis
Rhipicephalus appendiculatus - brown ear tick, vector of Theileriosis.
Source: PIADC

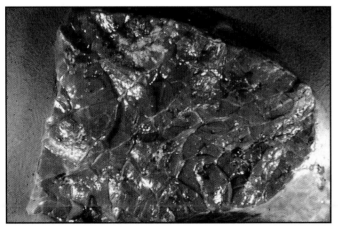

Theileriosis
Bovine, lung. The lung tissue is diffusely tan-brown, and lobules are noncollapsed and rubbery (interstitial pneumonia).
Source: PIADC

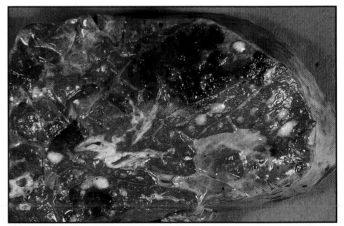

Theileriosis
Bovine, lung. Lung tissue is noncollapsed, contains multiple foci of hemorrhage, and there is fluid/foam within bronchi and interlobular septa.
Source: PIADC

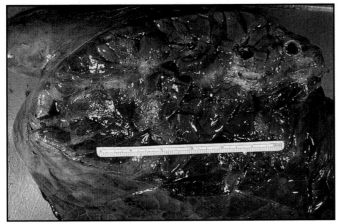

Theileriosis
Bovine, lung. The lobules are noncollapsed (rubbery) and diffusely tan-brown, and interlobular septa are markedly expanded due to edema and emphysema.
Source: PIADC

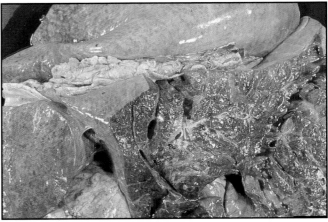

Theileriosis
Bovine, lungs. Lungs are diffusely noncollapsed, and there is moderate interlobular edema (interstitial pneumonia).
Source: PIADC

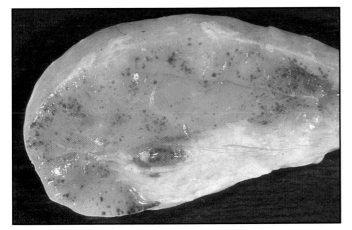

Theileriosis
Bovine, popliteal lymph node. The node is enlarged and diffusely pale, and contains numerous petechiae.
Source: PIADC

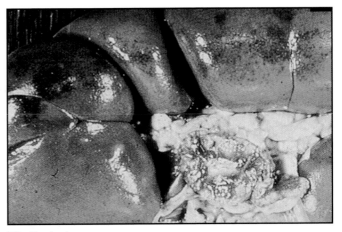

Theileriosis
Bovine, kidney. There are multiple petechiae on the surface of the cortex. The lymph node near the hilus is markedly enlarged.
Source: PIADC

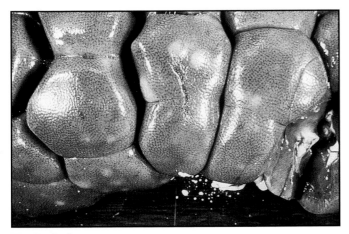

Theileriosis
Bovine, kidney. The multiple pale foci on the cortical surface are lymphoid infiltrates.
Source: PIADC

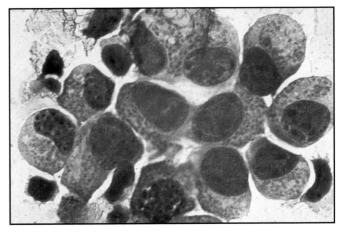

Theileriosis
Bovine lymphoblasts contain intracytoplasmic *Theileria parva*.
Source: PIADC

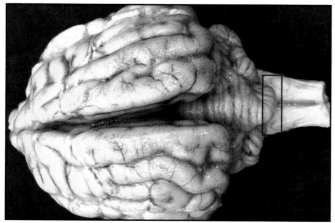

Transmissible Spongiform Encephalopathies
Brain. The red box indicates the region of the obex, the portion of the brainstem that is required for TSE diagnosis.
Source: Dr. S. Sorden, ISU CVM, VPTH

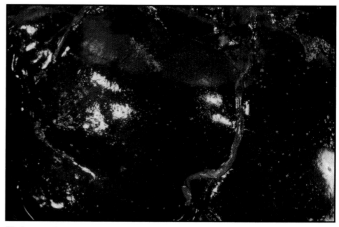

Tularemia
Beaver, liver. There are disseminated small pale foci of necrotizing hepatitis.
Source: Dr. G. Wobeser, CCWHC

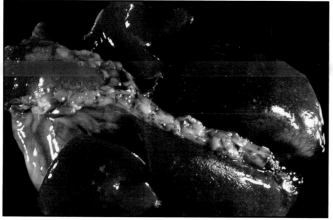

Tularemia
Cat, lung. Numerous <1 mm diameter pale foci are disseminated throughout all lung lobes.
Source: Dr. J. Nietfeld, KSU CVM

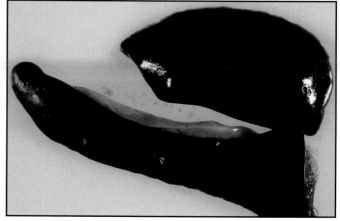

Tularemia
Cat, spleen and liver. Numerous ~1 mm diameter pale foci are disseminated throughout the spleen; fewer pale foci are discernible in the liver lobe.
Source: Dr. J. Nietfeld, KSU CVM

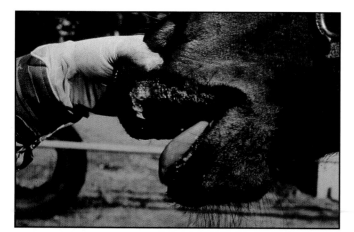

Vesicular Stomatitis
Equine, mouth. There is extensive erosion of the lip at the mucocutaneous junction.
Source: ISU CVM

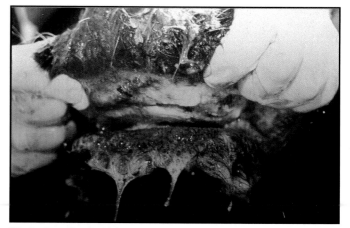

Vesicular Stomatitis
Bovine, mouth. There is extensive ulceration of the dental pad, and severe salivation.
Source: ISU CVM

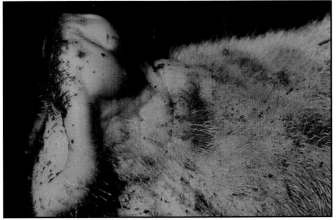

Vesicular Stomatitis
Porcine, skin. There is a large vesicle (bulla) on the dorsal snout.
Source: ISU CVM

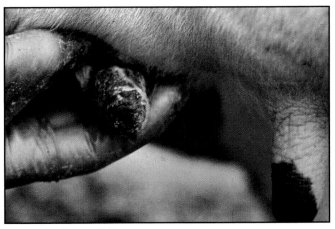

Vesicular Stomatitis
Bovine, skin. The distal teat is severely eroded and hemorrhagic.
Source: ISU CVM

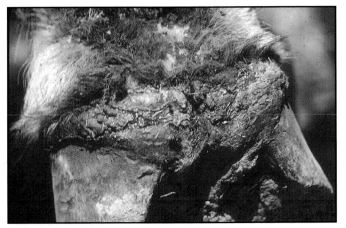

Vesicular Stomatitis
Bovine foot. The coronary band at the heels is thickened, multifocally eroded, and covered by dried necrotic exudate.
Source: PIADC.

Index

Page numbers in bold refer to fact sheets in Section 2; page numbers in bold and italics refer to disease images in Section 3.

103, 106, 107, 110
surveillance in FAD response 37
swine vesicular disease 88, 90, **232**, **286**

T

tapeworms 19
task forces and ICS 50
theileriosis —*Theileria parva* and
Theileria annulata **233**, **287**
ticks. *See* insect vectors; ticks; *See
also Boophilus spp, Amblyomma
spp, Ixodes spp, Dermacentor*
tortoises
example of portal of entry of FAD 12
Toxocara canis 18
example of maturation required for
infectivity 18
Toxoplasma gondii, example of vertical
transmission 15
transboundary disease 2
transmissible mink encephalopathy **235**
transmissible spongiform
encephalopathies (TSEs) 74, **235**,
289
emergence of 24
transmission of diseases
direct contact 15, 16, 18, 22, 23, 102
horizontal transmission 15, 16
iatrogenic transmission 16
indirect contact 15, 16, 22, 23
transovarial transmission 16, 17
transstadial transmission 17
vertical transmission 14, 16, 17
transovarial transmission 17
transplacental passage of pathogens 14.
See also vertical transmission
transstadial transmission
definition and examples of 17
definition of 16
trematodes (fluke)
example of indirect life cycle 19
trypanosomiasis **238**
TSEs. *See* transmissible spongiform
encephalopathies
tuberculosis **139**, **256**
tularemia **239**, **289**
Type 1 incident 36
Type 2 incident 36
Type 3 incident 35
Type 4 incident 35
Type 5 incident 35

U

U.S. animal imports in 2002 11
United States Department of Agriculture
(USDA) 1. *See also* Animal and

Plant Health Inspection Service
(APHIS)
Import Centers 28
Select Agent and Toxins list 9

V

vaccination in FAD response 37
variant Creutzfeldt Jakob Disease
(vCJD) 24
vCJD. *See* variant Creutzfeldt Jakob
Disease (vCJD)
vector controls in FAD response 38
vectors 11, 14, 17, 19, 21, 22. *See
also* biological vector, mechanical
vector, insect vector
definition 12
definition of biological 16
definition of mechanical 16
examples in transmission of disease 16
importation of disease 12
Venezuelan equine encephalomyelitis 157
vertical transmission 14
definition of 14
examples of 14–15
transovarial a form of 16, 17
vesicular exanthema of swine 88, 90
vesicular stomatitis 17, 88, 90, **240**, **289**
1980s outbreak described 17
as an example of transovarial
transmission 17
Veterinary Medical Assistance Teams
(VMATs) 45
deployment of 51
responsibilities during a disasters 51
veterinary response teams 51
ASPCA as part of 53
HSUS as part of 53
NAHERC 47
SARTs 52
VMATs 51
Veterinary Services (VS)
assistance from NAHERC 38
emergency management in response 32
intensive screwworm surveillance 106
responsibilities 28
role in recovery from an FAD 39
viral hemorrhagic disease of rabbits.
See rabbit hemorrhagic disease
viral hemorrhagic septicemia 242
visceral leishmaniasis. *See* leishmaniasis

W

Western equine encephalomyelitis 157
West Nile Encephalitis **244**
West Nile virus (encephalitis) 3, 21, 22
about WNV 109

continuing spread of the WNV 111
emerging disease 8
example of introduction into wildlife 3
in the US, 1999-2005 107–111
reasons for the declining case rate in
humans 111–112
response to the outbreak 110
US spread 3
vectors and the introduction into the
US 21
wild animals
as portals of entry 11–12, 61
wildlife
foreign animal diseases in 3, 12, 21,
22–23, 102–103, 107, 109, 110,
111
World Organization for Animal Health
3, 3–6, 4, 11, 23, 91, 92
List A and B definitions 4
notification of an FAD by a member
country 33
reportable disease list 5–6
World Trade Organization (WTO) 5

Z

zoo animals
foreign animal diseases in 108
zoonotic infections/diseases 8. *See
also* humans and non-human
primates; diseases of